Nephrology VOLUME I

PROCEEDINGS OF THE
Xth INTERNATIONAL CONGRESS OF NEPHROLOGY

Editor

Alex M. Davison

Associate Editors

J. D. Briggs · R. Green · J. Kanis
N. P. Mallick · A. J. Rees · D. Thomson

Baillière Tindall London Philadelphia Toronto
Sydney Tokyo

Baillière Tindall   24–28 Oval Road
W. B. Saunders   London NW1 7DX, England

West Washington Square
Philadelphia, PA 19105, USA

1 Goldthorne Avenue
Toronto, Ontario M8Z 5T9, Canada

ABP Australia Ltd, 44 Waterloo Road
North Ryde, NSW 2064, Australia

Harcourt Brace Jovanovich Japan Inc.
Ichibancho Central Building, 22–1 Ichibancho
Chiyoda-ku, Tokyo 102, Japan

First published 1988

TransMedica Europe Limited

This publication was produced by the TransMedica Conference Unit

Project Number: 0-88137-033-9

British Library Cataloguing in Publication Data

International Congress of Nephrology, 10th.
Nephrology.
1. Man. Kidneys. Diseases
I. Title. II. Davison, Alex M. (Alex Meikle). *1940–*
III. Briggs, J. Douglas
616.6′1

ISBN 0-7020-1312-9 v.1
ISBN 0-7020-1315-3 v.2

Printed and bound in Great Britain
At the University Press, Cambridge

FOREWORD

This book is the record of the 18 Guest Lectures and 30 Symposia presented at the Xth International Congress of Nephrology in London, July 1987. It does not pretend to be a comprehensive textbook of nephrology, but rather an update of the established advances which took place in the whole of nephrology during the period 1984–1987, and the position as seen by experts in each field last summer. Thanks to the hard work of our Editorial Board under the direction of Sandy Davison and Betty Dickens of TransMedica this very large book appears only months after the Congress whilst memories of it are still fresh. All of us owe them a large debt.

We would like to have included in this book the matter presented in the 30 Workshops which the Congress included. Sadly, we decided against this course, principally because it would have made the book too large and too expensive to produce. Other accessory reasons were first, the very large amount of work required in 1984 to summarize workshop material presented, which in retrospect those concerned felt had been excessive for the product achieved; and our desire not to inhibit discussion in the Workshops, by asking invited participants to present a manuscript beforehand or at the meeting.

We would like to thank the many contributors to this volume for their efforts and patience in producing the work which constitutes this volume; we hope all will enjoy and profit from their efforts.

Finally it is my sad task to record the loss we all sustained on September 29th 1987 when Frank Goodwin died. As Secretary of the Congress he had piloted it from the very beginnings in 1981, when the ISN accepted the application of the Renal Association to hold its congress in London. Many of the ideas and structures which made the Congress a success were his, and his alone.

J Stewart Cameron
President, Xth International Congress of Nephrology
London, United Kingdom

OFFICERS AND COMMITTEES
Xth INTERNATIONAL CONGRESS OF NEPHROLOGY
LONDON, ENGLAND, UNITED KINGDOM
26–31 July, 1987

OFFICERS

President	J S Cameron
Vice-Presidents	D N S Kerr
	D K Peters
Treasurers	A W Asscher
	N F Jones
Secretary	F J Goodwin

SCIENTIFIC PROGRAMME COMMITTEE

D N S Kerr, D K Peters, *Chairmen*
C G Winearls, *Secretary*
G M Aber, C Amiel (France), A W Asscher, T M Barratt, P H Baylis, J D Briggs, J S Cameron, W R Cattell, V Cattell, G R D Catto, C Chantler, R D Cohen, G A Coles, A M Davison, F G Epstein (USA), D J Evans, M El-Nahas, T G Feest, G Friedlander (France), I M Glynn, R Gokal, F J Goodwin, R Green, R Greger (FRG), D N S Kerr, N F Jones, G MacGregor, I MacIntyre, N P Mallick, M G McGeown, J F Moorhead, P N Morris, D K Peters, A J Rees, E Ritz (FRG), J R Salaman, J D Swales, K Thurau (FRG), C van Ypersele (Belgium), G F Viberti, J Walls, R H R White, R Wilkinson, D G Williams, O M Wrong

EDITORIAL COMMITTEE FOR PROCEEDINGS

A M Davison, *Editor*
Associate Editors
J D Briggs, R Green, J Kanis, N P Mallick, A J Rees, D Thomson

CONGRESS ADMINISTRATOR

S J White

PREFACE

These two volumes do not aspire to be a comprehensive review of nephrology but rather a reflection of current growing areas of interest including morphology, physiology and clinical management. It is based on the Guest Lectures and Symposia which formed the programme of the Xth International Congress of Nephrology which was held in London at the end of July 1987. Some chapters therefore are up-to-date reviews while others record laboratory, experimental or clinical experience in this ever advancing sphere of medicine. It is hoped that it will thus provide both a reference source and an insight into current developing concepts.

There are many people involved in the production of this text. Firstly I must thank the many contributors who provided their manuscripts within the very tight time schedule. Secondly to the Assistant Editors who undertook so ably the task of editing, proof reading and indexing in the few months after the Congress. It has been our hope that this has resulted in a uniformity of style and terminology which is difficult with an international authorship, and if any points have been overlooked we must apologize. In one area – that of units of measurement – the values have not been converted to a standard form but we do not think this will cause any confusion. To aid in speed of publication the contents have been indexed to the first page of the chapter in which they appear.

Finally, thanks are due to Mrs Gillian Tombs for her outstanding secretarial support and my most grateful thanks must go to Mrs Betty Dickens of Trans-Medica as without her expertise, good humour and common sense this text would not have been produced in this record time.

Alex M Davison
Editor
Leeds, United Kingdom

OFFICERS AND COUNCILLORS
OF THE INTERNATIONAL SOCIETY OF NEPHROLOGY
1981–1984

OFFICERS

President	D W Seldin, USA
Past President	G Richet, France
President Elect	K Thurau, FRG
Vice-President	R R Robinson, USA
Secretary-General	C Amiel, France
Treasurer	R W Schrier, USA
Editor	T E Andreoli, USA

ADVISORY COMMITTEE FOR THE 1987 CONGRESS

D W Seldin, USA, C Amiel, France, J S Cameron, UK, R J Glassock, USA, R R Robinson, USA, J Rodicio, Spain, R W Schrier, USA, K Ullrich, FRG, K Thurau, FRG, F J Goodwin, UK

COUNCILLORS

S Angielski	Poland, 1990*
R C Atkins	Australia, 1993
K Aukland	Norway, 1990
J Bergstrom	Sweden, 1987
V Bonomini	Italy, 1990
J S Cameron	UK, 1987
G d'Amico	Italy, 1993
V W Dennis	USA, 1993
J H Dirks	Canada, 1993
E J Dorhout Mees	The Netherlands, 1990
R J Glassock	USA, 1987
C W Gottschalk	USA, 1990
J-P Grünfeld	France, 1993
J Hamburger	France, lifetime
K Hierholzer	FRG, 1990
D N S Kerr	UK, 1993
R T McCluskey	USA, 1990
F C Rector Jr	USA, 1987
H Shigematsu	Japan, 1993
J Takeuchi	Japan, 1990
G Whittembury	Venezuela, 1990

*in office until

ACKNOWLEDGMENTS

The Congress Organizing Committee is most grateful to the following companies for their financial support of the Xth International Society of Nephrology Congress

Abbott Laboratories
Ames Laboratories
Amgen
Bayer UK Ltd
Baxter Travenol World Trade Corporation
Beechams
Bellco spa
British Telecom
Enka AG
E R Squibb and Sons Ltd
Gambro AB
Hospal Ltd
ICI plc
Jaguar Cars Ltd
Lederle International
Leo Laboratories
May and Baker
Merck Sharp and Dohme
Milner Laboratories
Ortho-Cilag Pharmaceutical Ltd
Ortho Pharmaceutical Corporation
Pfizer Ltd
Sandoz Products Ltd
Smith Kline and French Laboratories Ltd
Upjohn

CONTENTS
VOLUME I

Part XI – MESANGIAL PATHOPHYSIOLOGY

Part XII – MECHANISMS OF TUBULO-INTERSTITIAL NEPHRITIS

Part XIII – INHERITED RENAL DISEASES

Part XIV – DISORDERS OF SODIUM AND WATER EXCRETION

VOLUME II

Part XXI – ACUTE RENAL FAILURE

Part XXII – CHRONIC RENAL FAILURE

Part XXIII – RENAL BONE DISEASE AND ALUMINIUM

Part XXIV – ACQUIRED AND CONGENITAL CYSTIC DISEASE

Part XXV – PROGRESSIVE RENAL FAILURE

MORPHOLOGY OF THE KIDNEY

MORPHOLOGICAL ASPECTS OF GLOMERULAR FUNCTION

W Kriz, T Sakai*
with technical assistance of Hiltraud Hosser

Anatomisches Institut, Universität Heidelberg, FRG
**Faculty of Medicine, University of Tokyo, Japan*

The renal corpuscle is a very complex structure. It consists of a lobulated tuft of convoluted and anastomosing capillaries which – during development – is punched into the pouch-like commencement of the renal tubule. Thus, a fully developed renal corpuscle (Figure 1) is composed of a centrally located glomerulus (or 'glomerular tuft', since the entire renal corpuscle is now often termed 'glomerulus') and a membranous envelope called the glomerular capsule (Bowman's capsule). The latter has two parts, a visceral layer (podocyte layer) which covers the capillary tuft (thus becoming an integral part of the glomerular tuft) and the parietal layer which forms the outer wall of a renal corpuscle and, at its urinary pole, passes over into the proximal tubule epithelium. The space between both layers of the capsule is called the urinary space (Bowman's space); at the urinary pole it opens into the lumen of the proximal tubule.

At the interface between the derivatives of both primordia, i.e. between the capillary tuft and the epithelial envelope (the visceral layer of Bowman's capsule), the glomerular basement membrane is developed (Figures 1 and 2). It is of dual origin, both the epithelial podocytes and the invading endothelial cells contribute to its formation [1,2]. In a fully developed renal corpuscle, however, the glomerular basement membrane strictly follows the course of the visceral epithelium. Thus it is part of the membranous envelope that in total covers the capillary tuft. At the vascular pole, the glomerular basement membrane is reflected into the periglomerular basement membrane which underlies the parietal layer of Bowman's capsule. Thereby, an opening of Bowman's capsule is established which is bordered throughout its circumference by the collar created by the glomerular basement membrane/periglomerular basement membrane reflection. This opening corresponds to the vascular pole of the glomerulus. Through it the afferent arteriole enters and the efferent arteriole leaves the glomerular tuft.

The main function of the glomerulus is to produce a large volume of primary

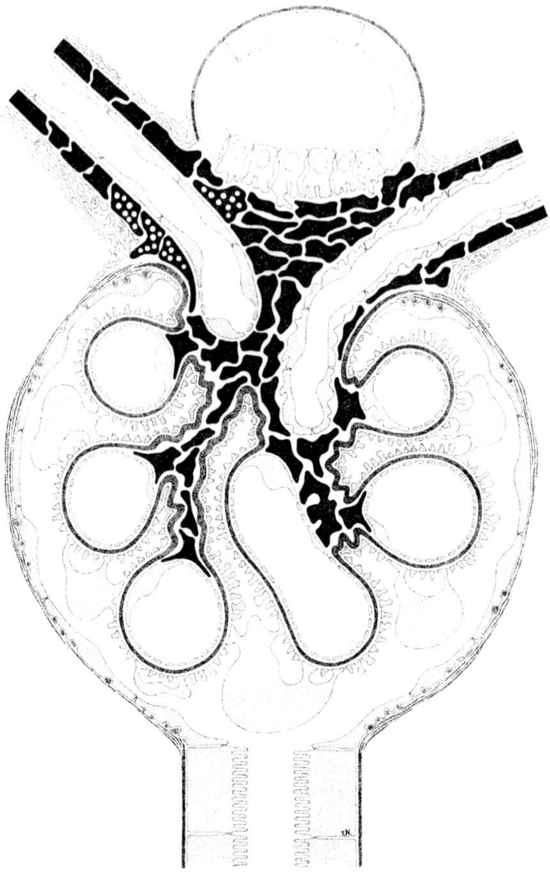

Figure 1. Schematic representation of the renal glomerulus and associated structures: not drawn to scale. All smooth muscle derived cells are shown in dark grey, i.e. the ordinary smooth muscle cells and granular cells of the afferent arteriole (left), the smooth muscle cells of the efferent arteriole (right), the extra- and intraglomerular mesangial cells. The latter together with the mesangial matrix (shown in white) establish the mesangium which has relationships to two structures; to the capillary endothelium (shown in pale grey) and to the glomerular basement membrane (shown in slightly darker grey). Note that the glomerular basement membrane has two parts: a pericapillary part which passes over into the perimesangial part at mesangial angles. At the vascular pole of the glomerulus the glomerular basement membrane is reflected into the periglomerular basement membrane, which is quite different in appearance exhibiting a multilayered structure. The collar of the glomerular basement membrane/periglomerular basement membrane reflection borders the opening in Bowman's capsule through which the extraglomerular mesangium passes over into the mesangium proper and both arterioles are connected to the capillary tuft.

All epithelial cells (parietal and visceral cells of Bowman's capsule, proximal and distal tubule cells including the macula densa) are shown in pale grey. Note the intimate relationships of the macula densa cells to the extraglomerular mesangium, which – like the mesangium – is composed of cells and an extracellular matrix (shown in white). The latter is continuous with the equally structured extracellular material underlying the endothelium of the efferent arteriole. See text for further explanation

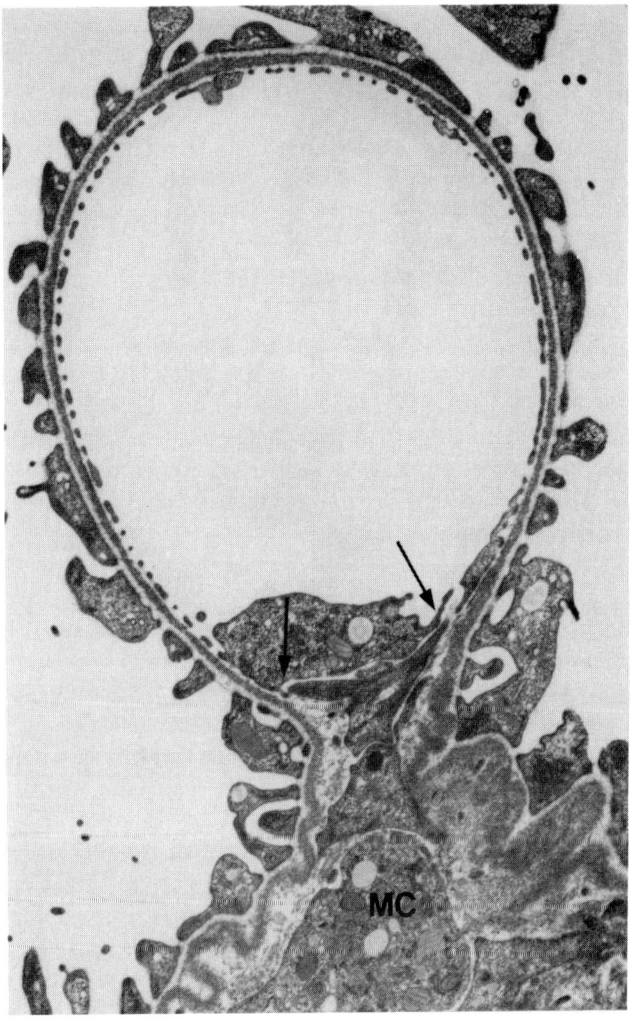

Figure 2. Cross sectional profile of a glomerular capillary together with its mesangium. The capillary endothelial tube is mainly composed of an extremely attenuated and fenestrated cytoplasm except for the cell body which is located towards the mesangium. The glomerular basement membrane is smooth and relatively thin in its pericapillary part and is wrinkled and of irregular thickness in its perimesangial part. The podocyte layer follows exactly the course of the glomerular basement membrane except its wrinkled part. A mesangial cell (MC) surrounded by the mesangial matrix sends a thick cytoplasmic process towards the capillary. From it, secondary tongue-like processes arise extending toward the mesangial angles (arrows). Unosmicated material (see Addendum); $\times \sim 16000$ (reduced for publication)

urine by ultrafiltration. This process is driven by the intracapillary hydraulic pressure (approximately 45 to 50mmHg in Munich Wistar rats [3]) which is much higher than in usual capillaries. The actual driving force of glomerular filtration is smaller, because the transmural oncotic pressure difference and the hydraulic pressure in Bowman's space oppose the intracapillary pressure. The tension in the wall of glomerular capillaries, however, is solely dependent on the hydraulic pressure difference, which amounts to about 35mmHg. Thus, we are dealing with a highly complicated structure which is continuously exposed to considerable distending forces exerted by the high hydraulic pressure in its centre. This article deals with the question of the specific structures that counterbalance the distending forces and guarantee the structural integrity of the renal corpuscle.

This question has to be considered first at the level of an individual glomerular capillary and secondly at the level of the entire corpuscle. It appears that the intraglomerular mesangial cells are the most important structures that support individual capillaries. The extraglomerular mesangial cells obviously maintain the complicated topography at the vascular pole. The parietal layer of Bowman's capsule must counterbalance the hydraulic pressure within the urinary space of Bowman's capsule.

Glomerular capillaries and mesangium

Glomerular capillaries are a specific type of blood vessel (Figure 2). Their wall is made up of an endothelial tube. A small strip of the outer circumference of this tube is in touch with the mesangium, which occupies the centre of a glomerular lobule. The glomerular basement membrane and the layer of podocytes do not belong to an individual capillary, but both together constitute a common surface cover wrapping the mesangium with its attached capillaries. Thus, the wall of glomerular capillaries has two portions (Figure 2): a *urinary portion* which bulges into Bowman's space and is covered by the glomerular basement membrane and by the visceral layer of Bowman's capsule (podocytes), and a much smaller *juxtamesangial portion* which consists of endothelium attached directly to the mesangium without even an underlying basement membrane.

At the points where the capillaries come into contact with the mesangium, the glomerular basement membrane and the podocyte layer deviate from a pericapillary course and cover the glomerular mesangium (Figures 2 and 3); these points have been called *mesangial angles* [4]. Therefore, two parts of the glomerular basement membrane and the podocyte layer have to be distinguished: a *pericapillary part* and a *perimesangial part*. The pericapillary part of the glomerular basement membrane (generally being of a fairly constant thickness in a given capillary profile) smoothly follows the outline of the capillary, whereas its perimesangial part is of irregular thickness and is frequently wrinkled. In the mesangium, two parts must also be distinguished (Figure 4a): a *juxtacapillary region* and a *sub-glomerular basement membrane region*.

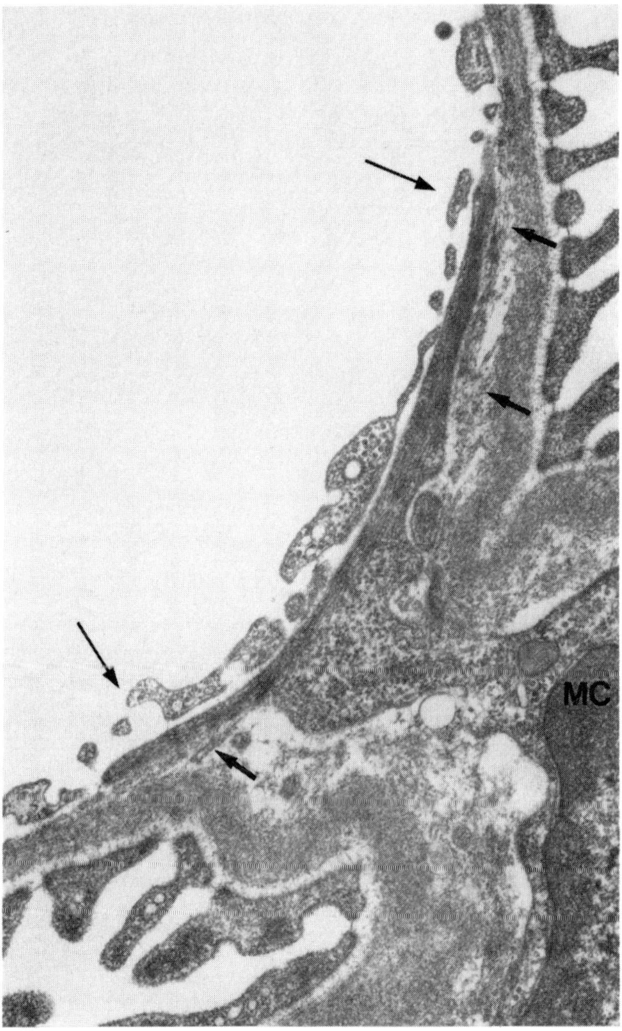

Figure 3. Electron micrograph of the juxtamesangial portion of a glomerular capillary including the juxtacapillary region of the mesangium and two opposing mesangial angles (long arrows). From the main process of the mesangial cell (MC) two tongue-like processes extend into the narrow space between the endothelium and the glomerular basement membrane at both mesangial angles. They are connected to the glomerular basement membrane by bundles of microfibrils (short arrows). Both tongue-like processes contain assemblies of microfilaments which appear to bridge the two opposing mesangial angles. Unosmicated material; × ~ 38000 (reduced for publication)

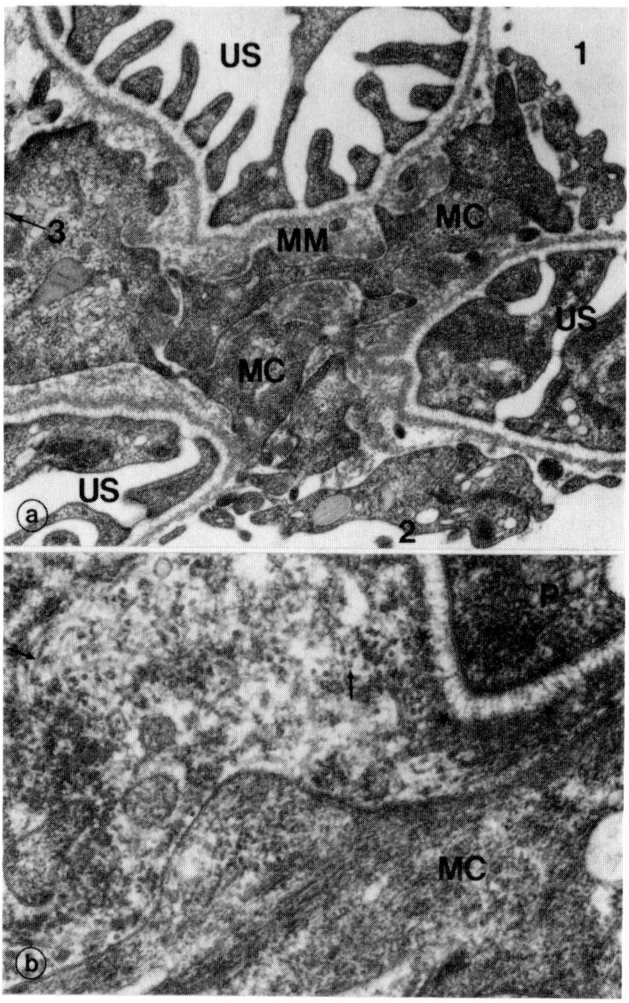

Figure 4. a) A survey view of the glomerular mesangium facing three capillaries (1, 2 and 3: the latter is not fully touched). The mesangium contains mesangial cells (MC) with many finger-like processes and the filamentous mesangial matrix (MM). Toward the urinary space (US) the mesangium is bordered by the perimesangial glomerular basement membrane and podocyte layer. Unosmicated material; × ~ 18000 (reduced for publication). b) Higher magnification of the mesangial matrix near to a mesangial angle. Individual microfibrils are seen en face or cross-sectioned (arrows). The glomerular basement membrane (marked by stars); MC=mesangial cell; P=podocyte. Unosmicated material; × ~ 65000 (reduced for publication)

The mesangium, which occupies the axial region of a glomerular lobule, consists of mesangial cells and the surrounding mesangial matrix (Figure 4a). Since their first description by Zimmermann in 1929 [5] and their ultrastructural characterization in the early sixties [6,7] the mesangial cells are widely believed to form a supporting framework which maintains the structural integrity of the glomerular tuft including its capillaries. Mesangial cells are quite irregular in shape with numerous cytoplasmic processes extending from the cell body. They contain, most densely within the processes, assemblies of microfilaments (actin bundles). From experiments in cell culture, mesangial cells are known to contract in response to a variety of vasoactive substances [8,9]. Therefore, it appears reasonable to suppose that the contractile properties of mesangial cells are responsible for active wall tension development which counteracts the distending forces of the intracapillary hydraulic pressure. However, an understanding of how mesangial cell contraction can be transferred to the capillary wall is lacking. The precise geometry of mesangial cells and their relationships to glomerular capillaries has not so far been investigated.

By applying the modified preservation technique for tissues to be studied by transmission electron microscopy (TEM: see addendum) we have recently found that mesangial cells are extensively connected with the glomerular basement membrane either directly or through microfibrils [4]. These connections, which appear to be mechanically strong, are found throughout the mesangial region; the mesangial matrix basically consists of densely interwoven microfibrils (Figure 4b). It is by this microfibrillar network that the entire perimesangial part of the glomerular basement membrane is fettered to mesangial cells. The wrinkles generally found in the perimesangial glomerular basement membrane appear to be the result of a basal tonic contraction of mesangial cells transferred to the glomerular basement membrane by microfibrils.

At mesangial angles, i.e. at the points where the glomerular basement membrane deviates from its pericapillary course and covers the mesangium, the mesangial cell–glomerular basement membrane connections are most prominent and are of a specific character (Figures 3 and 4a). The outer aspect of the juxtamesangial portion of each capillary, which can be viewed as a narrow strip extending in the longitudinal axis of the endothelial tube, is consistently associated with typically arranged mesangial cell processes. In a cross-sectional profile of a capillary such processes, arising from a more centrally located cell body, approach the capillary and give rise to secondary tongue-like processes which run towards the mesangial angles. Very frequently they extend into the narrowing space between the endothelium and the glomerular basement membrane, being either directly or indirectly connected via short microfibrils to the glomerular basement membrane. Other processes stay remote from the bend of the glomerular basement membrane at a mesangial angle but are connected to this bend by bundles of long microfibrils.

All these mesangial cell processes are stuffed with dense assemblies of contractile filaments which run in a tangential direction to the circular circumference of the capillaries (Figure 3). They appear to be anchored to the cytoskeleton in the parent process. In the case where a process is connected to the glomerular basement membrane by long microfibrils, the direction of the intracellular microfilaments is continued extracellularly to microfibrils which finally insert into the glomerular basement membrane in an oblique direction. At other places processes are found, which bridge the entire space between two mesangial angles, suggesting that the microfilament bundles almost directly connect the glomerular basement membrane from two opposing mesangial angles. All of these structures are arranged in such a way that contraction of mesangial cells can bring the glomerular basement membrane from opposing mesangial angles closer together.

In summary, these findings indicate that mesangial cells and the glomerular basement membrane are tightly connected with each other. From a functional point of view, both together appear to form a biomechanical unit capable of counterbalancing the distending forces of the high hydraulic intracapillary pressure. The contractility of mesangial cells is not in doubt; the glomerular basement membrane appears appropriate for its proposed relevance as a main skeletal element of the glomerulus. The dense meshwork of collagen type IV making up the lamina densa has been compared to a 'backbone' [10] and is thought to provide a remarkable firmness and tensile strength to the glomerular basement membrane [11,12].

From this point of view the glomerular basement membrane has two major functions in the glomerulus. It represents an important barrier within the glomerular filter and it serves as an elastic skeletal element of the capillary wall whose tension may be modulated by the contractility of mesangial cells. Possibly, this dual function will turn out to be the key to understanding how mesangial cell contraction or relaxation can influence the glomerular filtration coefficient and hence the glomerular filtration rate.

The glomerular vascular pole–extraglomerular mesangium

The specific relationships between mesangial cells and the glomerular basement membrane are obviously responsible for opposing the distending forces of the high intraglomerular pressure at the level of an individual capillary. A similar biomechanical relationship can be seen on a larger scale at the vascular pole of the renal corpuscle (Figures 1 and 5). At this point, the visceral layer of Bowman's capsule transforms into the parietal layer and the glomerular basement membrane is reflected into the periglomerular basement membrane, thereby forming an opening in Bowman's capsule mentioned in the beginning. This opening allows the entry and the exit of the afferent and efferent arterioles to and from the glomerular tuft, respectively. Furthermore, through this opening the glomerular mesangial cells pass out of the glomerular stalk to become extraglomerular mesangial cells. The afferent and efferent arterioles are located laterally

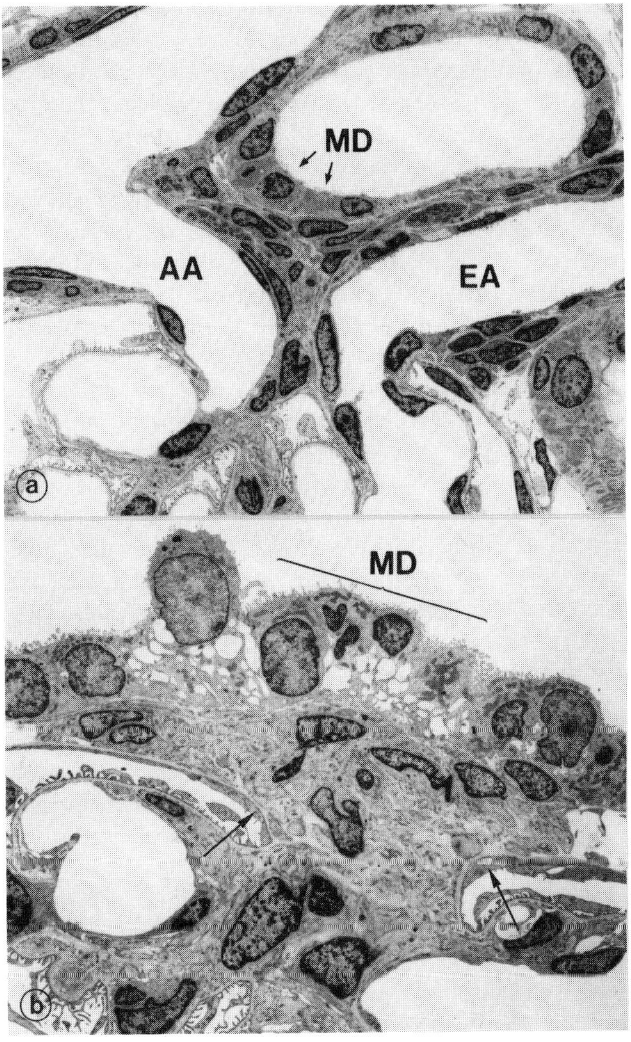

Figure 5. Sections through the glomerular vascular pole. In (a) the section plane runs through both the afferent (AA) and efferent (EA) arterioles. The extraglomerular mesangium is seen to fill the triangular space bordered by both arterioles and the macula densa (MD). It is continuous with the glomerular mesangium through a narrow stalk between both arterioles. In (b) a section through the vascular pole is shown running perpendicular to that in (a); thus the arterioles are not touched. The extraglomerular mesangium is seen as a solid group of cells which continues into the mesangium and is in close association with the macula densa (MD). On both sides, these cells cover the glomerular basement membrane/periglomerular basement membrane reflection (arrows) and are connected with the periglomerular basement membrane. Osmicated material (from cooperation with Dr Brigitte Kaissling); (a) × ~ 1250, (b) × ~ 2200 (reduced for publication)

in this elongated opening and the extra- and intraglomerular mesangial cells communicate predominantly through an area between both arterioles [13].

The extraglomerular mesangial cells are located within a triangular space bordered by the two glomerular arterioles and the macula densa of the thick ascending limb (Figure 5a). By reconstruction, extraglomerular mesangial cells of the rabbit kidney have been shown to be flat elongated cells which at both poles divide into two bunches of long cell processes [14]. They are piled up several layers deep, and the layers are arranged parallel to the base of the macula densa (Figures 5b and 6a). The cells nearest to the glomerular stalk and filling the deepest portion of the triangle are no longer parallel to the macula densa base; they extend – either with part of their cell body or at least with some processes – into the stalk of the glomerular tuft mixing there with mesangial cells [15].

Within a given layer the elongated extraglomerular mesangial cells all appear to point in the same direction. In adjacent layers, however, this primary direction of the cells is set at different angles. Even if precise data about the course of extraglomerular mesangial cells are lacking, they mostly appear to run straight across the angle between the two glomerular arterioles. In sections through the vascular pole following this direction it can be seen that their processes successively approach the periglomerular basement membrane to which they finally become anchored (Figure 6). Thus, the extraglomerular mesangial cells appear to bridge the two opposing sides of the middle part of the opening in Bowman's capsule, which is not occupied by the two arterioles. Other, more obliquely running extraglomerular mesangial cells interconnect the two glomerular arterioles. As a whole, the extraglomerular mesangium appears to be a closure device for the opening of Bowman's capsule. In the very centre of this opening the opposing parts of the glomerular basement membrane/periglomerular basement membrane reflection and the two glomerular arterioles are mechanically coupled to each other.

Thus, the extraglomerular mesangial cells have a similar topographical relationship to Bowman's capsule as intraglomerular mesangial cells have to glomerular capillaries. Although direct evidence is lacking, the extraglomerular mesangial cells – like intraglomerular mesangial cells – can be expected to be contractile for several reasons. Firstly, the extraglomerular mesangial cells contain a moderate amount of contractile microfilaments, mainly in their processes. Secondly, intimate structural similarities and topographical relationships are found among arteriolar smooth muscle cells, granular cells, intra- and extraglomerular mesangial cells suggesting that they have the same origin and are all variations of smooth muscle cells [16]. Extensively developed gap junctions among all of these cells support this idea [17–20].

An important component of the extraglomerular mesangium is the surrounding extracellular matrix [20] which appears to contribute essentially to the integrating function of the extraglomerular mesangial cells. Structurally, the

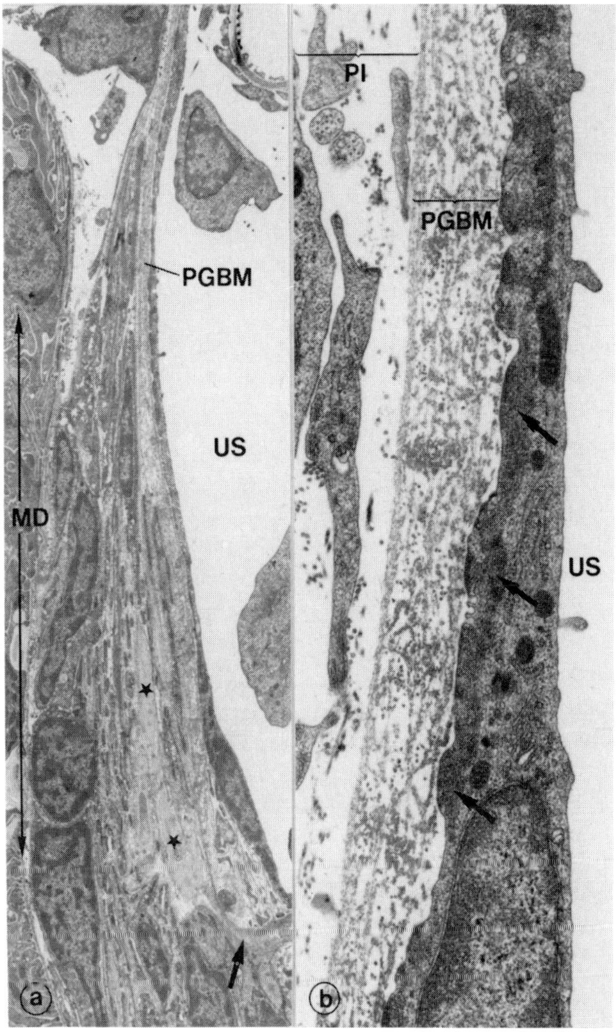

Figure 6. (a) Section through a glomerular vascular pole similar to that shown in Figure 5b. The extraglomerular mesangial cells with their plate-like processes are arranged in layers parallel to the base of the macula densa (MD). The lateral extensions of extraglomerular mesangial cells terminate and anchor at the periglomerular basement membrane (PGBM). The PGBM reflection is indicated by an arrow. US=urinary space. Some of the extraglomerular mesangial cells are less darkly stained (asterisks) than others. Unosmicated material; × ~ 4500 (reduced for publication).

(b) Middle part of the parietal layer of Bowman's capsule together with its underlying PGBM. Dense assemblies of microfilaments (arrows) are seen in the basal parts of a parietal cell. The PGBM is multilayered with extracellular fibrillar bundles. PI=periglomerular interstitium. Unosmicated material; × ~ 21000 (reduced for publication)

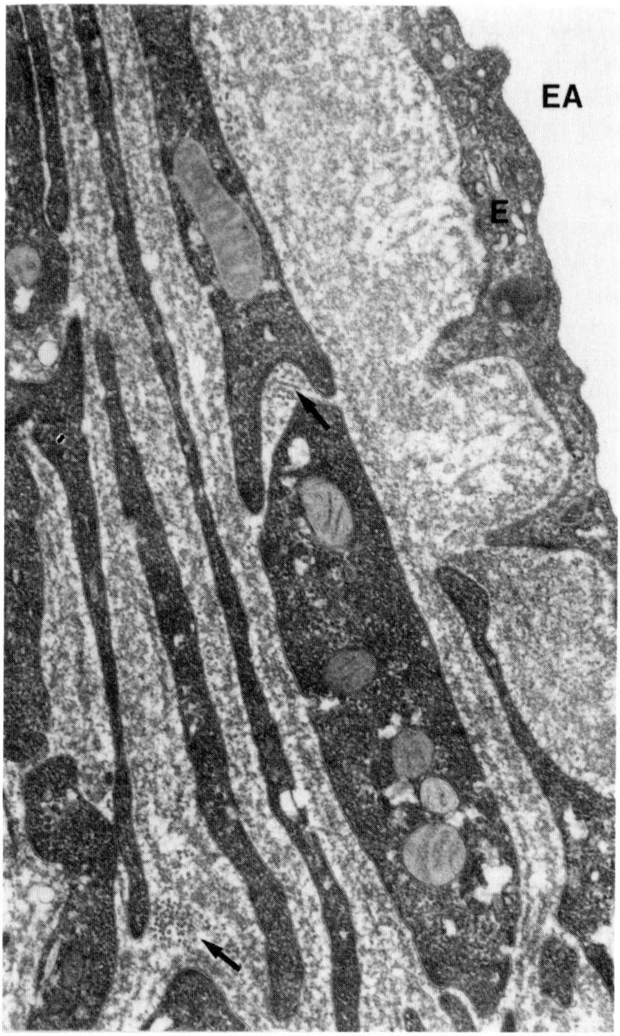

Figure 7. Extraglomerular mesangium near to an efferent arteriole (EA). The extracellular material between the extraglomerular mesangial cells is regularly arranged in sheets reflecting the plate-like shapes of the cell processes. At some places (arrows) microfibrils are encountered. The extraglomerular mesangial matrix is continuous with the extracellular matrix underlying the endothelium (E) of the efferent arteriole. Unosmicated material; × ~ 49000 (reduced for publication)

mesangial matrix of the glomerular tuft (as described above) consists of a network of microfibrils which appear to fetter the perimesangial part of the glomerular basement membrane to the contractile mesangial cells. At the vascular pole, within the stocking of the glomerular basement membrane/periglomerular basement membrane reflection, the mesangial matrix is continuous with the basement membrane-like extracellular material which surrounds the extraglomerular mesangial cells and which we call *extraglomerular mesangial matrix* (Figure 7). Structurally, this matrix is different from the mesangial matrix proper. Even though microfibrils have been found at many places in the extraglomerular matrix, this contrasts strongly with the dense microfibrils which are consistently seen within the mesangial matrix.

The extraglomerular matrix appears to be more regularly organized than the mesangial matrix (Figures 4b and 7) possibly reflecting the more regular shape and arrangement of the extraglomerular mesangial cells compared to intraglomerular mesangial cells. The extraglomerular matrix is often found to be organized in layers similar to basement membrane, but consisting of two or three dense layers separated by translucent laminae. This layered appearance can be interpreted as an adaptation to the narrow spaces between the plate-like cell processes of extraglomerular mesangial cells.

Even if generally thicker and often multilayered, the extraglomerular matrix material resembles the interposed basement membranes that connect individual smooth muscle cells to form a smooth muscle tunica (as, for instance, in the media of the afferent arteriole: Figure 7). We think, therefore, that this extracellular material between the extraglomerular mesangial cells also serves for the mutual mechanical coupling of extraglomerular mesangial cells. Moreover, at the periphery it couples the extraglomerular mesangial cells to the smooth muscle cells of the afferent and efferent arterioles, to granular cells, to the intraglomerular mesangial cells and possibly also to the macula densa cells. In addition this material mediates the connection of the extraglomerular mesangial cells to the periglomerular basement membrane.

Thus, any mechanical alteration, any movement (any active contraction, any passive distension) within the juxtaglomerular apparatus and related structures may be mechanically transmitted to all other structures. All these cells (except for the macula densa cells) are extensively coupled by gap junctions, so all the smooth muscle derived cells at the glomerular vascular pole appear to establish a contractile closure device for the glomerular vascular entrance. On the other hand, the overall tension in this system will depend on the intraglomerular pressure (or some equivalent of it) and this system will probably react to an increased tension by contraction. Furthermore, this arrangement may serve as some sort of a stretch transducer which signals changes in tension created by the intraglomerular pressure to more up- or down-stream located smooth muscle cells of the glomerular arterioles and to the granular cells of the afferent arteriole.

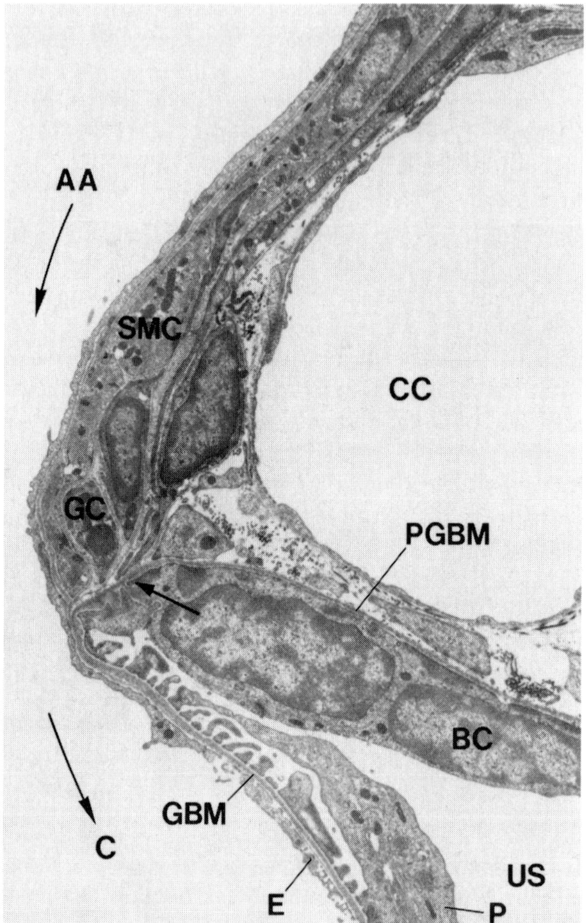

Figure 8. Transition of an afferent arteriole (AA) into an intraglomerular capillary (C). The media of the afferent arteriole including smooth muscle cells (SMC) and granular cells (GC) terminates just at the vessel entry into the glomerulus anchoring to the glomerular basement membrane/periglomerular basement membrane (GBM/PGBM) reflection (arrow). The glomerular capillary (C) is surrounded by the typical wall consisting of a fenestrated endothelium (E), the GBM and podocyte (P) layer. BC=Bowman's capsule, parietal layer; US=urinary space; CC=cortical capillary. Unosmicated material; × ~ 6800 (reduced for publication)

Glomerular vascular pole – afferent and efferent arterioles

The glomerular afferent and efferent arterioles enter and leave the glomerular tuft, respectively, located laterally in the elongated opening of Bowman's capsule (Figure 1). Just at its entry into the glomerular tuft, the afferent arteriole loses all its surrounding smooth muscle and granular cells which mostly anchor to the glomerular basement membrane/periglomerular basement membrane (Figure 8). Those smooth muscle and granular cells on the side towards the centre of the opening intermingle with extraglomerular mesangial cells. Again other smooth muscle and granular cells develop processes that enter alongside the afferent endothelial tube into the glomerular tuft mixing up with mesangial cells. Immediately after its entry, the endothelial tube of the afferent arteriole splits up into the first order branches which supply individual glomerular lobules.

The efferent arteriole behaves in a slightly different way (Figures 9–11). Frequently, the endothelial tube of the efferent arteriole is already established some distance within the glomerular tuft. At the exit level, the efferent arteriole receives a media which (at the very beginning) appears to consist, at least in part, of cell processes of extraglomerular mesangial cells that encircle the vessel like the smooth muscle cells proper; there is much branching of smooth muscle cells at this site [21]. Further downstream the efferent arteriole usually has a single-layered media.

There is a further conspicuous difference between the afferent and the efferent arteriole concerning the wall structure. The endothelium of the terminal portion of the afferent arteriole at the vascular pole is underlaid by a thin and smooth basement membrane which separates or connects the endothelium to the smooth muscle or granular cells of the media (Figure 8). As already mentioned, immediately after its entry into the glomerular tuft the afferent arteriole splits up into its lobular branches. In contrast, the efferent arteriole usually has an initial portion located some distance within the glomerular tuft. At its basal aspect the endothelium of the efferent arteriole is very irregular in appearance, exhibiting many invaginations and protrusions and is embedded into abundant extracellular matrix which resembles the extraglomerular mesangial matrix, even around the intraglomerular initial portion (Figures 10 and 11). Even after the emergence of the efferent arteriole from Bowman's capsule the intimate relationships between the extracellular matrix and the irregular basal aspect of the endothelium are maintained [22,23]. Thus, the endothelium of the outflow segment of the efferent arteriole (before and after the exit level from the glomerulus) has intimate relationships to the surrounding abundant extracellular matrix (Figure 7) – much different from the usual relationships of an arteriolar capillary endothelium to its underlying basement membrane. This extracellular material around the efferent arteriole is continuous with the intra- and extraglomerular mesangial matrix [24].

The functional relevance of this difference is unknown. One may, however, speculate that an overall (possibly a slight) contraction of the mesangium,

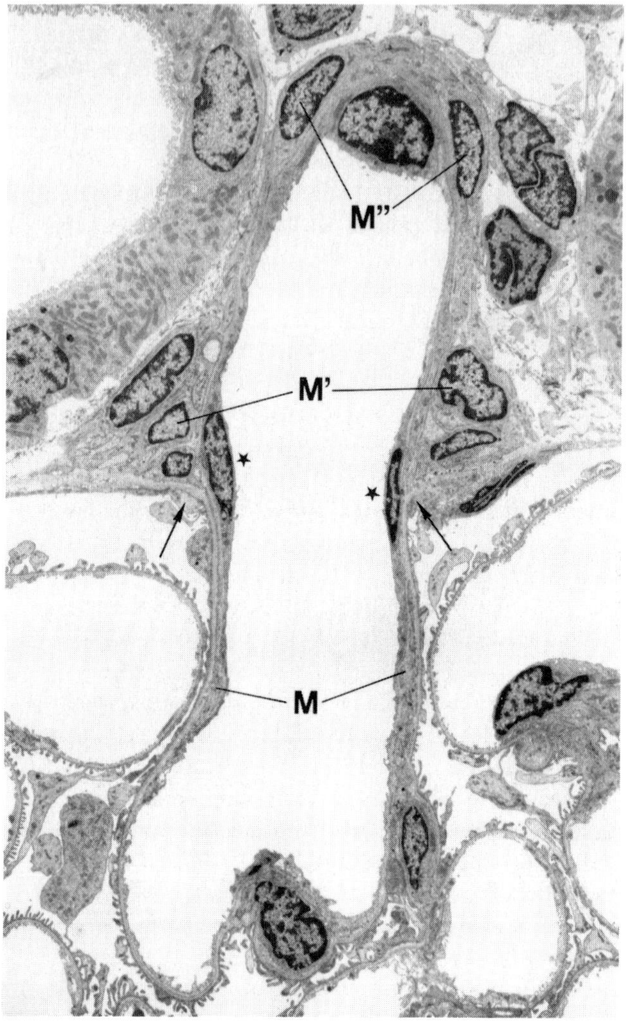

Figure 9. Outflow segment of an efferent arteriole consisting of an intraglomerular and an extraglomerular part. Just at the transition between both parts, the nuclei of two endothelial cells are found (asterisks). The wall of the intraglomerular part contains already a thin 'media' (M; made up of mesangial cell processes) found between the endothelial and the epithelial layers. Just after its exit the efferent arteriole appears to be surrounded by a thicker media (M'; made up here, at least in part, by extraglomerular mesangial cells) filling the corners between the endothelial tube and the parietal layer of Bowman's capsule at both sites. Downstream the media (M") is single layered made up of smooth muscle cells. Glomerular basement membrane/periglomerular basement membrane reflections are indicated by arrows. Routinely osmicated material; × ~ 2900 (reduced for publication)

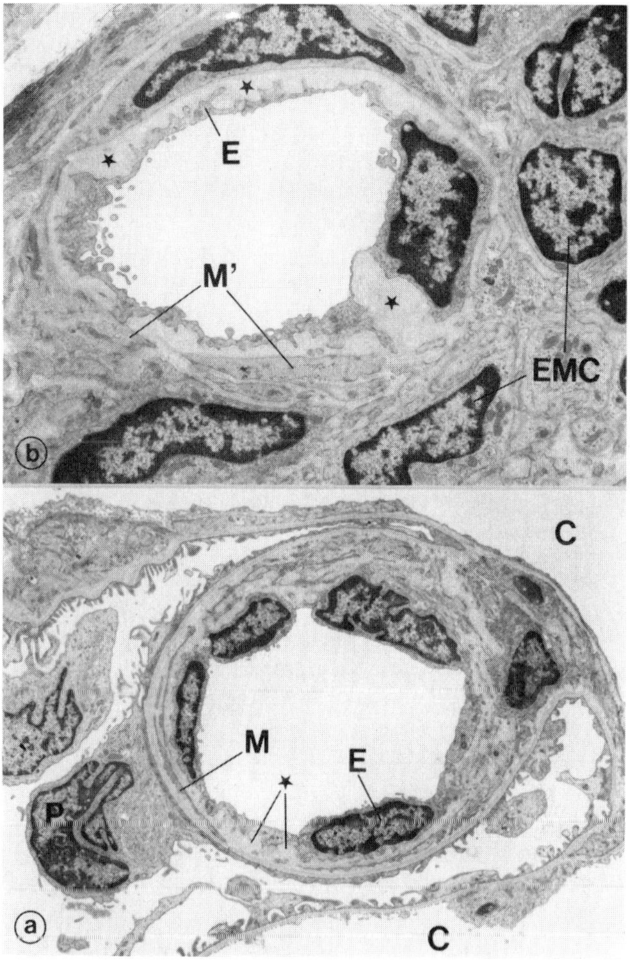

Figure 10. Cross sectional profiles of intraglomerular (a) and extraglomerular (b) parts of efferent arterioles. The intraglomerular efferent arteriole (a) is characterized by an irregularly shaped basal aspect of the endothelium associated with abundant extracellular material. This material together with sheet-like processes of mesangial cells establish a layer around the endothelial tube which may be compared to a media. The extracellular material filling the basal invaginations of the endothelium is marked by an asterisk. E=endothelium; M=media; C=glomerular capillary; P=podocyte.

The extraglomerular portion of the efferent arteriole (b) is outlined by a thin very irregularly elaborated endothelium underlayed by abundant extracellular material (asterisks). The endothelial tube is surrounded by a multilayered media (M') which is – in part at least – established by extraglomerular mesangial cells (EMC). Routinely osmicated material; (a) × ~ 3600, (b) × ~ 5800 (reduced for publication)

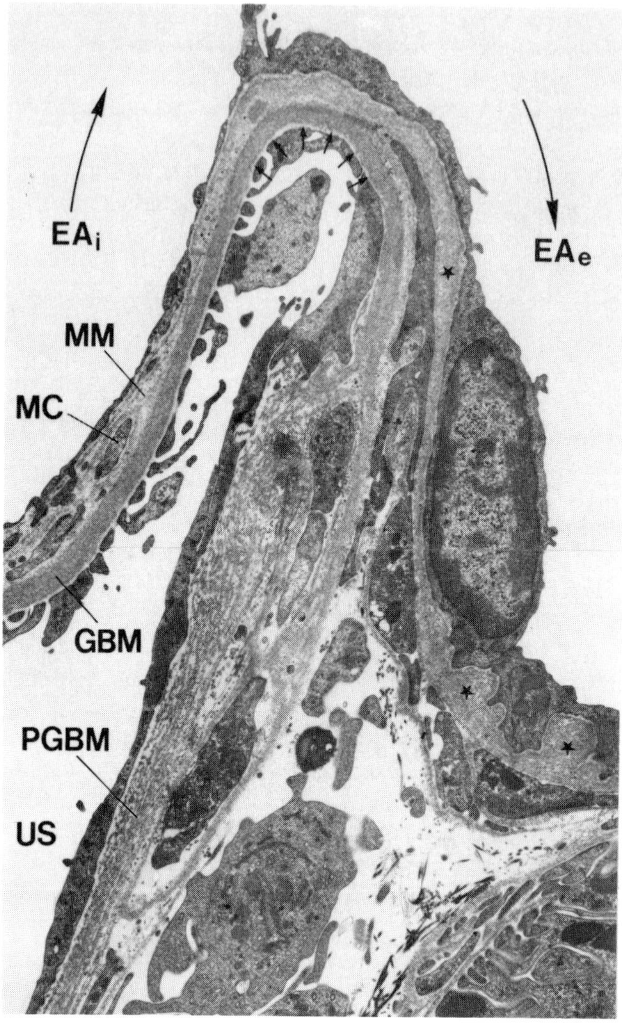

Figure 11. A survey view showing a glomerular basement membrane/periglomerular basement membrane reflection along the outflow segment of an efferent arteriole. Shortly after the reflection (shown by a sequence of arrows) the glomerular basement membrane splits up into several thin sheets which make up the periglomerular basement membrane. Note that the mesangial matrix found between the glomerular basement membrane and the endothelium of the intraglomerular part of the efferent arteriole (EAi) transforms into the extracellular material (asterisks) underlying the endothelium of the extraglomerular part of the efferent arteriole (EAe). GBM=glomerular basement membrane; MC=mesangial cell; MM=mesangial matrix; PGBM=periglomerular basement membrane; US=urinary space. Unosmicated material; X ~ 12700 (reduced for publication)

including the extraglomerular mesangium, will increase the interstitial pressure within this system and (via the extracellular matrix) be transferred to the efferent arteriole causing a slight compression of the endothelial tube. Thus, without affecting the afferent arteriole an overall contraction of intra- and extraglomerular mesangial cells of the vascular pole might cause a constriction of the effererent arteriole. In observations of the glomerular vessels in the split hydronephrotic kidney, the outflow segment of the efferent arteriole has been found to be strikingly narrow [25]. Whether this is an extreme adaptation to the non-filtering condition in this experimental model possibly mediated by the contraction of mesangial cells remains to be established.

In conclusion, the skeletal elements at the vascular pole of the glomerulus are arranged to interconnect the individual structures and to hold them together. In addition, this system appears to be actively involved in the regulation of glomerular blood flow. The details, even the structural details, are poorly understood. Aspects of the integration of the granular cells into this system and relationships to the macula densa have been excluded from this presentation.

Bowman's capsule

The parietal cell layer of Bowman's capsule, together with its underlying basement membrane, establish the outer wall of a renal corpuscle (Figure 1). This wall, as well, is exposed to distending forces exerted by the intraglomerular hydraulic pressure, or more precisely, by the hydraulic pressure difference between the urinary space and the periglomerular interstitium. There are both active and passive elements opposing this distending force.

The parietal cells of Bowman's capsule are stuffed with thick bundles of actin filaments running in all directions [26,27]. They are especially prominent at the vascular and the urinary pole (Figure 11) where they appear to run in a circular direction (suggested from the cross-sectioned appearance in meridional sections).

The passive component is represented by the periglomerular basement membrane, which has a very specific structure. As already mentioned, the periglomerular basement membrane develops from the glomerular basement membrane at the vascular pole and transforms to the tubular basement membrane at the urinary pole (Figure 11). The transition of the glomerular basement membrane into the periglomerular basement membrane is characterized by the splitting of the thick glomerular basement membrane into several sheets which together form the periglomerular basement membrane. Thus, the periglomerular basement membrane is a multilayered basement membrane composed of several dense layers which are separated by more translucent laminae (Figure 6b). It appears that within the individual sheets the network of the matrix is orientated in various directions. In sectional profiles through entire glomeruli, the periglomerular basement membrane may be found to be of very variable thickness, sometimes composed of five or six sheets, at other sites only of one sheet. We imagine that the entire structure in its three-dimensional appearance is a membranous envelope consisting (like the wicker-work of a basket) of thicker strands leaving thinner parts between. At many places, especially at the poles, the active and passive components, i.e. the intracellular assemblies of actin filaments and the extracellular filamentous material of the periglomerular basement membrane, are arranged in parallel.

At the vascular pole, the transitional region between the glomerular basement membrane and the periglomerular basement membrane is mechanically connected to the smooth muscle cells of the afferent and efferent arteriole and to the extraglomerular mesangial cells (Figures 8, 9 and 11). It appears that changes in the tension of the periglomerular basement membrane can be transferred to the extraglomerular mesangial cells as well as to granular cells and smooth muscle cells of the glomerular arterioles.

Addendum

This study is based on material from rats which for the most part has been prepared for transmission electron microscopy by a newly developed preservation technique. In this technique, the usual treatment with osmium is cut out but replaced by en-bloc staining with tannic acid and uranyl acetate (after various pretreatments). Dehydration is carried out in acetone at gradually decreasing temperatures [see 4]. Figures using this technique are 2, 3, 4, 6, 7, 8 and 11.

Acknowledgments

We are grateful to Ms Ingrid Ertel for photographic work, Mr Rolf Nonnenmacher for the excellent artwork and Ms Laura Winkel and Ms Helene Dehoust for secretarial help. The work is supported by Deutsche Forschungsgemeinschaft, Forschergruppe Niere, Heidelberg.

References

1 Sariola H, Peault B, La Douarin N et al. Extracellular matrix and capillary ingrowth in interspecies chimeric kidneys. *Cell Differ 1984; 15:* 43–52

2 Abrahamson DR. Origin of the glomerular basement membrane visualized after in vivo labeling of laminin in newborn rat kidney. *J Cell Biol 1985; 100:* 1988–2000

3 Brenner BM, Dworkin LD, Ichikawa I. Glomerular ultrafiltration. In Brenner BM, Rector FC, eds. *The Kidney*. Philadelphia: W B Saunders. 1986: 124–144

4 Sakai T, Kriz W. The structural relationship between mesangial cells and basement membrane of the renal glomerulus. *Anat Embryol 1987; 176:* 373–388

5 Zimmerman KW. Über den Bau des Glomerulus der menschlichen Niere. *Z Mikrosk Anat Forsch 1929; 18:* 520–552

6 Latta H, Maunsbach AB, Madden SC. The centrolobular region of the renal glomerulus studied by electron microscopy. *J Ultrastruct Res 1960; 4:* 455–472

7 Farquhar MG, Palade GE. Functional evidence for the existence of a third cell type in the renal glomerulus. Phagocytosis of filtration residues by a distinctive 'third' cell. *J Cell Biol 1962; 13:* 55–87

8 Kreisberg JI. Contractile properties of the glomerular mesangium. *Fed Proc 1983; 42:* 3053–3057

9 Foidart JB, Mahieu P. Glomerular mesangial cell contractility in vitro is controlled by an angiotensin-prostaglandin balance. *Mol Cell Endocrinol 1986; 47:* 163–173

10 Dousa TP. Glomerular metabolism. In Seldin DW, Giebisch G, eds. *The Kidney: Physiology and Pathophysiology*. New York: Raven Press. 1985: 645–667

11 Kanwar YS. Biology of disease. Biophysiology of glomerular filtration and proteinuria. *Lab Invest 1984; 51:* 7–21

12 Timpl R. Recent advances in the biochemistry of glomerular basement membrane. *Kidney Int 1986; 30:* 293–298

13 Frank M, Kriz W. Scanning electron microscopy studies of the vascular pole of the rat glomerulus. *Anat Rec 1982; 204:* 149–152

14 Spanidis A, Wunsch H, Kaissling B, Kriz W. Three-dimensional shape of a Goormaghtigh cell and its contact with a granular cell in the rabbit kidney. *Anat Embryol 1982; 165:* 239–252

15 Barajas L. The ultrastructure of the juxtaglomerular apparatus as disclosed by three-dimensional reconstructions from serial sections: the anatomical relationship between the tubular and vascular components. *J Ultrastruct Res 1970; 33:* 116–147

16 Rouiller C, Orci L. The structure of the juxtaglomerular complex. In Rouiller C, Muller AF, eds. *The Kidney: Morphology, Biochemistry, Physiology.* New York: Academic Press. 1971: 1–80

17 Taugner R, Schiller A, Kaissling B, Kriz W. Gap junctional coupling between the JGA and the glomerular tuft. *Cell Tissue Res 1978; 186:* 279–285

18 Pricam C, Humbert F, Perrelet A, Orci L. Gap junctions in mesangial and lacis cells. *J Cell Biol 1974; 63:* 349–354

19 Boll H-U, Forssmann WG, Taugner R. Studies on the juxtaglomerular apparatus. *Cell Tissue Res 1975; 161:* 459–469

20 Oberling C, Hatt PY. Etude de l'appareille juxtaglomerulaire du rat au microscope electronique. *Ann Anat Pathol 1960; 5:* 441–474

21 Gattone II VH, Luft FC, Evan AP. Renal afferent and efferent arterioles of the rabbit. *Am J Physiol 1984; 247:* F219–F228

22 Kriz W, Bachmann S. Pre- and postglomerular arterioles of the kidney. *J Cardiovasc Pharmacol 1985; 7 (Suppl 3):* S24–S30

23 Kriz W, Kaissling B. Structural organization of the mammalian kidney. In Seldin DW, Giebisch G, eds. *The Kidney: Physiology and Pathophysiology.* New York: Raven Press. 1985: 265–306

24 Schnabel E, Kriz W. Morphometric studies of the extraglomerular mesangial cell fluid in volume expanded and volume depleted rats. *Anat Embryol 1984; 170:* 217–222

25 Steinhausen M, Snoei H, Parekh N et al. Hydronephrosis: a new method to visualize vas afferens, efferens, and glomerular network. *Kidney Int 1983; 23:* 794–806

26 Newstead JD. Filaments in the renal parenchyma and interstitial cells. *J Ultrastruct Res 1971; 34:* 316–328

27 Andrews PM, Bates SD. Filamentous actin bundles in the kidney. *Anat Rec 1984; 210:* 1–9

NEPHRON HETEROGENEITY

J P Kokko

Emory University School of Medicine, Atlanta, Georgia, USA

Eighty years ago Peter [1] noted that not all nephrons are alike, but rather could be divided into two broad categories, based on their turning point in the medulla: nephrons that possess short loops (superficial nephrons) and ones that have long loops (juxtamedullary nephrons). In the last four decades there has been a systematic search for functional differences in different nephron segments. As a consequence of the development of in vivo micropuncture and in vitro microperfusion technices there has been an explosion of physiological information in the last two decades concerning the function of specific nephron segments. This functional difference has led to the division of each nephron into nine basic segments: proximal convoluted tubule, proximal straight tubule, descending limb of Henle, thin ascending limb of Henle, thick ascending limb of Henle, distal convoluted tubule, cortical collecting tubule, outer medullary collecting tubule and inner medullary collecting tubule. This functional segmentation of a specific nephron is known as *intranephron* or axial heterogeneity. It is clear that even within these nine primary segments further subsectional differences in function occur. Furthermore, since 1975 [2] we have also known that intrinsic tubular transport differences exist between proximal tubules of superficial as contrasted to juxtamedullary nephrons. This latter finding has led to the concept that is now known as *internephron* heterogeneity. Thus nephron heterogeneity exists at both inter- and intratubular levels. In general terms there exist corresponding morphological differences between specific nephron segments which form the basis of structural–functional relationships. Because of constraints of space this presentation will omit the consideration of vascular heterogeneity, but will review tubular heterogeneity in a sequential fashion.

Proximal convoluted tubule

The proximal convoluted tubule is divided into two sections: early and late. The early section (S_1) extend 1–3mm beyond the glomerulus and is morphologically different from the later section (S_2) [3–5]. While intrinsic differences exist between the S_1 and S_2 segments, these two segments also function differently as a consequence of the different composition of fluid flowing through each part.

The S_1 segments actively reabsorbs a number of intraluminal substituents. Many of these substances are reabsorbed completely or their concentrations are lowered significantly. The reabsorption of bicarbonate is most important with regard to change in composition of perfusing tubular fluid. Indeed, Walker et al [6] pointed out in 1941 that tubular fluid chloride concentration increased to an average of 1.4 times that of plasma within the first third of the proximal convoluted tubule. The mechanism of bicarbonate reabsorption is a complex subject that has been the subject of countless studies and numerous chapters. It is beyond the scope of this paper to review these studies but, in summary, the bicarbonate reabsorption occurs primarily due to H^+ secretion (Na/H exchange and probably electrogenic H^+ secretion) with subsequent formation of carbonic acid. Carbonic acid, in turn, may in part diffuse out of the tubule by nonionic diffusion or as CO_2, that is the product of dehydration of carbonic acid. This complex subject is beautifully reviewed in the recent work of Alpern, Warnock and Rector [7]. Nevertheless, with preferential reabsorption of bicarbonate and with secondary osmotic equilibration of water, the chloride concentration rises as originally pointed out by Walker et al [6] and subsequently confirmed by at least 17 studies [8]. The rise in chloride concentration occurs both in the early part of the superficial proximal convoluted tubule as well as the juxtamedullary proximal convoluted tubule [9].

Other active transport processes participate in the early proximal convoluted tubule to change the luminal composition of late proximal convoluted tubular fluid. Most glucose, aminoacids and a large part of phosphates are reabsorbed in the S_1 segment. These substrates are reabsorbed by Na coupled mechanisms driven by the Na gradient produced by basolateral Na/K-ATPase. Thus the fluid that enters the S_2 segment of the proximal convoluted tubule is different from glomerular filtrate in that it has a lower concentration of bicarbonate, glucose, aminoacids, phosphates and a higher concentration of chloride.

The transepithelial potential difference is different in S_1 versus S_2 segments. In early segments of both superficial and juxtamedullary nephrons, the transepithelial potential difference is lumen negative [9–13] due to electrogenic Na cotransport with various organic substrates. As the fluid courses through the S_2 segment then in superficial nephrons the potential difference becomes lumen positive due to a chloride diffusion potential [11,12,14,15]. However, if the findings of in vitro studies are extended to in vivo, then it can be argued that the lumen remains negative in S_2 of juxtamedullary nephrons because of lower chloride permeability [11]. The intrinsic permeability characteristics of various proximal convoluted tubule segments are summarized in Table I.

TABLE I. Relative transport characteristics of the different nephron segments

Modified from Kokko JP. Overview of renal physiology. In Kokko JP, Tannen RL, eds. *Fluids and Electrolytes.* Philadelphia: W B Saunders. 1986: 844. The summarized values may not be applicable to all species but reflect a consensus of data thus far obtained.

Segment	Permeability					Active transport process
	Osmotic water	Sodium	Chloride	Potassium	Urea	
Early superficial proximal convoluted tubule	+ + +	ND[1]	ND[1]	ND[2]	+ + +	Primary, Na[3]
Late superficial proximal convoluted tubule	+ + +	+ +	+ + +	+ +	+ + +	Secondary, glucose[3]
Early juxtamedullary proximal convoluted tubule	+ + +	ND[1]	ND[1]	ND[2]	+ + +	Secondary, aminoacids[3]
Late juxtamedullary proximal convoluted tubule	+ + +	+ + +	+ +	ND[2]	+ + +	Secondary, PO_4 [3]
Superficial pars recta	+ + +	+ +	+ + +	+	+	Primary, Na[4]
Juxtamedullary pars recta	+ + +	+ + +	+ +	+ + +	+ +	Secondary, H[4]
Thin descending limb of Henle[5]	+ + + +	+	+/−	+	0/+	0
Thin ascending limb of Henle	0	+ + + +	+ + + +	+ + + +	+ + +	0
Medullary thick ascending limb of Henle	0	+ + +	0/+	+	0/+	Secondary, Cl
Cortical thick ascending limb of Henle	0	+ +	0/+	+	+	Secondary, Cl
Distal convoluted tubule	0	0/+	0/+	+ +	0	Primary, Na Secondary, K, H
Cortical collecting duct	0 without ADH + + with ADH	0/+	+	0/+	0	Primary, Na, H Secondary, H, K
Outer medullary collecting duct	0 without ADH + + with ADH	0/+	0/+	+	0	Primary, H
Inner medullary collecting tubule 1	0 without ADH + + with ADH	0/+	0/+	0/+	+ +	Primary, Na
Inner medullary collecting tubule 2	0 without ADH + + with ADH	0/+	0/+	0/+	+ +	Primary, Na
Inner medullary collecting tubule 3	0 without ADH + + with ADH	0/+	0/+	0/+	+ + +	Primary, Na

1 Absolute permeability to Na and Cl has not been determined, but the early superficial and juxtamedullary proximal convoluted tubule are more permeable to Na than to Cl.

2 No data: absolute permeability to K in these segments of proximal tubules has not been determined, but in a study using random proximal convoluted tubules, the permeability coefficient for K was 4.8×10^{-5} cm/sec, which is equivalent to + + in relative terms.

3 Each of these active transport processes occurs in the four segments of proximal convoluted tubules summarized.

4 Both of these active transport processes occur in both superficial and juxtamedullary pars recta.

5 Values given are for the rabbit. Some species variation may exist – see text.

While active transport processes predominate in S_1 segments, driving forces due to electrochemical gradients contribute significantly to net fluid absorption in the S_2 segments. The magnitude of the passive reabsorption is a function of membrane permeability coefficients, fluid contact times and electrochemical gradients.

In summary, functional differences exist in early versus late proximal convoluted tubules because of intrinsic epithelial differences and due to differences in fluid that courses through these two sub-segments.

Proximal straight tubule

Proximal straight tubules are of variable length, depending upon whether their glomeruli are superficial or juxtamedullary. Both, however, descend through the outer stripe of the outer medulla. The early portion of the superficial proximal straight tubule contains a variable amount of S_2 epithelium while the medullary portion of proximal straight tubules of superficial and juxtamedullary tubules are made up of S_3 cells that are morphologically distinct from earlier S_2 cells [5]. The characteristics of proximal straight tubules can only be examined by in vitro microperfusion techniques. Both superficial and juxtamedullary nephron segments have been perfused with ultrafiltrate of serum, solutions simulating fluid that normally enters the proximal straight tubule and by other well-defined solutions that allow examination of specific membrane characteristics.

Over a dozen studies have noted that the net fluid reabsorptive capacity of the proximal straight tubule is roughly one-third of that of the proximal convoluted tubule [8]. Both active and passive transport processes contribute to the net fluid absorption. The active transport processes have significantly lower capacities than in the earlier proximal convoluted tubule. The reabsorption of bicarbonate occurs at roughly 25% the rate in proximal convoluted tubules and, like the proximal convoluted tubule, the reabsorptive rate is somewhat higher in the juxtamedullary proximal straight tubule as contrasted to superficial proximal straight tubules [16,17]. Also, the reabsorptive rates for glucose [18] and phosphate [19] are lower in proximal straight tubules as contrasted to the same length of proximal convoluted tubules. In addition, there seems to be a component of electrogenic Na reabsorption [2,20] that has been difficult to document in the proximal convoluted tubule.

The passive transport properties of the superficial and juxtamedullary proximal straight tubule show qualitative similar differences to those observed in the respective S_2 segments. These are reviewed in Table I.

Descending limb of Henle

The descending limb of Henle begins gradually at the junction of the outer and inner stripe of the outer medulla. Superficial nephrons have short descending limbs that have their bend near the outer–inner medullary junction, while juxtamedullary nephrons have long descending limbs that descend variable lengths down toward the papillary tip. While inter-species differences in the morphology of the descending limb of Henle exist [21], in general, short descending limbs of Henle are similar between species being composed of flat cells with deep intercellular short junctions [21–25]. However, while rabbit long descending limbs of Henle are similar to their superficial counterparts [26], many of the other species have long descending limbs of Henle where the early descending part has epithelium with shallow tight junctions with subsequent transition to epithelium similar to the superficial descending limbs [21,24,27]. These morphological differences suggest functional heterogeneity.

There exists no evidence to support the presence of active transport in any of the descending limb of Henle segments. Transepithelial potential difference is zero and the bidirectional fluxes for sodium and chloride are equivalent when these segments are perfused with fluid of similar composition to the bath [21,28].

While the descending limb of Henle is relatively impermeable to solutes (Table I) the short descending limb of Henle of a hamster is even less permeable to sodium and chloride while being somewhat more permeable to urea than the early portion of the long descending limb of Henle belonging to juxtamedullary nephrons [21].

Thin ascending limb of Henle

No morphological or functional differences have been noted along the thin ascending limb of Henle. The entire length of the thin ascending limb of Henle has similar flat epithelium with shallow tight junctions. Many investigators have attempted to show the presence of active transport across this segment, but, to date, no convincing evidence has been put forward to support its presence. When thin ascending limb of Henle of rabbit, rat and hamster are perfused in vitro with fluids similar to the bath there is: 1) no significant transepithelial potential difference; 2) no change in collected fluid osmolality; and 3) no differences in sodium or chloride unidirectional fluxes [29,30].

The thin ascending limb of Henle has interesting passive permeability characteristics being highly permeable to salt, moderately permeable to urea and impermeable to water (Table I).

Thick ascending limb of Henle

The thick ascending limb of Henle is composed of two sections: medullary and cortical. The cells of the medullary thick ascending limb of Henle are quite tall with an abrupt decrease in cell height in the cortical part. Both segments actively transport salt out of the lumen.

When segments of thick ascending limb of Henle are perfused in vitro it has been repeatedly demonstrated that the luminal potential is positive [8]. Initially it was thought that the lumen positive potential difference was the result of primary active chloride absorption [31,32], but more recent studies are most consistent with secondary active chloride transport in which two chloride ions are coupled to sodium and potassium [33–35]. The lumen positive potential difference is the result of cytoplasmic potassium diffusing back into the lumen [35]. While this transport process is present in both segments of the thick ascending limb of Henle it is interesting that heterogeneity exists in the response of this transport process to endogenous stimuli. Antidiuretic hormone (ADH) stimulates salt absorption across the cortical but not medullary thick ascending limb of Henle [36–39], while prostaglandin E_2 inhibits salt transport across the cortical but not medullary thick ascending limb [40].

The passive transport characteristics of the thick ascending limb of Henle are summarized in Table I.

Distal convoluted tubule

The micropuncturist's distal convoluted tubule no longer can be considered as an homogeneous segment. Indeed, four distinct morphological segments are evident. The first section beyond the macula densa has epithelium characteristics of the cortical thick ascending limb of Henle, the next component is a short bright segment that some call the true distal convoluted tubule; the third segment is granular in appearance, containing connecting and intercalated cells, while the fourth segment has characteristics of the cortical collecting tubule. While many investigators have contributed to the above view the reader is referred to an article by Imai and Nakamura [41] for a more detailed discussion.

Active transport characteristics should differ in each of the subsections of the distal convoluted tubule to correspond to the morphology. However, micro-puncture techniques cannot separate these subsections distinctly and in vitro technicques have not been used to compare systematically the function of each subsection. It has been shown there are differences in potential difference between the early and late micropuncture-accessible distal convoluted tubule [42]. The earliest part is either slightly lumen positive [43,44] or negative [42,45] but all agree that the potential difference becomes more negative at more distal puncture sites [42]. The origin of the early lumen positive potential difference may be similar to that in the cortical thick ascending limb while the origin of later lumen negative potential difference is mainly the result of primary active sodium absorption [46].

The entire length of the distal convoluted tubule seems to be relatively impermeable to solutes and water (Table I). Only the latter part increases its water permeability to antidiuretic hormone [47].

Cortical collecting tubule

The epithelial characteristics of the cortical collecting tubule begins prior to the junction of two surface distal tubules. It is composed of two primary cell types, dark (intercalated) and light (principal) cells. The ratio of dark to light cells progressively decreases from cortical surface to the cortico–medullary junction [48].

The cortical collecting tubule has a number of important physiological functions. Among its more important functions are: it absorbs sodium, secretes potassium, secretes hydrogen and regulates water absorption. Sodium absorption occurs by primary active electrogenic transport mechanisms, probably across the principal cells. This mechanism involves the passive entry of sodium across the luminal membrane, through conductive pathways, down its electrochemical gradient. The permeability of these pathways is under the partial control of aldosterone [49]. Once sodium gains access to the cell it acts as a substrate to increase the activity of Na/K-ATPase [49]. This active transcellular Na transport generates a lumen negative potential difference [50–52]. The lumen negative potential difference acts as a driving force for potassium secretion [52–54]. In addition, there appears to be an active potassium secreting mechanism across this segment [53,54]. Hydrogen secretion also is influenced by the potential difference. The more negative the lumen potential difference, the more acidic the lumen pH [55]. Of further interest is the observation that cortical collecting tubules can both reabsorb bicarbonate (if tubules are harvested from acidotic animals) or secrete bicarbonate (if harvested from alkalotic animals) [56–59]. The acid-base reabsorptive processes are thought to occur across the dark cells.

The cortical collecting tubule is relatively impermeable to solutes. It also is impermeable to water in the absence of antidiuretic hormone, but its water permeability increases in response to antidiuretic hormone (Table I).

Outer medullary collecting tubule

The outer medullary collecting tubule begins at the cortico–medullary junction and terminates at the junction of the outer and inner medulla. There is a continued decrease in the number of dark cells in this segment.

The transport functions of this segment are completely different from those of the cortical collecting tubule. This segment neither reabsorbs sodium nor secretes potassium [51]. However, it does have a lumen positive potential difference [51,59,60]. The lumen positive potential difference is the result of sodium independent hydrogen secretion [61].

The outer medullary collecting tubule like the cortical collecting tubule is impermeable to urea and water in the absence of antidiuretic hormone. Water but not urea permeability increases in response to antidiuretic hormone (Table I).

Inner medullary collecting duct

The term inner medullary collecting duct should not be used synonymously with the term papillary collecting duct [62]. Madsen and Tisher [62] indicate that it is more accurate to use the nomenclature of outer third ($IMCT_1$), middle third ($IMCT_2$) and inner third ($IMCT_3$) to divide the inner medullary collecting duct into subsegments. Their view is based on morphological observations and recent theoretical [63] and physiological [64] studies strongly support this axial subsectioning.

Mathematical considerations have suggested that active NaCl absorption from the inner medullary collecting tubule is important for renal conservation of NaCl. Indeed, micropuncture [65,66] and microperfusion [67] studies have shown that sodium and chloride can be absorbed actively without the generation of significant transepithelial potential difference.

The passive permeability characteristics of the inner medullary collecting tubule are interesting (Table I). Sands and Knepper [64] have shown that there exists axial heterogeneity with respect to urea permeability. $IMCT_1$ has a finite but low urea permeability with a transition to high urea permeability in the $IMCT_3$. This thus becomes an important source of inner medullary interstitial urea concentration.

In summary, each of the nine major nephron segments has unique and differing transport characteristics. While the proximal tubules absorb quantitatively the greatest amount of salt and water, the more distal tubular segments are important in the fine tuning of salt, water and acid-base homeostasis. The unique topographic location and specific transport properties of the renal tubules allow for the integrated and interdependent operation of the various nephron segments that participate in the function of the counter-current multiplication system.

References

1 Peter K. *Untersuchungen über Bau und Entwickelung der Niere.* Jena: Gustav Fischer. 1909: 1–358pp

2 Kawamura S, Imai M, Seldin DW, Kokko JP. Characteristics of salt and water transport in superficial and juxtamedullary straight segments of proximal tubules. *J Clin Invest 1975; 55:* 1269–1277

3 Maunsbach AB. Observations on the segmentation of the proximal tubule in the rat kidney: comparison of results from phase contrast, fluorescence, and electron microscopy. *J Ultrastruct Res 1966; 16:* 239–258

4 Kaissling B, Kriz W. Structural analysis of the rabbit kidney. In *Advances in Anatomy: Embryology and Cell Biology, Vol 56.* Berlin: Springer Verlag. 1979: 13

5 Woodhall PB, Tisher CC, Simonton CA, Robinson RR. Relationship between para-aminohippurate secretion and cellular morphology in rabbit proximal tubules. *J Clin Invest 1978; 61:* 1320–1329

6 Walker AM, Bott PA, Oliver J, McDonnell MC. The collection and analysis of fluid from single nephrons of the mammalian kidney. *Am J Physiol 1941; 134:* 580–595

7 Alpern RJ, Warnock DJ, Rector FC. Renal acidification mechanisms. In Brenner BM, Rector FC, eds. *The Kidney.* Philadelphia: W B Saunders. 1986: 206–250

8 Kokko JP, Jacobson HR. Renal chloride transport. In Seldin DW, Giebisch G, eds. *The Kidney: Physiology and Pathophysiology.* New York: Raven Press. 1985: 1097–1117

9 Jacobson HR. Characteristic of volume reabsorption in rabbit superficial and juxtamedullary proximal convoluted tubules. *J Clin Invest 1979; 63:* 410–418

10 Burg M, Patlak C, Green N, Villey D. Organic solutes in fluid absorption by renal proximal convoluted tubules. *Am J Physiol 1976; 231:* 627–637

11 Jacobson HR, Kokko JP. Intrinsic differences in various segments of the proximal convoluted tubule. *J Clin Invest 1976; 57:* 818–825

12 Kokko JP. Proximal tubule potential difference: dependence on glucose HCO_3^-, and amino acids. *J Clin Invest 1973; 52:* 1362–1367

13 Kokko JP, Rector FC Jr. Flow dependence of transepithelial potential difference in isolated perfused segments of rabbit proximal convoluted tubule. *J Clin Invest 1971; 50:* 2745–2750

14 Barratt LJ, Rector FC, Kokko JP, Seldin DW. Factors governing the transepithelial potential differences across the proximal tubule of the rat kidney. *J Clin Invest 1974; 53:* 454–464

15 Frömter E, Kinne R. Free-flow potential profile along rat kidney proximal tubule. *Pfluegers Arch 1974; 351:* 69–83

16 McKinney TD, Burg MB. Bicarbonate and fluid absorption by renal proximal straight tubules. *Kidney Int 1977; 12:* 1–8

17 Neumann KH, Rector FC. Mechanisms of NaCl and water reabsorption in the proximal convoluted tubule of rat kidney. *J Clin Invest 1976; 58:* 1110–1118

18 Tune B, Burg MB. Glucose transport by proximal renal tubules. *Am J Physiol 1971; 221:* 580–585

19 Dennis VW, Woodhall PB, Robinson RR. Characteristics of phosphate transport in isolated proximal tubules. *Am J Physiol 1976; 231:* 979–985

20 Schafer JA, Troutman SL, Watkins ML, Andreoli TE. Volume absorption in the pars recta: I. "Simple" active Na+ transport. *Am J Physiol 1978; 234:* F332–F339

21 Imai M, Hayashi M, Araki M. Functional heterogeneity of the descending limbs of Henle's loop. I. Internephron heterogeneity in the hamster kidney. *Pfluegers Arch 1984; 402:* 385–392

22 Dietrich HJ, Barrett JM, Kriz W, Bulhoff JP. The ultrastructure of the thin loop limbs in the mouse kidney. *Anat Embryol 1975; 147:* 1–13

23 Schwartz MM, Karnovsky MJ, Venkatachalam MA. Regional membrane specialization in the thin limbs of Henle's loops as seen by freeze-fracture electron microscopy. *Kidney Int 1979; 16:* 577–589

24 Schwartz MM, Venkatachalam MA. Structural differences in thin limbs of Henle: physiological implications. *Kidney Int 1974; 6:* 193–208

25 Barrett JM, Kriz W, Kaissling B, de Rouffignac C. The ultrastructure of the nephrons of the desert rodent *(Psammonys obesus)* kidney. I Thin limbs of Henle of short-looped nephrons. *Am J Anat 1978; 151:* 487–498

26 Kaissling B, Kriz W. Structural analysis of rabbit kidney. *Adv Anat Embryol Cell Biol 1979; 56:* 1–123

27 Bachman S, Kriz W. Histotopography and ultrastructure of the thin limbs of the loop of Henle in the hamster. *Cell Tissue Res 1982; 225:* 111–127

28 Kokko JP. Sodium chloride and water transport in the descending limb of Henle. *J Clin Invest 1970; 49:* 1838–1846

29 Imai M, Kokko JP. Sodium, chloride, urea, and water transport in the thin ascending limb of Henle. *J Clin Invest 1974; 53:* 393–402

30 Imai M. Function of the thin ascending limbs of Henle of rats and hamsters perfused in vitro. *Am J Physiol 1977; 232:* F201–F209

31 Rocha AS, Kokko JP. Sodium chloride and water transport in the medullary thick ascending limb of Henle. Evidence for active chloride transport. *J Clin Invest 1973; 52:* 612–623

32 Burg M, Green N. Function of the thick ascending limb of Henle's loop. *Am J Physiol 1973; 224:* 659–668

33 Greger R. Coupled transport of Na^+ and Cl^- in the thick ascending limb of Henle's loop of rabbit nephron. *Scand J Audiol 1981 (Suppl); 14:* 1–15

34 Greger R. Cation selectivity of the isolated perfused cortical thick ascending limb of Henle's loop in the rabbit kidney. *Pfluegers Arch 1981; 390:* 30–37

35 Greger R, Schlatter E. Presence of luminal K, a prerequisite for active NaCl transport in the cortical thick ascending limb of Henle's loop of rabbit kidney. *Pfluegers Arch 1981; 392:* 92–94

36 Sasaki S, Imai M. Effects of vasopressin on water and NaCl transport across the in vitro perfused medullary thick ascending limbs of Henle's loop of mouse, rat and rabbit kidneys. *Pfluegers Arch 1980; 383:* 215–221

37 Hall DA, Varney DM. Effect of vasopressin on electrical potential difference and chloride transport in mouse medullary thick ascending limbs of Henle's loop. *J Clin Invest 1980; 66:* 792–802

38 Hebert SC, Culpepper RM, Andreoli TE. NaCl transport in mouse medullary thick ascending limbs. II. ADH enhancement of transcellular NaCl cotransport: origin of the transepithelial voltages. *Am J Physiol 1981; 241:* F432–F442

39 Hebert SC, Culpepper RM, Andreoli TE. NaCl transport in mouse medullary thick ascending limbs. I. Functional nephron heterogeneity and ADH-stimulated NaCl cotransport. *Am J Physiol 1981; 241:* F412–F431

40 Stokes JB. Effect of prostaglandin E_2 on chloride transport across the rabbit thick ascending limb of Henle. *J Clin Invest 1979; 64:* 495–502

41 Imai M, Nakamura R. Function of distal convoluted and connecting tubules studied by isolated nephron fragments. *Kidney Int 1982; 22:* 465–472

42 Wright FS. Increasing magnitude of electrical potential along the renal distal tubule. *Am J Physiol 1971; 220:* 624–638

43 Allen GG, Barratt LJ. Electrophysiology of the early distal tubule: further observations on electrode techniques. *Kidney Int 1981; 19:* 24–35

44 Barratt LJ, Rector FC, Kokko JP et al. Transepithelial potential difference profile of the distal tubule of the rat kidney. *Kidney Int 1975; 8:* 368–375

45 Hayslett J, Boulpaep EL, Kashgarian M, Giebisch G. Electrical characteristics of the mammalian distal tubule. Comparison of Ling, Gerard and macroelectrodes. *Kidney Int 1977; 12:* 324–331

46 Almeida AJ, Burg MB. Sodium transport in rabbit connecting tubule. *Am J Physiol 1982; 243:* F330–F334

47 Woodhall PB, Tisher CC. Response of the distal tubule and cortical collecting duct to vasopressin in the rat. *J Clin Invest 1973; 52:* 3065–3108

48 Stokes JB, Tisher CC, Kokko JP. Structural-functional heterogeneity along the rabbit collecting tubule. *Kidney Int 1975; 14:* 585–593

49 Petty KJ, Kokko JP, Marver D. Secondary effect of aldosterone on Na-K-ATPase activity in the rabbit cortical collecting tubule. *J Clin Invest 1981; 68:* 1514–1521

50 Gross JB, Imai M, Kokko JP. A functional comparison of the cortical collecting tubule and the distal convoluted tubule. *J Clin Invest 1975; 55:* 1284–1294

51 Stokes JB, Ingram MJ, Williams AD, Ingram D. Heterogeneity of the rabbit collecting tubule: localization of mineralocorticoid hormone action to the cortical portion. *Kidney Int 1981; 20:* 340–347

52 O'Neil RG, Helman SI. Transport characteristics of renal collecting tubules: influences of DOCA and diet. *Am J Physiol 1977; 233:* F544–F558

53 Stokes JB. Potassium secretion by the cortical collecting tubule: relation to sodium absorption, luminal sodium concentration, and transepithelial voltage. *Am J Physiol 1981; 241:* F395–F407

54 Wingo CS, Kokko JP, Jacobson HR. Effects of in vitro aldosterone on the rabbit cortical collecting tubule. *Kidney Int 1985; 28:* 51–57

55 Koeppen BM, Helman SI. Acidification of luminal fluid by the rabbit cortical collecting tubule perfused in vitro. *Am J Physiol 1982; 242:* F35–F47

56 McKinney TD, Burg MB. Bicarbonate transport by rabbit cortical collecting tubules. Effect of acid and alkali loads in vivo on transport in vitro. *J Clin Invest 1977; 60:* 766–768

57 McKinney TD, Burg MB. Bicarbonate absorption by rabbit cortical collecting tubules in vitro. *Am J Physiol 1978; 234:* F141–F145

58 McKinney TD, Burg MB. Bicarbonate secretion by rabbit cortical collecting tubules in vitro. *J Clin Invest 1978; 61:* 1421–1427

59 Lombard WE, Kokko JP, Jacobson HR. Bicarbonate transport in cortical and outer medullary collecting tubules. *Am J Physiol 1983; 244:* F239–F296

60 Stone DK, Seldin DW, Kokko JP, Jacobson HR. Anion dependence of rabbit medullary collecting duct acidification. *J Clin Invest 1983; 71:* 1505–1508

61 Stone DK, Seldin DW, Kokko JP, Jacobson HR. Mineralocorticoid modulation of rabbit medullary collecting duct acidification: a sodium independent effect. *J Clin Invest 1983; 71:* 77–83

62 Madsen KM, Tisher CC. Structural-functional relationships along the distal nephron. *Am J Physiol 1986; 250:* F1–F15

63 Chandhoke PS, Saidel GM, Knepper MA. Role of inner medullary collecting duct NaCl transport in urinary concentration. *Am J Physiol 1985; 249:* F688–F697

64 Sands JM, Knepper MA. Urea permeability of mammalian inner medullary collecting duct system and papillary surface epithelium. *J Clin Invest 1987; 79:* 138–147

65 Higashihara E, DuBose TD, Kokko JP. Direct examination of chloride transport across papillary collecting duct of the rat. *Am J Physiol 1978; 235:* F219–F226

66 Stein JM, Osgood RW, Kunai RT. Direct measurement of papillary collecting duct sodium transport in the rat. *J Clin Invest 1976; 58:* 767–773

67 Rocha AS, Kudo LH. Water, urea, sodium, chloride, and potassium transport in the in vitro perfused papillary collecting duct. *Kidney Int 1982; 22:* 485–491

RENAL CIRCULATION

REGULATION OF PRE- AND POST-GLOMERULAR RESISTANCES VISUALIZED IN THE SPLIT HYDRONEPHROTIC KIDNEY

M Steinhausen, F G Holz, N Parekh

I. Physiologisches Institut, Universität Heidelberg, FRG

Pre- and post-glomerular resistances have been extensively analysed using filtration fraction data or direct measurements of glomerular pressure [1–3]. Furthermore, estimates of the intravascular pressure proximal to the afferent arteriole have been obtained by using stop-flow techniques on glomerular circulation [4–6], and by direct measurements in kidney preparations with their surface layers removed [7,8]. Local vessel reactions have been investigated in glomeruli grafted to the hamster cheek pouch [9] as well as in microperfused isolated renal vessels [10] and single juxtamedullary nephrons [11].

Micropuncture methods do not permit precise localization of the sites where renal vascular responses occur. The problem with transplanted glomeruli lies in the incomplete renal vascular system which lacks the larger pre- and post-glomerular vessels. The disadvantage of isolated renal vascular perfusion is a loss of neural control and an absence of the physiological vessel tone. Therefore, we have developed the split hydronephrotic kidney [12] which allows investigation of the whole renal vascular system by intravital-microscopy techniques. The circulation of the kidney and the neural control remains intact. However, since long-term ureteral ligation induces atrophy of the tubular system, it is a non-filtering kidney. In comparison with the filtering kidney the vascular system is morphologically unchanged, only podocytes and mesangial cells within the glomerulus show slight structural aberrations [13]. Nevertheless, total renal blood flow of the hydronephrotic kidney is less than that in normal kidneys, possibly due to a long-lasting adaptation mechanism, which is poorly understood.

Figure 1 shows diagrammatically the structures that can be seen. Changes of the luminal diameters were measured between the arcuate arteries and the welling point [14].

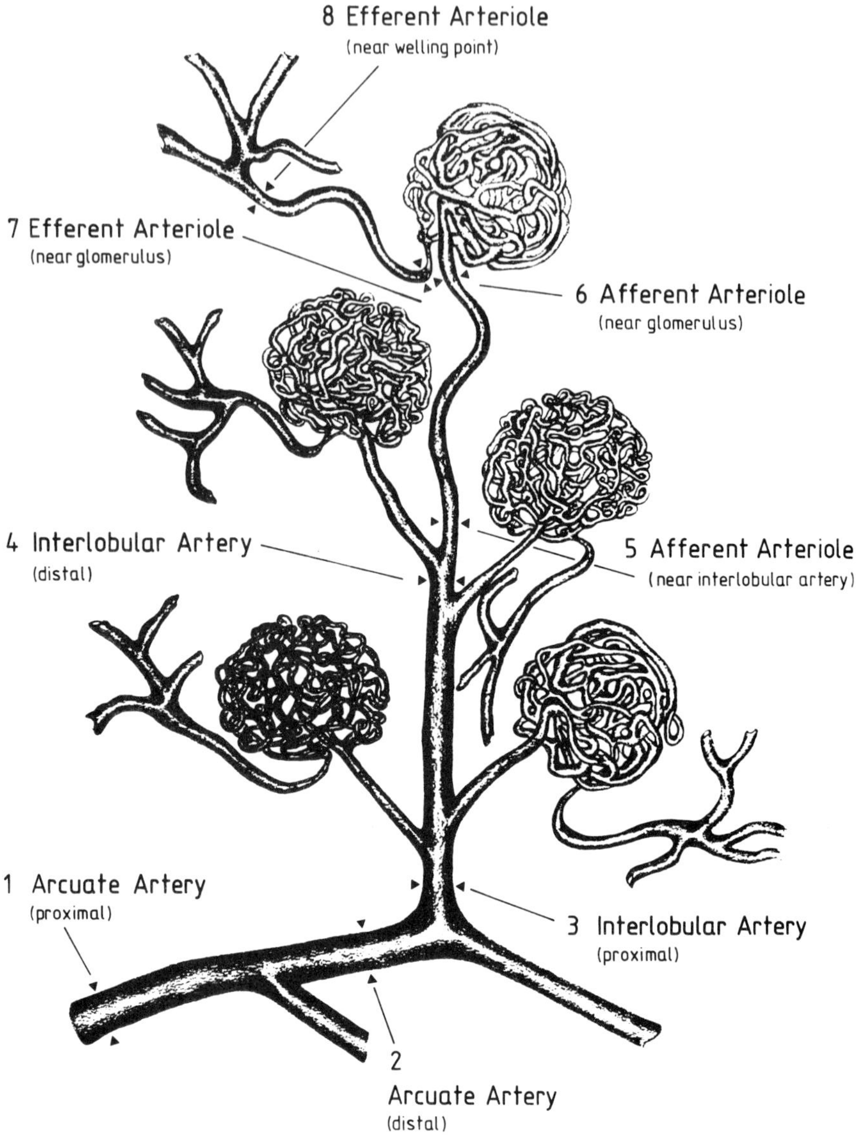

Figure 1. A schematic diagram of visible renal vessels in the hydronephrotic kidney. Sites used for measurements of vessel diameters are marked

Localization of angiotensin II effects on the renal vasculature

The glomerular pressure changes after intravenous administration of angiotensin II which were seen during micropuncture experiments were interpreted by Myers et al [15] to be predominantly due to post-glomerular vasoconstriction. A pre-glomerular constriction which was also found in this study could be largely abolished by reducing the systemic pressure to the pre-infusion value by clamping the aorta above the renal artery. Blantz et al [16] and Steiner and Blantz [3] concluded from their micropuncture experiments that angiotensin II constricts both pre- and post-glomerular vessels. In isolated perfused kidneys angiotensin II showed no pre-glomerular vasoconstriction [17,18], whereas in experiments where vessel diameters were measured from casts of the vascular system after in vivo fixation distinct pre-glomerular vasoconstrictions were obvious [19].

In the split hydronephrotic kidney we found [20] that locally applied angiotensin II, which does not influence systemic blood pressure, exerted a dose dependent pre- and post-glomerular vasoconstriction (Figure 2). Also during intravenous angiotensin II infusion we could show a pre- and post-glomerular vasoconstriction (Figure 3). In these experiments the renal perfusion pressure was reduced by clamping the aorta above the renal arteries and controlling the renal arterial blood pressure to pre-angiotensin II levels. Thus, it was demonstrated that angiotensin II causes a pre-glomerular vasoconstriction, and the rise in systemic blood pressure during angiotensin II infusion augments the pre-glomerular constriction by only about one-third of the total effects.

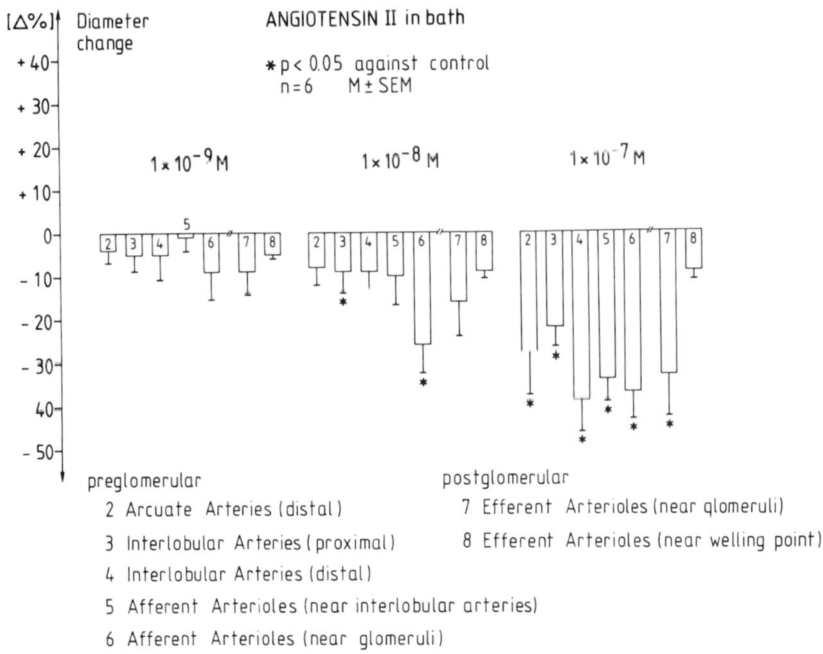

Figure 2. Relative change of diameter in renal vessels due to locally applied angiotensin II [based on 20]

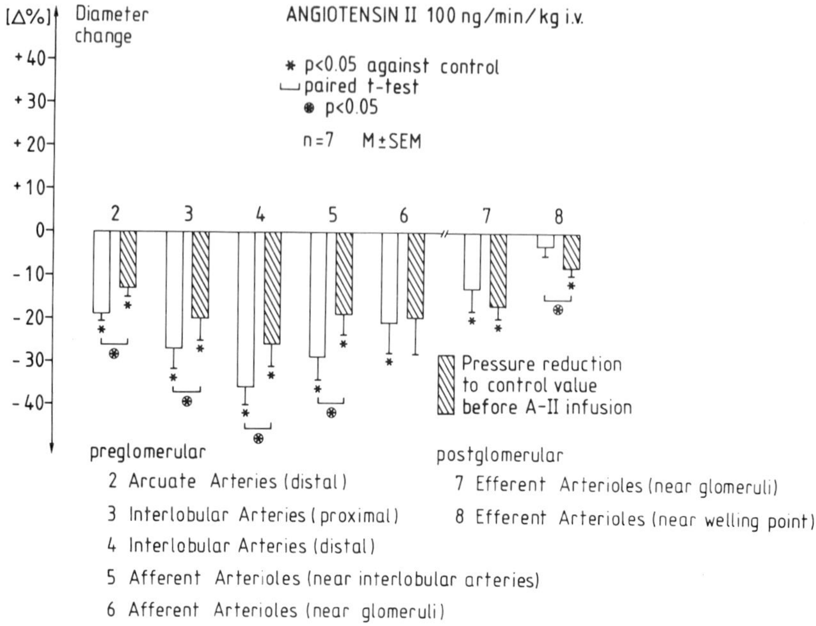

Figure 3. Relative change of diameter in renal vessels during intravenous infusion of angiotensin II at systemic renal perfusion pressure and after reducing the renal perfusion pressure to pre-infusion systemic values [based on 20]

Interestingly, the segment of the afferent arteriole closest to the glomerulus did not dilate with increasing pressure. In another series of experiments concerned with renal autoregulation, we confirmed that without angiotensin II infusion the part of the afferent arteriole nearest to the glomerulus does not respond to increased pressure. It is in this part of the afferent arteriole that the major production of renin has been demonstrated histochemically [13]. Furthermore, we could show that endogenous angiotensin II contributes to the pre- and post-glomerular vascular resistances, at least in anaesthetized rats under our experimental conditions. The angiotensin II antagonist Saralasin induced obvious vascular effects after local application (Figure 4) [21]. In these experiments a dose dependent vasodilation in pre- and post-glomerular vessels could be measured. Again, the part of the afferent arteriole with a high renin content near to the glomerulus did not respond, even though local angiotensin II application showed contractility of this segment (Figure 2).

Localization of dopamine effects on the renal vascular system

From systemic dopamine administration it is well known that dopamine at low concentrations decreases renal vascular resistance, whereas at high doses it induces an increase in renal vascular resistance [22,23]. Dopaminergic neurons

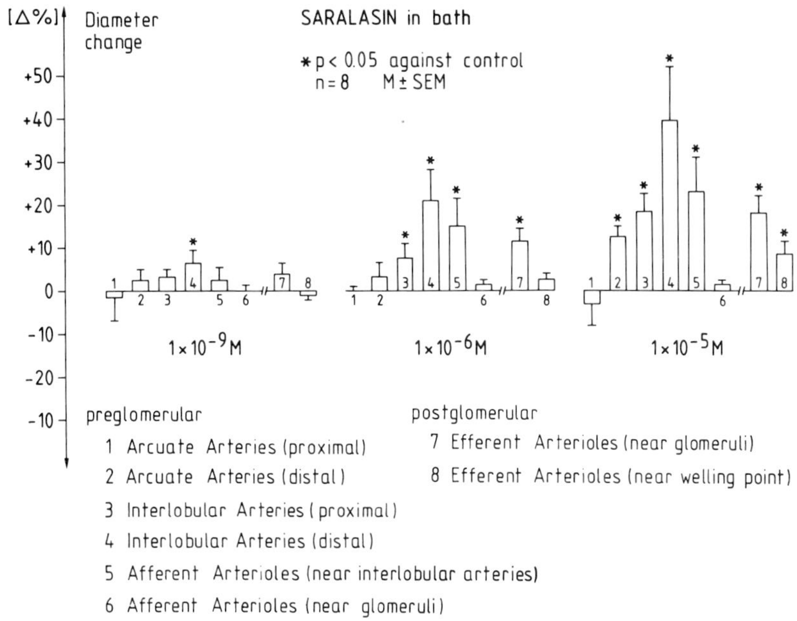

Figure 4. Relative change of diameter in renal vessels during local application of Saralasin [based on 21]

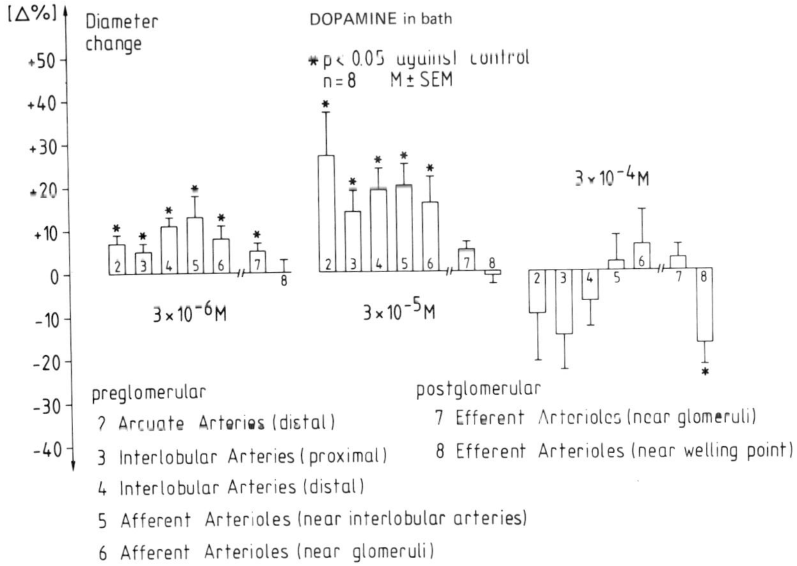

Figure 5. Relative change of diameter in renal vessels during local application of dopamine [based on 14]

have been found in the kidney [24,25], but the contribution of endogenous dopamine to the control of renal blood flow is still controversial. We investigated the site of action of exogenous dopamine [14]. At low dopamine concentration (10^{-6}M) a pre- and post-glomerular vasodilation was observed (Figure 5). In contrast, higher local dopamine concentrations (10^{-4}M) induced a vasoconstriction. After pre-treatment with haloperidol, dopamine did not cause dilatation to any pre- or post-glomerular vascular segment, but the constriction seen with higher concentrations of dopamine was not abolished. Pre-treatment with phentolamine and propranolol enhanced the dilator response of dopamine on the pre- and post-glomerular vessels (except at the afferent arterioles near to glomeruli and the efferent arteriole near welling points) and abolished the vasoconstrictory effect found at the high dopamine concentrations.

Localization of the effect of atrial natriuretic peptide on the renal vasculature
The mechanism by which atrial natriuretic peptide induces natriuresis is still controversial [26]. Renal vascular resistance is decreased by atrial natriuretic peptide in the isolated kidney as well as in the intact animal, especially if the vascular resistance is increased prior to atrial natriuretic peptide administration. In other experiments renal blood flow was not increased by atrial natriuretic peptide and sometimes even reduced. Lowering perfusion pressure by suprarenal aortic clamping prevents the rise of glomerular filtration rate on atrial natriuretic peptide administration and blunts the natriuretic response, suggesting that vascular events are involved in the natriuresis [27]. Figure 6 shows the effect of locally administered atrial natriuretic peptide on the vascular system of the hydronephrotic kidney [28]. In these experiments a dose dependent vasodilatation was found only in the pre-glomerular vessels. In contrast, high concentrations of atrial natriuretic peptide induced a significant post-glomerular vasoconstriction. These results suggest that the increase in glomerular filtration pressure following atrial natriuretic peptide in micropuncture studies [26] is due to a pre-glomerular vasodilation in combination with post-glomerular vasoconstriction.

Localization of autoregulatory pressure response on the renal vascular system
Autoregulatory responses of the split hydronephrotic kidney were quantified in a separate study [Steinhausen M, Blum K, Endlich KH et al. *Kidney Int:* submitted for publication]. In this study luminal diameters of the arcuate artery, interlobular artery, afferent and efferent arteriole were measured microscopically, and the glomerular blood flow was determined by the dual slit technique. Renal perfusion pressure was reduced by graded clamping of the abdominal aorta and downstream pressure was measured in the femoral artery. With pressure reduction from 118 to 95mmHg pre-glomerular vessels dilated 5–10% (except for the distal afferent arteriole) and glomerular blood flow was maintained. Further reduction in perfusion pressure to 71mmHg and then to

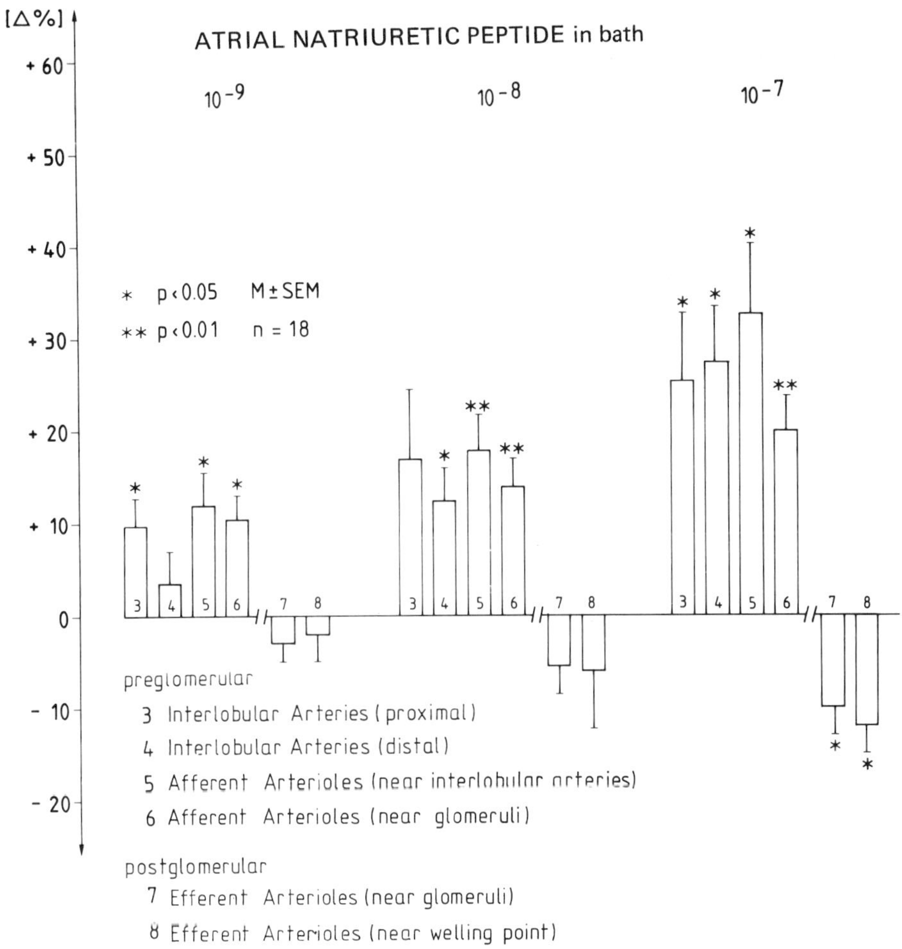

Figure 6. Relative change of diameter in renal vessels during local application of rat atrial natriuretic peptide (rANP) [based on 28]

43mmHg gave additional dilation of the pre-glomerular vessels but there was also a decrease in flow. This is in good agreement with previous studies which had found a lower limit to highly efficient autoregulation in the anaesthetized rat at about 80–95mmHg [29–31].

It is often hypothesized that tubuloglomerular feedback may be involved in renal autoregulation. For falls in blood pressure similar to those above, Schnermann et al [31] found that 50% of the autoregulation in the intact kidney was due to the feedback system. However, we found complete glomerular blood flow autoregulation in a non-filtering and hence a non-feedback controlled kidney. Further investigation is needed to settle this controversy.

Summary

The split hydronephrotic kidney allows localization of the changes in diameter within the renal vascular system. In this preparation vasoactive substances to be investigated can be applied not only systemically but also locally to the tissue bath. In this paper the different sites of actions for angiotensin II, dopamine, atrial natriuretic peptide and for autoregulatory responses are demonstrated. This facilitates explanations about the causes of glomerular pressure changes.

Acknowledgments

Excellent technical assistance was given by R Dussel. The work was supported by the German Research Foundation (DFG, Forschergruppe Niere).

References

1 Brenner BM, Rector FC. *The Kidney.* Philadelphia: W B Saunders. 1976

2 Ofstad J, Aukland K. Renal circulation. In Seldin DW, Giebisch G, eds. *The Kidney: Physiology and Pathophysiology.* New York: Raven Press. 1985: 471–496

3 Steiner RW, Blantz RC. Acute reversal by saralasin of multiple intrarenal effects of angiotensin II. *Am J Physiol 1979; 237:* F386–F391

4 Hammerstein K. *Straudrucke in Quellpunkten der Nierenrinde von Ratten.* MD Thesis: University of Heidelberg. 1974

5 Källskog Ö, Lindbom LO, Ulfendahl H, Wolgast M. Regional and single glomerular blood flow in the rat kidney prepared for micropuncture. A methodological study. *Acta Physiol Scand 1975; 94:* 145–153

6 Steinhausen M, Parekh N, Zimmerhackl B. Pathophysiology of acute renal failure. In Gessler, ed. *Acute Renal Failure.* Basel: Karger. 1982: 9–22

7 Aukland K, Heyeraas TK, Naess G. Capillary pressure in deep and superficial glomeruli of the rat kidney. *Acta Physiol Scand 1977; 101:* 418–427

8 Heyeraas KJ, Aukland K. Interlobular arterial resistance: influence of renal arterial pressure and angiotensin II. *Kidney Int 1987; 31:* 1291–1298

9 Gilmore JP, Cornish KG, Rogers SD, Joyner WL. Direct evidence for myogenic autoregulation of the renal microcirculation in the hamster. *Circ Res 1980; 47:* 226–250

10 Edwards RM. Response of isolated renal arterioles to acetylcholine, dopamine and bradykinin. *Am J Physiol 1985; 248:* F183–F189

11 Rosivall L, Navar LG. Effects of renal hemodynamics of intraarterial infusion of angiotensin I and II. *Am J Physiol 1983; 225:* F181–F187

12 Steinhausen M, Snoe H, Parekh N et al. Hydonephrosis: a new method to visualize vas afferens, efferens and glomerular network. *Kidney Int 1983; 23:* 794–806

13 Bührle CP, Nobiling N, Hackental E et al. Ultrastructure, renin status, contractile and electrophysiological properties of the afferent arteriole in the rat hydronephrotic kidney. *Virchows Arch 1986; 410:* 31–42

14 Steinhausen M, Weis S, Fleming JT et al. Responses of in vivo renal microvessels to dopamine. *Kidney Int 1986; 30:* 361–370

15 Myers BD, Deen WM, Brenner BM. Effects of norepinephrine and angiotensin II on the determinants of glomerular ultrafiltration and proximal tubule reabsorption in the rat. *Circ Res 1975; 37:* 101–110

16 Blantz RC, Konnen KS, Tucker BJ. Angiotensin II effect upon glomerular microcirculation and ultrafiltration coefficient of the rat. *J Clin Invest 1976; 57:* 419–434

17 Davalos M, Frega NS, Saker B, Leaf A. Effect of exogenous and endogenous angiotensin II in the isolated perfused rat kidney. *Am J Physiol 1987; 235:* F605–F610

18 Frega NS, Davalos M, Leaf A. Effect of endogenous angiotensin on the efferent glomerular arteriole of rat kidney. *Kidney Int 1980; 18:* 323–327

19 Wilson SK. The effects of angiotensin II and norepinephrine on afferent arterioles in the rat. *Kidney Int 1986; 30:* 895–905

20 Steinhausen M, Sterzel RB, Fleming JT et al. Acute and chronic effects of angiotensin II in the vessels of the split hydronephrotic kidney. *Kidney Int 1987; 31 (Suppl 20):* S64–S73

21 Steinhausen M, Kücherer H, Parekh N et al. Angiotensin II control of the renal microcirculation: effect of blockade by saralasin. *Kidney Int 1986; 30:* 56–61

22 Goldberg LI. Cardiovascular and renal actions of dopamine: potential clinical applications. *Pharmacol Rev 1979; 24:* 1–29

23 Chapman BJ, Horn MN, Robertson MG. Dopamine induced vasodilatation in the rat kidney. *J Physiol 1987; 275 (Abstract):* 24

24 Bell C, Lang WJ. Neural dopaminergic vasodilator control in the kidney. *Nature 1973; 246:* 27–29

25 Dinerstein RJ, Vannice J, Henderson RC et al. Histofluorescent techniques provide evidence of dopamine containing neuronal elements in canine kidney. *Science 1979; 205:* 497–499

26 Schnermann J, Marin-Grez M, Briggs JP. Filtration pressure response to infusion of atrial natriuretic peptides. *Pfluegers Arch 1986; 406:* 237–239

27 Burnett JC Jr, Opgenorth TJ, Granger JP. The renal action of atriuretic peptide during control of glomerular filtration. *Kidney Int 1986; 30:* 16–19

28 Marin-Grez M, Fleming JT, Steinhausen M. Atrial natriuretic peptide causes preglomerular vasodilation and post-glomerular vasoconstriction in rat kidney. *Nature 1986; 324 (6096):* 473–476

29 Arendshorst WJ, Finn WF, Gottschalk CW. Autoregulation of blood flow in the rat kidney. *Am J Physiol 1975; 228:* 127–133

30 Källskog Ö, Lindbom LO, Ulfendahl H, Wolgast M. The pressure flow relationship of different nephron populations in the rat. *Acta Physiol Scand 1975; 94:* 289–300

31 Hope A, Clausen G, Rosivall L. Total and local renal blood flow and filtration in the rat during reduced renal arterial blood pressure. *Acta Physiol Scand 1981; 113:* 455–463

32 Schnermann J, Briggs JP. Function of the juxtaglomerular apparatus: local control of glomerular hemodynamics. In Seldin DW, Giebisch G, eds. *The Kidney: Physiology and Pathophysiology.* New York: Raven Press. 1985: 669–697

INTRARENAL FORMATION OF ANGIOTENSIN II AND ITS EFFECT ON RENAL HAEMODYNAMICS

L Rosivall, R Taugner*, L G Navar†

Semmelweis University Medical School, Budapest, Hungary,
**University of Heidelberg, Heidelberg, FRG,*
†Nephrology Research and Training Center, University of Alabama at Birmingham, Birmingham, Alabama, USA

Introduction

Several recent studies have demonstrated the existence of all the components of the renin-angiotensin system in different tissues including kidney, brain, adrenal glands, testis and arterial wall [1–3]. There is also an increasing amount of evidence demonstrating intrarenal formation of angiotensin II and its involvement in the regulation of renal function [4]. As far as the kidney is concerned, these findings suggest a modification of the original concepts of Goormaghtigh [5], described 50 years ago, which postulated that the renin-angiotensin system participates in the local regulation of glomerular circulation by the "state of filling or the physicochemical composition of the urine" in the part of the distal tubule forming the macula densa. Studies in comparative physiology suggest that the renin-angiotensin system appears early in phylogeny and helps to regulate glomerular haemodynamics. Perhaps this action is its original, primitive function.

There may be different mechanisms for production of angiotensin II that affects vascular, glomerular, tubular and medullary structures. Angiotensin II may be generated either extrarenally or intrarenally, extravascularly or intravascularly. Because of this complexity, it is not possible to make a clear-cut distinction between the effects of the angiotensin formed at different sites even under experimental conditions. This paper focuses only in the intrarenal formation of angiotensin II and on the difference between the contribution to the control of renal haemodynamics by the circulating and the locally formed angiotensin II.

Intrarenal conversion of angiotensin I to angiotensin II

Angiotensin converting enzyme has been demonstrated in certain regions in the kidney [6], and it is clear that conversion of angiotensin I to angiotensin II occurs within the kidney since infusion of angiotensin I into the kidney elicits a local vasoconstriction that may be inhibited by receptor blockers or converting enzyme inhibitors [4]. The extent of angiotensin conversion capability of the kidney has remained somewhat uncertain, however. In a recent study, we quantified the intrarenal conversion of angiotensin I to angiotensin II using injections of tracer doses of ^{125}I-labelled angiotensin I into the renal artery and measuring the labelled peptides in the renal venous effluate with high voltage paper electrophoresis [7]. The average conversion of ^{125}I-angiotensin I to ^{125}I-angiotensin II during a single passage through the kidney was 22±2% at the control blood flow; this conversion ratio remained unchanged during a reduction in renal blood flow (Figure 1). Since circulating concentrations of angiotensin I are at least as high as arterial angiotensin II concentrations [7,8], these results indicate that a substantial fraction of the intrarenally formed angiotensin II could be derived from systemically delivered angiotensin I.

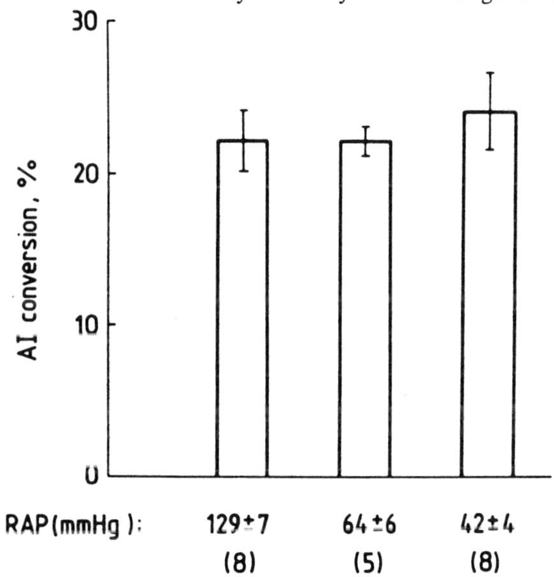

Figure 1. Intrarenal conversion of ^{125}I-angiotensin I to ^{125}I-angiotensin II at normal and reduced renal arterial pressures (RAP) calculated from ^{125}I-labelled angiotensin I, angiotensin II and metabolites measured in the renal venous effluate by high-voltage paper electrophoresis after injection of tracer doses of ^{125}I-angiotensin I into the renal artery. % conversion = ^{125}I-angiotensin II (^{125}I-angiotensin I + ^{125}I-angiotensin + ^{125}I-peptide metabolite). This may represent the minimum conversion rate because it takes no account of the fraction of the metabolites that may have first undergone conversion to angiotensin II prior to degradation

Determination of intrarenal angiotensin II formation under conditions of normal and enhanced renin secretion

Previous studies have not been able to determine the net intrarenal formation of angiotensin II from arteriovenous angiotensin II concentration differences because the concentration of angiotensin II in renal venous blood was lower than that in arterial blood due to a high intrarenal angiotensin II degradation rate [7,9]. Use of angiotensin II concentrations in renal lymph as recommended by Bailie et al [10] or in renal tissue as proposed by Mendelsohn [11] has had only limited application since these techniques do not permit a quantitative determination of changes in angiotensin II formation in response to specific manipulations. Furthermore, lymph angiotensin II concentrations are difficult to interpret since continued angiotensin II formation probably occurs during the relatively slow transit of fluid along the lymphatic channels.

In a recent study, we attempted to assess the amount of intrarenally formed angiotensin II in renal venous blood as compared with the amount which could be attributed to angiotensin II delivered by the systemic circulation that escaped degradation [12]. In each experiment, arterial and renal venous concentrations of angiotensin II were measured under control conditions and during enhanced renin release elicited by reductions in renal arterial pressure. Then the angiotensin II degradation rate was determined from the arterial–renal venous angiotensin II concentration difference during a period of angiotensin II infusion in the presence of angiotensin converting enzyme inhibitors. The average percentage of angiotensin II degradation was 89±2%. By applying the degradation data to observations obtained prior to converting enzyme inhibition, it was possible to predict the venous angiotensin II concentration due to systemically delivered angiotensin II that was not degraded by the kidney. Subtraction of this value from the total venous angiotensin II concentration yielded the component in the renal venous blood that was added by the kidney. The net renal angiotensin II generation rate was then estimated from the product of renal plasma flow and the corrected renal venous angiotensin II concentration.

The estimated renal angiotensin II generation rate averaged 44±11ng/min per gram of kidney weight under control conditions, increasing to 83±13ng/min per gram with reduced renal arterial pressure (69±1mmHg). There was a significant correlation between the renin secretion rate and the angiotensin formation rate when all data at control and reduced pressure were pooled (Figure 2).

Although this method allows an estimation of angiotensin II generation by the kidney, this estimate takes no account of angiotensin II formed within the kidney and degraded before it reaches the renal vascular compartment. Nor is it possible to determine the source of the angiotensin I (endogenously generated or systemically delivered) utilized by the kidney to generate angiotensin II. It does, however, provide a valuable means for estimating the minimum change in local angiotensin II formation rate under different conditions.

Microtopographical localization of intrarenal angiotensin II generation by an electrophysiological technique

With different sodium intakes angiotensin II concentrations measured in renal lymph and tissue are much higher than can be accounted for by the angiotensin

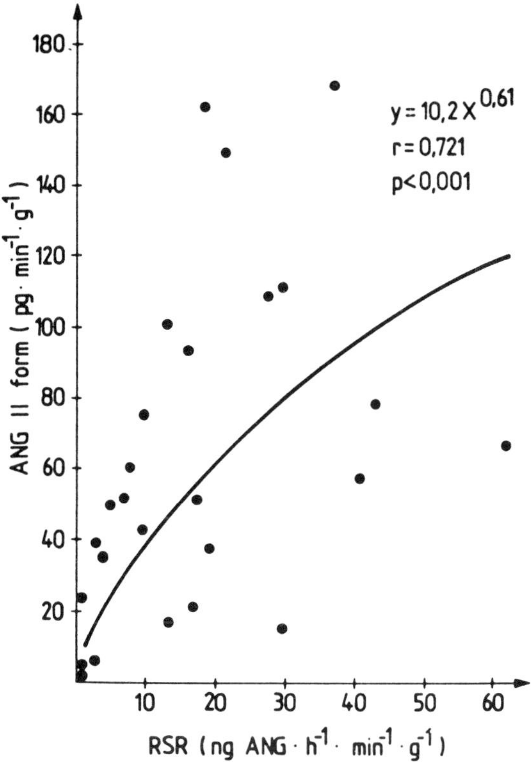

Figure 2. Correlation between renin secretion and intrarenal angiotensin II formation rate calculated from all the data measured at control and reduced renal arterial pressures (n=26, r=0.720, p<0.001)

II content in the circulating blood, so it is assumed that there is significant extravascular angiotensin II formation [10,11]. Juxtaglomerular granulated cells of hydronephrotic mouse kidney depolarize in response to angiotensin II [13]. We have used this model to test for extravascular angiotensin II formation from its precursors – artificial renin substrate (Tetradecapeptide) and angiotensin I [14]. Juxtaglomerular epithelioid cells exhibiting a resting membrane potential of about -75mV were depolarized not only by angiotensin II, but also by administration of angiotensin I or artificial renin substrate to the superfusate (Figure 3). All these responses were completely blocked by saralasin. As opposed to saralasin, several converting enzyme and renin inhibitors only diminished but generally did not abolish the action of angiotensin I and renin substrate.

The observation that depolarization of epithelioid cells in response to angiotensin I was completely blocked by saralasin, an angiotensin II receptor blocker, indicates an intrarenal conversion of angiotensin I to angiotensin II. This interstitially generated angiotensin II may have an effect in the immediate vicinity

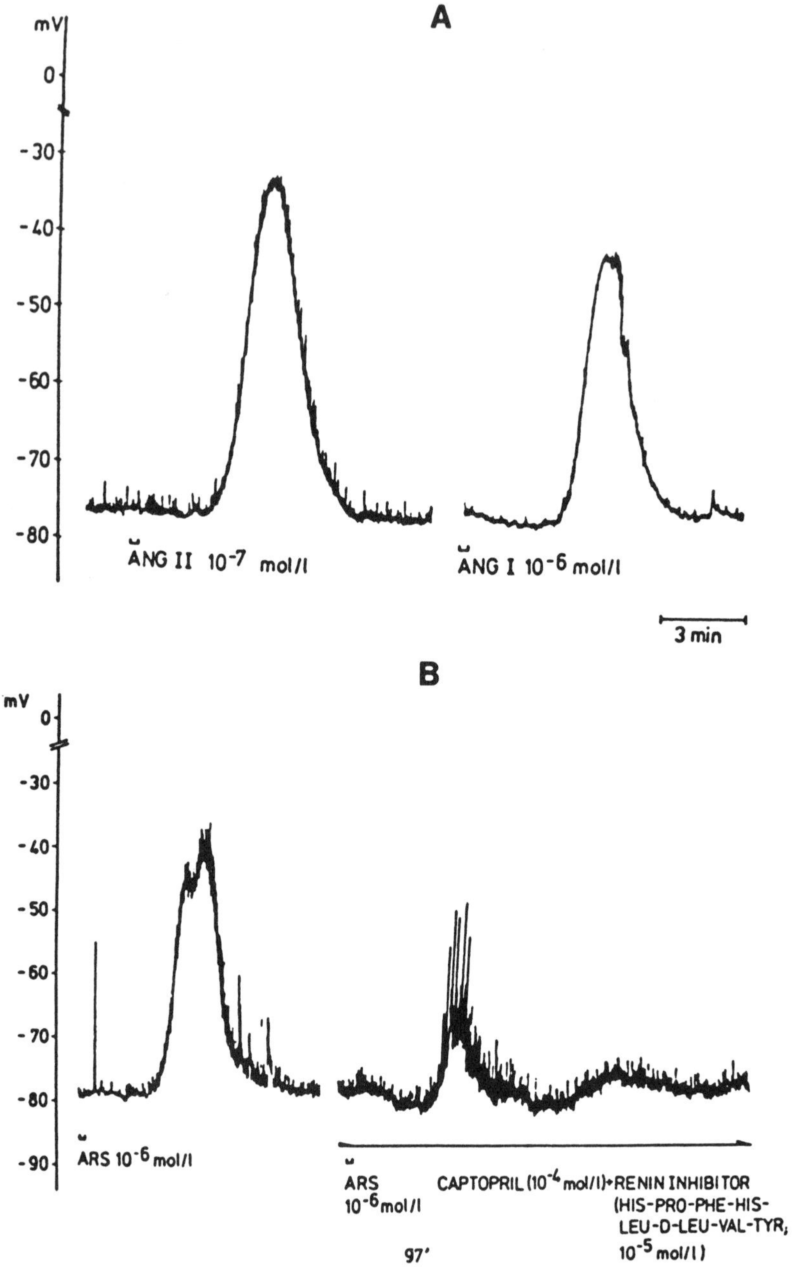

Figure 3. Reversible repolarization of epithelioid cells of the hydronephrotic mouse kidney afferent arteriole upon the administration of angiotensin II, angiotensin I and artificial renin substrate (ARS) into the superfusate (panels A and B). The doses and exposition times are depicted on the figure. Note that the effect of ARS is not abolished by captopril plus renin inhibitor (panel B)

of its formation or it may reach intrarenal arteries through periarterial spaces as suggested recently by Kriz [15]. The possibility of interstitial conversion is also supported by the recent immunocytochemical localization of converting enzyme to the area of basolateral membranes of proximal tubules in the kidney [16]. The variable effects of renin and converting enzyme inhibitors on the depolarization induced by renin substrate and angiotensin I, respectively, suggests an alternative pathway for angiotensin II generation in renal tissue; one that is not dependent on renin and converting enzyme. These findings are in agreement with data showing angiotensin II generation by cathepsin B, trypsin, kallikrein, tonin etc [17].

Effects of intrarenally converted angiotensin II on glomerular filtration rate

Although several approaches have been used to assess the effects of locally formed angiotensin II on renal haemodynamics, most have attempted to unmask the pre-existing influence of angiotensin II by evaluating responses to angiotensin blockers such as converting enzyme inhibitors or angiotensin II receptor antagonists. The variability observed in the responses of glomerular filtration rate to these agents under different experimental conditions has led to conflicting interpretations of the role of intrarenally formed angiotensin II on glomerular dynamics [1,18–21]. The response to angiotensin II blockade, however, results from reduced effects of both circulating and intrarenally formed angiotensin II as well as changes in other hormones, such as prostaglandins and the kallikrein-kinin system [1,4].

Observations of intrarenal blood flow distribution suggested the existence of subtle differences between the effects of intrarenally-converted and circulating angiotensin II [22]. In addition the capacity of the kidney to convert angiotensin I to angiotensin II [7] is such that circulating angiotensin I may effectively contribute to the effects of angiotensin II on renal haemodynamics. In recent experiments, we studied the effects of increased intrarenally converted angiotensin II, induced by intrarenal arterial angiotensin I infusion, on glomerular haemodynamics and compared them with effects due to increased delivery of circulating angiotensin II [23]. The experiments were performed on anaesthetized dogs kept on a normal or on a high sodium diet. In both groups of animals intrarenal arterial angiotensin I infusion significantly decreased the glomerular filtration rate even at a low dose with the high sodium diet. None of the changes in glomerular filtration rate following angiotensin II were statistically significant from zero even though the dose was shown to be equiconstrictor (Figure 4). The glomerular filtration rate reducing effect of angiotensin I infusion indicates that angiotensin I can be converted to angiotensin II sufficiently early within the renal vasculature to have effects on either preglomerular or glomerular structures, but in any case before reaching the postglomerular arteriole.

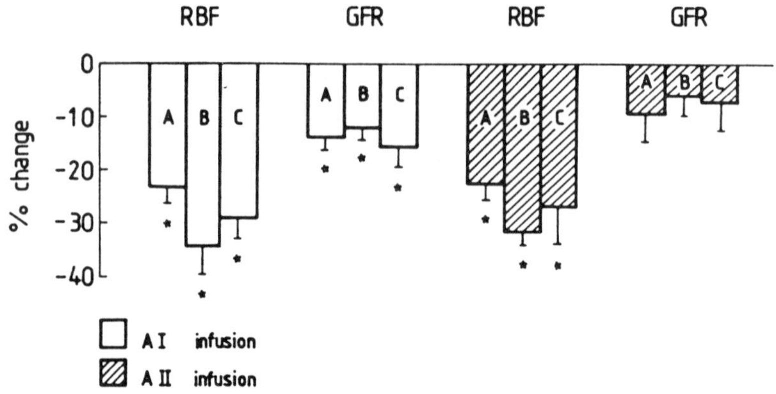

Figure 4. Comparison of relative changes in renal blood flow (RBF) and glomerular filtration rate (GFR) values during intrarenal arterial infusion of angiotensin I and angiotensin II in equiconstrictor doses (verified by the equivalent changes in the RBF under different experimental conditions.) A:normal sodium group (8) angiotensin I dose=1.80±0.49μg/min, angiotensin II=0.48±0.08μg/min. B=high sodium group (5) angiotensin I dose=3.31±0.42μg/min; angiotensin II 1.07±0.23μg/min. C=high sodium group (11) angiotensin I dose=1.15±0.04μg/min; angiotensin II 0.28±0.05μg/min. Note the more consistent effect of angiotensin I on GFR. The significance of the change from zero is indicated *p<0.05

The site of the effects of intrarenally converted angiotensin II

The intrarenal sites of angiotensin II induced increases in renal vascular resistance has been extensively studied by different methods [19,24–28]. These experiments have produced conflicting data in that some studies have indicated preferential postglomerular effects while others have shown effects on both pre- and postglomerular resistances. Because of our observations showing the effects of angiotensin I infusion in decreasing glomerular filtration rate, micropuncture studies were conducted in dogs that had been sodium loaded to reduce the activity of the endogenous renin-angiotensin system [29]. Experiments were performed at reduced renal arterial pressures (91±3mmHg) to minimize the tubuloglomerular feedback induced overestimation of glomerular capillary pressure as estimated from the stop-flow pressure [4]. Intrarenal arterial angiotensin I infusions induced similar reductions in renal blood flow and glomerular filtration rate to those discussed before, and decreased single-nephron glomerular filtration rate (38%), proximal tubular pressure (26%), and peritubular capillary pressure (49%). Neither glomerular capillary pressure nor effective filtration pressure were significantly reduced during angiotensin I infusion (Figure 5). The reduction in glomerular filtration rate was mainly a consequence of the decreases in glomerular filtration coefficient (44%) and glomerular plasma flow (55%) due to almost parallel increases in preglomerular and efferent arteriolar resistances.

The exact mechanism by which angiotensin II can alter the glomerular

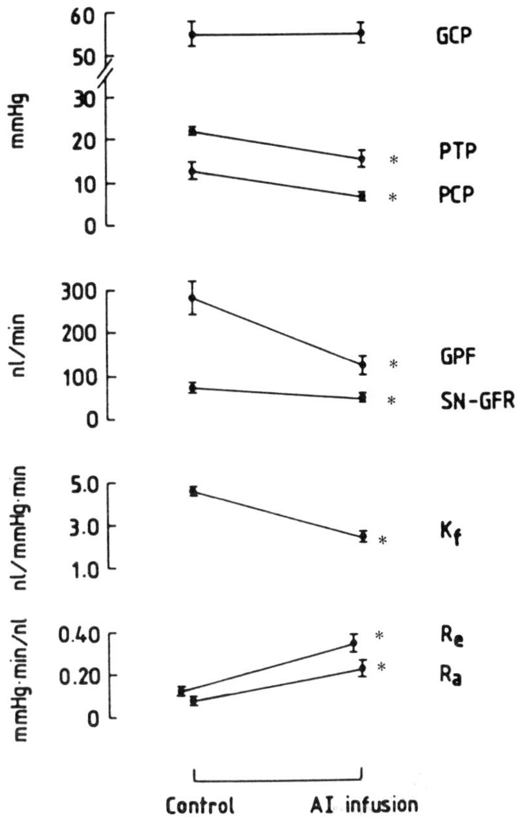

Figure 5. Effects of intrarenally converted angiotensin II on glomerular dynamics. GCP= glomerular capillary pressure; PTP=proximal tubular pressure; PCP=peritubular capillary pressure; GPF=glomerular plasma flow; SN-GFR=single-nephron glomerular filtration rate; K_f=glomerular filtration coefficient; R_e and R_a=efferent arteriolar and preglomerular resistances; *=$p<0.05$

filtration coefficient is unclear. A number of studies have noted the presence of angiotensin II receptors on the mesangial cells of glomeruli [30,31] and mesangial cells have been reported to contract in response to angiotensin II [32,33]. A recent morphological study has demonstrated the existence of a biomechanical unit composed of glomerular basement membrane and mesangial cells, and suggested that this unit is capable of changing the geometry of glomerular capillaries [34]. Thus it is reasonable to assume that changes in the filtration barrier induced by angiotensin II are mainly due to the alteration of the surface area. Angiotensin converting enzyme is present in the glomerulus [6], and locally formed angiotensin II may achieve a high concentration in the interstitium of the glomerular mesangium. It is worth mentioning, however, that in one study, changes were not observed in glomerular capillary diameter or in the number of perfused capillaries during angiotensin II infusions at least in the hydronephrotic kidney preparation [36].

The exact localization of the effect of angiotensin II in the preglomerular vessels is also unclear. There are studies which suggest that most of the vasoconstriction due to angiotensin II effect appears in the interlobular and proximal afferent arteriolar part of the vessels [27,28], while other studies suggest rather uniform [24] or highly localized late proximal effects [25]. On the basis of the findings of a recent study it is proposed that the juxtaglomerular part of the preglomerular arteriole is not contractile since it has been demonstrated that the renin-positive granulated cells are myosin negative [37]. It is possible, however, that functionally important pre- and postglomerular resistance elements may reside within the glomerular corpuscle in the form of angiotensin II sensitive intraglomerular mesangial cells surrounding the arterioles at their junction with the glomerular capillaries [33].

Conclusions

In this presentation, recent studies of the intrarenal formation of angiotensin II and of the effects of intrarenally formed angiotensin II on glomerular haemodynamics are reviewed. It has been demonstrated that the kidney has a large capacity to convert angiotensin I to angiotensin II, which suggests that circulating angiotensin I may also contribute to the effects of angiotensin II on renal haemodynamics. An electrophysiological method is presented as a tool to study the site of intrarenal angiotensin conversion, and with this technique the existence of interstitial conversion of angiotensin I to angiotensin II was shown in the vicinity of the juxtaglomerular apparatus. The results obtained with this method also suggest a non-renin and non-converting enzyme pathway of angiotensin II generation in renal tissue.

With another method it is possible to measure how much angiotensin II is formed within the kidney under the conditions of normal and increased renin secretion rate. These data demonstrate a substantial formation of angiotensin II in the kidney under control conditions and a correlation between the renin secretion and intrarenal angiotensin II formation. This method is also a novel tool for studying the relation of angiotensin II formation to the changes in renal haemodynamics or tubular function during various physiological conditions.

Studies on the effects of intrarenal conversion of angiotensin I demonstrate that the local generation of angiotensin II takes place within the kidney vasculature early enough to decrease glomerular function. Micropuncture studies have shown that intrarenally converted angiotensin II decreases single-nephron glomerular filtration rate as a consequence of the reduction in glomerular filtration coefficient as well as in glomerular plasma flow, the latter being due to the concomitant increase in both preglomerular and postglomerular resistances.

Acknowledgments

These studies were supported by Hungarian Research Foundation grant OTKA 207, by German Research Foundation within Forschegruppe Niere/Heidelberg, and by US Public Health Service Grants HL-18426, HL-25451 and HL-22544.

References

1 Navar LG, Rosivall L. Contribution of renin-angiotensin system to the control of intrarenal haemodynamics. *Kidney Int 1984; 25:* 857–868

2 Ganten D, Hatchinson JS, Schelling P et al. The isorenin angiotensin systems in extrarenal tissues. *Clin Exp Pharmacol Physiol 1976; 3:* 103–126

3 Levens NR. Control of intestinal absorption by renin-angiotensin system. *Am J Physiol 1985; 249 (Gastrointest Liver Physiol 12):* G3–G15

4 Navar LG, Evan AP, Rosivall L. Microcirculation of the kidneys. In Mortillaro A, ed. *The Physiology and Pharmacology of Microcirculation, Vol 1.* New York: Academic Press. 1983: 394–488

5 Goormaghtigh N. L'appareil neuro-myo-arterial juxtaglomerulaire du rein; ses reactions en pathologie et ses rapports avec le tube urinifere. *CR Soc Biol 1937; 124:* 293–296

6 Taugner R, Ganten D. The localization of converting enzyme in kidney vessels of the rat. *Histochemistry 1982; 75:* 191–201

7 Rosivall L, Rinder DF, Champion J et al. Intrarenal angiotensin I conversion at normal and reduced renal blood flow in the dog. *Am J Physiol 1983; 245 (Renal Fluid Electrolyte Physiol 14):* F408–F415

8 Abe Y, Okohar T, Kishimoto T, Yamamoto K. Intrarenal role of renin-angiotensin system in the regulation of renal haemodynamics. *Jpn J Pharmacol 1979; 29:* 325–333

9 Oparil S, Bailie MD. Mechanism of renal handling of angiotensin II in the dog. *Circ Res 1973; 33:* 500–507

10 Bailie MD, Rector FC Jr, Seldin DW. Angiotensin II in renal arterial and renal venous plasma and renal lymph in the dog. *J Clin Invest 1971; 50:* 119–126

11 Mendelsohn FAO. Evidence for the local occurrence of angiotensin II in rat kidney and its modulation by dietary sodium intake and converting enzyme inhibition. *Clin Sci 1979; 57:* 173–179

12 Rosivall L, Narkates AJ, Oparil S, Navar LG. De novo intrarenal formation of angiotensin II during control and enhanced renin secretion. *Am J Physiol (Renal Fluid Electrolyte Physiol):* in press

13 Bührle CP, Scholz H, Hackenthal E et al. Epithelioid cells: membrane potential changes induced by substances influencing renin secretion. *Mol Cell Endocrinol 1986; 45:* 37–47

14 Bührle CP, Rosivall L, Taugner R. Intrarenal generation of angiotensin II evaluated by an electrophysiological technique. *Am J Physiol (Renal Fluid Electrolyte Physiol):* in press

15 Kriz W. A periarterial pathway for intrarenal distribution of renin. *Kidney Int 1987; 31 (Suppt 20):* S51–S56

16 Bruneval P, Hinglais N, Alhenc-Gelas et al. Angiotensin I converting enzyme in human intestine and kidney. Ultrastructural immunohistochemical localization. *Histochemistry 1986; 85:* 73–80

17 Genest J. Angiotensin-forming enzymes from extrarenal source. In Doyle AE, Bearn AG, eds. *Hypertension and the Angiotensin System.* New York: Raven Press. 1984: 93–107

18 Lohmeier TE, Cowley AW, Trippodo NC et al. Effects of endogenous angiotensin II on renal sodium excretion and haemodynamics. *Am J Physiol 1977; 233 (Renal Fluid Electrolyte Physiol 2):* F388–F395

19 Navar LG, Jirakulsomchok D, Bell D et al. Influence of converting enzyme inhibition on renal haemodynamics and glomerular dynamics in sodium restricted dogs. *Hypertension 1982; 4:* 58–68

20 Carmines PK, Rosivall L, Till MF, Navar LG. Renal haemodynamic effects of captopril in anaesthetized sodium-restricted dogs. Relative contribution of prostaglandin stimulation and suppressed angiotensin activity. *Renal Physiol 1983; 6:* 281–287
21 Rosivall L, Youngblood P, Navar LG. Renal autoregulatory efficiency during angiotensin converting enzyme inhibition in dogs on low sodium diet. *Renal Physiol 1986; 9:* 18–28
22 Britton SL. Intrarenal vascular effects of angiotensin I and angiotensin II. *Am J Physiol 1981; 240 (Heart Circ Physiol 9):* H914–H919
23 Rosivall L, Navar LG. Effects on renal haemodynamics of intra-arterial infusions of angiotensins I and II. *Am J Physiol 1983; 245 (Renal Fluid Electrolyte Physiol 14):* F181–F187
24 Carmines PK, Morrison TK, Navar LG. Angiotensin II effects on microvascular diameters of in vitro blood-perfused juxtamedullary nephrons. *Am J Physiol 1986; 251 (Renal Fluid Electrolyte Physiol 20):* F610–F618
25 Casellas D, Carmines PK, Navar LG. Microvascular reactivity of in vitro perfused juxtamedullary nephron from rats. *Kidney Int 1985; 28:* 752–759
26 Edwards RM. Segmental effects of norepinephrine and angiotensin II on isolated renal microvessels. *Am J Physiol 1983; 244 (Renal Fluid Electrolyte Physiol 13):* F526–F534
27 Steinhausen M, Kücherer H, Parekh N et al. Angiotensin II control of the renal microcirculation. Effect of blockade by saralasin. *Kidney Int 1986; 30:* 56–61
28 Steinhausen M, Sterzel RD, Fleming JT et al. Acute and chronic effects of angiotensin II on the vessels of the split hydronephrotic kidney. *Kidney Int 1987; 31 (Suppl 20):* S64–S73
29 Rosivall L, Carmines PK, Navar LG. Effects of renal arterial angiotensin I infusion on glomerular dynamics in sodium replete dogs. *Kidney Int 1984; 26:* 263–268
30 Mendelsohn FAO, Dunbar M, Allen A et al. Angiotensin II receptors in the kidney. *Federation Proc 1986; 45:* 1420–1425
31 Osborne MJ, Droz B, Meyer P, Morell F. Angiotensin II: renal localization in glomerular mesangial cells by autoradiography. *Kidney Int 1975; 8:* 245–254
32 Ausiello DA, Kreisberg JI, Roy C, Karnovszky MJ. Contraction of cultured rat glomerular mesangial cell after stimulation with angiotensin II and arginine vasopressin. *J Clin Invest 1980; 65:* 754–760
33 Kreisberg JI. Contractile properties of the glomerular mesangium. *Federation Proc 1983; 42:* 3053–3057
34 Sakai T, Kriz W. The structural relationship between mesangial cells and basement membrane of the renal glomerulus. *Anat Embryol:* in press
35 Latta H, Fligiel S. Mesangial fenestrations, sieving, filtration, and flow. *Lab Invest 1985; 52:* 591–598
36 Zimmerhackl B, Parekh N, Kücherer H, Steinhausen M. Influence of systematically applied angiotensin II on the microcirculation of glomerular capillaries in the rat. *Kidney Int 1985; 27:* 17–24
37 Taugner R, Rosivall L, Bührle CP, Gorschel-Stewart U. Myosin content and vasoconstrictive ability of the proximal and juxtaglomerular (renin positive) segment of the afferent arteriole. *Cell Tissue Res 1987; 248:* 579–588

HUMORAL AND NEURAL REGULATION OF GLOMERULAR FUNCTION

V Kon, T Yoshioka, K F Badr, A Yared, I Ichikawa

Vanderbilt University School of Medicine, Nashville, Tennessee, USA

Kinetics of glomerular filtration

Blood flow to any organ is controlled by the resistance of the arterioles immediately upstream to the capillary bed. Alteration in resistance of arterioles affects not only flow but also pressure within the capillaries, so the vasomotor tone of the arterioles has an important regulatory rôle for fluid movement across the capillary bed. In addition to this precapillary sphincter, or afferent arteriole, the glomerular circulatory system of the kidney is unique as it also possesses a postcapillary sphincter, namely, the efferent arteriole (Figure 1). This arrangement of resistance vessels permits a range of responses, depending on the site of the change in vasomotor tone. For example, a preferential increase in afferent arteriolar resistance (R_A) tends to precipitate a greater fall in the rate of glomerular filtration within each nephron than in the rate of glomerular plasma flow (Q_A); this occurs because an increase in pre-glomerular resistance

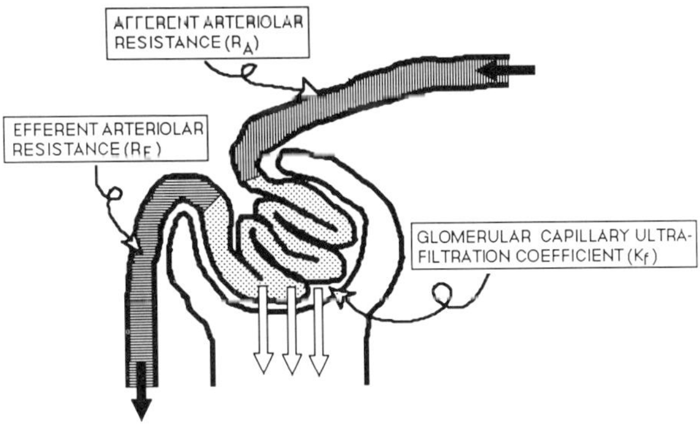

Figure 1. Schematic presentation of the three effector sites for humoral and neural actions within the glomerular microcirculatory system in modulating glomerular filtration and sieving functions

decreases both Q_A and glomerular capillary pressure (P_{GC}), both of which are determinants of single nephron glomerular filtration rate. A contrasting pattern is seen with a selective increase in efferent arteriolar resistance (R_E) when, although the predicted decline in Q_A may be identical to that seen with increased afferent arteriolar resistance, single nephron glomerular filtration rate remains constant, or even increases; this occurs because the P_{GC} upstream to the site of vasoconstriction tends to rise rather than fall, thereby achieving an increased ultrafiltration pressure and a higher filtration fraction.

A third site for intrarenal control of glomerular filtration rate has recently become evident. When either the hydraulic conductivity to water or the filtering surface area of the glomerular capillary is selectively reduced there is a diminished glomerular capillary ultrafiltration coefficient (K_f) and this results in a decreased glomerular filtration rate without a change in P_{GC} or Q_A. Technological advances in the early 1970s [1] now permit assessment of these three distinct effector sites within the glomerular circulation of mammals. Micropuncture measurements of pressures and flows at various sites of the glomerular circulation [1] allows precise descriptions of the process of ultrafiltration and so permit assessment of the contribution of these other sites under a variety of experimental conditions. This article discusses several of the recent experimental findings which delineated the important involvement of each of these three sites in modulating glomerular function in health and disease.

Glomerular capillary ultrafiltration coefficient

Many hormones affect the rate of glomerular plasma flow. It has been known for some time that infusion of potent vasodilators such as prostaglandin E_1, bradykinin, acetylcholine, and histamine cause large increases in renal blood flow [2–5]. The puzzling observation was that the increased blood flow was not accompanied by an elevation in glomerular filtration rate. To gain more insight into the filtration process under these circumstances, micropuncture measurements were made during infusion of mildly vasodilator doses of histamine [6]. Single nephron glomerular filtration rate was essentially unchanged, despite a 25% increase in glomerular plasma flow, Q_A. The elevated plasma flow reflected a reduction in pre- and post-glomerular arteriolar resistances, particularly in the pre-glomerular vessels. It was concluded that the histamine-induced increase in glomerular plasma flow was offset by a profound fall in the glomerular capillary ultrafiltration coefficient, K_f. These observations are particularly relevant to the regularly observed circumstance where spontaneous or therapeutic renal vasodilation is not accompanied by improvement in glomerular filtration rate, e.g. absence of elevation in glomerular filtration rate despite a rise in renal blood flow, as in acute renal failure. Subsequent micropuncture studies showed that other hormones, including angiotensin II, vasopressin, parathyroid hormone, prostaglandins, thromboxane and leukotriene D_4 [7–12], are also capable of reducing the ultrafiltration coefficient.

There has been renewed interest in the potential contribution of renal nerves to regulation of glomerular filtration rate. Direct stimulation or reflex activation of renal nerves is known to cause renal vasoconstriction [13]. Recent micropuncture studies by Kon et al [14] examined the effects of electrical stimulation of renal nerves on the process of glomerular ultrafiltration. It was found that single nephron glomerular filtration rate fell by more than 50% in response to high frequency stimulation. There was profound vasoconstriction in both pre- and post-glomerular arterioles, evidenced by a marked fall in Q_A. The comparable

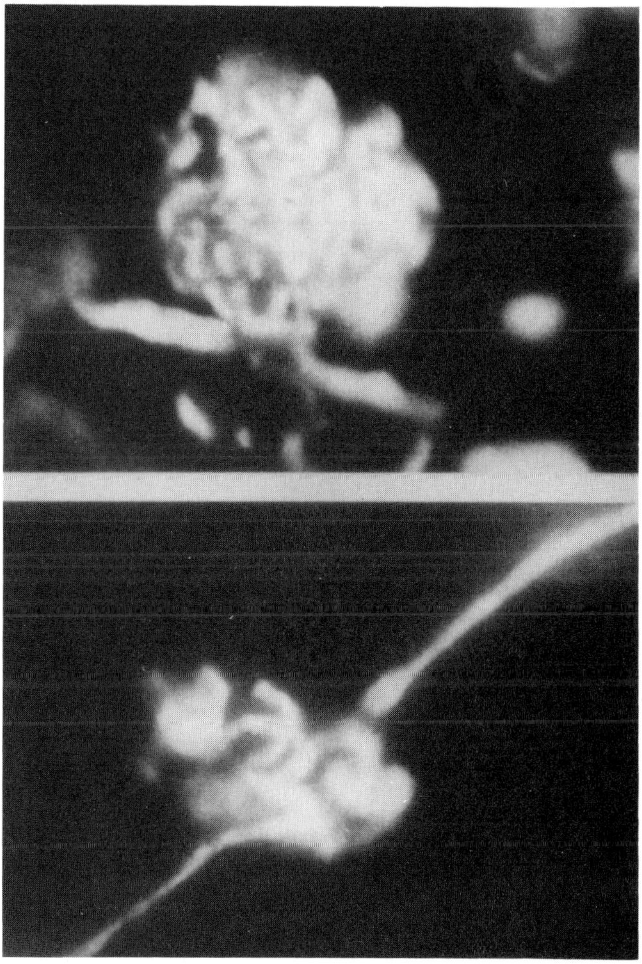

Figure 2. Glomeruli from left (top) and right (bottom) silicone-injected kidneys of the same rat that were perfusion-fixed during electrical stimulation of the right renal nerves. Reprinted with permission from *Fed Proc 1983; 42:* 3075–3079 [15]

degree of vasoconstriction in pre- and post-glomerular arterioles resulted in essentially stable values of P_{GC}. Values for K_f fell markedly, on average, by more than 70% from baseline values. Morphological studies [15] also demonstrated glomerular changes in response to direct stimulation of renal nerves. Kidneys were perfusion-fixed while the right renal nerves were selectively stimulated. The kidneys were then perfused with silicone rubber (Figure 2). When the silicone casts were examined, only large diameter glomerular capillaries of the stimulated kidney were still patent, contrasting with the many fine capillary tufts that were open on the contralateral non-stimulated kidney. The obliteration of glomerular capillary tufts in the stimulated kidney is consistent with the dramatic reduction in the filtering surface area, which may account for the more than 70% reduction in the value of K_f found in functional studies of renal nerve stimulation.

It is now well established that the kidney is a richly innervated organ [16]. Electronmicroscopic and immunohistochemical studies show nerve endings in direct contact with various tubular as well as vascular structures, including afferent and efferent arterioles and the mesangial cells. This anatomic relationship permits direct interaction between the adrenergic nervous system and mesangial cells which contain intracellular contractile myofilaments [17]. Recent studies by Kon and Karnovsky [18] directly examined the response of mesangial cells to the sympathetic neurotransmitter, noradrenaline. Cells were grown on plastic Petri dishes and studied on the day following the first passage. The mesangial cells were directly observed under a phase microscope and the images recorded on a time-lapse video recorder. Noradrenaline (10^{-6} M) reduced the length and diameter of cellular extensions and increased the cellular density (Figure 3). Cellular planar area, measured with an electronic planimeter was decreased by noradrenaline from $2.72 \pm 0.45 \times 10^3 mm^2$ (mean ± SEM) to $2.52 \pm 0.45 \times 10^3 mm^2$ ($p < 0.001$ paired 't' test). This decrease could be appreciated at five minutes and reached a maximum at about 20 minutes from addition of noradrenaline. It was further found that replacement of the noradrenaline-containing culture medium with a noradrenaline-free medium returned the planar area towards baseline in every cell examined, 2.47 ± 0.43 versus $2.61 \pm 0.40 \times 10^3 mm^2$ ($p < 0.005$). There was no change in cellular configuration over a 45–60 minute period in mesangial cells if the initial bathing medium contained no noradrenaline. Overall, it appears that noradrenaline can reversibly induce changes in mesangial cell configuration which are consistent with cellular contraction and this suggests an important rôle of mesangial contractility as a relay between nerve stimulation and glomerular capillary obliteration.

Micropuncture studies performed during the last decade showed that a variety of low glomerular filtration rate states are characterized by a low level of K_f. These include congestive heart failure, acute and chronic volume depletion, protein malnutrition, certain forms of glomerulonephritis and minimal change disease, ureteral obstruction, renal hypertension, renal vein constriction and

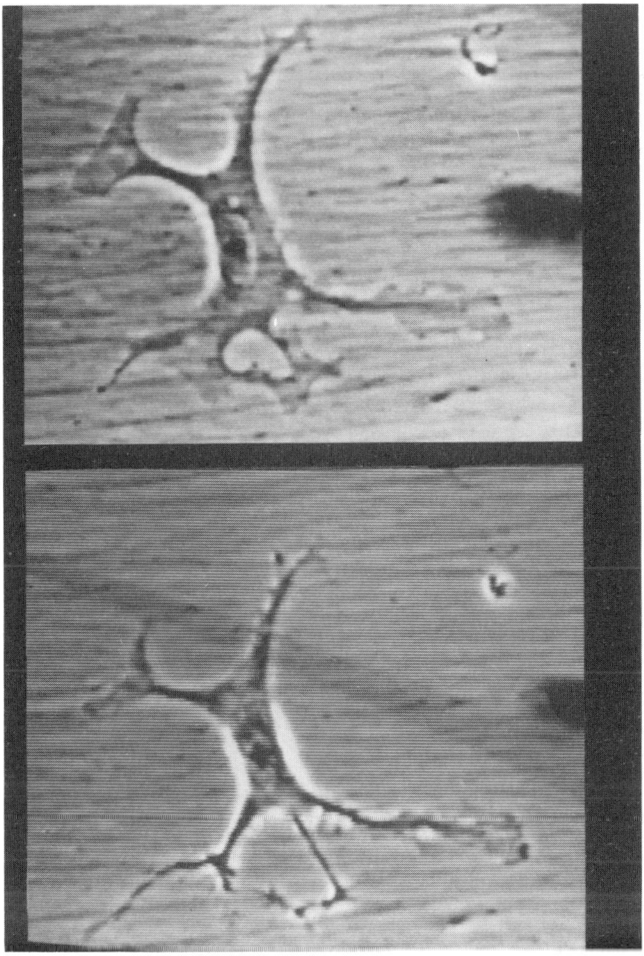

Figure 3. Mesangial cell configuration observed under a phase microscope (top). ×1000 – reduced for publication. The same cell after adding noradrenaline, 10^{-6} M (bottom)

some forms of acute renal failure such as from gentamicin and uranyl nitrate [8,19–35]. In many of these conditions, humoral and neural contributions to the low level of K_f have been identified by using specific hormonal inhibitors or by denervation. For example, glomerular dynamics of Munich-Wistar rats several hours after intravenous injection of rabbit anti-rat glomerular basement membrane antibody, are characterized by a low single nephron glomerular filtration rate, compared to normal rats [19,34]. This hypofiltration was attributed to a reduction of both K_f and Q_A. The low level of Q_A, in turn, is due to increased afferent and efferent arteriolar resistances. When anti-glomerular basement membrane antibody was given to rats treated with the highly specific leukotriene D_4 receptor antagonist SK&F 104353, the large reduction in K_f

observed in rats given anti-glomerular basement membrane antibody alone was absent [34]. Although this leukotriene D_4 antagonist had no effect on R_A, R_E or Q_A, its protective effect on K_f was sufficient to prevent the reduction in single nephron glomerular filtration rate. This highly localized protective action of leukotriene D_4 antagonist might indicate a major functional rôle for intra-glomerularly-released leukotriene D_4 derived from the infiltrating leucocytes inherent in the pathophysiology of this form of glomerulonephritis.

Afferent arteriolar resistances

The afferent arteriole, or precapillary sphincter, is not unique to the kidney but present in a variety of organ systems. As in many other organs, the renal afferent arteriole plays a crucial rôle in autoregulation of renal blood flow, a mechanism which maintains homeostasis of organ blood flow rate in the face of changes in systemic blood pressure. Dilatation and constriction of the afferent arteriole are also important for maintenance of glomerular filtration rate. As discussed above, afferent arteriolar resistance changes, along with R_E and K_f, in response to several vasoactive substances, i.e. histamine and leukotriene D_4. Although there are a number of substances capable of changing R_A, atrial natriuretic peptide has recently become the focus of investigations. As will be discussed, this is because atrial natriuretic peptide has been found to have a selective vasodilatory action on afferent arterioles [36]. Therefore, unlike other renal vasodilators, it potentially has a glomerular filtration rate improving ability which is of particular importance in acute renal failure. In a micropuncture study [36], administration of synthetic atrial natriuretic peptide, Auriculin, led to a significant reduction in R_A, whereas R_E increased and K_f remained unaffected. These actions of atrial natriuretic peptide on glomerular microvasculature were accompanied by a significant elevation in P_{GC}. Since Q_A remained unchanged, the rise in P_{GC} was solely responsible for the increase in single nephron glomerular filtration rate.

Efferent arteriolar resistances

The glomerulus is the only organ with a postcapillary sphincter. Recent micropuncture studies have demonstrated the importance of this microvascular arrangement in the homeostasis of glomerular function. As already discussed, the kidney has a regulatory system which maintains blood flow in the face of fluctuating perfusion pressures, a phenomenon called autoregulation of blood flow. Experimental reduction of renal perfusion pressure in normal rats from 110 to 75mmHg result in reduction of Q_A by only 15% of its baseline value [37]; single nephron glomerular filtration rate also fell by 15%. The absence of a profound reduction in Q_A despite a drastic fall in renal perfusion pressure, was attributed to a reduction in afferent arteriolar resistance, R_A, by 25% of its baseline. In addition, the efferent arteriolar resistance, R_E increased. This increase is crucially important in preventing an otherwise profound fall in P_{GC}.

Despite systemic circulatory derangement in extracellular fluid volume depletion and congestive heart failure, glomerular filtration rate is remarkably well preserved. However, both conditions are known to predispose to pre-renal azotaemia in the event of even relatively minor hypotensive episodes. Recent micropuncture studies [37] have given new insights into this phenomenon. In rat models of both acute extracellular fluid volume depletion and congestive heart failure, experimental reduction of renal perfusion pressure caused a modest fall in Q_A which was comparable to that found in normal rats. These similar and relatively small changes in Q_A were attributed to reduction in afferent arteriolar resistances, which were of similar magnitude in the three groups studied: extracellular fluid volume depletion, congestive heart failure and normal control. However, single nephron glomerular filtration rate fell markedly in rats with acute extracellular fluid volume depletion and congestive heart failure but not in normal animals. In normal rats R_E increased and contributed towards preserving single nephron glomerular filtration rate, but in the pathophysiological groups efferent arteriolar resistances decreased, resulting in a profound fall in P_{GC}, which, in turn, accounted for the fall in single nephron glomerular filtration rate. Overall, these experiments suggest that maintenance of glomerular filtration rate during reduced perfusion pressure requires maintenance of both glomerular plasma flow rate and glomerular capillary pressure, which are mediated primarily by reduction in R_A and increase in R_E, respectively (Figure 4). Other

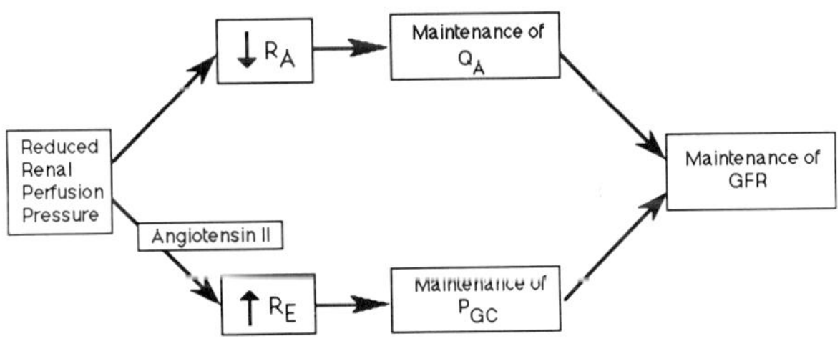

Figure 4. Autoregulatory adjustments made within the glomerular microcirculatory system in maintaining glomerular filtration rate (GFR) during reduction in renal perfusion pressure. The maintenance of GFR is accomplished by a reduction in afferent arteriolar resistance (R_A) and efferent arteriolar constrictive response to locally released angiotensin II. These changes serve to preserve glomerular plasma flow rate (Q_A) and glomerular capillary hydraulic pressure (P_{GC}), respectively

studies [38] have indicated that the increase in R_E is mediated by angiotensin II. The lack of response of the efferent arteriole to reduction in renal perfusion pressure during acute extracellular fluid depletion or congestive heart failure occurs because even without reduction in perfusion pressure angiotensin II is *already* acting maximally to preserve a high glomerular filtration rate; further increases in angiotensin II have no effect [37].

Kinetics of glomerular sieving function

It is important to recognize that vasomotor tone of the glomerular microvascular tree affects not only glomerular filtration rate but also glomerular sieving function. In rats mean systemic arterial pressure was unaffected during acute, partial renal vein constriction, but an elevation in renal venous pressure from two to 15mmHg led to a rise in intravascular pressure at every level of renal cortical microcirculation [33]. The elevation in pressure was greatest at the glomerular capillary; the average increase in P_{GC} was 14mmHg. Whereas afferent arteriolar resistances remained largely unaffected, efferent arteriolar resistances increased more than two-fold during renal vein constriction and this significant rise in R_E, contributed to the accentuated rise in P_{GC}. It is known that renal renin release is markedly enhanced during any impedence of renal venous outflow [39], so in animals with renal vein constriction the action of angiotensin II was inhibited by an infusion of Saralasin. This led to a reduction in P_{GC} to almost control levels despite continued renal vein constriction, which was associated with a profound fall in R_E, while R_A once again remained essentially unaffected. This, indicates that renal vein constriction-induced fall in glomerular plasma flow rate and the rise in P_{GC} were not merely due to the mechanical resistance created at the renal vein, but rather, due primarily, to an increase in R_E caused by the enhanced action of endogenous angiotensin II.

Figure 5 summarizes the results of measurements of clearance of neutral dextrans, having effective molecular radii between 20 and 58Å, in rats treated in identical fashion to those of the renal vein constriction experiments above [33]. As can be seen, the sieving coefficients, or fractional clearance of dextran (dextran clearance rate/inulin clearance rate), of relatively small molecules (20 to 44Å) were essentially unchanged from control to renal vein constriction, whereas the sieving coefficients of larger dextran molecules were substantially elevated. These changes in glomerular sieving function were accompanied by a dramatic increase of urinary protein excretion on average from 11 to 106mg/24 hours. The middle curve shows that Saralasin infusion during renal vein constriction returned the sieving profile and urinary protein excretion toward the normal pattern. Again, the sieving coefficients for the small molecules were essentially unaffected; however, a reduction in the coefficient for larger dextrans was evident during Saralasin infusion.

A recent mathematical analysis of the size selective function of the glomerular capillary wall in a variety of experimental conditions led to the conclusion that there exists two distinctive populations of functional pores on the capillary wall [40]. One type is small but numerous and primarily determines the hydraulic conductance being virtually impermeable to large molecules; the other type is large in size but few in number, and freely permeable to large molecules, thereby determining the transcapillary passage of large molecules. Using various measurements of glomerular microcirculatory dynamics and dextran clearances obtained in our renal vein constriction study [33], we calculated the pore radius of the

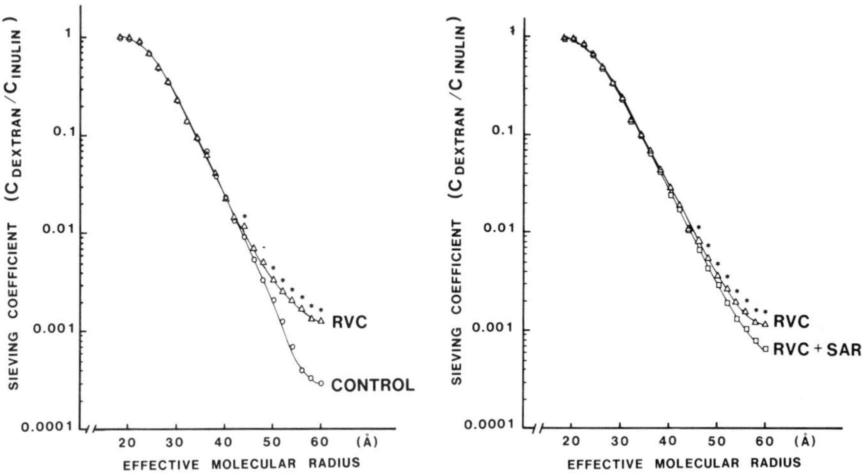

Figure 5. Semilogarithmic presentation of the relationship between the effective molecular radius of the dextran and the sieving coefficient of dextran. Left: values for baseline period (Control=open circles) and those during partial renal vein constriction (RVC= open triangles). The values of sieving coefficient, molecular radii greater than 44Å (except for 46Å) are significantly elevated during renal vein constriction. Right: values for renal vein constriction period (open triangles) and those during renal vein constriction with superimposed Saralasin treatment (RVC+SAR, open squares). Those values of molecular radii greater than 46Å are significantly decreased during Saralasin infusion. * indicates statistical significance at $p<0.05$. Reprinted with permission from *Kidney Int* 1986; 30: 538–545 [33]

small pores and large-to-small pore population ratio. These calculations indicated that endogenous angiotensin II released during renal vein constriction reduces the total pore area without affecting small pore radius, thereby reducing net hydraulic conductance of the glomerular capillary; large-to-small pore population was increased, accounting for the attenuation of the size selective function of the glomerular capillary wall during renal vein constriction. The large-to-small pore population ratio varied in close association with the level of glomerular capillary pressure, so it was concluded that angiotensin II, by raising glomerular capillary pressure via its potent constrictor action on efferent arteriole, may expose new, large non-size selective pores on the glomerular capillary. Thus, angiotensin II appears to affect not only glomerular filtration via its action on the mesangium but also affects the glomerular sieving function via its vasoconstrictive influence on the efferent arteriole. Loss of size selective function of the glomerular capillary wall secondary to high glomerular capillary pressure has recently been noted in rat models of glomerulonephritis [41] and progressive chronic renal failure [42]. These preliminary studies indicate that mechanisms other than angiotensin II may be involved in these two conditions.

Summary

Using recent experimental data we have discussed the rôle of various humoral and neural influences in glomerular filtering and sieving function via their actions on the three effector sites of the glomerular microcirculatory system, namely afferent and efferent arterioles and the glomerular mesangium.

Acknowledgments

The authors are grateful to Ms Marye Yeomans for secretarial assistance. Dr Kon is a recipient of the American Heart Association Clinician Scientist Award and Dr Ichikawa is a recipient of the Established Investigatorship Award from the American Heart Association.

These studies were supported by Public Health Service Grants DK-37868 and 37869, and American Heart Association AHA-820424.

References

1 Brenner BM, Troy JL, Daugharty TM. The dynamics of glomerular ultrafiltration in the rat. *J Clin Invest 1971; 50:* 1776–1780

2 Johnston HH, Hertzog JP, Lauler DP. Effect of prostaglandin E_1 on renal hemodynamics, sodium and water excretion. *Am J Physiol 1967; 213:* 939–946

3 Baer PG, Navar LG, Guyton AC. Renal autoregulation, filtration rate and electrolyte excretion during vasodilation. *Am J Physiol 1970; 219:* 619–625

4 Stein JH, Congbalay RC, Karsh DL et al. The effect of bradykinin on proximal tubular sodium reabsorption in the dog: evidence for functional nephron heterogeneity. *J Clin Invest 1972; 51:* 1709–1721

5 Strandhoy JW, Ott CE, Schneider EG et al. Effects of prostaglandin E_1 and E_2 on renal sodium reabsorption and Starling forces. *Am J Physiol 1974; 226:* 1015–1021

6 Ichikawa I, Brenner BM. Mechanisms of action of histamine and histamine antagonists on the glomerular microcirculation in the rat. *Circ Res 1979; 45:* 737–745

7 Blantz RC, Konnen KS, Tucker BJ. Angiotensin II effects upon the glomerular microcirculation and ultrafiltration coefficient of the rat. *J Clin Invest 1976; 57:* 419–434

8 Ichikawa I, Brenner BM. Evidence for glomerular actions of ADH and dibutyryl cyclic AMP in the rat. *Am J Physiol 1977; 233:* F102–F117

9 Baylis C, Deen WM, Myers BD, Brenner BM. Effects of some vasodilator drugs on transcapillary fluid exchange in renal cortex. *Am J Physiol 1976; 230:* 1148–1158

10 Ichikawa I, Purkerson ML, Yates J, Klahr S. Dietary protein intake conditions the degree of renal vasoconstriction in acute renal failure caused by ureteral obstruction. *Am J Physiol 1985; 249:* F54–F61

11 Ichikawa I, Humes HD, Dousa TP, Brenner BM. Influence of parathyroid hormone on glomerular ultrafiltration in the rat. *Am J Physiol 1978; 234:* F393–F401

12 Badr KF, Brenner BM, Ichikawa I. Effects of leukotriene D_4 on glomerular dynamics in the rat. *Am J Physiol:* in press

13 Katz MA, Shear L. Effect of renal nerves on renal hemodynamics. I. Direct stimulation and carotid occlusion. *Nephron 1975; 14:* 246–256

14 Kon V, Ichikawa I. Effector loci for renal nerve control of cortical microcirculation. *Am J Physiol 1983; 244:* F545–F553

15 Ichikawa I, Kon V. Glomerular mesangium as an effector locus for the tubuloglomerular feedback system and renal sympathetic innervation. *Fed Proc 1983; 42:* 3075–3079

16 Barajas L, Wang P, Powers K, Nishio S. Identification of renal neuroeffector junctions by electron microscopy of reembedded light microscopic autoradiograms of semithin sections. *J Ultrastruct Res 1981; 77:* 379–385

17 Kreisberg JI, Karnovsky MJ. Characterization of rat glomerular cells in vitro. In Cummings NB, Michael AF, Wilson CB, eds. *Immune Mechanisms in Renal Disease.* New York: Plenum. 1982

18 Kon V, Karnovsky MJ. Norepinephrine reversibly decreases planar surface area of rat mesangial cells. *Kidney Int 1987; 31:* 424

19 Blantz RC, Tucker BJ, Wilson CB. The acute effects of antiglomerular basement membrane antibody on the process of glomerular filtration in the rat. *J Clin Invest 1976; 58:* 899–911

20 Ichikawa I, Brenner BM. Local intrarenal vasoconstrictor-vasodilator interactions in mild partial ureteral obstruction. *Am J Physiol 1979; 236:* F131–F140

21 Blantz RC, Tucker BJ, Gushwa LC et al. Glomerular immune injury in the rat: the influence of angiotensin II and α-adrenergic inhibitors. *Kidney Int 1981; 20:* 452–461

22 Schor N. Ichikawa I, Brenner BM. Glomerular adaptations to chronic dietary salt restriction or excess. *Am J Physiol 1980; 238:* F428–F436

23 Steiner RW, Tucker BJ, Blantz RC. Glomerular hemodynamics in rats with chronic sodium depletion. Effect of Saralasin. *J Clin Invest 1974; 64:* 503–512

24 Ichikawa I, Purkerson ML, Klahr S et al. Mechanism of reduced glomerular filtration rate in chronic malnutrition. *J Clin Invest 1980; 65:* 982–988

25 Baylis C, Rennke HG, Brenner BM. Mechanisms of the defect in glomerular ultrafiltration associated with gentamicin administration. *Kidney Int 1977; 12:* 344–353

26 Schor N, Ichikawa I, Rennke HG et al. Pathophysiology of altered glomerular function in the amino-glycoside-treated rats. *Kidney Int 1981; 19:* 288–296

27 Ichikawa I, Hoyer JR, Seiler MW, Brenner BM. Mechanism of glomerulotubular balance in the setting of heterogeneous glomerular injury. Preservation of a close functional linkage between individual nephrons and surrounding microvasculature. *J Clin Invest 1982; 69:* 185–198

28 Ichikawa I, Rennke HG, Badr KF et al. Role for intrarenal mechanisms in mediating salt retention in experimental nephrotic syndrome. *J Clin Invest 1983; 71:* 91–103

29 Ichikawa I, Ferrone RA, Duchin KL et al. Relative contributions of vasopressin and angiotensin II to the altered renal microcirculatory dynamics in two-kidney Goldblatt hypertension. *Circ Res 1983; 53:* 592–602

30 Ichikawa I, Pfeffer JM, Pfeffer MA et al. Role of angiotensin II in the altered renal function of congestive heart failure. *Circ Res 1984; 55:* 669–675

31 Yared A, Kon V, Ichikawa I. Mechanism of preservation of glomerular perfusion and filtration during acute extracellular fluid volume depletion. Importance of intrarenal vasopressin-prostaglandin interaction for protecting kidneys from constrictor action of vasopressin. *J Clin Invest 1985; 75:* 1477–1487

32 Kon V, Yared A, Ichikawa I. The role of renal sympathetic nerves in mediating hypoperfusion of renal cortical microcirculation in experimental congestive heart failure and acute ECF volume depletion. *J Clin Invest 1985; 76:* 1913–1920

33 Yoshioka T, Mitarai T, Kon V et al. Role for angiotensin II in an overt functional proteinuria. *Kidney Int 1986; 30:* 538–545

34 Badr KF, Gung A, Schreiner GF et al. Reversal of antiglomerular basement membrane-antibody-induced fall in the glomerular ultrafiltration coefficient by leukotriene D4 antagonist SK&F 104353. *Kidney Int 1987; 31:* 363

35 Blantz RC. The mechanism of acute renal failure after uranyl nitrate. *J Clin Invest 1975; 55:* 621–635

36 Dunn BR, Ichikawa I, Pfeffer JM et al. Renal and systemic hemodynamic effects of synthetic atrial natriuretic peptide in the anesthetized rat. *Circ Res 1986; 237:* 237–246

37 Yoshioka T, Yared A, Ichikawa I. Impaired autoregulation of GFR in systemic circulatory derangement: a predisposing factor for prerenal azotemia. *Kidney Int 1987; 31:* 293

38 Ichikawa I, Brenner BM. Importance of efferent arteriolar vascular tone in the regulation of proximal tubule fluid reabsorption and glomerulotubular balance in the rat. *J Clin Invest 1980; 65:* 1192–1201

39 Kishimoto R, Maekawa M, Miyazaki K et al. Effects of renal venous pressure elevation on renal hemodynamics, urine formation and renin release. *Jpn Circ J 1972; 36:* 439–448

40 Deen WM, Bridges CR, Brenner BM, Myers BD. Heteroporous model of glomerular size-selectivity: application to normal and nephrotic humans. *Am J Physiol 1985; 249:* F374–F389

41 Yoshioka T, Rennke HG, Salant DJ et al. Role of abnormally high transmural pressure in the permselectivity defect of glomerular capillary wall: a study in early passive Heymann nephritis. *Circ Res:* in press

42 Ichikawa I, Shiraga H, Yoshida Y et al. Basis for lack of correlation between changes in glomerular structure and permselectivity in individual nephrons in chronic renal disease. *Kidney Int 1987; 31:* 424

RENAL MEDULLARY MICROCIRCULATION AND RENAL WATER AND SOLUTE HANDLING

L B Zimmerhackl

Philipps University, Marburg, FRG

Interest in the medullary microcirculation has increased considerably during recent years. Two major events have played leading rôles: the introduction of video-microscopy into the renal laboratory and the discovery of the atrial natriuretic peptide. The first event improved the investigation of blood flow in the inner medulla of small laboratory animals; the second phenomenon stimulated interest due to reports that medullary blood flow may mediate the natriuretic effect of atrial natriuretic peptide.

The rôle of the medullary microcirculation in the model of countercurrent exchange has not been completely evaluated, but it may have three major functions. Firstly, according to the mathematical urinary concentrating model put forward mainly by Stephenson [1], it may serve as a nephrovascular coupler. Following mass balance principles fluid that has been reabsorbed by tubular cells has to be removed from the medulla at the same rate. The medulla probably has no lymphatic vessels that are able to transport considerable volumes [2]. Extravascular routes for fluid removal have been described; nevertheless their quantitative rôle for fluid transport are of minor importance [3]. Therefore the only major structures remaining for fluid transfer are the vasa recta [4]. For fluid reabsorption the following equation holds true at every level of the renal medulla [1]:

$$T_{H_2O} = Q_{Blood}(AVR) - Q_{Blood}(DVR) \qquad \text{Equation 1}$$

where T_{H_2O} is volume of fluid reabsorbed from tubular structures within the medulla, Q_{Blood} (DVR) is total blood inflow to descending vasa recta (DVR) and Q_{Blood} (AVR) is total blood outflow from ascending vasa recta (AVR). Thus, the volume of fluid that can be removed by the vasa recta may limit the volume of fluid reabsorbed from medullary tubular portions of the nephron.

Secondly, using the same mathematical concept just mentioned [1], the medullary microcirculation may influence solute transport:

$$T(S) = Q_{Blood}(AVR) \times C(S)_{AVR} - Q_{Blood}(DVR) \times C(S)_{DVR} \qquad \text{Equation 2}$$

where T(S) is the mass of solute removed from the medulla by vasa recta and C(S) stands for concentration of solute in ascending (AVR) and descending vasa recta (DVR) respectively.

Thirdly, the microcirculation has to supply the substrates necessary for medullary tubular cells to generate metabolic energy. Considerable information has been gained in recent years regarding the metabolism of tubular cells [5]. Studies which investigate the links between metabolism and the medullary microcirculation are rare, however [4].

The first two rôles of the medullary microcirculation (in solute and water transport) have been re-examined in recent years. In this paper we will focus on results obtained by modern video-microscopic and micropuncture techniques [4,6–8].

The medullary microcirculation during antidiuresis

Originally Thurau, Ullrich and co-workers described an association between urinary osmolality and medullary blood flow [9,10]. At high medullary blood flow levels urine to plasma ratio of osmolality (U/P_{Osm}) was low and at low medullary perfusion U/P_{Osm} was high. Using mass balance principles Stephenson [1] concluded that high perfusion rates cause diminution of the interstitial solute concentration in the medulla which, in turn, reduces the reabsorption of water in the loop of Henle and from collecting duct structures. This phenomenon was named 'medullary washout'. In the following years many groups tried to evaluate the influence of medullary blood flow on urinary concentration. However, these studies were hampered by the fact that any experimental disturbance might influence other driving forces of tubular reabsorption, as for example interstitial pressure.

In order to find out whether medullary blood flow influences the ability to concentrate urine under physiological conditions of antidiuresis we designed a study in rodents [11].

Infusion of physiological doses of arginine vasopressin into chronically water diuretic rats caused a significant reduction in vasa recta blood flow in the papilla (Figure 1A). Total renal blood flow and glomerular filtration rates were unaltered during the experimental period. Urinary osmolality increased from hypotonic values to hypertonic values, around 700mOsm/kg H_2O, within 60 minutes (Figure 1A). This increase in osmolality was probably due to arginine vasopressin-associated water reabsorption. It should be noted that chronic water diuresis causes considerable washout of urea from the medullary interstitium, and to achieve higher urinary osmolalities requires restitution of significant urea concentrations in the renal medulla which takes several hours; full restitution may require days [12].

In a second group of animals we inhibited the vasoactive action of arginine

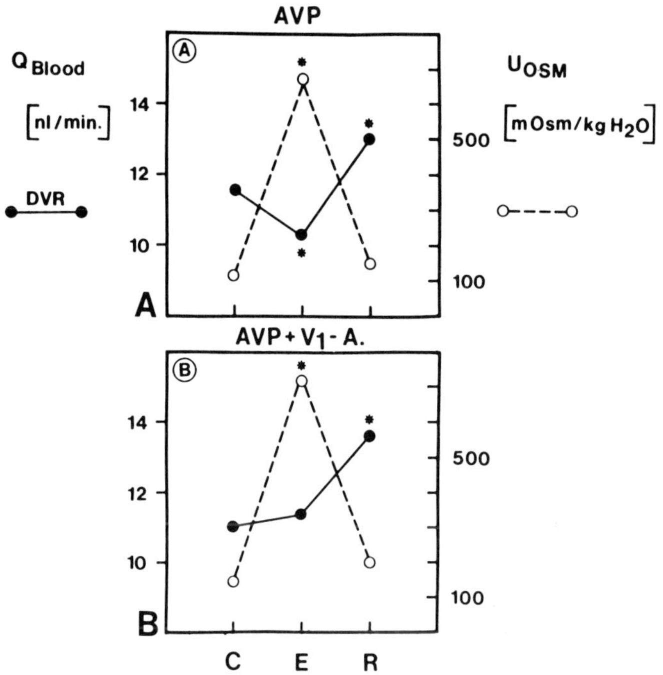

Figure 1. A. Influence of arginine vasopressin (AVP) on blood flow in descending vasa recta (Q_{Blood}) and urinary osmolality (U_{Osm}). C=control period; E=experimental period; R=recovery. *denotes significant difference from the control period. Adapted from [11]. B. Vasa recta blood flow during the infusion of AVP and the vasoactive antagonist (V_1-A). For abbreviations see above. Adapted from [11]

vasopressin using the pharmacological antagonist $d(CH_2)_5Tyr(Me)AVP$, a so-called V_1 antagonist (V_1-A). The action of arginine vasopressin on V_1 receptors, which is responsible for the effects of arginine vasopressin on blood vessels, is thought to be mediated through increases in intracellular calcium concentration and is related to phosphatidyl-inositol metabolism. The addition of V_1-A to the infusion did indeed inhibit the decrease in papillary blood flow. Urinary osmolality however, was as high as in the arginine vasopressin group. These experiments indicate that the acute increase in urinary osmolality caused by arginine vasopressin does not depend on medullary perfusion, at least under physiological conditions.

That medullary blood flow follows simple mass balance principles, could be demonstrated in additional experiments [8,13]. Paradoxically total water reabsorption in the papilla is higher during water diuresis than during antidiuresis. In 1971 Jamison designed an experiment to measure total water reabsorption in papillary collecting ducts using inulin as a marker for fluid reabsorption [14]. Fractional water reabsorption in water diuresis averaged 2.2% of the filtered water, while in antidiuresis the volume of reabsorption in collecting ducts decreased to 0.6% of filtered water. According to equation 1 this should also be reflected in the volume removed by vasa recta from the papilla. The volume of fluid removed from the papilla by vasa recta increased significantly during water diuresis and decreased in antidiuresis. These studies demonstrated that the mass balance of fluid movement is preserved in the medulla and can be studied with modern video-microscopic methods [4,5,8,11,13].

The medullary microcirculation during atrial natriuretic peptide-induced natriuresis

Atrial natriuretic peptide causes profound natriuresis [15]. Several modes of action have been proposed [15–18]. Decreases in pre-glomerular resistance and increases in efferent glomerular resistance leading to increased glomerular filtration rate and increased tubular loads have been described [17,18]. In addition, effects on tubular reabsorption of solute have been found as well [19]. An attractive hypothesis was put forward by Sonnenberg and co-workers who found an increase in medullary blood flow during atrial natriuretic peptide infusion [15].

They proposed that natriuresis was a consequence of interstitial washout of solutes (see equation 2). Their results, however, depended on the use of the albumin accumulation technique which does not permit studies of the development of microcirculatory changes with respect to time [8]. Therefore, Kiberd et al [20] studied the time dependent course of the natriuresis and medullary blood flow in rats. In this study sodium excretion increased almost immediately after atrial natriuretic peptide infusion as shown in Figure 2A. Simultaneously vasa recta blood flow was determined by video-microscopy. Within four minutes after initiation of the atrial natriuretic peptide infusion sodium excretion had more than tripled compared to the control animals (Figure 2B). Vasa recta blood flow remained unaltered during the initial period (Figures 2A and B). Forty-five minutes later, however, vasa recta blood flow and urine flow increased significantly. Increased blood flow associated with increased diuresis may be explained by the observations of Jamison et al [14] that fluid reabsorption from the collecting duct is greater during diuresis; this 'extra' fluid reabsorption is then transported by the vasa recta increasing blood flow. These results, therefore, do not support the view that medullary solute washout by vasa recta is the primary cause of atrial natriuretic peptide-induced natriuresis.

In summary, the medullary microcirculation is an important contributor to the countercurrent solute and water exchange. The passive removal of fluid and solute from the medulla by the medullary microcirculation is a prerequisite for the function of nephrovascular coupling. This rôle of the microcirculation in the process of urinary concentration during water diuresis and arginine vasopressin-related antidiuresis is well established. However, whether acute changes in medullary blood flow significantly affect medullary interstitial solute concentration and thus influence tubular reabsorption is still open to question.

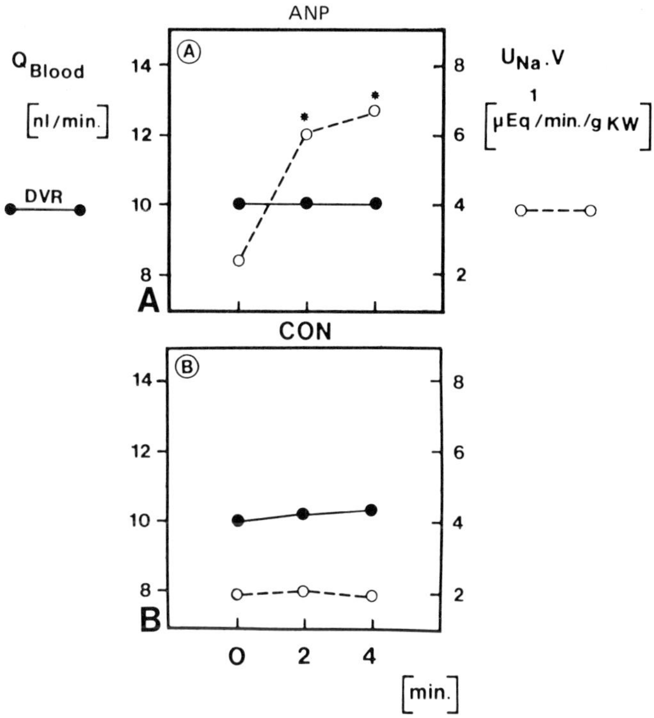

Figure 2. Effect of atrial natriuretic peptide (ANP) on vasa recta blood flow and urinary sodium excretion ($U_{Na}V$) at time 0, 2 and 4 minutes after initiation of ANP. *denotes significant difference from time 0. Adapted from [20].
B. Time control. Adapted from [20]

It is, furthermore, unclear to what extent changes in medullary blood flow influence tubular solute transport and hence urinary solute excretion, at least under physiological conditions. Atrial natriuretic peptide causes natriuresis by mechanisms other than medullary interstitial solute washout.

Acknowledgments

Research from the author's laboratories which is cited in the article was supported by National Institute of Health Grants 5-RO1-AM 18077, RT32 07357, The American Heart Association Grant 81-712, the German Research Foundation ZI 269/1-1 and SFB 'cardiovascular system'. Dr Zimmerhackl was a recipient of the Hoechst-Roussel Pharmaceutical Inc/National Kidney Foundation fellowship and of a stipendiary from the German Research Foundation.

Professors R L Jamison, C R Robertson and M Steinhausen gave invaluable support during the course of the studies cited and Professors M Brandis, C Reiger and R L Jamison assisted in discussing this manuscript.

References

1 Stephenson JL. Models of urinary concentrating mechanism. *Kidney Int 1987; 31:* 648–661

2 Jamison RL, Kriz W. *Urinary Concentrating Mechanism: Structure and Function.* New York: Oxford University Press. 1982

3 Bargman J, Leonard SL, McNeely E et al. Examination of transepithelial exchange of water and solute in the rat renal pelvis. *J Clin Invest 1984; 74:* 1860–1870

4 Zimmerhackl LB, Robertson CR, Jamison RL. The medullary microcirculation. *Kidney Int 1987; 31:* 641–647

5 Wirtensohn G, Guder WG. Renal substrate metabolism. *Physiol Rev 1986; 66:* 469–497

6 Gussis GL, Jamison RL, Robertson CR. Determination of erythrocyte velocities in the mammalian inner renal medulla by a video velocity tracking system. *Microvasc Res 1979; 18:* 370–383

7 Holliger C, Lemely KV, Schmitt SL et al. Direct determination of vasa recta blood flow in the rat renal papilla. *Circ Res 1983; 53:* 401–413

8 Zimmerhackl B, Dussel R, Steinhausen M. Erythrocyte flow and dynamic hematocrit in the renal papilla of the rat. *Am J Physiol 1985; 249:* F898–F902

9 Thurau K. Renal hemodynamics. *Am J Med 1964; 36:* 698–719

10 Ullrich KJ, Pehling G, Espinar-La Fuente. Wasser- und Elektrolytfluss im vascularen Gegenstromsystem des Nierenmarkes. *Pfluegers Arch 1961; 273:* 562–572

11 Zimmerhackl B, Robertson CR, Jamison RL. Effect of arginine vasopressin on renal medullary blood flow. *J Clin Invest 1985; 76:* 770–778

12 Gellai M, Silverstein J, Hwang JC et al. Influence of vasopressin on renal hemodynamics in conscious Brattleboro rats. *Am J Physiol 1984; 246:* F819–F827

13 Zimmerhackl, Robertson CR, Jamison RL. Fluid uptake in the renal papilla by vasa recta estimated by two methods simultaneously. *Am J Physiol 1985; 248:* F347–F353

14 Jamison RL, Buerkert J, Lacy F. A micropuncture study of collecting tubule function in rats with hereditary diabetes insipidus. *J Clin Invest 1971; 50:* 2444–2452

15 Borenstein HB, Cupples WA, Sonnenberg H, Veress A. The effect of a natriuretic atrial extract on renal haemodynamics and urinary excretion in anesthetized rats. *J Physiol (Lond) 1983; 334:* 133–140

16 Dunn BR, Troy JL, Ichikawa I, Brenner BM. Effect of atrial natriuretic peptides on hydraulic pressures in the rat renal papilla, implications for ANP-induced natriuresis. *Kidney Int 1986; 29:* 382A

17 Huang CL, Lewicki J, Johnson LK, Cogan MG. Renal mechanisms of action of rat atrial natriuretic factor. *J Clin Invest 1985; 75:* 769–773

18 Marin-Grez MJ, Fleming JT, Steinhausen M. Atrial natriuretic peptide causes preglomerular vasodilatation and post-glomerular vasoconstriction in rat kidney. *Nature 1986; 324:* 473–476

19 Sonnenberg H, Honrath U, Chong CK, Wilson DR. Atrial natriuretic factor inhibits sodium transport in medullary collecting ducts. *Am J Physiol 1986; 250:* F963–F966

20 Kiberd BA, Larson TS, Robertson CR, Jamison RL. The effect of atrial natriuretic peptide on vasa recta blood flow in the rat. *Am J Physiol:* in press

EFFERENT ARTERIOLE: THE MAIN TARGET VESSEL FOR SOME RENAL VASOCONSTRICTORS?

J Heller, V Horáček, S Kamarádová

Institute for Clinical and Experimental Medicine, Prague, Czechoslovakia

The rate of ultrafiltration for a single glomerulus is equal to the product of the mean net driving pressure (P_{UF}, being the difference between the mean glomerular transcapillary hydraulic (P) and oncotic (π) pressure gradients) and the ultrafiltration coefficient (K_f). The availability of a strain of Wistar rats that possess glomeruli on the cortical surface which enable direct puncture of glomerular capillaries has made it possible to estimate the forces governing glomerular ultrafiltration [1]. In the dog, no glomeruli can be seen on the cortical surface. Therefore, a technique of removal of a very thin layer of the cortex has been developed enabling direct puncture of glomerular capillaries [2]. Estimation of single nephron glomerular filtration rate (from end-proximal fluid collection and ^{3}H-inulin concentration), single nephron filtration fraction (from ^{131}I albumin measurements in arterial and efferent arteriolar blood), and hydraulic pressures in glomerular and peritubular capillaries and the proximal tubule, made it possible to calculate all the forces determining the rate of ultrafiltration. In recent years, it has become apparent that this rate is greatly influenced by various vasoactive substances or hormones produced both inside and outside the kidney [see 3]. The purpose of this study is to describe the influence of some of these substances on glomerular haemodynamics in the dog kidney.

Methods

Beagles (11–15kg bodyweight) of both sexes were used. The dogs were fed a standard pellet diet and the amount was determined according to bodyweight. Usually, sodium intake was 4mmol · kg bodyweight^{-1} · day^{-1}. Food and water were withdrawn 24 hours prior to the experiment. Animals were anaesthetized with pentobarbital, femoral vessels and ureters were cannulated, the left kidney was exposed via flank incision and immobilized in a holder. A thin layer (0.5mm) of the outermost layer of the cortex was removed from an area of approximately 1 x 2 sq cm; the area exposed was continuously superfused with Tyrode solution at 38°C. In addition to the measurement already detailed (vide supra), ^{3}H-inulin or exogenous creatinine clearance was measured and renal blood flow estimated by electromagnetic flowmeter. A thin curved needle was introduced into the renal artery; 0.1ml · min^{-1} of isotonic saline or the experimental solution was infused via this needle. The methodology is described in detail elsewhere [2,4,5].

Influence of angiotensin II on glomerular haemodynamics

A major unresolved question is whether angiotensin II constricts the efferent or both the efferent and afferent arterioles. To study this, dogs were fed a diet containing 12mmol sodium · kg bodyweight^{-1} · day^{-1} for at least three weeks prior to the experiment [6]. One group of dogs had an intravenous infusion of a converting enzyme inhibitor, SQ 14,225, 15μg · kg bodyweight^{-1}; in Group 2 either indomethacin (1mg · kg bodyweight^{-1} · min^{-1}) or aspirin (5mg · kg bodyweight^{-1} · min^{-1}) was also infused over a five minute period. As the effect of both cyclo-oxygenase inhibitors was similar, the results are pooled and for convenience called the indomethacin group. In both groups, after stabilization angiotensin II was infused into the renal artery at a rate of 1ng · kg bodyweight^{-1} · min^{-1}. This infusion changed neither the mean blood pressure nor contralateral kidney function. A decrease in single nephron glomerular filtration rate and single nephron blood flow was observed in both groups; with cyclo-oxygenase inhibitors, the decreases were significantly higher than without them. It is clear from Figure 1 that angiotensin II infusion increased total arteriolar resistance (R_T which is calculated as the sum of afferent (R_A) and efferent (R_E) resistances) in both groups, the increase being steeper in the

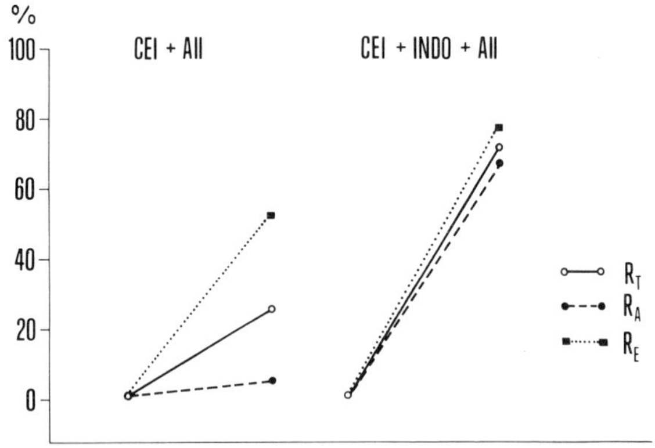

Figure 1. Percentage changes in renal arteriolar afferent (R_A), efferent (R_E) and total (R_T=R_A+R_E) resistances in dogs after intrarenal arterial infusion of 1ng · kg^{-1} · min^{-1} of angiotensin II during concomitant infusion of converting enzyme inhibitor (CEI) (SQ 14,225, 15μg · kg^{-1} · min^{-1} i.v.) – Group 1 (left), and CEI plus indomethacin (1mg · kg^{-1} · min–^{1} for 5 minutes) – Group 2 (right)

indomethacin group. Whereas in Group 1, the increase in R_T was caused almost entirely by an increase in R_E, with a very small, but still significant, increase in R_A, in the indomethacin group, the increase was due to an approximately equal increase in R_A and R_E. These results show that in the absence of blockage of prostanoid synthesis, intrarenal infusion of a very small amount of angiotensin II, in dogs with maximal suppression of endogenous angiotensin II formation, increased R_E preferentially, whereas this preference disappears in the presence of their blockage. These findings provide indirect evidence for attenuation by prostanoids of the normal constrictor activity of angiotensin II on afferent arterioles.

Although Schnerman et al [7] had postulated that some of the increase in R_A was due to a tubuloglomerular feedback mechanism this was recently excluded in experiments on non-filtering kidneys [8]. The mechanism by which prostanoids inhibit angiotensin II constriction of the afferent arteriole is unclear.

Rôle of leukotrienes

In the kidneys of rats and pigs, the most frequent effect of leukotrienes C_4 or D_4 is vasoconstriction [9–12]. In the dog, however, exogenous leukotrienes produce either only mild vasoconstriction [13] or no response [14], or even vasodilation [15,16]. Use of inhibitors of leukotriene synthesis, however, provide indirect evidence for a rôle of leukotrienes in control of renal circulation [17,18]. Receptors with a high affinity for LTC_4 have been found in rat glomeruli [19] and mesangial cells from rat glomeruli in culture contract after addition of leukotrienes; this contraction can be inhibited by a number of putative leukotriene antagonists [15]. We studied glomerular and whole kidney variables in beagles fed 4mmol sodium · kg bodyweight^{-1} · day^{-1}. Saralasin, phentolamine, 1-penicillamine-2-0-methyltyrosine-8-arginine-vasopressin (a V_1 receptor antagonist) and SCH 23390 (a DA_1 receptor antagonist) were infused into the renal artery, and indomethacin and aprotinin intravenously (Group 1). In Groups 2 and 3, two chemically different leukotriene antagonists, FPL 55712 and LY 171883, were infused into the renal artery during the fourth period of experiments.

In comparison to Group 1, there was an increase in total kidney (40% in Group 1 and 33% in Group 3) as well as single nephron glomerular blood flow (46% and 31%, respectively), accompanied by a decrease in total kidney (16% and 17%) as well as single nephron glomerular filtration rate (25% in both groups). The fall in total kidney filtration fraction amounted to 36% and 41%, respectively, and to 45% and 41%, respectively, in corresponding single nephron values (Figure 2). No changes in proximal tubular and peritubular capillary hydraulic pressures were observed; directly measured glomerular capillary pressure decreased by 10% and 12%, respectively. As shown in Figure 3, a decrease in R_T by 34% and 23%, respectively, was caused by a comparatively higher decrease in efferent (44% and 34%, respectively) than afferent (26% and 15%, respectively)

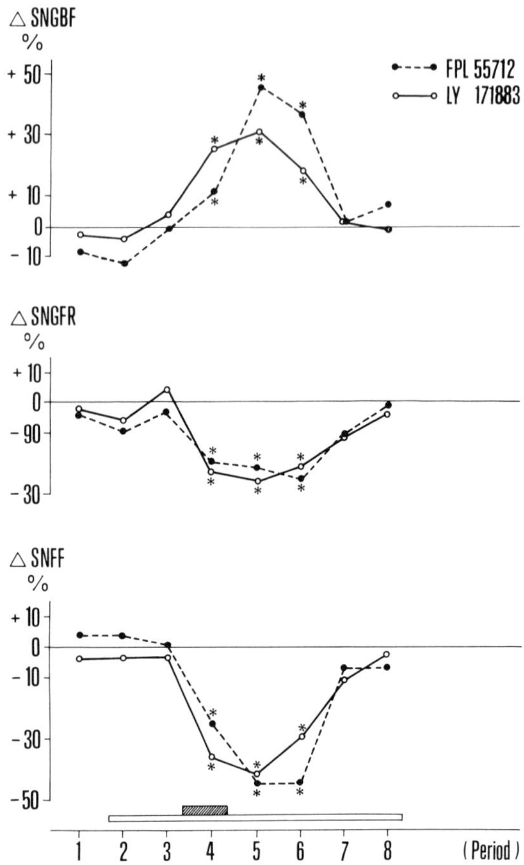

Figure 2. Percentage changes in single nephron glomerular blood flow (SNGBF), glomerular filtration rate (SNGFR) and filtration fraction (SNFF) in dogs infused with two putative leukotriene antagonists (FPL 55712 or LY 171883). The white bar represents the duration of infusion of Saralasin, phentomalamine, V_1 and DA_1 antagonists into the renal artery, and indomethacin and aprotinin intravenously, while the hatched bar is the duration of leukotriene antagonist infusion into the renal artery

arteriolar resistance values. No change in the filtration coefficient, K_f, was detected. Except for the effects on K_f, these results are a mirror image of the results of Badr et al [20] in rats infused with LTD_4 into the renal artery. If we assume that both leukotriene antagonists are specific for leukotriene receptors in the kidney, our data indicate some preferential efferent constriction due to the leukotriene in anaesthetized mildly surgically stressed dog. This constriction could be either a direct effect of leukotrienes or be mediated by some other vasoconstrictor substance. Such a hypothetical mediator could not be angiotensin II, a catecholamine, vasopressin or a thromboxane.

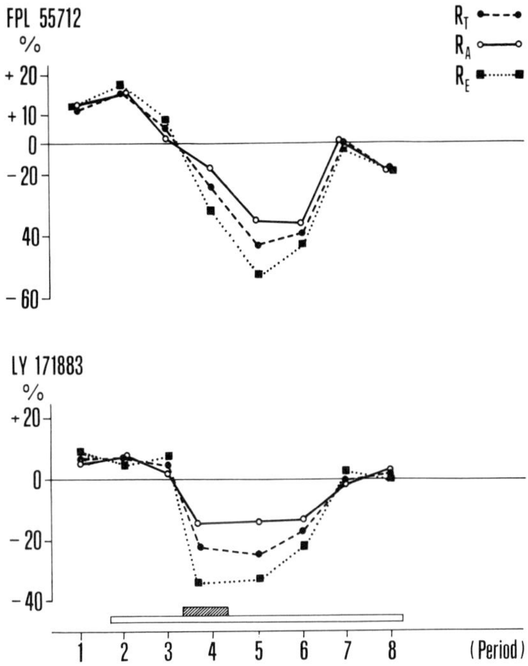

Figure 3. Percentage changes in renal arteriolar resistances after infusion of two putative leukotriene antagonists, FPL 55712 and LY 171883. For explanation see legends to Figures 1 and 2

A possible rôle of thromboxanes

In recent years, evidence has accumulated for a vasoconstrictor action of thromboxanes on the kidney in various pathological states [21–24]. Substantial evidence exists that thromboxanes are formed in the kidney [25,26]. However, the question whether they could play a rôle in glomerular haemodynamics in a relatively 'normal' situation, as in our model of anaesthetized mildly surgically stressed dog, has not been answered. Therefore, in experiments similar to those with leukotrienes, except that no infusion of indomethacin was given, we infused a highly selective thromboxane receptor antagonist, SQ 27427 [27] into the renal artery. As shown in Figures 4 and 5, the results are very similar to those obtained with both leukotriene antagonists: an increase in renal blood flow (and single nephron glomerular blood flow) accompanied by a decrease in glomerular filtration rate (and single nephron glomerular filtration rate). The decrease in R_E was greater than that in R_A. In other dogs, LY 171883 (the leukotriene antagonist) was added to the intrarenal arterial infusion of Saralasin, phentolamine, 1-penicillamine-2-0-methyltyrosine-8-arginine vasopressin and SCH 23390; infusing SQ 27427 in these dogs led to practically identical results as in the dogs without LY 171883. Thus, thromboxanes seem to constrict the

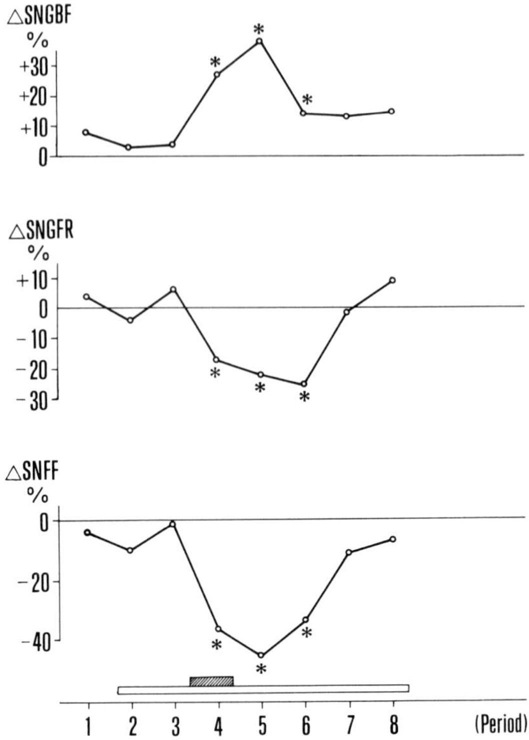

Figure 4. Percentage changes in SNGBF, SNGFR and SNFF in dogs after intrarenal infusion of a putative thromboxane antagonist, SQ 27427 (hatched bar). For explanation see legend to Figure 2

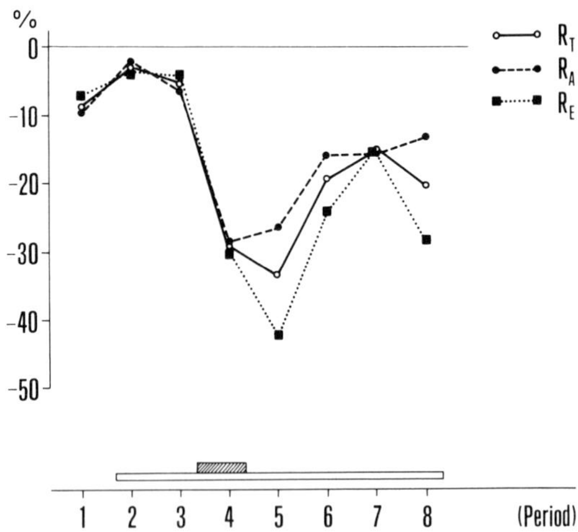

Figure 5. Percentage changes in renal arteriolar resistances after infusion of a putative thromboxane antagonist, SQ 27427 (hatched bar) into the renal artery. For explanation see legends to Figures 1 and 2

efferent arteriole preferentially; this constriction is not mediated by angiotensin II, catecholamines, vasopressin or leukotrienes.

Influence of pharmacological doses of atrial natriuretic peptide

In the dog, atrial natriuretic peptide infused into the renal artery consistently increases renal blood flow, glomerular filtration rate, and sodium and water excretion when administered at hundreds of ng · kg bodyweight^{-1} · min^{-1}; if a lower amount (tens of nanograms) is infused, no change in renal haemodynamics is observed while natriuresis and diuresis are still present [28–30]. To study changes in single nephron haemodynamics, we infused dogs treated as described above with 0.3μg · kg bodyweight^{-1} · min^{-1} of atrial natriuretic peptide into the renal artery. More than a 1000% increase in sodium excretion and an approximately 600% increase in water excretion were observed. Total kidney renal blood flow increased by 27%, glomerular filtration rate by 52% leading to an increase in filtration fraction by 23%. The corresponding single nephron values were 14%, 26%, and 12% respectively, all significantly lower than total kidney values indicating a redistribution of blood flow within the kidney towards the deeper cortical areas. As shown in Figure 6, R_T fell slightly after atrial natriuretic peptide infusion. Whereas R_A fell steeply, R_E was increased. These data could be interpreted as afferent dilation plus efferent constriction, a highly improbable dual effect for a single hormone. Since atrial natriuretic peptide is commonly described as a vasodilator [31,32], the efferent constriction is probably mediated by some other substances which, however, could not be angiotensin II, catecholamine, vasopressin, or thromboxane. These unexpected results are in accord with similar findings of Dunn et al [32] in rats and Marin-Grez et al [33] in

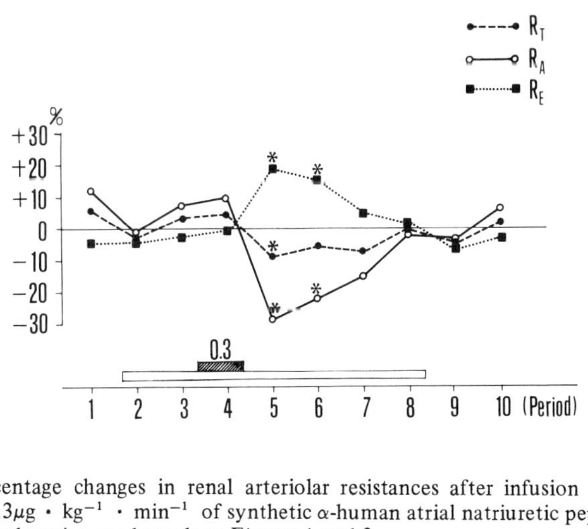

Figure 6. Percentage changes in renal arteriolar resistances after infusion into the renal artery of 0.3μg · kg^{-1} · min^{-1} of synthetic α-human atrial natriuretic peptide (hatched bar). For explanation see legends to Figures 1 and 2

hydronephrotic rat kidney preparation. A much lower dose, 0.03μg · kg body-weight^{-1} · min^{-1}, evoked significant diuresis and natriuresis without any change in renal haemodynamics. Both doses used are highly unphysiological and the significance of the changes is not clear.

In summary, angiotensin II, leukotrienes, thromboxane and even atrial natriuretic peptide at a high dose, all constrict the efferent arteriole preferentially or exclusively. The antagonists of leukotrienes and thromboxane are regarded as highly specific and suggest a direct action of leukotrienes and thromboxane on the arteriole; it is not certain whether there is a common mechanism leading to preferential efferent constriction.

References

1 Baylis C, Brenner BM. The physiologic determinants of glomerular ultrafiltration. *Rev Physiol Biochem Pharmacol 1978; 80:* 1–46

2 Heller U, Horáček V. Comparison of directly measured and calculated glomerular capillary pressure in the dog kidney at varying perfusion pressure. *Pfluegers Arch 1980; 385:* 253–258

3 Dworkin LD, Ichikawa I, Brenner BM. Hormonal modulation of glomerular function. *Am J Physiol 1983; 244:* F95–F105

4 Heller J, Horáček V. Autoregulation of superficial nephron function in the allo-perfused dog kidney. *Pfluegers Arch 1979; 382:* 99–104

5 Heller J, Horáček V. Kidney function during decreased perfusion pressure due to aortic clamping and hemorrhagic hypotension: a single nephron study in dog kidney. *Renal Physiol 1984; 7:* 90–101

6 Heller J, Horáček V. Angiotensin II: preferential efferent constriction? *Renal Physiol 1986; 9:* 357–365

7 Schnermann J, Briggs JP, Weber PC. Tubuloglomerular feedback, prostaglandins, and angiotensin in the autoregulation of glomerular filtration rate. *Kidney Int 1984; 25:* 53–64

8 Olsen M, Hall JE, Montani J-P et al. Interaction between renal prostaglandins and angiotensin II in controlling glomerular filtration in the dog. *Clin Sci 1987; 72:* 429–436

9 Allen D, Wassermann M, Gellai M. Dissociation of renal blood flow and cardiac output with acute leukotriene administration. *Kidney Int 1986; 29:* 379A

10 Eimerl J, Sirén A-L, Feuerstein G. Systemic and regional hemodynamic effects of leukotrienes D_4 and E_4 in the conscious rat. *Am J Physiol 1986; 251:* H700–H709

11 Badr KF, Baylis C, Pfeffer JM et al. Renal and systemic hemodynamic responses to intravenous infusion of leukotriene C_4 in the rat. *Circ Res 1984; 54:* 492–499

12 Piper PJ, Stanton AWB, McLeod LJ. The actions of leukotrienes C_4 and D_4 in the porcine renal vascular bed. *Prostaglandins 1985; 29:* 61–73

13 Plante GE, Hebert RL, Maheux P et al. Leukotriene D_4 affects the renal transport of ions. In Braquet P et al, eds. *Prostaglandins and Membrane Ion Transport.* New York: Raven Press. 1984: 271–280

14 Chapnick BM. Divergent influences of leukotrienes C_4, D_4, and E_4 on mesenteric and renal blood flow. *Am J Physiol 1984; 246:* H518–H524

15 Simonson MS, Dunn MJ. Leukotriene C_4 and D_4 contract rat glomerular mesangial cells. *Kidney Int 1986; 30:* 524–531

16 Secrest JR, Olsen EJ, Chapnick BM. Leukotriene D_4 relaxes canine renal and superior mesenteric arteries. *Circ Res 1985; 57:* 323–329

17 Hartupee D, Passmore J. Role of leukotrienes in the control of urine osmolality. *Kidney Int 1986; 29:* 335A

18 Tannenbaum J, Womack A, Toto R. Evidence that non-cyclo-oxygenase derived arachidonic acid (AA) metabolites alter renal hemodynamics and sodium reabsorption in intact dogs. *Kidney Int 1985; 27:* 299A

19 Ballermann BJ, Lewis RA, Corey EJ et al. Identification and characterization of leukotriene C_4 receptors in isolated rat renal glomeruli. *Circ Res 1985; 56:* 324–330
20 Badr KF, Brenner BM, Wassermann M et al. Evidence for local glomerular actions of leukotriene D_4 (LTD_4). *Kidney Int 1986; 29:* 328A
21 Purkerson ML, Joist JH, Yates J et al. Inhibition of thromboxane-synthesis ameliorates the progressive kidney disease of rats with subtotal renal ablation. *Proc Natl Acad Sci USA 1985; 82:* 193–197
22 Saneri GGN, Masotti G, Castellani S. Pathophysiology of renal prostaglandins. *Contr Nephrol 1985; 49:* 156–172
23 Lefer AM. Eicosanoids as mediators of ischemia and shock. *Fed Proc 1985; 44:* 275–280
24 Ichikawa I, Purkerson M, Yates J et al. High protein diet augments renal vasoconstriction induced by bilateral ureteral obstruction (BUO). *Kidney Int 1984; 25:* 231A
25 FitzGerald GA, Oates JA. Selective and nonselective inhibition of thromboxane formation. *Clin Pharmacol Therap 1984; 35:* 633–640
26 Kawasaki A, Needleman P. Contribution of thromboxane to renal resistance changes in the isolated perfused hydronephrotic rabbit kidney. *Circ Res 1982; 50:* 486–490
27 Greenberg R, Steinbacher TE, Harris DN et al. Thromboxane receptor antagonist properties of SQ 27,427 in the anesthetized guina pig. *Europ J Pharmacol 1984; 103:* 19–24
28 Yukimura T, Ito K, Takenega T. Renal effects of a synthetic α-human atrial natriuretic polypeptide (α-hANP) in anesthetized dogs. *Europ J Pharmacol 1984; 103:* 363–366
29 Salazar FJ, Fiksen-Olsen MJ, Opgenorth TJ et al. Renal effects of ANP without changes in glomerular filtration rate and blood pressure. *Am J Physiol 1986; 251:* F532–F536
30 Burnett JC Jr, Opgenorth TJ, Granger JP. The renal action of atrial natriuretic peptide during control of glomerular filtration. *Kidney Int 1986; 30:* 16–19
31 Oshima T, Currie MG, Geller DM et al. An atrial peptide is a potent renal vasodilator substance. *Circ Res 1984; 54:* 612–616
32 Dunn BR, Ichikawa I, Pfeffer JM et al. Renal and systemic hemodynamic effects of synthetic atrial natriuretic peptide in the anesthetized rat. *Circ Res 1986; 59:* 237–246
33 Marin-Grez M, Fleming JT, Steinhausen M. Atrial natriuretic peptide causes preglomerular vasodilatation and post-glomerular vasoconstriction in rat kidney. *Nature 1986; 324:* 473–476

EICOSANOIDS AND THE CONTROL OF RENAL FUNCTION

THE ROLE OF LIPOXYGENASE PRODUCTS OF ARACHIDONATE METABOLISM IN THE CONTROL OF GLOMERULAR FUNCTIONS

R Ardaillou, L Baud, Dominique Chansel, Josée Sraer

INSERM 64, Hôpital Tenon, Paris, France

The lipoxygenase products of arachidonic acid (C20:4) were initially identified in inflammatory cells [1] and their main activities were related to the inflammatory process [2]. In fact, cells other than monocyte-macrophages, platelets and polymorphonuclear leucocytes can synthesize lipoxygenase products, and functions in addition to chemotaxis, chemokinesis and alteration of vascular permeability have been attributed to them [3]. Moreover, following the initial description of the hydroperoxy- and hydroxy-derivatives, new metabolites such as leukotrienes and lipoxins were described and endowed with specific functions. The glomerulus is a capillary network submitted to a local regulation by autacoids. In addition, immunological glomerular injury results in the infiltration of glomeruli by bone marrow-derived cells. It has been repeatedly demonstrated that prostaglandins and thromboxane which represent the metabolites of C20:4 through the cyclo-oxygenase pathway play a major rôle in the control of the glomerular microcirculation and in glomerular injury in experimental glomerulonephritis [4]. Thus it was logical to investigate the influence on the glomerular functions of the products of lipoxygenase activity which is the second main pathway of conversion of C20:4.

Synthesis of lipoxygenase products by glomeruli in health and diseases

Murine and human glomeruli convert arachidonic acid (C20:4) through the cyclo-oxygenase and the lipoxygenase pathways. This has been demonstrated using freshly isolated glomeruli and cultured glomerular cells. We [5] and others [6,7] have identified hydroxyeicosatetraenoic acids (HETE) in the glomeruli. Rat glomeruli produce essentially 12-HETE [5–7]. They can also synthesize 15-HETE but only in the presence of high concentrations of substrate. At low C20:4 concentrations, human glomeruli synthesize equivalent amounts of 12- and 15-HETE, but in smaller quantities than rat glomeruli. Cultured epithelial [6] and mesangial [8] glomerular cells also synthesize 12-HETE. These results demonstrate that the production of HETEs by isolated glomeruli is due essentially to the resident glomerular cells and not to platelets or leucocytes entrapped in the glomerular capillaries. Another argument in favour of this assumption derives from the study of experimental glomerulonephritis. Lianos et al [7] have reported that 12-HETE synthesis was markedly enhanced in glomeruli from rats with nephrotoxic serum nephritis. It is highly likely that 12-HETE originates in this model from glomerular cells and not from the invading blood cells since polymorphonuclear leucocytes synthesize essentially 15- and 5-HETE which were not found. 12-HETE could be produced by the platelets present in the microthrombi but platelet depletion induced by antiplatelet antiserum administration did not modify glomerular 12-HETE synthesis. Because of these results, it is now largely accepted that the glomerular cells possess 12- and 15-lipoxygenase activities.

In contrast, the problem of whether glomeruli also have 5-lipoxygenase activity and can synthesize leukotrienes has not yet been resolved. We [5] and others [6] did not detect any substantial amount of radiolabelled 5-HETE after incubation of normal intact glomeruli with radiolabelled C20:4. However, in further studies an increased synthesis of leukotrienes was demonstrated in experimental models of glomerulonephritis. Lianos [9] studied rats with nephrotoxic serum glomerulonephritis. In this model, LTB_4 but not LTC_4 synthesis was transiently enhanced in the glomeruli at the early stage of the disease. Lianos and Noble [10] also reported similar transient LTB_4 synthesis during active and passive Heymann nephritis. In contrast with these results, Rahman et al [11] were unable to measure detectable levels of LTB_4 in glomeruli from control rats and rats with nephrotoxic serum glomerulonephritis, but the animals were studied at later periods of the disease. LTB_4 production by glomeruli was increased in another model of glomerulonephritis obtained by administration of cationic bovine gammaglobulin. This form of glomerulonephritis represents a model of membranous nephropathy devoid of cellular infiltration. Moreover, glomerular synthesis of LTB_4 was also enhanced in irradiated rats with a more than 85% reduction in polymorphonuclear leucocyte count. Therefore, it is likely that LTB_4 originated from the glomerular cells themselves. These studies demonstrate that rat glomeruli can synthesize LTB_4 upon appropriate stimulation and thus that they possess the two enzymes necessary to convert C20:4 into LTB_4, 5-lipoxygenase and hydrolase. More recently [12] using two different systems of radiometric reverse high performance liquid chromatography (HPLC) we could detect small amounts of sulphidopeptide leukotrienes in homogenized rat glomeruli incubated with $[^{14}C]$C20:4 in the presence of reduced glutathione. In fact, the amounts produced were negligible when compared with those of 12- and 15-HETE. A small but distinct peak of 5-HETE was also observed (Figure 1). We confirmed its presence using straight phase HPLC with a system allowing clear separation of 12-, 15- and 5-HETEs. Another major problem is the difficulty of separating the leukotrienes from their biologically

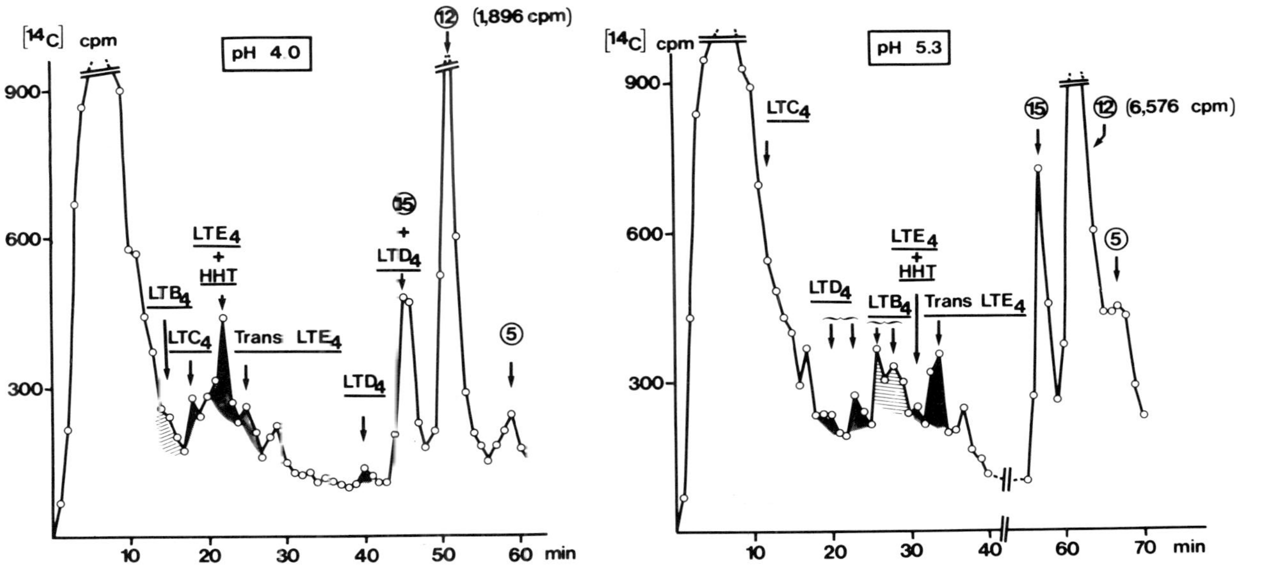

Figure 1. Reverse phase high performance liquid chromatography of glomeruli incubated with [^{14}C]C20:4. Two eluent systems were used: 1-methanol : H_2O : acetic acid, 58 : 32 : 0.08 (v/v), pH 4 (left); 2-methanol : H_2O : acetic acid, 65 : 35:0.02 (v/v), pH 5.3 (right). The flow rate was 1.2ml/min in both systems. The retention times of authentic standards are indicated by arrows

inactive isomers. For example, the two main isomers of LTB_4, all-trans LTB_4 and 5S, 12S-HETE comigrate with LTB_4 in most systems of HPLC and cross-react with the anti-LTB_4 antibodies. The best method of identification would be gas chromatography-mass spectrometry associated with biological assay. Unfortunately, the synthetic rates of leukotrienes in the glomeruli are too low to permit such techniques to be utilized.

Metabolism of lipoxygenase products in glomeruli

We have examined the in vitro metabolism of exogenously added [^{3}H] leukotrienes to rat glomeruli. Homogenized as well as intact glomeruli converted LTC_4 into LTE_4 and, to a smaller extent, into LTD_4 [13]. In contrast there was no conversion of LTB_4 to its two main metabolites, 20-OH LTB_4 and 20-COOH LTB_4 (Figure 2). This indicates that rat glomeruli possess both enzymes necessary to metabolize LTC_4 into its further products, γglutamyl transpeptidase and dipeptidase, whereas they do not contain ω-hydroxylase. This is noteworthy because the metabolism of both classes of leukotrienes is basically different. The processing of LTC_4 into LTD_4 and LTE_4 by peptide cleavage is a bioconversion from one active mediator to another as LTD_4 possesses, in many respects, the same potency as LTC_4 and LTE_4, although generally less potent, does have agonist properties. In contrast, 20-OH LTB_4 and 20-COOH LTB_4 are devoid of any biological activity. Thus glomerular cells are not well equipped to protect themselves from the noxious effects of leukotrienes. Only local production of H_2O_2 by stimulated mesangial cells [8] or infiltrating polymorphonuclear leucocytes or macrophages, via production of hypochlorous acid in the presence of myeloperoxidase, could result in inactivation of sulphidopeptide leukotrienes after formation of sulphoxides.

Effects of the lipoxygenase products on the glomerular functions

The lipoxygenase products, regardless of their glomerular or extraglomerular origin, modify the glomerular functions in several aspects. They act on the glomerular microcirculation either directly or via their effect on the local synthesis of renin. They play a rôle in the glomerular inflammation process and, finally, they stimulate the proliferation of glomerular cells (Figure 3).

Lipoxygenase products and glomerular microcirculation

The effects of leukotrienes on the glomerular microcirculation have been studied both in vivo and in vitro. Badr et al [14] using micropuncture techniques have studied glomerular haemodynamics in Munich-Wistar rats after intravenous injection of LTD_4. Precautions (Saralasin administration, replacement of plasma volume loss, partial aortic constriction to maintain constancy of renal perfusion pressure) were taken to evaluate only the direct glomerular effects of LTD_4. Under these conditions, LTD_4 administration caused an increase of efferent but not afferent arteriolar resistance with consequent fall in glomerular plasma

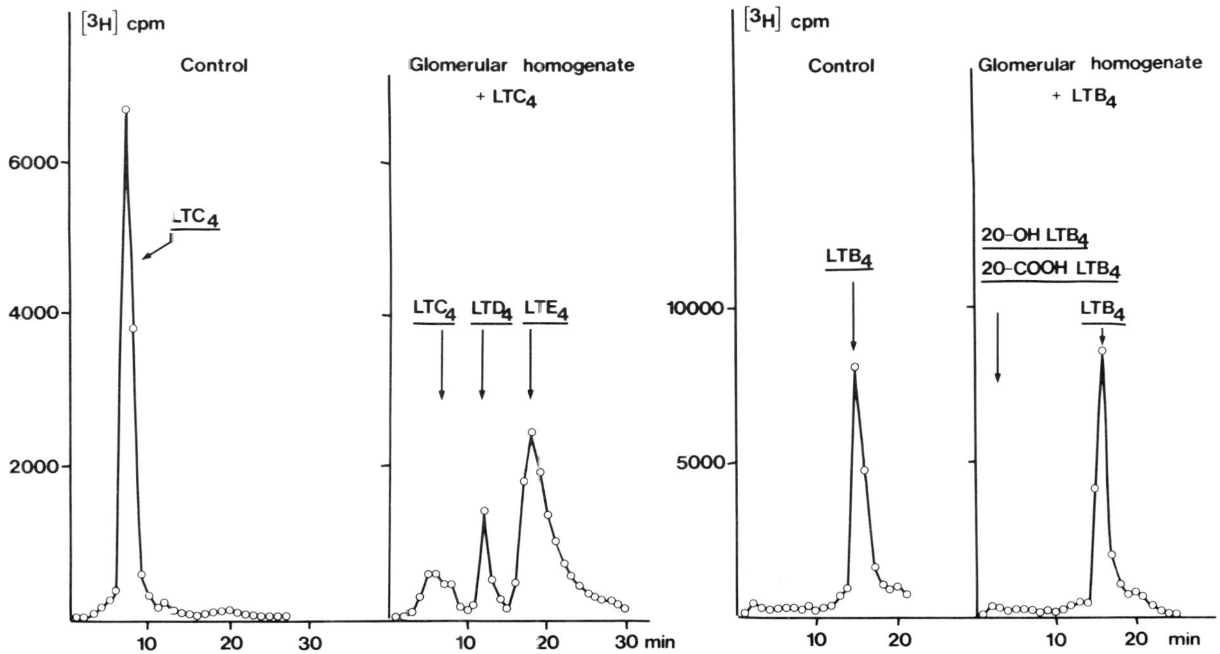

Figure 2. Reverse phase high performance liquid chromatography of [^{3}H] LTC_4 (left) and [^{3}H] LTB_4 (right) in buffer or in the presence of a glomerular homogenate. The retention times of authentic standards are indicated by arrows

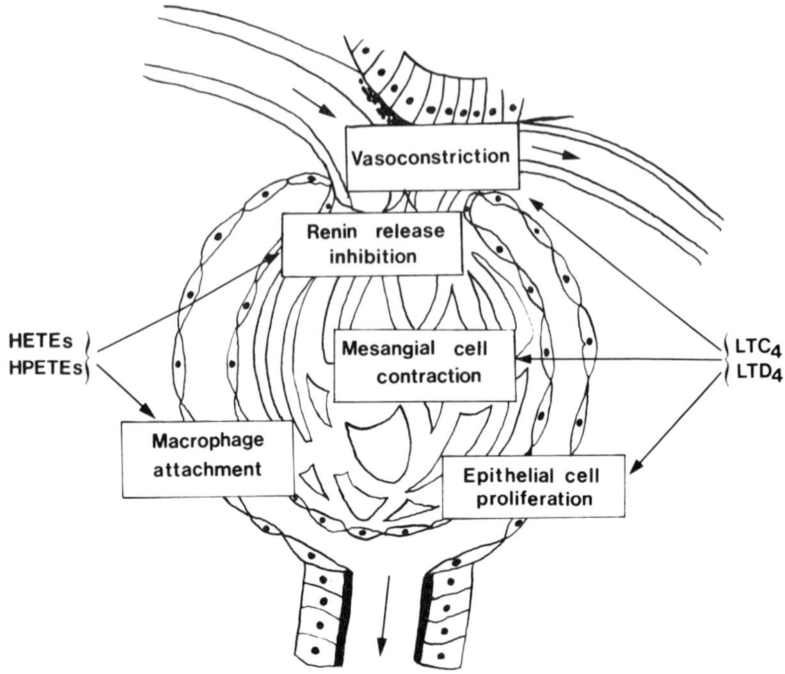

Figure 3. Effects of HETEs, HPETEs, and leukotrienes on glomerular functions

flow rate and rise in glomerular capillary pressure. Single nephron glomerular filtration rate fell due to combined reductions in glomerular plasma flow and glomerular ultrafiltration coefficient (Kf). These results demonstrate the local glomerular constrictor effect of LTD_4. In vitro studies suggested that the decrease of Kf could be attributed to contraction of glomerular mesangial cells. Barnett et al [15] reported that both LTC_4 and LTD_4 at $1\mu M$ produced a fall of 10–14% in the surface area of isolated glomeruli comparable to what has been observed previously with other vasoconstrictor agents such as angiotensin II (AII), arginine vasopressin (AVP) and platelet aggregation factor (PAF). The effects of both agonists was dose- and time-dependent. It is likely that the shape change represented cell contraction because rapid increases in wrinkling of the mobile surface of the mesangial cells grown on a flexible silicone rubber support were observed. Dunn and Simonson [16] obtained similar results. Using image analysis microscopy they measured the number of contracting mesangial cells and the cross-sectional areas of these cells in the presence of increasing doses ($1nM-1\mu M$) of LTC_4 and reported a dose-dependent decrease (16–23%) in the surface area of approximately 30% of the cells. Contraction started at 5 minutes and was maximum between 10–20 minutes. In contrast to AII, AVP and PAF, sulphidopeptide

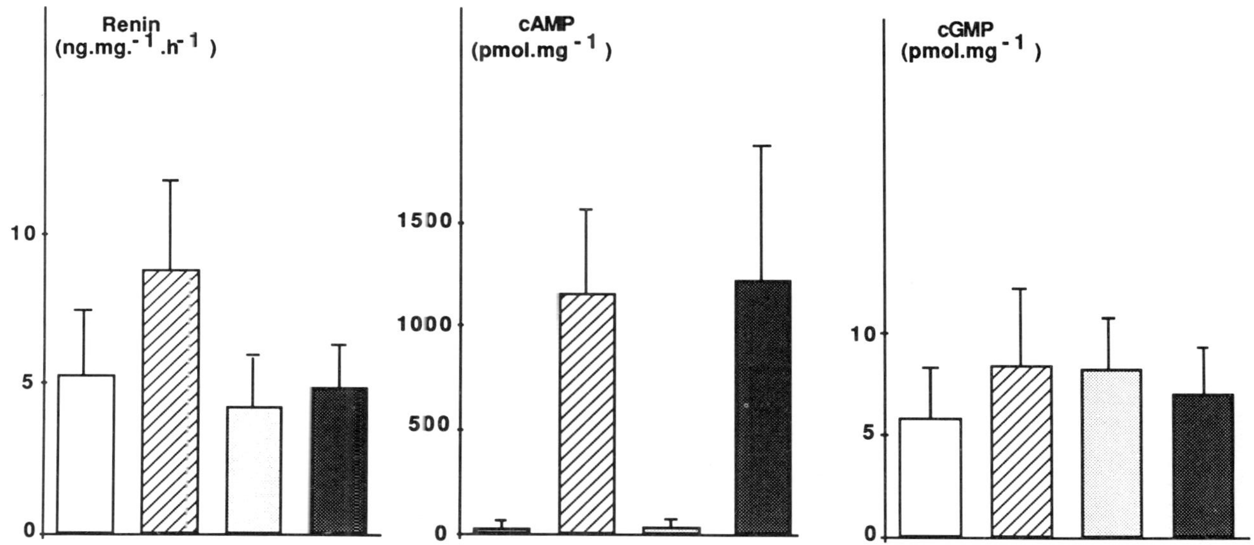

Figure 4. Renin (left), cyclic AMP (middle) and cyclic GMP (right) productions by human cultured mesangial cells under basal conditions (open bars), in the presence of 100μM PGE_2 (cross-hatched bars), 0.1μM 12-HETE (light bars) or the latter two in combination (dark bars). Renin activity was measured in the medium after trypsin activation and thus represented total renin. Means ± SEM of six individual experiments (different preparations) are given

leukotrienes did not stimulate PGE_2 production by rat mesangial cells [15]. It is thus probable that their cellular mode of action is different from those of the other vasoconstrictor agents. HPETEs have also been shown to induce a dose-dependent reduction of the surface area of human cultured visceral epithelial cells. 5- and 12-HPETE were active whereas their hydroxyderivatives, 5- and 12-HETE had no effect [17].

Lipoxygenase products may also act indirectly on the glomerular microcirculation via their effects on the local renin production. 12-HETE at 0.1μM did not modify basal renin production but it inhibited PGE_2-stimulated renin production in human mesangial cells. The mechanism of this effect has not been yet unravelled. 12-HETE did not change either basal and PGE_2-stimulated production of endogenous cyclic AMP. Like PGE_2, it had no effect on endogenous cyclic GMP (Figure 4). Therefore, it may be hypothesized that 12-HETE acts via a change in intracellular calcium which is considered, together with cyclic AMP and GMP, to be a second messenger of renin secretion.

Lipoxygenase products and glomerular inflammation

The role of lipoxygenase products in glomerular inflammation is suggested indirectly by experiments utilizing inhibitors of the lipoxygenase pathway. With such pharmacological agents we could demonstrate that lipoxygenase products interfered with the attachment of macrophages to glomeruli [18] and the oxidative burst induced in mesangial cells by phagocytosis of opsonized particles [8].

^{3}H-uridine-labelled rat macrophages have been incubated with rat glomeruli in an incubation medium devoid of plasma. Binding of macrophages to glomeruli increased with the amount of glomerular protein and the number of macrophages, temperature, time of incubation, and was a saturable process [18]. Macrophage adherence depended on glomerular lipoxygenase but not cyclo-oxygenase activity since preincubation of glomeruli with nordihydroguaiaretic acid (NDGA) or with two other inhibitors of the lipoxygenase pathway, eicosatetraynoic acid (ETYA) and phenidone was inhibitory whereas preincubation with indomethacin was ineffective. Therefore, enhanced glomerular lipoxygenase activity as reported in experimental glomerulonephritis [7] could represent a novel stimulus for macrophage accumulation in glomeruli independent of the plasma components such as complement and fibrin. Furthermore, a lipid extract which was prepared from the incubation medium of the glomeruli and contained the oxygenated metabolites of C20:4 stimulated the production of prostanoids (TXB_2, 6-keto $PGF_{1\alpha}$ and PGD_2) and 12-HETE by macrophages. The factor responsible for this effect is not C20:4 which was excluded from the extract but probably a lipoxygenase product since stimulation of macrophages by glomeruli was blunted by pretreatment of glomeruli with NDGA but not indomethacin. 12-HETE which is the main product of the lipoxygenase pathway synthesized in the glomeruli and which has also been shown to stimulate leukotriene synthesis in polymorphonuclear leucocytes [19]. In favour of this hypothesis, is the fact that authentic 12-HPETE, at a concentration in the range of what is produced by isolated glomeruli under basal conditions, stimulated prostaglandin synthesis in macrophages. 15-HPETE was also stimulatory whereas the corresponding hydroxy derivatives were inactive. We also observed that the lipid extract prepared from the macrophage-conditioned medium inhibited the production of 12-HETE by the glomeruli [20]. Taken together, these results suggest the following hypothesis: lipoxygenase products of glomerular origin influence adhesion of monocyte-macrophages to glomeruli. In parallel, they stimulate prostaglandin synthesis by macrophages. This increased production of prostaglandins may, in turn, inhibit the synthesis of 12-HPETE by glomeruli and thus limit adherence of macrophages.

Lipoxygenase products play also a rôle in the biochemical events associated with the phagocytosis of serum-treated zymosan (STZ) by cultured rat mesangial cells [8]. Under these conditions, the cells exhibited an oxidative burst with increased synthesis of superoxide anion ($O_2^{\bar{}}$) and hydrogen peroxide (H_2O_2). Incubation with STZ markedly stimulated the release of C20:4 from its phospholipid stores and its transformation into 12-HETE. Two lipoxygenase inhibitors, ETYA and phenidone, inhibited STZ-stimulated H_2O_2 production without modifying the phagocytic process as shown by the absence of any effect on the uptake of ^{125}I-STZ by the mesangial cells. In contrast, indomethacin did not produce any effect [8] and exogenous PGE_2 decreased H_2O_2 production by phagocytosing mesangial cells in a concentration-dependent manner [21]. Taken together, these results demonstrate opposing effects of cyclo-oxygenase and of the lipoxygenase products on the oxidative burst associated with phagocytosis in the mesangial cells.

Lipoxygenase products and proliferation of the glomerular cells

Sulphidopeptide leukotrienes promote glomerular cell proliferation. Dose-dependent (1–100nM) stimulation of [^{3}H] thymidine incorporation, an index of cell proliferation was observed in cultured human glomerular epithelial cells incubated with LTC_4 and LTD_4, but not with LTB_4. The response was 248% and 172% of control values at 100nM LTC_4 and LTD_4 respectively and the effect of sulphidopeptide leukotrienes was abolished by FPL 55712 [22]. LTC_4 and LTD_4 increased in parallel the cell number which confirmed that thymidine incorporation reflected increased cell proliferation. This biological effect of sulphidopeptide leukotrienes could be related to the presence of high affinity binding sites for LTC_4 on human glomerular epithelial cells [22]. [^{3}H] LTC_4 bound rapidly at 8°C to these cells. There was a plateau after 40 minutes' incubation. Maximum specific binding was 70–90% of total binding and was totally reversible with addition of an excess of unlabelled LTC_4. The equilibrium dissociation constant was 220nM. LTD_4 and LTE_4 also displaced [^{3}H] LTC_4 from its receptors with ED_{50} values that were two orders of magnitude higher than for LTC_4. In this study, as in that of Ballermann et al [23] who characterized LTC_4 receptors in isolated rat renal glomeruli, specific binding could be demonstrated only at low temperature (4–8°C) and in the presence of inhibitors of γ-glutamyltranspeptidase activity such as the L-serine borate complex. This confirms that the enzymes metabolizing LTC_4 are very active in the glomeruli. LTC_4 stimulated also the proliferation of rat mesangial cells [16]. Thus, LTC_4 in addition to being a vasoactive agent for glomerular mesangial cells is also a mitogen as demonstrated for epidermal growth factor and platelet-derived growth factor which exhibit both properties [24,25].

We tried in further experiments with cultured human fibroblasts to analyse the mechanism of action of LTC_4 on cell proliferation [26]. LTC_4-induced cell growth was observed only when PGE_2 synthesis was blocked by indomethacin. However, LTC_4 modified neither [^{3}H] C20:4 release from prelabelled fibroblasts nor PGE_2 production by fibroblasts. These results suggest that the basal production of PGE_2 by fibroblasts was sufficient to inhibit LTC_4-induced DNA synthesis in these cells. Thus, the initiation and development of the fibrotic process in the different tissues could depend in part on the balance between prostaglandin and leukotriene production.

Conclusions

Lipoxygenase products are formed in the glomeruli both by the resident glomerular cells and the invading blood cells, and both types of cells cooperate in the metabolism of C20:4. The local synthesis of lipoxygenase products is enhanced in several forms of glomerulonephritis but a precise link between this event and proteinuria has not yet been established. Specific inhibitors of synthesis and antagonists at the receptor or post-receptor level which could be used both in vitro and in vivo will represent essential tools to precisely further characterize the rôle of the lipoxygenase products on the glomerular functions in health and disease.

References

1 Borgeat P, Hamberg M, Samuelsson B. Transformation of arachidonic acid and homolinolenic acid by rabbit polymorphonuclear leukocytes. *J Biol Chem 1976; 251:* 7816–7820

2 Goetzl J, Woods JM, Gorman RR. Stimulation of human eosinophil and neutrophil polymorphonuclear leukocyte chemotaxis and random migration by 12-L-hydroxy-5,8,10,14-eicosatetraenoic acid. *J Clin Invest 1977; 59:* 179–183

3 Ardaillou R, Baud L, Sraer J. Leukotrienes and other lipoxygenase products of arachidonic acid synthesized in the kidney. *Am J Med 1986; 81 (Suppl 2B):* 12–22

4 Schlondorff D, Ardaillou R. Prostaglandin and other arachidonic acid metabolites in the kidney. *Kidney Int 1986; 29:* 108–119

5 Sraer J, Rigaud M, Bens M et al. Metabolism of arachidonic acid via the lipoxygenase pathway in human and murine glomeruli. *J Biol Chem 1983; 258:* 4325–4330

6 Jim K, Hassid A, Sun F, Dunn MJ. Lipoxygenase activity in rat kidney glomeruli, glomerular epithelial cells and cortical tubules. *J Biol Chem 1982; 257:* 10294–10299

7 Lianos EA, Rahman MA, Dunn MJ. Glomerular arachidonate lipoxygenation in rat nephrotoxic serum nephritis. *J Clin Invest 1985; 76:* 1355–1359

8 Baud L, Hagege J, Sraer J et al. Reactive oxygen production by cultured rat glomerular mesangial cell during phagocytosis is associated with stimulation of lipoxygenase activity. *J Exp Med 1983; 158:* 1836–1852

9 Lianos EA. Leukotrienes (LT) synthesis in nephrotoxic serum nephritis (NSN): role of complement (C) and polymorphonuclear leukocytes (PMNL). *Clin Res 1986; 34:* 972A (Abstr)

10 Lianos EA, Noble B. Glomerular arachidonate 5-lipoxygenation in active (A) and passive (B) Heymann nephritis (HN). *Kidney Int 1987; 31:* 277 (Abstr)

11 Rahman MA, Nakazawa M, Emancipator SN, Dunn MJ. Increased leukotriene B_4 (LTB_4) synthesis in immune injured rat glomeruli. *Kidney Int 1986; 29:* 343 (Abstr)

12 Sraer J, Bens M, Ardaillou R, Sraer JD. Sulfidopeptide leukotriene biosynthesis and metabolism by rat glomeruli and papilla. *Kidney Int 1986; 29:* 346 (Abstr)

13 Sraer J, Bens M, Oudinet JP, Ardaillou R. Bioconversion of leukotriene C_4 by rat glomeruli and papilla. *Prostaglandins 1986; 31:* 909–921

14 Badr KF, Brenner BM, Wasserman M, Ichikawa I. Evidence for local glomerular actions of leukotriene D_4. *Kidney Int 1986; 29:* 328 (Abstr)

15 Barnett R, Goldwasser P, Scharschmidt LA, Schlondorff D. Effects of leukotrienes on isolated rat glomeruli and cultured mesangial cells. *Am J Physiol 1986; 250:* F838–F844

16 Simonson MS, Dunn MJ. Leukotriene C_4 and D_4 contract rat glomerular mesangial cells. *Kidney Int 1986; 30:* 524–531

17 Lacave R, Delarue F, Rondeau E, Sraer JD. 5- and 12-hydroperoxyeicosatetraenoic cids promote contraction of cultured glomerular visceral epithelial cell. *Kidney Int 1986; 27:* 339 (Abstr)

18 Baud L, Sraer J, Delarue F et al. Lipoxygenase products mediate the attachment of rat macrophages to glomeruli in vitro. *Kidney Int 1985; 27:* 855–863

19 Maclouf J, Fruteau de Laclos B, Borgeat P. Stimulation of leukotriene biosynthesis in human blood leukocytes by platelet-derived 12-hydroperoxy-icosatetraenoic acid. *Proc Natl Acad Sci (USA) 1982; 79:* 6042–6046

20 Sraer J, Baud L, Bens M et al. Glomeruli cooperate with macrophages in converting arachidonic acid to prostaglandins and hydroxyeicosatetraenoic acids. *Prostaglandins Leukotrienes Med 1984; 13:* 67–74

21 Baud L, Perez J, Ardaillou R. Dexamethasone and hydrogen peroxide production by mesangial cells during phagocytosis. *Am J Physiol 1986; 250:* F596–F604

22 Baud L, Sraer J, Perez J et al. Leukotriene C_4 binds to human glomerular epithelial cells and promotes their proliferation in vitro. *J Clin Invest 1985; 76:* 374–377

23 Ballerman BJ, Lewis RA, Corey EJ et al. Identification and characterization of leukotriene C_4 receptors in isolated rat renal glomeruli. *Circ Res 1985; 56:* 324–330

24 Mene P, Abboud HE, Dubyak GR et al. Platelet-derived growth factor modulates contraction and cytosolic free calcium in cultured mesangial cells. *Kidney Int 1987; 31:* 175 (Abstr)

25 Tsivitse P, Abboud HE, Saunders C, Knauss TC. Effect of epidermal growth factor on cultured mesangial cells. *Kidney Int 1987; 31:* 184 (Abstr)

26 Baud L, Perez J, Denis M, Ardaillou R. Modulation of fibroblast proliferation by sulfidopeptide leukotrienes: effect of indomethacin. *J Immunol 1987; 138:* 1190–1195

ACTIONS AND SECOND MESSENGERS OF THROMBOXANE A_2 AND PROSTAGLANDINS IN CULTURED RAT MESANGIAL CELLS

P Menè, G R Dubyak, M J Dunn

Case Western Reserve University, Cleveland, Ohio, USA

Since the first report of contraction of cultured rat mesangial cells by the vasoactive peptides, angiotensin II and arginine vasopressin [1], considerable evidence has been provided that a variety of biologically active compounds, including platelet activating factor [2], histamine [3], leukotrienes [4,5], and platelet-derived growth factor [6] modify, in vitro, mesangial cell morphology and size. Hormonal actions on the mesangium may in turn affect renal haemodynamics via a reduction of filtration surface area or by altering glomerular perfusion patterns, with resulting changes of the ultrafiltration coefficient, K_f. Recent studies have also focused on agents that inhibit mesangial contractility, providing evidence that intracellular cyclic adenosine and guanosine monophosphates stimulated by isoproterenol [8] or dopamine [8] and atriopeptins or nitroprusside [9], respectively, modulate the resting tone of the cells as well as responses to angiotensin II.

Freshly isolated human and rat glomeruli undergo a rapid reduction of size upon stimulation with angiotensin II, possibly mediated by mesangial cell contraction [10]. Similar responses are elicited by the vasoconstrictor metabolite of arachidonic acid, thromboxane A_2 [10,11]. Since enhanced synthesis of thromboxane A_2, along with other prostaglandins, characterizes several inflammatory kidney diseases, including nephrotoxic serum nephritis [12], ureteral obstruction [13], and renal allograft rejection [14], and may contribute to impaired renal haemodynamics, we recently studied the effects of thromboxane A_2 on the morphology of cultured rat mesangial cells, reporting dose-dependent, specific contractile responses, inhibitable by selective thromboxane A_2-receptor antagonists [15]. Contraction was accompanied by rapid release of PGE_2 into the culture media. In the present work, we focused on the identification of a biochemical mechanism of action of thromboxane A_2, investigating its effects on a phospholipase C/intracellular Ca^{2+} signalling system that mediates the actions of thromboxane A_2 in platelets and other cells [16]. On the other hand, vasodilator prostaglandins such as PGE_2, synthesized by mesangial cells, and PGI_2, a product of endothelium, act via stimulation of cAMP [17] in other cell types. We therefore hypothesized that these agents would modulate mesangial contractile responses to thromboxane A_2, and sought to analyse their effects employing a dual approach: 1) blockade of PGE_2 synthesis by pretreatment of the cells with cyclo-oxygenase inhibitors, and 2) addition of exogenous PGE_2/PGI_2 while measuring intracellular cyclic adenosine monophosphate (cAMP) levels.

Methods

Cell culture
Mesangial cell lines isolated and grown as previously described [5,15] were employed in subcultures two through eight. Growth medium was PRMI 1640 supplemented with 17% fetal bovine serum, 100U/ml penicillin, 100μg/ml streptomycin, 5μg/ml insulin, 5μg/ml transferrin, 5ng/ml selenium. Free cytosolic Ca^{2+} ($[Ca^{2+}]^i$), PGE_2 synthesis and intracellular cAMP accumulation were measured in confluent monolayers. Contraction experiments were performed on non-confluent cells 36 hours after plating at low density on glass chamber-slides.

Morphometric analysis
Computer-assisted image analysis microscopy was employed as described elsewhere [5,15]. Phase contrast photomicrographs at 200X of sparsely seeded cells before and after stimulation with the agents to be tested were subjected to computer analysis for surface measurement after digitization on an electronic grid. Experimental medium was Krebs-Henseleit-Hepes buffer (KHH), pH 7.4, supplemented with 0.2% (w/v) fatty acid-free bovine serum albumin. All agents employed were prepared in KHH from the outset, when preincubation was required, or added after obtaining three basal pictures of the cells at five minute intervals.

Photomicrographs were then taken at 5, 10, 20, 30 and 40 minutes, and compared to the average cross-sectional area of each individual cell in the triplicate basal measurements. Cross-sectional area profiles for each cell studied throughout the entire incubation were averaged to obtain the time course of contraction in responding cells. Contraction was defined by a reduction of cross-sectional area >8% at any time after addition of the agonist, on the basis of preliminary evaluation of spontaneous fluctuations of cell size and instrumental error [15].

Chemicals
The PGH_2/thromboxane A_2 analogue U-46619 (9,11-dideoxy-9α,11α-epoxymethano-prostaglandin $F_{2\alpha}$) and PGE_2 were obtained from Upjohn (Kalamazoo Mi), The stable PGI_2 analogue Iloprost (carbacyclin) was a kind gift of Berlex,

Wayne NJ. All prostaglandins were tested for contractile activity and only U-46619 was found to be effective at concentrations between 1nM and 1μM. In further studies the cells were preincubated with increasing concentrations of PGE_2 and Iloprost, to examine a possible inhibitory effect on U-46619-induced contraction. Three structurally unrelated nonsteroidal anti-inflammatory drugs (NSAIDs), indomethacin, meclofenamate and piroxicam were used to inhibit mesangial cyclo-oxygenase activity. In all cases the NSAIDs were added 10 minutes prior to addition of U-46619. Cell viability upon exposure to each agent was evaluated by Trypan Blue exclusion (0.1%, diluted 1:1 in KHH buffer), at the end of 40 minute incubations with or without U-46619.

Measurement of $[Ca^{2+}]^i$

$[Ca^{2+}]^i$ was measured by spectrofluorometry in confluent monolayers of mesangial cells grown on Aclar plastic coverslips and loaded with the fluorescent Ca^{2+} probe fura-2 acetoxymethylester for 40 minutes at 37°C. Following a 20 minute wash in serum-free RPMI 1640 without fura-2, monolayers were kept on ice until used. Fluorescence was monitored continuously with a Johnson Biomedical Instrumentation spectrofluorometer [18] at 339nm excitation and 500nm emission wavelengths, after rewarming the monolayers in a quartz cuvette containing KHH at 37°C under continuous stirring. At the end of each experiment maximal fluorescence was determined by saturating the dye with a rapid elevation of $[Ca^{2+}]^i$ induced by the Ca^{2+} ionophore, ionomycin, 40μM. Ca^{2+} was then dissociated from fura-2 by chelating extracellular Ca^{2+} with 7.5mM ethyleneglycol-bis-(β-amino-ethyl ether)N,N'-tetraacetic acid (EGTA) at a slightly alkaline pH to obtain minimal fluorescence. $[Ca^{2+}]^i$ was then calculated by standard equations [19].

Radioimmunoassays (RIA)

Effective inhibition of mesangial PGE_2 production was evaluated at the end of 15 minute incubations by direct measurement in the medium, employing established RIA techniques, without prior extraction [20]. Results were corrected for the protein content of each well, measured by a modification of Lowry's technique [21], and expressed as percentage inhibition of basal and arachidonic acid-stimulated PGE_2 synthesis. Intracellular cAMP was measured by RIA after three minute incubations with PGE_2, U-46619 and Iloprost in the presence of 0.1mM isobutylmethylxanthine (IBMX) followed by extraction in 0.1N HCl for two hours at room temperature [22]. Results were noramlized for cell protein.

Results

Figure 1 shows representative morphometric experiments in which cultured mesangial cells were stimulated with U-46619 or its vehicle in the absence or presence of one of three structurally different NSAIDs at concentrations chosen

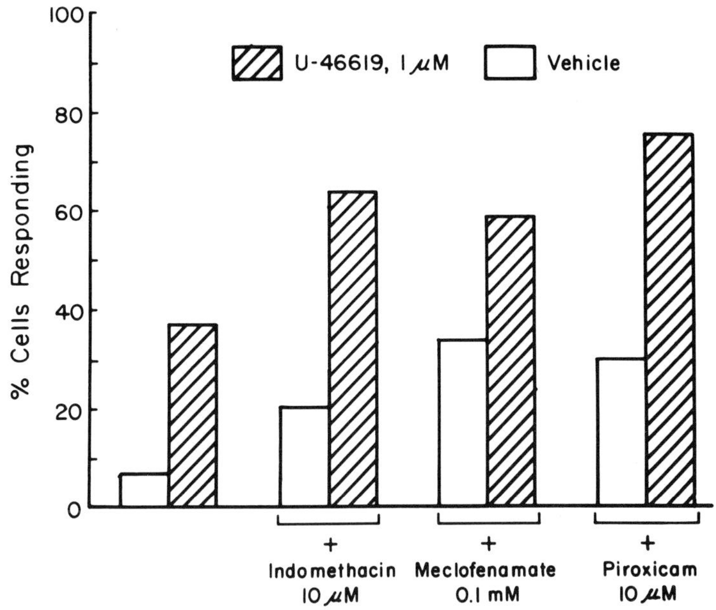

Figure 1. Enhancement of U-46619-induced contraction of cultured rat mesangial cells by NSAID. Open bars=control incubations without U-46619; hatched bars=U-46619 + vehicle (left) or each NSAID. Representative experiments, percent cells responding during 40 minute incubations

on the basis of effective prostaglandin synthesis inhibition (indomethacin 10μM, 98.0 and 95.0% of basal and stimualted PGE_2 synthesis respectively; meclofenamate 0.1mM, 96.7 and 88.4%). Control incubations with each NSAID resulted in marked increases of the percentage of cells spontaneously contracting, a phenomenon generally negligible during 40 minute observations in KHH without agonists, in which <7% of the cells contract. U-46619-induced contraction was similarly enhanced by all three NSAIDs, with 60 to 120% increments of the number of cells responding as compared to U-46619 alone. No signs of cell toxicity were evidenced by Trypan Blue vital staining (control incubations, 6.3% of the cells stained after one minute, U-46619 5.9%, indomethacin 5.1%, meclofenamate 7.9%, piroxicam 7.5%).

In the experiments presented in Figure 2, the addition of exogenous PGE_2 or Iloprost, 1μM, markedly inhibited responses to U-46619, an effect that was also mimicked by excess arachidonic acid, the substrate for cyclo-oxygenase that is rapidly metabolized to PGE_2 by rat mesangial cells. PGE_2 also reversed the enhancement of contraction by indomethacin, indicating that inhibition of PGE_2 synthesis rather than cell toxicity is indeed the major mechanism underlying this action of NSAIDs.

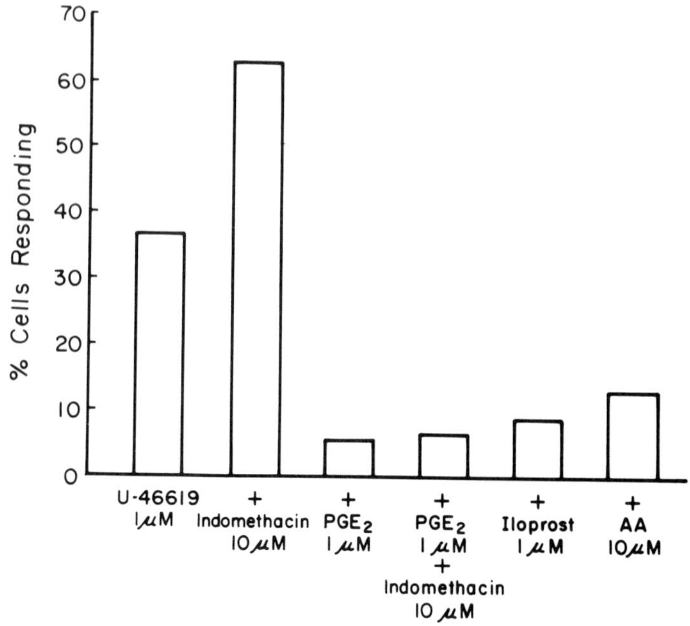

Figure 2. Inhibition of U-46619-induced contraction of cultured rat mesangial cells by PGE_2, Iloprost or arachidonic acid (AA), in the presence or absence of indomethacin. Representative experiments, percent cells responding during 40 minute incubations

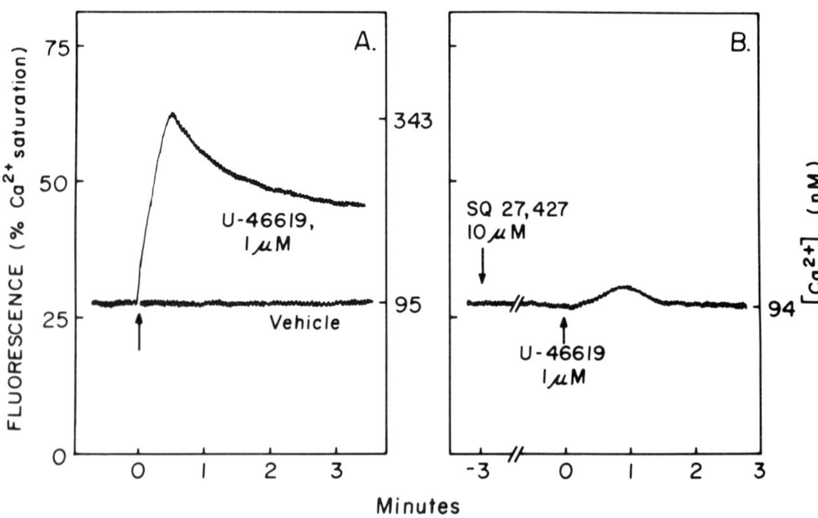

Figure 3. Stimulation of $[Ca^{2+}]i$ by U-46619 in monolayers of fura-2 loaded, cultured rat mesangial cells. Panel A=1µM U-46619 or vehicle added at time 0 (arrow); panel B=1µM U-46619 added after three minute preincubation with the thromboxane A_2-receptor antagonist SQ 27,427

In further studies, we aimed at the identification of an intracellular mechanism of action for vasoconstrictor and vasodilator prostanoids in mesangial cells. We therefore measured $[Ca^{2+}]^i$ and intracellular cAMP accumulation in response to U-46619, PGE_2 and Iloprost. Figure 3A shows representative tracings of $[Ca^{2+}]^i$ responses to U-46619 at the final concentrations employed in the contraction studies. The addition of U-46619 stimuated a rapid rise of $[Ca^{2+}]^i$, that immediately declined to sustained, steady-state levels maintained for >10 minutes. Basal $[Ca^{2+}]^i$ levels, found to be constantly regulated at approximately 100nM, were not affected by the vehicle of U-46619 (0.01% ethanol in KHH) or by addition of U-46619 after pretreatment of the cells for three minutes with the thromboxane A_2-receptor antagonist SQ 27,427, 10μM (Figure 3B). Angiotensin II, arginine vasopressin and $PGF_{2\alpha}$-induced $[Ca^{2+}]^i$ transients were not affected by SQ 27,427 (not shown), thus indicating specificity of responses to U-46619. While PGE_2 showed quantitatively minor and inconstant Ca^{2+} responses, Iloprost did not stimulate $[Ca^{2+}]^i$ at concentrations as high as 0.1mM. On the other hand, both PGE_2 and Iloprost stimulated dose-dependent, rapid elevations of intracellular cAMP (Figure 4). This effect was not shared by U-46619 (not shown), pointing to independent signal transduction mechanisms for eicosanoids with opposite functional effects on the glomerular mesangium.

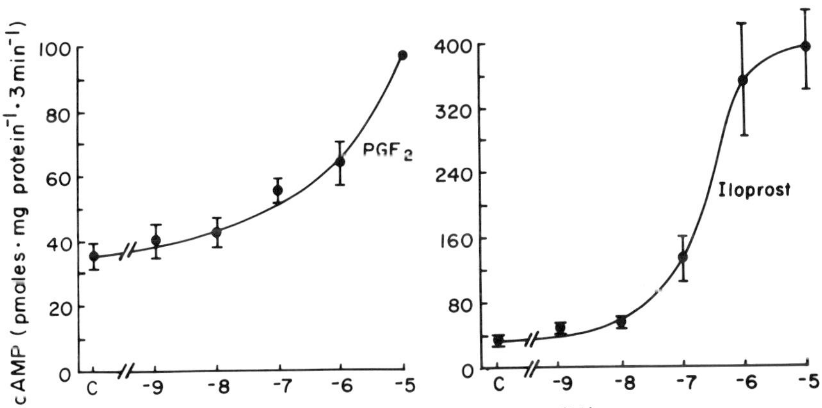

Figure 4. Stimulation of intracellular cAMP accumulation by PGE_2 and Iloprost in cultured rat mesangial cells. Three minute incubations in the presence of 0.1mM isobutylmethylxanthine

Discussion

Taken together with our earlier observations on the contractile effects of thromboxane A_2 and endoperoxide analogues [15], the present data support the hypothesis of a specific receptor for thromboxane A_2 in rat mesangial cells that is coupled to contractility via a phospholipase C/$[Ca^{2+}]^i$ signal transduction system. On the other hand, vasodilator prostanoids may inhibit contractility in response to various agonists, including thromboxane A_2, via stimulation of cAMP, with separate receptors both coupled to adenylate cyclase or, possibly, a common receptor with different affinity constants for PGE_2 and PGI_2. An interplay between vasoconstrictor and vasodilator prostanoids is further demonstrated by the rôle of endogenous prostaglandin synthesis, unmasked by inhibition of mesangial cyclo-oxygenase with NSAIDs. Our experimental design with three structurally unrelated drugs rules out possible cyclo-oxygenase-independent effects, such as an interference with adenylate cyclase and phosphodiesterase activities of Ca^{2+} gating at the cell membrane level. Piroxicam, in particular, was chosen because of published evidence that this newer, non-carboxylic NSAID lacks the effects on Ca^{2+} transport previously described for indomethacin and meclofenamate [23,24]. Inhibition of basal and stimulated PGE_2 synthesis was invariably associated with enhanced contractile responses, as well as perturbed resting morphology of the cells in control incubations. This points to a tonic, modulatory effect of endogenously produced PGE_2, that could subsequently bind to membrane receptors to control intracellular cAMP levels. Such autocrine function may also be supplemented by paracrine effects of prostaglandins released by other resident cells of the kidney glomerulus, i.e. endothelial and epithelial cells, whose major arachidonic acid metabolites are PGI_2 and PGE_2, respectively [25]. Bone marrow-derived cells can also contribute relevant amounts of vasoactive prostanoids, with effects on glomerular smooth muscle, including the mesangium [11,12]. It is of interest that mesangial arachidonic acid metabolism yields mostly 'relaxant' prostaglandins, which may counteract the effects of multiple inflammatory mediators locally released by blood-borne cells in glomerular inflammation, such as platelet activating factor, histamine, serotonin, and platelet-derived growth factor [26].

The presence of distinct intracellular mediators for prostaglandins in mesangial cells is consistent with earlier work in platelets [27] and smooth muscle [17], in which hormonal inhibition is generally mediated by an elevation of intracellular cAMP, whereas activation of cytoskeletal and contractile responses is controlled by a rise of $[Ca^{2+}]^i$ [16,28]. Some overlap between the two signal transduction pathways was observed in mesangial cells only for PGE_2, a relatively weak stimulus of both cAMP and $[Ca^{2+}]^i$; a functional prevalence of the vasodilator effects of cAMP is indicated by the lack of contractile potency at concentrations as high as $1 \mu M$. Based on the present and previous studies, it is tempting to speculate that stimulation of $[Ca^{2+}]^i$ by U-46619 is the result of receptor-mediated activation of phospholipase C with breakdown of membrane polyphosphoinositides and release of inositol (1,4,5)-triphosphate ($InsP_3$) and diacylglycerol [28,29]. The former is thought to release Ca^{2+} from intracellular stores; subsequent opening of surface divalent ion channels allows for enhanced entry and sustained resetting of basal $[Ca^{2+}]^i$. This represents a permissive condition for the activation of certain enzymes such as myosin light chain kinase, a key regulator of contractile protein interaction. Diacylglycerol, on the other hand, is the substrate for phospholipase A_2 and diglyceride lipases that are responsible for arachidonic acid release and enhanced prostaglandin production upon stimulation of this biochemical pathway. This may therefore be the source of elevated PGE_2, as described in our earlier study on thromboxane A_2/endoperoxide analogues [15]. While our data indicate a functional antagonism between $[Ca^{2+}]^i$ and cAMP at the level of integrated responses, that is the contraction/relaxation process, it remains to be established whether interactions exist at earlier steps in the generation of intracellular signals, e.g. receptor-enzyme coupling or biosynthesis of second messengers.

In conclusion, modulation of mesangial contractility by arachidonic acid metabolites is an experimental model for the study of their rôle in the control of glomerular microcirculation. An imbalance between constrictor stimuli and a prostaglandin-dependent negative feedback system could contribute to the increased vascular resistances and filtration dysfunction that follow administration of NSAID in chronic glomerular disease [30,31]. On the other hand, selective pharmacological manipulation of deranged arachidonic acid metabolism with enzyme inhibitors or receptor antagonists may provide substantial benefits in the management of acute and chronic glomerular disease.

Acknowledgments

Supported by National Heart, Lung and Blood Institute Grant HL-22563.

P Menè is the recipient of research fellowships from the American Heart Association, Northeast Ohio Affiliate, and from Consiglio Nazionale delle Ricerche of Italy.

The excellent technical assistance of Michael Simonson, Cheryl Subjoc, Edith Hanzmann and Raymond McDermott is gratefully acknowledged.

References

1 Ausiello DA, Kreisberg JI, Roy C, Karnovski MJ. Contraction of cultured rat glomerular cells of apparent mesangial origin after stimulation with angiotensin II and arginine vasopressin. *J Clin Invest 1980; 65:* 754–760

2 Schlondorff DJ, Satriano JA, Hagege J et al. Effect of platelet activating factor on prostaglandin E_2 synthesis, arachidonic acid release and contraction of cultured rat mesangial cells. *J Clin Invest 1984; 73:* 1227–1231

3 Sedor JR, Abboud HE. Histamine modulates contraction and cyclic nucleotides in cultured rat mesangial cells. *J Clin Invest 1985; 75:* 1679–1689

4 Barnett R, Goldwasser P, Scharschmidt LA, Schlondorff D. Effects of leukotrienes on isolated rat glomeruli and cultured mesangial cells. *Am J Physiol 1986; 250 (Renal fluid Electrolyte Physiol 19):* F838–F844

5 Simonson MS, Dunn MJ. Leukotriene C_4 and D_4 contract rat glomerular mesangial cells. *Kidney Int 1986; 30:* 524–531

6 Menè P, Abboud HE, Dubyak GR et al. Effects of platlet-derived growth factor on inositol phosphates, cytosolic calcium and contraction of mesangial cells. *Am J Physiol 1987; 253 (Renal Fluid Electrolyte Physiol 22):* in press

7 Kreisberg JI, Venkatachalam MA, Radnik RA, Patel PY. Role of myosin light-chain phosphorylation and microtubules in stressfiber morphology in cultured mesangial cells. *Am J Physiol 1985; 249 (Renal Fluid Electrolyte Physiol 18):* F227–F235

8 Barnett R, Singhal PC, Scharschmidt LA, Schlondorff D. Dopamine attenuates the contractile response to angiotensin II in isolated rat glomeruli and cultured mesangial cells. *Circ Res 1986; 59:* 529–533

9 Appel RG, Wang J, Simonson MS, Dunn MJ. A mechanism by which atrial natriuretic factor mediates its glomerular actions. *Am J Physiol 1986; 251 (Renal Fluid Electrolyte Physiol 20):* F1036–F1042

10 Scharschmidt LA, Douglas JG, Dunn MJ. Angiotensin II and eicosanoids in the control of glomerular size in rat and human. *Am J Physiol 1986; 250 (Renal Fluid Electrolyte Physiol 19):* F348–F356

11 Scharschmidt LA, Lianos E, Dunn MJ. Arachidonate metabolites and the control of renal function. *Fed Proc 1983; 42:* 3058–3063

12 Lianos EA, Andres GA, Dunn MJ. Glomerular prostaglandin and thromboxane synthesis in rat nephrotoxic serum nephritis. Effects on renal hemodynamics. *J Clin Invest 1983; 72:* 1439–1448

13 Morrison AR, Nishikawa K, Needleman P. Unmasking of thromboxane A_2 synthesis by ureter obstruction in the rabbit kidney. *Nature (Lond) 1977; 269:* 259–260

14 Coffman TM, Yarger WE, Klotman PE. Functional role of thromboxane production by acutely rejecting renal allografts in rats. *J Clin Invest 1985; 75:* 1242–1248

15 Menè P, Dunn MJ. Contractile effects of TxA_2 and endoperoxide analogues on cultured rat glomerular mesangial cells. *Am J Physiol 1986; 251 (Renal Fluid Electrolyte Physiol 20):* F1029–F1035

16 Brace LD, Venton DL, LeBreton GC. Thromboxane A_2/prostaglandin H_2 mobilizes calcium in human blood platelets. *Am J Physiol 1985; 249 (Heart Circ Physiol 18):* H1–H2

17 Oliva D, Noé A, Nicosia S et al. Prostacyclin-sensitive adenylate cyclase in cultured myocytes: differences between rabbit aorta and mesenteric artery. *Eur J Pharmacol 1984; 105:* 207–213

18 Dubyak GR, De Young MB. Intracellular Ca^{2+} mobilization activated by extracellular ATP in Ehrlich ascites tumor cells. *J Biol Chem 1985; 260:* 10653–10661

19 Grynkiewicz G, Poenie M, Tsien RY. A new generation of Ca^{2+} indicators with greatly improved fluorescence properties. *J Biol Chem 1985; 260:* 3440–3450

20 Scharschmidt LA, Dunn MJ. Prostaglandin synthesis by rat glomerular mesangial cells in culture. *J Clin Invest 1983; 71:* 1756–1764

21 Markwell MK, Haas SM, Bieber LL, Tolbert NE. A modification of the Lowry procedure to simplify protein determination in membrane and lipoprotein samples. *Anal Biochem 1978; 87:* 206–210

22 Brooker G, Harper JF, Terasaki WL, Moylan RD. Radioimmunoassay of cyclic AMP and cyclic GMP. In Brooker G, Greengard P, Robison GA, eds. *Advances in Cyclic Nucleotide Research, Vol 10.* New York: Raven Press. 1979: 1–33

23 Wiseman EH. Pharmacologic studies with a new class of nonsteroidal anti-inflammatory agents – the oxicams – with special reference to piroxicam (Feldene). *Am J Med 1982; 72:* 2–8

24 Burch RM, Wise WC, Halushka PV. Prostaglandin-independent inhibition of calcium transport by nonsteroidal anti-inflammatory drugs: differential effects of carboxylic acids and piroxicam. *J Pharmacol Exp Ther 1983; 227:* 84–91

25 Kreisberg JI, Karnovsky MJ, Levine L. Prostaglandin production by homogeneous cultures of rat glomerular epithelial and mesangial cells. *Kidney Int 1982; 22:* 355–359

26 Cameron JS. Platelets in glomerular disease. *Ann Rev Med 1984; 35:* 175–180

27 Gorman RR, Bunting S, Miller OV. Modulation of human platelet adenylate cyclase by prostacyclin (PGX). *Prostaglandins 1977; 13:* 377–388

28 Smith JB. Angiotensin-receptor signalling in cultured vascular smooth muscle cells. *Am J Physiol 1986; 250 (Renal Fluid Electrolyte Physiol 19):* F759–F769

29 Berridge MJ. Inositol trisphosphate and diacylglycerol as second messengers. *Biochem J 1984; 220:* 345–360

30 Dunn MJ. Nonsteroidal antiinflammatory drugs and renal function. *Ann Rev Med 1984; 35:* 411–428

31 Ciabattoni G, Cinotti GA, Pierucci A et al. Effects of sulindac and ibuprofen in patients with chronic glomerular disease. Evidence for the dependence of renal function on prostacyclin. *N Engl J Med 1984; 310:* 279–283

ATRIAL NATRIURETIC PEPTIDE AND OTHER NATRIURETIC SUBSTANCES

ATRIAL NATRIURETIC PEPTIDE

A J de Bold, Mercedes L de Bold, Martha M Ruben de Campione

Heart Institute Research Centre, Ottawa Civic Hospital, Ottawa, Ontario, Canada

Introduction

Atrial natriuretic peptide is a group of peptides initially discovered in the atria of rat hearts. These peptides interact in a number of ways with mechanisms involved in the control of blood pressure and volume, and so play a rôle in homeostasis. In rat atrial tissue, the cardiocytes have features associated with both contractile and secretory cells (Figure 1). The latter elements include the specific atrial granules. These granules possess morphological and cytochemical characteristics usually associated with granules which are known to store polypeptide hormones [1]. It is in these granules that atrial natriuretic peptide is stored.

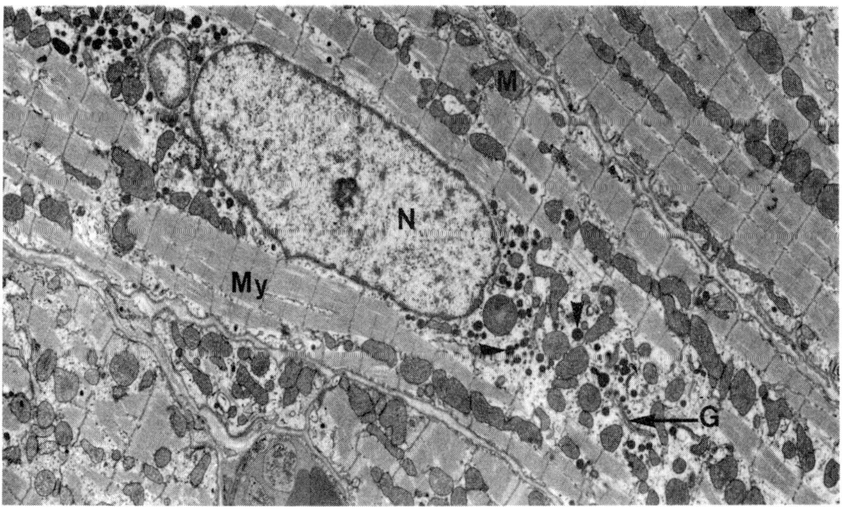

Figure 1. Transmission electronmicroscopy of rat atrial cardiocyte. Specific atrial granules (arrow-heads) and Golgi (G) complex are seen at the nuclear pole. Nucleus (N); myofibrils (My); mitochondria (M). × 5000 – reduced for publication

The secretory-like characteristics of atrial cardiocytes are not unique to rats, but are found in all mammals, and in both the atria and ventricles of non-mammalian vertebrates and elasmobranchs. Atrial natriuretic peptides have also been localized using biochemical, immunocytochemical and hybridization histochemical techniques in organs other than the heart [2], particularly in central and peripheral nervous tissues [3].

Atrial natriuretic peptide was so named after the observation that crude atrial extracts injected intravenously into rats induce four very powerful effects: diuresis, natriuresis, lowering of blood pressure and increase in haematocrit [4], all of which had a rapid onset.

Chemical structure

The first homogeneous preparation of an atrial natriuretic peptide was obtained in 1983 [5] from chromatographic fractions of atrial extracts. Four groups of fractions containing natriuretic activity were found. From one of these fractions a 28 aminoacid residue peptide containing a disulphide bridge was isolated, sequenced and proven to have the same biological properties as atrial natriuretic peptide. This peptide is referred to as cardionatrin I (CI) (Figure 2).

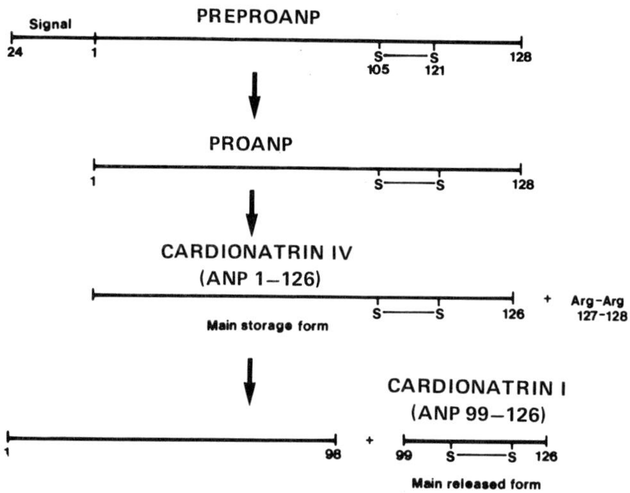

Figure 2. Rat atrial natriuretic peptide (ANP) is synthesized as a 152 aminoacid preproANP. The polypeptide is cleaved at the amino terminal losing the 24 aminoacid 'signal peptide'. The proANP molecule is further cleaved at the carboxy terminal end losing two Arg at positions 127–128 generating cardionatrin IV (ANP 1–126) which is the main form of ANP encountered in specific atrial granules. Further processing generates cardionatrin I (ANP 99–126) which is the main circulating form of cardionatrin

Shortly thereafter, several other sequences were communicated [6–11], including the human counterpart to the rat peptide which was shown to differ from it by only one aminoacid residue.

The major proportion of natriuretic activity is stored in the atria as a polypeptide referred to as cardionatrin IV (CIV) with a molecular weight considerably higher than the 28 aminoacid CI. This suggested a precursor-product relationship that has been confirmed through biochemical and molecular cloning studies [6,7,12,13] which showed that atrial natriuretic peptide is translated as a pre-prohormone of 151 (human) or 152 (rat) residues [14,15]. The amino terminal 25 (human) or 24 (rat) aminoacid sequence contains several hydrophobic residues thought to act as a 'signal peptide' which is cleaved as the nascent polypeptide moves across the microsomal membrane [13–16] (Figure 3).

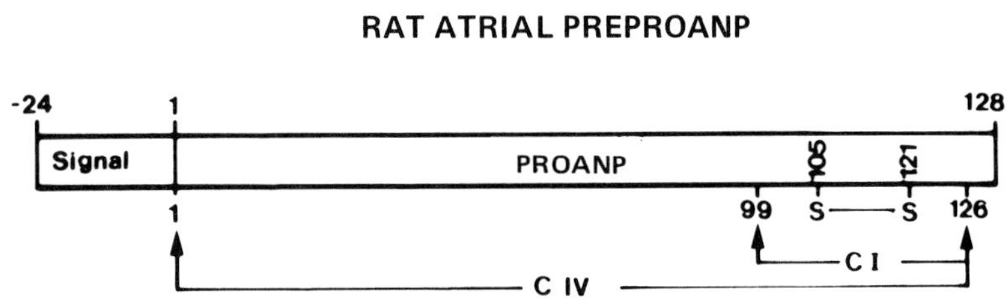

Figure 3. Schematic representation of proANP showing cardionatrin IV (CIV), the storage form of ANP and cardionatrin I (CI), the main molecular form present in plasma and in vitro atrial perfusates

The proANP molecule so generated contains the 126 residues cardionatrin IV (ANP 1–126) [13,17,18] which is the major storage form in atrial cardiocytes while the 28 residues carboxy terminal peptide-cardionatrin I (ANF 99–126) is the major circulating form [6,7,19,20] (Figure 3).

Genetic control of atrial natriuretic peptide

Complementary DNA clones (cDNA) specific for rat or human atrial natriuretic peptide have been isolated from cDNA libraries after hybridization with oligonucleotide probes predicted from the aminoacid sequence or after selecting for atrial specific mRNAs [13–15, 21–24]. The homology in nucleotide sequence between species has enabled the use of human or rat cDNA probes to isolate and characterize atrial natriuretic peptide cDNA from other species [25].

The sequence of the precursor mRNA – as deduced from the cDNA – shows that cardionatrin I is located at the 3′ end followed by the termination codon and by the 3′ untranslated region [21]. Although initial attempts to detect atrial natriuretic peptide mRNA in tissues other than cardiac atria were essentially unsuccessful [21,22,26], recent studies have shown detectable atrial natriuretic peptide mRNA and peptides in ventricles, pituitary and lungs [23,27,28]. The abundance of atrial natriuretic peptide specific mRNA in atria has been estimated between 0.5% to 3% of total RNA [21,25]. Atrial natriuretic peptide mRNA in extra atrial tissues has been detected at levels of 1–2% of those found in atrial tissues [3,24,28]. The meaning of the latter findings is not clear but, because of the large mass of some organs (ventricles, lungs), they might contribute significantly to the circulating pool of atrial natriuretic peptide.

Control of mRNA

Because of the presumptive rôle of atrial natriuretic peptide in cardiovascular homeostasis, changes in water and electrolyte balance should be expected to change the levels of mRNA in the atria. Nakayama et al [21] examined the effect of two and four days of water deprivation on atrial natriuretic peptide mRNA levels in rat atria and found lower levels than in controls after two and four days without water. Similar results were reported by Zisfein et al [17] who reported 28% reduction of atrial natriuretic peptide mRNA in volume-depleted rats after five days of water restriction but no change in the levels of immunoreactive atrial natriuretic peptide. Tadross et al [29] analysed the degree of cardiocyte granularity, atrial natriuretic peptide atrial content, plasma values and the ratio of atrial natriuretic peptide mRNA to actin mRNA in rats as a function of age, water deprivation or sodium overload. It was found that in normal animals, granularity increases with age and corresponds to changes in atrial natriuretic peptide stores. This association was not found in other situations: atrial natriuretic peptide storage, synthesis and release were found to be depressed following water deprivation while there was an increase in granularity, which was probably artefactual and due to tissue dehydration and shrinkage. In sodium overload, on the other hand, there is a decrease in granularity, and a non-significant decrease in storage. Nevertheless, mRNA synthesis increased and plasma atrial natriuretic peptide levels were not changed.

Local regulation of transcription of atrial natriuretic peptide mRNA seems to be different in the various tissues. Atrial levels, for example, are 2000-fold greater than in the hypothalamus [30]. Some experimental manoeuvres leading to changes in water and electrolyte balance appear to affect differently cardiac and brain atrial natriuretic peptide stores [31,32].

DNA mapping

DNA hybridization studies have shown that there is only one copy of the gene in human or rat genome [33,34]. The human atrial natriuretic peptide gene has been placed on chromosome 1 while the mouse gene has been found in chromosome 4 [35]. Mullins et al [36] mapped the gene in the mouse in a region close to the position previously determined for cribiform degeneration, a recessive mutation which includes in its phenotype an abnormal electrolyte distribution. This finding suggests a possible connection in the expression of atrial natriuretic peptide.

Atrial natriuretic peptide cDNA clones have been used to probe genomic libraries and to isolate plasmids containing genomic atrial natriuretic factor DNA [25,33,34,37]. Human and rat genes are formed by three exons separated by two introns. The first exon contains the AUG codon, 5′ untranslated sequences, the 24–25 residue signal peptide and 16 aminoacids following the signal peptidase cleavage site. The second exon has the information for the atrial natriuretic polypeptide up to the penultimate aminoacid in human or up to the third last aminoacid in rats. The latter are coded in the third exon as are the stop codon and 3′ untranslated sequences. Altogether the human gene spans about 2 kilobases and has the basic structure of an eukaryotic protein coding gene [33,37]. The second intron of the human gene (about 1050 base pairs) contains two complete 300 base pair sequences 70–86% homologous to the consensus Alu family sequence [38]. A single nucleotide change at the end of the coding sequence of the human with respect to the rat sequence converts an arginine codon (CGA) into a stop codon (UGA) and makes the human peptide two aminoacids (2 Arg) shorter.

Nemer et al [39,40] and Frossard et al [41,42] reported polymorphisms in the human gene for the enzymes Kpn I, Xho I, Taq I and Bgl II. These polymorphisms are considered representatives of allelic variations in the human population.

Differences in the polypeptide aminoacid sequence of proANP occur only at position 17 (86.5% homology) for rat and human. The nucleotide homology in the same region is 85.4% [37]. Differences between both species are much bigger at the signal peptide coding region and in non-coding sequences. The 5′ flanking sequences of the human, rat and mouse atrial natriuretic peptide genes are highly conserved [25]. An 11 base pair sequence has been identified [23] in this region which is almost identical to the SV40 (Simian Virus 40) enhancer (9/11ths for the human and rat and 8/11ths for the mouse [25,43]. These sequences may play a rôle in causing the high level of atrial-specific transcription of the atrial natriuretic peptide gene. A potential glucocorticoid-receptor binding site has been reported in the second intron of the human and rat gene [25,44, 45]. To investigate whether human atrial natriuretic peptide is responsive to glucocorticoids Iwai et al [46] transfected L cells with a plasmid carrying the 3.5 kilobase Bam fragment containing the human atrial natriuretic peptide gene. Two transformed colonies expressing the human atrial natriuretic peptide were isolated; both showed a decrease in the amount of atrial natriuretic peptide mRNA detected after treatment with dexamethasone. In vivo, in contrast, others [45] have shown that after dexamethasone treatment of normal and water-deprived rats there was a significant increase in atrial natriuretic peptide mRNA from 1.5–2.0-fold. It is evident that more in vitro studies are necessary to elucidate the rôle played by glucocorticoids in atrial natriuretic peptide mRNA transcription.

Atrial processing of atrial natriuretic peptide

Atrial peptides are processed by the atria. ANP 1–126 or cardionatrin IV is the main storage form of atrial natriuretic peptide in atrial granules [13,47] while the released form of atrial natriuretic peptide and that circulating in plasma is ANP 99–126 or cardionatrin I [19,48]. These results are summarized in Figure 3. Interestingly, cardiocytes in culture release cardionatrin IV, suggesting that the procedure of cell isolation impairs processing [49]. Atrial natriuretic peptide-like peptides isolated from the hypothalamus [30,31], however, have molecular weights considerably smaller than those present in atria. This finding suggests differences in processing between heart and brain.

Atrial natriuretic peptide receptors

Atrial natriuretic peptide receptors have been identified in several target tissues, including vascular smooth muscle, lungs, adrenal zona glomerulosa cells, and in the central nervous system [50–53]. The number of receptors in the target organs has been reported to vary in response to fluid balance showing a reciprocal relationship between plasma atrial natriuretic peptide concentrations and receptors [52]. Water deprivation depresses plasma concentrations and increases receptor numbers in kidney and adrenal cortex. On the other hand, increased values of circulating atrial natriuretic peptide in salt-loaded rats have been reported to decrease receptor levels. Binding to vascular, renal and adrenal receptors has been shown to activate particulate guanylate cyclase and to increase intracellular cGMP [54–56]. Recent studies have shown the existence of at least two kinds of receptors. One type is coupled to the particulate guanylate cyclase and is related to the biological effects of atrial natriuretic peptide in the different target organs [56,57]; the other kind of receptor seems to be mostly related to removal of atrial natriuretic peptide from the circulation [57]. Both receptors migrate as a single band with a molecular weight of 120,000–136,000 daltons on SDS polyacrylamide gels in the absence of reducing agents. The addition of reducing agents induces the shifting of the uncoupled receptor band to the 61,000 dalton position, while the coupled receptor remains as a 136,000 dalton band [58–60]. Work done with truncated atrial natriuretic peptide analogues also show two kinds of receptors: one population binds parent and truncated analogues with high affinity, the other increases cGMP in response to native atrial natriuretic peptide [59,61]. Deletion of aminoacids from the carboxyl and/or amino termini of the peptides diminish their ability to increase cGMP levels. Analogues lacking the carboxyl-terminal phe-arg-tyr tripeptide were found to be 100- to 1000-fold less potent in increasing intracellular levels of cGMP than the parent compound [59]. On the other hand, the *binding* of these peptides is only 1–5-fold weaker than the original compounds. Furthermore, analogues that bind to receptors and fail to induce any cGMP response do not antagonize or modulate an increase in cGMP produced by unaltered atrial natriuretic peptide compounds [59]. Guanylate cyclase-coupled receptors seem to be less abundant and their number is independent of blood concentrations of atrial natriuretic peptide. They seem to bind only native atrial natriuretic peptide, while the substantially more abundant uncoupled receptors are related to circulating atrial natriuretic peptide concentrations and seem to bind native and truncated froms almost as effectively [59,60,62].

The persistent association of atrial natriuretic peptide binding activity and particulate guanylate cyclase activity after extensive purification led Kuno et al [60] to postulate that the atrial natriuretic peptide coupled receptor and particulate guanylate cyclase are parts of a single transmembrane glycoprotein. The receptor domain would be located on the extracellular surface of the cells while the catalytic domain for cGMP synthesis would be located on the intracellular surface. The activation of particulate guanylate cyclase by atrial natriuretic peptide in target tissues such as kidney or adrenals [55, 60,62,63] is followed by a marked elevation of cGMP in plasma and urine. Intracellular elevation of cGMP levels is thought to activate cGMP-dependent protein kinases, which in turn regulate the functions of some cellular proteins by phosphorylation [64]. Cyclic GMP has been reported to interfere with calcium fluxes [61,65] and in smooth muscle, inhibition of calcium mobilization by cGMP could possibly explain the vasorelaxant action of atrial natriuretic peptide.

Atrial natriuretic peptide release

Atrial natriuretic peptide is released from the atria into the circulation through a process presumed to be exocytotic release. There is some morphological evidence [66–68] for such a mechanism, but it is clear that more investigation is needed because morphologically, exocytosis of atrial granules is a very rare event. There is unequivocal evidence that an increased rate of release from atrial cardiocytes is observed following atrial stretch in vitro [19,48,69–71] or in vivo following elevation of right or left atrial pressure and central venous pressure brought about by a variety of means [72–74]. The contribution of atrial receptors and autonomic innervation is less clear. In vitro, some investigators have reported that adrenaline, isoprenaline, arginine vasopressin and acetylcholine significantly stimulate release [75–78] while others [78,79] have found either no effect or even a reduction in atrial natriuretic peptide secretion rate. A similar controversy exists with in vivo studies. Kihara et al [80] showed that the atrial natriuretic peptide release induced by isotonic volume expansion in rats was not altered by chronic guanethidine treatment, and Ledsome et al [81] reported that bilateral vagotomy did not prevent the rise in plasma atrial natriuretic peptide levels in dogs with mitral obstruction. Others [82], however, have found that in pithed rats, cardiac denervation blocks release induced by acute volume loading thus suggesting that neuronal influences might affect release in this situation.

Intracellular stimuli

The intracellular signals controlling the kinetics of CI release are still poorly understood. Studies on in vitro static preparations [76] and in the perfused Langendorff heart [77] suggest that atrial natriuretic peptide release is a process modulated by muscarinic cholinergic stimulation which in turn activates the phosphoinositol system. In this system, inositol triphosphate and diacylglycerol would act as the second messengers in the stimulus-secretion coupling of atrial cardiocytes. In addition, studies with the calcium ionophores A23187 and Bay K8644 suggest that an increase in intracellular free calcium stimulates CI release [77,83–85]. These results have been confirmed by some [84,85] but not others. In our laboratory we have found that in vitro perfusion of spontaneously beating rat atria with media containing EGTA significantly stimulates the basal release of atrial natriuretic peptide. Similarly, if calcium is omitted from the media, the basal release is significantly augmented [86]. To further explore the effect of calcium on basal release, rat atria were perfused with EGTA followed by perfusion with 1.25mM calcium. Reintroduction of calcium caused inhibition of the augmented atrial natriuretic peptide release induced by EGTA within three minutes of perfusion as the atrial mechanical activity was restored. Atrial natriuretic peptide levels continued to decrease gradually and stabilized during the last five minutes of perfusion. Saint-Come and Fray [87] obtained similar results with a Langendorff heart preparation after EGTA perfusion.

Rôle of myocyte activity

In our preparation stretching the atria by changing load from 0.2g to 5.0g tension significantly stimulated the release of atrial natriuretic peptide. The stretch-coupled secretory response was evident in the presence and absence of calcium. In the absence of calcium mechanical activity of the atria ceased but the release of atrial natriuretic peptide under these conditions was significantly augmented [86]. These experiments showed that atrial beating is not necessary for atrial cardiocytes to release atrial natriuretic peptide and that the basal release, unlike most other endocrine systems, is stimulated by decreasing rather than increasing extracellular calcium. Recently others [88] have observed that release induced by increasing extracellular osmolality is also independent of calcium.

The stretch-coupled and basal atrial natriuretic peptide release was also investigated in non-paced and paced rat left atrium and human atrial trabeculae obtained from patients undergoing coronary bypass surgery. The quiescent rat left atrium and the human atrial trabeculae responded with a significant release after stretching of the atrial muscle, confirming our previous observations in whole atria or auricles.

Increasing the frequency of atrial contraction has been reported to increase release [89]. However, under physiological conditions, the heart rate accelerates with hypotension or volume depletion. To elucidate the rôle of pacing on atrial natriuretic peptide release, rat left atria and human atrial trabeculae were paced at 0.1, 0.2, 0.5, 1.0 and 2 Hz with 10ms electrical pulses at 50% threshold voltage. It was found that the rate of contraction did not affect the release of atrial natriuretic peptide. An increase was observed only at the start of pacing when the atrial muscle developed tension. If calcium were involved in the release process, depolarization would facilitate the entry of calcium into atrial cardiocytes and, as in other endocrine organs, increase release. Depolarization with high potassium (49mM) in the presence of calcium (1.25mM) failed to enhance atrial natriuretic peptide release suggesting that release is a process independent of calcium. Similar results have been reported by others [88,90]. These observations point to a dissociation between stretch-coupled secretion and contraction which seems to assist atrial cardiocytes to accomplish their dual function of contraction and secretion.

Actions of atrial natriuretic peptide

In addition to the biological effects of atrial natriuretic peptide described above, several less apparent effects have been found in recent years. These include endocrinological interactions, e.g. the ability to inhibit aldosterone secretion and synthesis and a possible rôle in the regulation of renin secretion. The hypotensive effect has been demonstrated to be, at least in part, due to its ability to relax vascular smooth muscle and also partly due to the ability of the peptide to decrease intravascular volume by increasing vascular permeability [see review 47]. The fact that even major increases in haematocrit are not followed by reflex increases in heart rate has been attributed to inhibition of cardiopulmonary chemoreceptors [91]. A possible effect on antidiuretic hormone secretion remains unsettled. The presence of atrial natriuretic peptide in the peripheral nervous system as well as those areas of the brain concerned with cardiovascular regulation, hint at a rôle for this peptide as a modulator of neuronal function.

The mechanisms by which atrial natriuretic peptide produces its natriuretic and diuretic effects are controversial, a particular point of contention being the relative contribution to the brisk diuresis and natriuresis of haemodynamic changes versus a tubular sodium transport effect. There is general agreement in that atrial natriuretic peptide does not affect Na/K-ATPase; several other lines of investigation have virtually unanimously shown no effect on sodium transport in various isolated epithelia or tubular nephron segments. On the other hand, there is ample evidence showing profound changes in renal haemodynamics. Renal blood flow may increase or decrease. The latter follows systemic injection of atrial natriuretic peptide that reduces mean arterial pressure. The observed effect on renal vasculature seems to depend on the initial status of the vasculature; infusions reduce renal vascular resistance when there is pre-existing vasoconstriction, but have little effect under other circumstances [92]. An increase in glomerular filtration rate plays a major rôle in the mechanism resulting in diuresis and natriuresis. The increase in glomerular filtration rate seems to be partly due to efferent vasoconstriction leading to an increase in glomerular capillary hydrostatic pressure. Redistribution of blood flow to deeper nephrons, accompanied by a decrease in inner-medullary tonicity might contribute to the observed natriuretic property.

The renal haemodynamic changes following injection may not be sufficient to account for the observed natriuresis. Acetylcholine produces the same changes in inner cortical blood flow as atrial natriuretic peptide but the degree of urinary sodium excretion does not approach that induced by atrial natriuretic peptide. Furthermore, studies using proximal tubule brush-border membrane vesicles, have provided some support regarding a direct effect in decreasing proximal tubular sodium reabsorption linked to bicarbonate or phosphate transport [93]. Specific atrial natriuretic peptide receptors have been demonstrated in kidney epithelia and in a kidney-derived epithelial cell line [93–97].

References

1 de Bold AJ, Raymond JJ, Bencosme SA. Atrial specific granules of the rat heart: light microscopic staining and histochemical reactions. *J Histochem Cytochem 1978; 26:* 1094–1102

2 Gardner DG, Deschepper CF, Ganong WF et al. Extra-arterial expression of the gene for atrial natriuretic factor. *Proc Natl Acad Sci USA 1986; 83:* 6697–6701

3 Gardner DG, Vlasuk GP, Baxter JD et al. Identification of atrial natriuretic factor gene transcripts in the central nervous system of the rat. *Proc Natl Acad Sci USA 1987; 84:* 2175–2179

4 de Bold AJ, Borenstein HB, Veress AT, Sonnenberg H. A rapid and potent natriuretic response to intravenous injection of atrial myocardial extract in rats. *Life Sci 1981; 28:* 89–94

5 de Bold AJ, Flynn TG. Cardionatrin I – a novel heart peptide with potent diuretic and natriuretic properties. *Life Sci 1983; 33:* 297–302

6 Flynn TG, de Bold ML, de Bold AJ. The amino acid sequence of an atrial peptide with potent diuretic and natriuretic properties. *Biochem Biophys Res Commun 1983; 117:* 859–865

7 Currie MG, Geller DM, Cole BR et al. Purification and sequence analysis of bioactive atrial peptides (atriopeptins). *Science 1984; 223 (4631):* 67–69

8 Kangawa K, Fukuda A, Minamino N, Matsuo H. Purification and complete amino acid sequence of beta-rat atrial natriuretic polypeptide (beta-rANP) of 5,000 daltons. *Biochem Biophys Res Commun 1984; 119:* 933–940

9 Seidah NG, Lazure C, Chretien M et al. Amino acid sequence of homologous rat atrial peptides: natiuretic activity of native and synthetic forms. *Proc Natl Acad Sci USA 1984; 81:* 2640–2644

10 Thibault G, Garcia R, Cantin M et al. Primary structure of a high Mr form of rat atrial natriuretic factor. *FEBS Lett 1984; 167:* 351–356

11 Kangawa K, Matsuo H. Purification and complete amino acid sequence of alpha-human atrial natriuretic polypeptide (alpha-hANP). *Biochem Biophys Res Commun 1984; 118:* 131–139

12 Trippodo NC, Ghai RD, MacPhee AA, Cole FE. Atrial natriuretic factor: atrial conversion of high to low molecular weight forms. *Biochem Biophys Res Commun 1984; 119:* 282–288

13 Flynn TG, Davies PL, Kennedy BP et al. Alignment of rat cardionatrin sequences with the preprocardionatrin sequence from complementary DNA. *Science 1985; 228 (4697):* 323–325

14 Seidman CE, Duby AD, Choi E et al. The structure of rat preproatrial natriuretic factor as defined by a complementary DNA clone. *Science 1984; 225 (4659):* 324–326

15 Maki M, Takayanagi R, Misono KS et al. Structure of rat atrial natriuretic factor precusor deduced from cDNA sequence. *Nature 1984; 309 (5970):* 722–724

16 Blobel G, Dobberstein B. Transfer of proteins across membranes. 1. Presence of proteolitically processed and unprocessed nascent immunoglobulin light chain on membrane-bound ribosomes of murine myeloma. *J Cell Biol 1975; 67:* 835–851

17 Zisfein JB, Matsueda GR, Fallon JT et al. Atrial natriuretic factor: assessment of its structure in atria and regulation of tis biosynthesis with volume depletion. *J Mol Cell Cardiol 1986; 18:* 917–929

18 Kangawa K, Tawaragi Y, Oikawa S et al. Identification of rat gamma atrial natriuretic polypeptide and characterization of the cDNA encoding its precursor. *Nature 1984; 312 (5990):* 152–155

19 Lang RE, Ganten D, Luft FC et al. Atrial natriuretic factor – a circulating hormone stimulated by volume loading. *Nature 1985; 314 (6008):* 264–266

20 Schwartz D, Geller DM, Manning PT et al. Ser-Leu-Arg-Arg-Atriopeptin III: the major circulating form of atrial peptide. *Science 1985; 229:* 397–400

21 Nakayama K, Ohdubo H, Hirose T et al. mRNA sequence for human cariodilatin-atrial natriuretic factor precursor and regulation of precursor mRNA in rat atria. *Nature 1984; 310 (5995):* 654–656

22 Yamanaka M, Greenberg B, Johnson L et al. Cloning and sequence analysis of the cDNA for the rat atrial natriuretic factor precursor. *Nature 1984; 309:* 719–722

23 Oikawa S, Imai M, Ueno A et al. Cloning and sequence analysis of cDNA encoding a precursor for human atrial natriuretic polypeptide. *Nature 1984; 309 (5970):* 724–726

24 Zivin RA, Condra JH, Dixon RA et al. Molecular cloning and characterization of DNA sequences encoding rat and human atrial natriuretic factors. *Proc Natl Acad Sci USA 1984; 81:* 6325–6329

25 Seidman C, Bloch K, Klein K et al. Nucleotide sequences of the human and mouse atrial natriuretic factor gene. *Science 1984; 226:* 1206–1209

26 Seidman C, Block K, Zisfein J et al. Molecular studies of the atrial natriuretic factor gene. *Hypertension 1985; 7 (Suppt I):* 131–134

27 Saper CB, Standaert DG, Currie MG et al. Atriopeptin-immunoreactive neurons in the brain: presence in cardiovascular regulatory areas. *Science 1985; 227:* 1047–1049

28 Gardner DG, Deschepper CF, Baxter JD. The gene for the atrial natriuretic factor is expressed in the aortic arch. *Hypertension 1987; 9:* 102–106

29 Tadross OE, Sarda IR, de Bold AJ. Relation between atrial-specific granules and cardionatrin synthesis and storage in the rat. In Brenner BM, Laragh JH, eds. *Biologically Active Atrial Peptides.* New York: Raven Press. 1987: 158–162

30 Glembotski CC, Wildey GM, Gibson TR. Molecular forms of immunoactive atrial natriuretic peptide in the rat hypothalamus and atrium. *Biochem Biophys Res Commun 1985; 129:* 671–678

31 Tanaka I, Misono KS, Inagami T. Atrial natriuretic factor in rat hypothalamus, atria and plasma: determination by specific radioimmunoassay. *Biochem Biophys Res Commun 1984; 124:* 663–668

32 Samson WK. Dehydration-induced alterations in rat brain vasopressin and atrial natriuretic factor immunoreactivity. *Endocrinology 1985; 117:* 1279–1281

33 Nemer M, Chamberland M, Sirois D et al. Gene structure of human cardiac hormone precursor, pronatriodilatin. *Nature 1984; 312 (5995):* 654–656

34 Argentin S, Nemer M, Drouin J et al. The gene for rat atrial natriuretic factor. *J Biol Chem 1985; 260:* 4568–4571

35 Yang-Feng T, Floyd-Smith G, Nemer M et al. The pronatriodilatin gene is located on the distal short arm of human chromosome 1 and on mouse chromosome 4. *Am J Hum Genet 1985; 37:* 1117–1128

36 Mullins J, Zeng Q, Gross K. Mapping of the mouse atrial natriuretic factor gene. Evidence for tight linkage to the Fv-1 locus. *Hypertension 1987; 9:* 518–521

37 Greenberg BD, Bencen GH, Selhamer JJ et al. Nucleotide sequence of the gene encoding human atrial natriuretic factor precursor. *Nature 1984; 312 (5995):* 656–658

38 Deininger PL, Jolly DJ, Rubin CM et al. Base sequence studies of 300 nucleotide renatured repeated human DNA clones. *J Mol Biol 1981; 151:* 17–33

39 Nemer M, Sirois D, Drouin J. Taq I polymorphism at the 3' end of the human pronatriodilatin gene (hPND). *Nucleic Acids Res 1986; 14:* 8696

40 Nemer M, Sirois D, Drouin J. XhoI polymorphism at the human pronatriodilatin (hPND) gene locus. *Nucleic Acids Res 1986; 14:* 8696

41 Frossard PM, Coleman RT. Human atrial natriuretic peptides (ANP) gene locus: Bgl I RFLP. *Nucleic Acids Res 1986; 14:* 9223

42 Frossard PM, Gonzalez PA, Greenberg B et al. Bgl II dimorphism at the human atrial natriuretic peptide (ANP) gene locus. *Nucleic Acids Res 1986; 14:* 5121

43 Khoury G, Gruss P. Enhancer elements. *Cell 1983; 33:* 313–314

44 Renkawitz R, Schutz G, von der Ahe D, Beato M. Sequences in the promotor region of the sequence of the chicken lysozyme gene required for steroid regulation and receptor binding. *Cell 1984; 37:* 503–510

45 Gardner DG, Hane S, Trachewsky et al. Atrial natriuretic peptide mRNA is regulated by glucocorticoids in vivo. *Biochem Biophys Res Commun 1986; 139:* 1047–1054

46 Iwai N, Matsunaga M, Ogawa K et al. Regulated expression of human atrial natriuretic polypeptide gene in mouse L cells. *Biochem Biophys Res Commun 1987; 144:* 402–408

47 de Bold AJ. Atrial natriuretic factor: a hormone produced by the heart. *Science 1985; 230:* 767–770

48 de Bold AJ, de Bold ML, Sarda IR. Functional-morphological studies on in vitro cardionatrin release. *J Hypertension 1986; 4 (Suppt 2):* 53–57

49 Glembotski CC, Gibson TR. Molecular forms of immunoactive atrial natriuretic peptide released from cultured rat atrial myocytes. *Biochem Biophys Res Commun 1985; 132:* 1008–1017

50 Hirata Y, Tomita M, Yoshimi H, Ikeda M. Specific receptors for atrial natriuretic factor (ANF) in cultured vascular smooth muscle cells of rat aorta. *Biochem Biophys Res Commun 1984; 125:* 562–568

51 Quirion R, Dalpe M, Dam TV. Characterization and distribution of receptors for the atrial natriuretic peptides in mammalian brain. *Proc Natl Acad Sci USA 1986; 83:* 174–178

52 Lynch DR, Braas KM, Snyder SH. Atrial natriuretic factor in rat kidney, adrenal gland, and brain: autoradiographic localization and fluid balance dependent changes. *Proc Natl Acad Sci USA 1986; 83:* 3357–3361

53 Vandlen RL, Arcuri KE, Napier MA. Identification of a receptor for atrial natriuretic factor in rabbit aorta membranes by affinity cross-linking. *J Biol Chem 1985; 260:* 10889–10892

54 Winquist RJ, Faison EP, Waldman SA et al. Atrial natriuretic factor elicits an endothelium-independent relaxation and activates particulate guanylate cyclase in vascular smooth muscle. *Proc Natl Acad Sci USA 1984; 81:* 7661–7666

55 Waldman SA, Rapoport RM, Murad F. Atrial natriuretic factor selectively activates particulate guanylate cyclase and elevates cyclic GMP in rat tissues. *J Biol Chem 1984; 259:* 14332–14334

56 Huang CL, Ives HE, Cogan MG. In vivo evidence that cGMP is the second messenger for atrial natriuretic factor. *Proc Natl Acad Sci USA 1986; 83:* 8015–8018

57 Scarborough R, McEnroe G, Kang L et al. Receptor interaction of atrial natriuretic peptide ring deletion analogs. *Proc 2nd Annual Meeting Am Soc Hypertension.* 1987: 190

58 Takayanaigi R, Misono KS, Snajdar RN et al. Purification and characterization of guanylate cyclase-coupled and uncoupled atrial natriuretic factor receptors from bovine adrenal cortex. *Proc 2nd Annual Meeting Am Soc Hypertension.* 1987: 188

59 Scarborough RM, Schenk DD, McEnroe GA et al. Truncated atrial natriuretic peptide analogs. Comparison between receptor binding and stimulation of cyclic GMP accumulation in cultured vascular smooth muscle cells. *J Biol Chem 1986; 261:* 12960–12964

60 Kuno T, Andresen JW, Kamisaki Y et al. Co-purification of an atrial natriuretic factor receptor and particulate guanylate cyclase from rat lung. *J Biol Chem 1986; 261:* 5817–5823

61 Murad F. Cyclic guanosine monophosphate as a mediator of vasodilation. *J Clin Invest 1986; 78:* 1–5

62 Hamet P, Tremblay J, Pang SC et al. Effect of native and synthetic atrial natriuretic factor on cyclic GMP. *Biochem Biophys Res Commun 1984; 123:* 515–527

63 Grezer R, Hein JM, Schutte B, Weil J. Cellular mechanisms of action of atrial natriuretic factor. *Klin Wochenschr 1987; 65 (Suppt VIII):* 109–114

64 Lincoln TH, Johnson RM. Possible role of cyclic-GMP-dependent protein kinase in vascular smooth muscle function. *Adv Cyclic Nucl Protein Phosphor Res 1984; 17:* 285–296

65 Meyer-Lehnert H, Tsai P, Schier RW. Atrial natriuretic factor (ANF) inhibits arginine vasopressin-stimulated Ca^{2+} fluxes and cell contraction in vascular smooth muscle cells. *Klin Wochenschr 1987; 65 (Suppt VIII):* 115–121

66 Page E, Goings GE, Power P, Upshaw-Early J. Ultrastructural features of atrial peptide secretion. *Am J Physiol 1986; 251:* H340–H348

67 Theron JJ, Biaggio R, Meyer AC, Boekkooi S. Ultrastructural observations on the maturation and secretion of granules in atrial myocardium. *J Mol Cell Cardiol 1978; 10:* 567–572

68 Sugawara M. Ultrastructural evidence for exocytotic release of atrial natriuretic polypeptide in the rat atrial muscle with the use of the tannic acid method. *Biomed Res 1987; 8:* 9–17

69 Dietz JR. Release of natriuretic factor from rat heart-lung preparation by atrial distension. *Am J Physiol 1984:* R1093–R1096

70 Kabayama Y, Fukamachi Y, Kamisaki T, Tanaka H. Stimulation by volume expansion of atrial natriuretic peptide release from perfused rat heart. *Peptides 1987; 8:* 256–260

71 Agnoletti G, Rodella A, Ferrari R, Harris P. Release of atrial natriuretic peptide-like immunoreactive material during stretching of the rat atrium in vitro. *J Mol Cell Cardiol 1987; 19:* 217–220

72 Ledsome JR, Wilson N, Rankin AJ, Courneya CA. Time course of release of atrial natriuretic peptide in the anaesthetized dog. *Can J Physiol Pharmacol 1986; 64:* 1017–1022

73 Pettersson A, Ricksten SE, Towles AC et al. Effect of blood volume expansion and sympathetic denervation on plasma levels of atrial natriuretic factor (ANF) in the rat. *Acta Physiol Scand 1985; 124:* 309–311

74 McKenzie J, Tauaka I, Inagaui T et al. Alterations in atrial and plasma atrial natriuretic factor (ANF) content during development of hypoxia-induced pulmonary hypertension in the rat. *Proc Soc Exp Biol Med 1984; 12:* 783–784

75 Sonnenberg H, Krebs RF, Veress AT. Release of atrial natriuretic factor from incubated rat heart atria. *IRCS Med Sci 1984; 12:* 783–784

76 Sonnenberg H, Veress AT. Cellular mechanism of release of atrial natriuretic factor. *Biochem Biophys Res Commun 1984; 124:* 443–449

77 Ruskoaho H, Toth M, Lang RE. Atrial natriuretic peptide secretion: synergistic effect of phorbol ester and A23187. *Biochem Biophys Res Commun 1985; 133:* 581–588

78 Arjamaa O, Vuolteenaho O. Sodium ion stimulates the release of atrial natriuretic polypeptides (ANP) from rat atria. *Biochem Biophys Res Commun 1985; 132:* 375–281

79 Hattor T, Hashimoto K, Inove H et al. Effect of α and β-adrenergic agonists and antagonists on atrial natriuretic peptide secretion in vitro. In Brenner BM, Laragh JH, eds. *Biologically Active Atrial Peptides.* New York: Raven Press. 1987: 149–151

80 Kihara M, Nakao K, Morii N et al. Responses of plasma atrial natriuretic polypeptide to isotonic volume expansion in conscious spontaneously hypertensive and chronically guanethidine-treated rats. *J Hypertension 1986; 4:* S321–S324

81 Ledsome JR, Wilson N, Courneya CA, Rankin AJ. Release of atrial natriuretic peptide by atrial distension. *Can J Physiol Pharmacol 1985; 63:* 739–742

82 Eskay R, Zukowska-Grojec Z, Heas M et al. Circulating atrial natriuretic peptides in conscious rats: regulation of release by multiple factors. *Science 1986; 232:* 630–639

83 Saito Y, Nakao K, Morii N et al. Bay K8644, a voltage-sensitive calcium channel agonist, facilitates secretion of atrial natriuretic polypeptide from isolated perfused rat heart. *Biochem Biophys Res Commun 1986; 138:* 1170–1176

84 Ruskoaho H, Toth M, Gauteu D et al. The phorbol ester induced atrial natriuretic peptide secretion is stimulated by Forskolin and Bay K8644 and inhibited by 8-Bromo-cyclic GMP. *Biochem Biophys Res Commun 1986; 139:* 266–274

85 Masuda H, Nagai K, Kangawa K, Matsuo H. Atrial natriuretic peptide secretion from the isolated rat atria. In Brenner BM, Laragh JH, eds. *Biologically Active Atrial Peptides.* New York: Raven Press. 1987: 170–173

86 de Bold ML, de Bold AJ. Atrial stretch-secretion coupling and immunoreactive cardionatrin release in vitro: effect of Ca^{2+} and EGTA. In Brenner BM, Laragh JH, eds. *Biologically Active Atrial Peptides.* New York: Raven Press. 1987: 173–175

87 Saint-Come CM, Fray SCS. Direct effects of right atrial pressure on release of atrial natriuretic peptide from isolated rat heart. In Brenner BM, Laragh JD, eds. *Biologically Active Atrial Peptides.* New York: Raven Press. 1987: 162–165

88 Gibbs D. Noncalcium-dependent introduction of in vitro atrial natriuretic factor release by extracellular osmolality. *Endocrinology 1987; 120:* 194–197

89 Schiebinger RJ, Lindeu J. Effect of atrial contraction frequency on atrial natriuretic peptide secretion. *Am J Physiol 1986; 251:* H1095–H1099

90 Baertschi AJ, Hausmaninger C, Walsh RS et al. Hypoxia-induced release of atrial natriuretic factor (ANF) from the isolated rat and rabbit heart. *Biochem Biophys Res Commun 1986; 140:* 427–433

91 Ackerman U, Irizawa TG, Milojevic S, Sonnenberg H. Cardiovascular effects of atrial extracts in anaesthetized rats. *Can J Physiol Pharmacol 1984; 62:* 819–826

92 Maack T, Kleinert HD. Renal and cardioascular effects of atrial natriuretic factor. *Biochem Pharmacol 1986; 35:* 2057–2064

93 Hammond TG, Yusufi AN, Knox FG, Dousa TP. Administration of atrial natriuretic factor inhibits sodium-coupled transport in proximal tubules. *J Clin Invest 1985; 75:* 1983–1989

94 Cantiello HF, Ausiello DA. Atrial natriuretic factor and cGMP inhibit amiloride-sensitive Na+ transport in the cultured renal epithelial cell line, LLC-PK1. *Biochem Biophys Res Commun 1986; 134:* 852–860

95 Napier MA, Vandlen RL, Alberts-Schonberg G et al. Specific membrane receptors for atrial natriuretic factor in renal and vascular tissues. *Proc Natl Acad Sci USA 1984; 81:* 5946–5950

96 Inui K, Saito H, Matsukawa Y et al. Specific binding activities and cyclic GMP responses by atrial natriuretic polypeptide in kidney epithelial cell line (LLC PK1). *Biochem Biophys Res Commun 1985; 132:* 253–260

97 Hori R, Inue K, Saito H et al. Specific receptors for atrial natriuretic polypeptide on basolateral membranes isolated from rat renal cortex. *Biochem Biophys Res Commun 1985; 129:* 773–779

FUNCTIONAL PROPERTIES OF ATRIAL NATRIURETIC PEPTIDE AND ITS RECEPTORS

T Maack

Cornell University University Medical College, New York, NY, USA

Introduction

Atrial natriuretic peptide is a polypeptide hormone with broad actions directed at the regulation of salt excretion, plasma volume and vascular resistance. The first two parts of this article provide a brief review of the renal and systemic actions of atrial natriuretic peptide and its rôle in plasma volume regulation. For more detailed reviews and bibliography on these subjects the reader is directed to references 1 to 5. The last part of the article summarizes our recent evidence on the physiological rôle of atrial natriuretic peptide receptors, including the discovery of specific clearance receptors involved in the modulation of plasma levels of atrial natriuretic peptide.

Effect of atrial natriuretic peptide on renal function

Overall renal haemodynamic and natriuretic actions

In 1982, soon after the discovery by de Bold et al [6] that administration of crude atrial extract leads to a brisk diuresis and natriuresis in intact anaesthetized rats, we examined the effects of a semi-purified atrial extract in a functioning, isolated, perfused rat kidney preparation [7]. Addition of atrial extract to the perfusate led to a marked diuresis, natriuresis and kaliuresis. Furthermore, atrial extract increased glomerular filtration rate, despite a slight but significant increase in renal vascular resistance; there was a major increase in filtration fraction. This combination of events suggested that atrial natriuretic peptide constricts preferentially the efferent glomerular arteriole. Removal of calcium from the perfusate abolished the actions of atrial extract on renal haemodynamic and excretory functions. The data in the isolated kidney demonstrated for the first time that the natriuretic activity of atrial natriuretic peptide is due to its direct action on the kidney on which it has major haemodynamic effects. On the basis of these results and from the fact that the isolated kidney has a washed-out inner medulla, we concluded that the natriuretic effect is due at least in part to a combination of an increase in filtered load of sodium (increase in glomerular filtration rate) and a decrease in inner-medullary hypertonicity [1,3–5,7].

The experiments in the isolated kidney provided further insights as to the renal vascular actions of atrial natriuretic peptide [7]. In control isolated kidneys which have a low renal vascular resistance, atrial natriuretic peptide had a slight vasoconstrictive effect. However, in kidneys preconstricted with hormonal (norepinephrine, angiotensin, vasopressin) or non-hormonal (ouabain, tetracain) agents, atrial natriuretic peptide had a marked vasorelaxant effect tending to return renal vascular resistance to control levels. Thus, atrial natriuretic peptide did not behave as such classical renal vasodilators as bradykinin or acetylcholine but as a strong antagonist of renal vasoconstriction, with weak agonist (vasoconstrictive) effects of its own.

The overall effects of crude and semi-purified atrial extract described above were confirmed using synthetic atrial peptides in in vitro preparations and in experimental animals and humans [1–5]. In steady-state conditions, infusion of atrial peptides increase glomerular filtration rate, filtration fraction, water, sodium and potassium excretion and decreases inner-medullary tonicity. In intact animals, atrial natriuretic peptide has similar effects on renal vascular resistance to those in the isolated kidney. These depend on the initial vascular tone and are geared towards returning vascular resistance towards normal levels [1–5]. Although some investigators claim that there may be a dissociation between the renal haemodynamic and natriuretic actions of atrial natriuretic peptide in intact animals and humans, our studies indicate that, in steady-state conditions, such dissociation does not occur [3–5]. Nevertheless, atrial natriuretic peptide has been said to affect tubular mechanisms in the proximal or distal nephron, particularly in inner-medullary collecting ducts [8,9].

Sites of mechanisms of renal actions

Figure 1 depicts schematically the possible sites of renal action of atrial natriuretic peptide. Atrial natriuretic peptide increases glomerular filtration rate and decreases inner-medullary hypertonicity. The increase in glomerular filtration rate is due to an increase in glomerular hydrostatic pressure brought about by an increase in 'efferent' vasoconstriction or by a combination of 'efferent' constriction and 'afferent' dilation [7,10–12]. Atrial natriuretic peptide may also increase glomerular hydraulic permeability [12]. The reason for the decrease in inner-medullary hypertonicity is unknown [3–5].

Whatever the exact mechanism, a decrease in inner-medullary hypertonicity magnifies the natriuretic effect of an increase in load to the papillary descending limb of Henle's loop and there is a decrease in passive abstraction of water in the descending limb and consequently of sodium in the thin ascending limb [3–5,7]. As a result, there is an increase in water and sodium load to the base

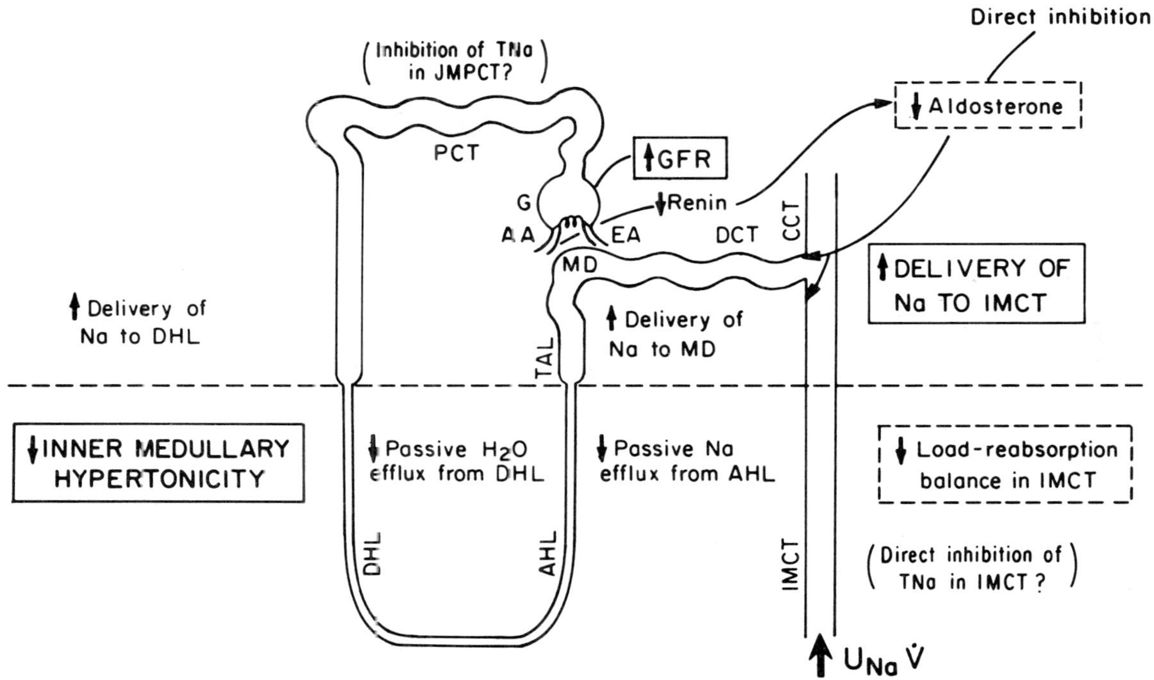

Figure 1. Sites of action of atrial natriuretic peptide in the kidney. See text for description. Abbreviations: G=glomerulus; AA=afferent ateriole; EA=efferent arteriole; PCT=proximal convoluted tubule; JMPCT=PCT of juxta-medullary nephrons; DHL=descending limb of Henle's loop; AHL=thin ascending limb of Henle's loop; TAL=thick ascending limb of Henle's loop; MD=macula densa; DCT=distal convoluted tubule; CCT=cortical collecting duct; IMCT=inner-medullary (papillary) collecting duct; ↑=increase; ↓=decrease

of the inner-medullary collecting duct. This phenomenon is observed regularly during the administration of atrial natriuretic peptide [9]. Thus, increase in glomerular filtration rate, decrease in inner-medullary tonicity and increase in load to the base of the papillary collecting duct are important mechanisms of the natriuretic effect of atrial natriuretic peptide [1–5].

In addition, atrial natriuretic peptide may decrease proximal tubular reabsorption of sodium [8]. Since free flow micropuncture studies or studies in isolated perfused proximal tubules of the rabbit show a lack of effect of atrial natriuretic peptide on proximal fluid and electrolyte reabsorption, it has been postulated that this effect occurs in proximal tubules of juxta-medullary nephrons which are remote from direct puncture study [8]. At present it cannot be concluded unequivocally that atrial natriuretic peptide decreases proximal reabsorption.

Following the initial observation of Sonnenberg et el [9] that atrial natriuretic peptide infusion leads to a disruption of load-to-reabsorption balance in papillary collecting ducts, several investigators postulated an important rôle for this phenomenon among the natriuretic actions of atrial natriuretic peptide [9, 13–15]. Recent studies indicate that atrial natriuretic peptide increases cGMP in isolated papillary collecting ducts and in a suspension of purified papillary collecting duct cells [13,14]. However, there is controversy as to the mechanism by which atrial natriuretic peptide may disrupt load-to-reabsorption balance in papillary collecting ducts. Increase in passive permeability to sodium [9], decrease in amiloride-sensitive sodium reabsorption [13] or increase in NaCl co-transport from blood to lumen [15] have been invoked but not confirmed as causes of such disruption.

Finally, atrial natriuretic peptide inhibits aldosterone secretion both by a direct action on the adrenal and by decreasing renal renin secretion [8,16]. Distal nephron sodium reabsorption must decrease as a consequence, at least during chronic elevation of plasma atrial natriuretic peptide [see ref 5 for a review of the possible mechanisms by which atrial natriuretic peptide decreases renin and aldosterone secretion].

From the schema in Figure 1 and the description above, it is clear that atrial natriuretic peptide has multiple effects on the kidney and that further work is needed to elucidate the intricacies of its mechanisms and of the quantitative contribution of each effect to the eventual natriuretic action. However, the renal haemodynamic effects of atrial natriuretic peptide and its effect of increasing sodium load to the distal nephron are well documented and have important theoretical and practical implications which are briefly described below.

Physiological and pathophysiological consequences

Reduction of renal perfusion pressure prior to ('early clamp') or during ('late clamp') continuous infusion of atrial natriuretic peptide practically abolishes its natriuretic action in dogs and rats [3–5,17,18]. This finding, confirmed by other investigators [for review see refs 3–5], has several important implications:

1. It demonstrates that the renal haemodynamic effects of atrial natriuretic peptide are a major component of its natriuretic actions and that alterations in renal haemodynamics may override any direct effect of atrial natriuretic peptide on the renal tubule.
2. It explains the effectiveness of atrial natriuretic peptide as a natriuretic agent in diseases accompanied by a reduction in renal perfusion such as congestive heart failure or some renal diseases. In these pathological conditions the human kidney behaves as does the clamped kidney in experimental animals.
3. Since a 'late' renal clamp does not impede the natriuresis of acute saline expansion in rats, our finding that this experimental manoeuvre blocks the natriuretic action of atrial natriuretic peptide strongly suggests that atrial natriuretic peptide is *not* an important mediator of acute saline diuresis. However, atrial natriuretic peptide may be a mediator of natriuresis in acute or chronic iso-oncotic plasma expansion [17].

Since an increase in sodium load to the distal nephron is a basic mode by which atrial natriuretic peptide increases sodium excretion, compensatory sodium reabsorption more distally will blunt its effect. Indeed, in spite of marked natriuresis, absolute sodium reabsorption as well as sodium reabsorption in each of the nephron segments studied so far, including papillary collecting ducts, is increased during administration of atrial natriuretic peptide [1,3–5,9]. In this condition an important distal compensatory mechanism could be an increase in sodium reabsorption via amiloride-sensitive sodium channels. Our recent studies demonstrate that this is the case since, as will be summarized below, amiloride markedly potentiates the natriuretic effect of atrial natriuretic peptide and abolishes its kaliuretic action.

In isolated rat kidneys perfused with 10^{-6} M amiloride, addition of a maximally effective dose of ANP_{1-28} (10^{-7} M) increased sodium excretion to a level which was approximately threefold the sum of the natriuretic effect of 10^{-6} M amiloride alone + 10^{-7} M ANP_{1-28} alone. Furthermore, in the presence of amiloride the kaliuretic response to atrial natriuretic peptide was completely abolished [19]. The potentiation of the natriuretic effect of atrial natriuretic peptide and abolition of its kaliuretic action in the isolated kidney was also demonstrable at doses of amiloride as low as 10^{-8} M and at physiological concentrations of atrial natriuretic peptide (10^{-11}) [Suzuki M, Almeida FA, Maack T, unpublished results].

This recent finding demonstrates conclusively that increase in load to the distal nephron is a major mode by which atrial natriuretic peptide increases sodium excretion in the isolated perfused rat kidney. In addition, this finding opens the possibility of combining amiloride and atrial natriuretic peptide therapeutically, so as to increase the natriuretic action of the hormone and abolish its kaliuretic effect.

Systemic effects of atrial natriuretic peptide: intravascular volume homeostasis

Overall systemic effects

Figure 2 depicts schematically some of the major systemic effects of atrial natriuretic peptide. In addition to its blood pressure lowering effect, infusion of atrial peptides leads to a major decrease in plasma volume by shifting fluid from intravascular to interstitial compartment in the systemic circulation [20]. This action, which explains in great part the blood pressure lowering action of atrial natriuretic peptide in normotensive animals, highlights what is probably its major

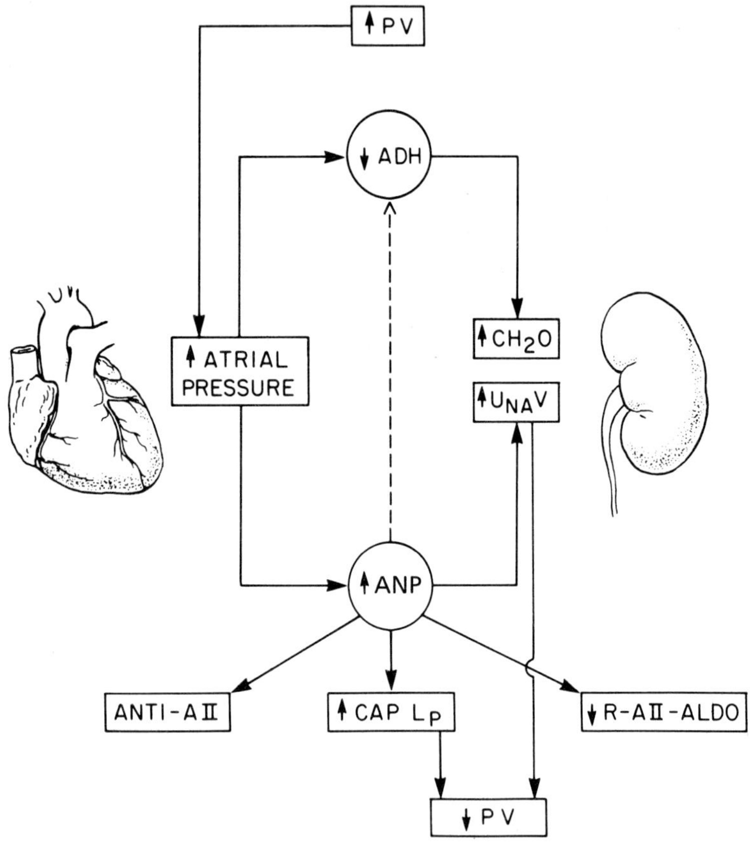

Figure 2. Atrial natriuretic peptide systemic actions and the regulation of plasma volume. See text for description. Abbreviations: PV=plasma volume; ADH=antidiuretic hormone; AII=angiotensin II; CAP L_p=capillary hydraulic permeability; R=renin; ALDO=aldosterone; $U_{Na}V$=excretion rate of sodium; C_{H_2O}=free water clearance; ↑=increase; ↓=decrease

homeostatic rôle. Atrial natriuretic peptide interacts with other hormonal systems involved in the regulation of fluid volume and blood pressure, particularly with the renin-angiotensin aldosterone system of which it is a powerful inhibitor [6]. In addition, atrial natriuretic peptide counteracts the most important actions of angiotensin II by inhibiting: 1) angiotensin-induced vasoconstriction; 2) angiotensin stimulation of aldosterone secretion; and 3) the central dipsinogenic effect of angiotensin. In this section I will consider briefly the effects of atrial natriuretic peptide on plasma volume. Other systemic and central actions of atrial natriuretic peptide and its interactions with other hormonal systems are covered in a recent review [5].

Mechanisms of blood pressure lowering effect

Since the initial experiments with atrial extract it became established that atrial natriuretic peptide decreases blood pressure and increases haematocrit in normotensive animals [6]. This phenomenon was thought to be an indirect consequence of its diuretic action [6]. Then after the discovery of the vasoactive properties of atrial natriuretic peptide, it was assumed that the blood pressure lowering effect of atrial natriuretic peptide was due to peripheral vasorelaxation [1,2]. However, measurements of cardiovascular functions did not confirm this assumption. In normotensive conditions, atrial natriuretic peptide does not decrease total peripheral resistance (TPR) but rather decreases cardiac output [4,5]. It is only in experimental models of hypertension characterized by high vascular tone (e.g. renin-dependent hypertension) that atrial natriuretic peptide decreases TPR towards control values [5]. Therefore, the effects of atrial natriuretic peptide on TPR depend on the initial systemic vascular tone and do not explain the blood pressure lowering effects of atrial natriuretic peptide in normotensive animals.

Effects on plasma volume and capillary hydraulic permeability

Several hypotheses were raised to explain the decrease in cardiac output, including a direct negative inotropic action and/or venodilatory effects of atrial natriuretic peptide [5]. There is no evidence for these mechanisms at present. On the other hand, we suggested that the decrease in cardiac output may be due at least in part to a decrease in plasma volume brought about by an atrial natriuretic peptide-induced shift of fluid from the intravascular to the interstitial compartment [16].

Definitive proof was obtained in experiments in nephrectomized rats [20]. In these experiments intravenous infusion of ANP_{1-28} led to an approximately 7% increase in haematocrit and a 14% decrease in plasma volume as measured by radiolabelled albumin distribution volume. The decrease in plasma volume could be accounted for entirely by efflux of fluid from capillaries without a concomitant increase in permeability to albumin. Consequently, we postulated that the increase in efflux of fluid from the systemic circulation was due to an increase in capillary hydraulic permeability [20]. Recent direct studies by Huxley et al [21] in capillaries of the frog mesenterium strongly indicate that this is the case. In this preparation, with Starling forces kept at constant levels, high concentrations of atrial natriuretic peptide led to a fourfold increase in capillary hydraulic permeability.

The effect of atrial natriuretic peptide on capillary hydraulic permeability is consistent with the widespread localization of specific binding sites of atrial natriuretic peptide in the vascular endothelium. Furthermore, cultured endothelial cells respond to atrial natriuretic peptide by increasing cGMP to a greater extent than any other cell type tested to date [22,23]. Consequently, it is reasonable to assume that cGMP is a major mediator of the effects of atrial natriuretic peptide on the capillary endothelium. In this regard it is of interest that nitrites do not increase cGMP in cultured endothelial cells or shift fluid from the intravascular to the interstitial compartment, when administered to nephrectomized rats at doses which produced a similar decrease in blood pressure as atrial natriuretic peptide [20].

Physiological and pathophysiological consequences

Regulation of plasma volume is perhaps the foremost homeostatic rôle of atrial natriuretic peptide in the mammalian organism. Under normal conditions this rôle is accomplished by regulating renal excretion of salt and by regulating capillary hydraulic permeability. Increases in plasma volume raise atrial pressure and, hence, the secretion of atrial natriuretic peptide [5]. The consequent increase in sodium excretion and efflux of fluid from systemic capillaries tend to return plasma volume to control levels. Even in conditions in which the kidney is unresponsive to the natriuretic effect of atrial natriuretic peptide such as congestive heart failure (see above), the hormone may still be effective in maintaining plasma volume homeostasis by its action in increasing capillary hydraulic permeability. To some extent, then, plasma volume homeostasis may be accomplished at the cost of an increase in systemic interstitial fluid volume. Perhaps the oedema in congestive heart failure is due partly to the elevated plasma levels of atrial natriuretic peptide in this condition [4]. It is noteworthy that, in normal conditions, an increase in hydraulic permeability in lung capillaries will tend to favour reabsorption rather than efflux of fluid in view of the negative balance of Starling forces in the pulmonary circulation. Consequently, atrial natriuretic peptide may have a major homeostatic rôle in regulating systemic plasma volume at the same time that it protects the interstitial pulmonary volume.

Physiological rôle of atrial natriuretic peptide receptors

High affinity binding sites of atrial natriuretic peptide are widely distributed in several tissues, including kidney cortex, adrenal, endothelial and vascular smooth muscle cells [22–25]. In these target tissues, atrial natriuretic peptide causes large increases in cGMP the probable second messenger of its actions [23]. However, studies in cultured endothelial and vascular smooth muscle cells established that a significant proportion of the high affinity binding sites of atrial natriuretic peptide is not coupled to the generation of cGMP [22,23]. Recently, we presented evidence demonstrating that a major function of these receptors – which we named C-ANF receptors – is to remove atrial natriuretic peptide from the circulation [26].

Renal receptors

Studies in the isolated rat kidney perfused with a near physiological solution, demonstrated that the kidney cortex contains more than 95% of the total renal binding sites of atrial natriuretic peptide [27]. These receptors, localized in glomerular and vascular structures of the kidney cortex, have a very high affinity for ANP_{1-28}, the biologically active form of circulating endogenous atrial natriuretic peptide (K_d, app. 50pM) [27]. Consequently, there is receptor occupancy at physiological concentrations of the hormone. The papillae contain less than 2% of the total renal binding sites of atrial natriuretic peptide and the affinity of these receptors is lower than that in the cortex (K_d, app. 300pM) [27].

Studies in the isolated kidney demonstrated that there is an excellent agreement between the specific binding curves of ANP_{1-28} in the kidney cortex and the dose response curves of all the known renal effects of the peptide in this preparation [27]. Indeed, the effects of atrial natriuretic peptide on glomerular filtration rate, sodium excretion and the other measured functional parameters were detectable at near physiological concentrations of the hormone (10^{-11}M) and the ED_{50} of these effects was similar to the K_d of atrial natriuretic peptide binding to the kidney cortex. This indicates that the binding affinity of ANP_{1-28} closely estimates the physiological affinity of the biological receptors of atrial natriuretic peptide in the kidney cortex. However, as will be described below, only a minority of the high affinity binding sites of ANP_{1-28} in kidney cortex mediate the known renal effects of the hormone.

Clearance receptors (C-ANF receptors)

The issue of the rôle of the majority of the renal receptors of atrial natriuretic peptide was addressed by using a ring deleted analogue of atrial natriuretic peptide (C-ANP_{4-23}) whose aminoacid sequence is depicted in Figure 3. This analogue binds extensively to endothelial, vascular smooth muscle and glomerular mesangial cells in culture but does not generate cGMP or antagonize the cGMP-generating effect of biologically active ANP_{1-28} in these cells [28,29]. Recent studies by Lewicki et al [28] demonstrated that C-ANP_{4-23} binds only to one class of atrial natriuretic peptide receptors, the 60kDa receptor, whereas ANP_{1-28} binds both to the 60kDa and the 120kDa receptor. The latter is the cGMP coupled receptor (B-ANF receptor) and probably mediates the biological effects

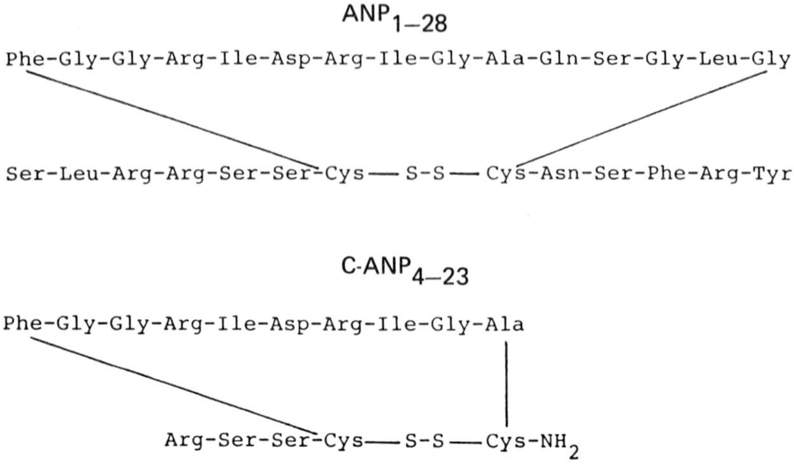

Figure 3. Aminoacid sequence of ANP_{1-28} and C-ANP_{4-23}. ANP_{1-28} is the endogenous biologically active form of atrial natriuretic peptide. C-ANP_{4-23} is a truncated synthetic analogue of atrial natriuretic peptide used to unveil the presence of clearance receptors of atrial natriuretic peptide. See text for description

of atrial natriuretic peptide [30]. The 60kDa receptor was recently purified, sequenced, cloned, and expressed in *Xenopus* oocytes [28].

In the isolated rat kidney preparation, C-ANP_{4-23} binds with high affinity to more than 95% of the specific binding sites of biologically active ANP_{1-28} in whole kidney tissue and kidney cortex and to approximately 60% of the binding sites of ANP_{1-28} in the renal papilla [26]. Even at maximal occupancy of binding sites, the analogue is devoid of any known renal action and does not antagonize or potentiate any of the known renal haemodynamic and natriuretic effects of ANP_{1-28} [26]. On the basis of these results we concluded that the overwhelming majority of atrial natriuretic peptide receptors in whole kidney tissue and kidney cortex are biologically silent since they do not mediate any of the known renal actions of the hormone [26]. Several lines of evidence demonstrated that the major rôle of C-ANF receptors is to serve as clearance receptors (C-ANF receptors) and in this manner remove endogenous atrial natriuretic peptide from the circulation:

1. Blockage of C-ANF receptors by administration of C-ANP_{4-23} to intact conscious or anaesthetized rats markedly increased plasma levels of endogenous immunoreactive (ir)ANP in a reversible manner [26].
2. Contrary to its ineffectiveness in the isolated kidney, administration of C-ANP_{4-23} to anaesthetized rats led to a reversible increase in natriuresis and a decrease in blood pressure which accompanied pari passu the changes in plasma levels of endogenous irANP [26].

3. Administration of C-ANP_{4-23} to rats markedly reduced the volume of distribution and metabolic clearance rate of administered ^{125}I-ANP_{1-28} [30].

4. Finally, in anaesthetized rats, C-ANP_{4-23} inhibited in a dose-related manner the appearance of ^{125}I-monoiodotyrosine in plasma after the administration of ^{125}I-ANP_{1-28} [30].

C-ANF receptors: physiological and therapeutic implications

Although the above evidence does not rule out that C-ANF receptors may mediate some unknown action of atrial natriuretic peptide, it demonstrates unequivocally that they are involved in the removal of atrial natriuretic peptide from the circulation. Clearance receptors are well defined entities as far as circulating glycoproteins and lipoproteins are concerned but, to my knowledge, this is the first evidence of the presence of a separate class of clearance receptors for a peptide hormone. Some of the possible implications of this novel finding are briefly described below.

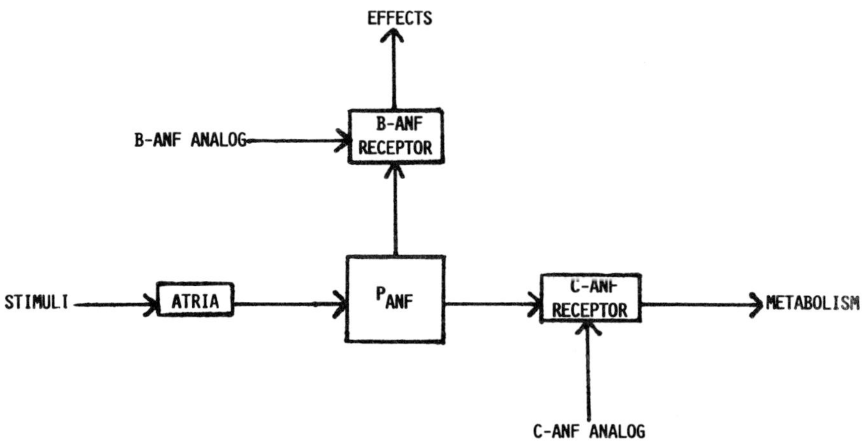

Figure 4. Biological (B) and clearance (C) receptors of atrial natriuretic peptide. B-ANF receptors are the minority of total receptor population of atrial natriuretic peptide and mediate its biological effects. C-ANF receptors are the overwhelming majority of the total atrial natriuretic effect receptors and are involved in the removal of atrial natriuretic peptide from the circulation and its eventual metabolism. C-ANF receptors act as a hormonal buffer system to modulate plasma levels of atrial natriuretic peptide. Analogues which bind only to C-ANF receptors increase plasma levels of endogenous atrial natriuretic peptide (P_{ANP}) by decreasing its metabolic clearance rate. See text for further description

As depicted schematically in Figure 4, plasma levels of atrial natriuretic peptide are determined by the balance between the secretion and metabolic clearance rates of the hormone. Our studies demonstrate that the latter is essentially mediated by binding of atrial natriuretic peptide to C-ANF receptors. These receptors are responsible for the very large volume of distribution and the high metabolic clearance rate of atrial natriuretic peptide. On the other hand, B-ANF receptors which constitute a minority of the specific binding sites of atrial natriuretic peptide, mediate the biological effects of the hormone. Observed discrepancies between binding of atrial peptide and generation of cGMP [22, 23] are likely due to the presence of the very large proportion of C-ANF in relationship to B-ANF receptors [26]. Consequently, these discrepancies do not necessarily imply that cGMP cannot be the sole mediator of the biological action of atrial natriuretic peptide.

The discovery of C-ANF receptors has important implications for studies on receptor regulation. Indeed, down regulation of C-ANF receptors would have physiological consequences which are exactly opposite to those of down regulation of B-ANF receptors. The former would have a positive impact since it would decrease removal of atrial natriuretic peptide from the circulation and, consequently, plasma levels of atrial natriuretic peptide would tend to increase (Figure 4). On the other hand, down regulation of B-ANF receptors would have a negative effect by decreasing the end-organ actions of the hormone.

A potential therapeutic implication of the discovery of C-ANF receptors is that administration of analogues such as C-ANP$_{4\text{-}23}$, which bind to these receptors but not to B-ANF receptors, leads to an increase in plasma levels of endogenous atrial natriuretic peptide [26]. One obvious advantage of such an approach is that the structural requirements of atrial peptides for binding to C-ANF receptors are far less stringent than those for binding to B-ANF receptors. Consequently, the task of developing therapeutically useful analogues may be greatly simplified.

Probably, the most important implication of our finding is that C-ANF receptors may act as a hormonal buffer system to modulate plasma levels of atrial natriuretic peptide. The physiological rôle of such function is far from clear but it is hoped that future research in this area will bring exciting new avenues for the understanding of the homeostasis of atrial natriuretic peptide and perhaps that of other peptide hormones.

Acknowledgments
Research supported by NIH grant AM14241 and by a grant from California Biotechnology Inc, Mountain View, CA, USA.

References

1 Maack T, Camargo MJF, Kleinert HD et al. Atrial natriuretic factor: structure and functional properties. *Kidney Int 1985; 27:* 607–615

2 Needleman P, Adams SP, Cole BR et al. Atriopeptins as cardiac hormones. *Hypertension 1985; 7:* 469–482

3 Maack T. Atrial natriuretic factor: a physiological link between the heart and the kidney. In Bromm B, Lubbers DW, eds. *Physiologie Aktuell, Vol 2.* Stuttgart: Gustav Fisher Verlag. 1986: 59–85

4 Maack T, Kleinert HD. Renal and cardiovascular effects of atrial natriuretic factor. *Biochem Pharmacol 1986; 35:* 2057–2064

5 Atlas SA, Maack T. Effects of atrial natriuretic factor on the kidney and the renin-angiotensin-aldosterone system. In Rosenblatt M, Jacobs JW, eds. *Endocrinology and Clinics of North America, Vol 16: Atrial Natriuretic Factor.* Philadelphia: WB Saunders. 1987: 107–144

6 de Bold AJ, Borenstein HB, Veress AT et al. A rapid and potent natriuretic response to intravenous injection of atrial myocardial extract in rats. *Life Sci 1981; 28:* 89–94

7 Camargo MJF, Kleinert HD, Atlas SA et al. Ca-dependent hemodynamic and natriuretic effects of atrial extract in the isolated rat kidney. *Am J Physiol 1984; 246:* F447–F456

8 Burnett JC Jr, Granger JP, Opgenorth TS. Effects of synthetic atrial natriuretic factor on renal function and renin release. *Am J Physiol 1984; 247:* F863–F866

9 Sonnenberg H, Honrath U, Chong CK et al. Atrial natriuretic factor inhibits sodium transport in medullary collecting ducts. *Am J Physiol 1986; 250:* F963–F966

10 Huang CL, Lewicki J, Johnson LK et al. Renal mechanism of action of atrial natriuretic factor. *J Clin Invest 1985; 75:* 769–773

11 Dunn BR, Ischikawa I, Pfeffer SM et al. Renal and systemic hemodynamic effects of synthetic atrial natriuretic peptide in the anesthetized rat. *Circ Res 1986; 59:* 237–246

12 Fried TA, McCoy RN, Osgood RW et al. Effect of atriopeptin II on determinants of glomerular filtration rate in the in vitro perfused dog glomerulus. *Am J Physiol 1986; 250:* F1119–F1122

13 Zeidel MI, Seifter JL, Lear S et al. Atrial peptides inhibit oxygen consumption in kidney medullary collecting ducts. *Am J Physiol 1986; 251:* F379–F383

14 Nogoguchi H, Knepper MA, Manganiello VC. Effects of atrial natriuretic factor on cyclic guanosine monophosphate and cyclic adenosine monophosphate accumulation in microdissected nephron segments from rats. *J Clin Invest 1987; 79:* 500–507

15 Rocha AS, Kudo IM. Direct effect of atrial natriuretic factor (ANF) on Na, Cl and H_2O in papillary collecting ducts. *Abstracts Xth Int Congress Nephrology.* London. 1987: 218

16 Maack T, Marion DN, Camargo MJF et al. Effects of auriculin (atrial natriuretic factor) on blood pressure, renal function, and the renin-aldosterone system in dogs. *Am J Med 1984; 77:* 1069–1075

17 Camargo MJF, Atlas SA, Maack T. Role of increased glomerular filtration rate in atrial natriuretic factor-induced natriuresis in the rat. *Life Sci 1986; 38:* 2397–2404

18 Sosa RE, Volpe M, Marion DN et al. Relationship between renal hemodynamic and natriuretic effects of atrial natriuretic factor. *Am J Physiol 1986; 250:* F520–F524

19 Suzuki M, Almeida FA, Maack T. Amiloride potentiates the maximal natriuretic effects of ANF and abolishes its kaliuretic action in isolated perfused rat kidney. *Abstract Second World Congress of Biologically Active Atrial Peptides.* New York. 1987: 213

20 Almeida FA, Suzuki M, Maack T. Atrial natriuretic factor increased hematocrit and decreases plasma volume in nephrectomized rats. *Life Sci 1986; 39:* 1193–1199

21 Huxley VH, Tucker VL, Verburg KM, Freeman RH. Increased capillary hydraulic conductivity induced by atrial natriuretic peptide. *Circ Res 1987; 60:* 304–307

22 Scarborough RM, Schenk BB, McEnroe GA et al. Truncated atrial natriuretic peptide analogs. *J Biol Chem 1986; 261:* 12960–12964

23 Murad F. Cyclic guanosine monophosphate as a mediator of vasodilation. *J Clin Invest 1986; 78:* 1–5

24 Napier MA, Vandlen RL, Albert-Schonberg G et al. Specific membrane receptors for atrial natriuretic factor in renal and vascular tissues. *Proc Natl Acad Sci USA 1985; 81:* 5946–5950

25 Jacobs JW, Vlasuk GP, Rosenblatt M. Atrial natriuretic factor receptors. In Rosenblatt M, Jacobs JW, eds. *Endocrinology and Clinics of North America, Vol 16: Atrial Natriuretic Factor.* Philadelphia: W B Saunders. 1987: 63–68

26 Maack T, Suzuki M, Almeida FA et al. Physiological role of silent receptors of atrial natriuretic factor. *Science.* In press

27 Suzuki M, Almeida FA, Nussenzveig D et al. Binding and functional effects of atrial natriuretic factor in isolated rat kidney. *Am J Physiol [Renal Fluid Electrolyte Physiol]*. In press

28 Lewicki JA, Scarborough R, Fuller F et al. Pharmacological and biochemical studies of ANF receptor subpopulations. *Abstract Second World Congress of Biologically Active Atrial Peptides.* New York. 1987: 187

29 Nussenzveig D, Scarborough R, Lewicki J, Maack T. Clearance receptors of atrial natriuretic factor (C-ANF receptors) in isolated glomeruli and mesangial cells in culture. *Abstract 20th Congress of the American Society of Nephrology.* Washington DC. 1987. In press

30 Almeida FA, Suzuki M, Scarborough R et al. C-ANF receptors are specific binding sites involved in the metabolic clearance rate and modulation of plasma levels of ANF. *Abstract Second World Congress of Biologically Active Atrial Peptides.* New York. 1987: 187

Editorial note. The term atrial natriuretic peptide has been used throughout this publication. In this paper the author has specifically named a receptor C-ANF receptor – see under 'Clearance receptors (C-ANF receptors)' – so the abbreviation ANF for atrial natriuretic factor has been kept.

NATRIURETIC FACTORS OTHER THAN ATRIAL NATRIURETIC PEPTIDE

H E de Wardener

Charing Cross and Westminster Medical School, London, United Kingdom

There is little doubt that, in addition to the atrial natriuretic peptide, the plasma contains other natriuretic substances, changes in the physiological concentration of which induce changes in urinary sodium excretion. One of these appears to be MSH which I will come back to at the end of this account.

Once a substance has been identified the direction of events has a certain logic and is relatively circumscribed. On the other hand, when trying to isolate and structure an active but elusive substance circulating in the plasma, progress is apt to be disorderly and tortuous. Unless one is working in the same field, it may be difficult to discern what is going on. I think a glance at the history of the subject helps understanding.

The earliest experiments which suggested that the plasma could acquire natriuretic properties were performed by expanding the volume of body fluids with large amounts of saline [1]. The inconvertible evidence which demonstrated that the plasma contains at least one natriuretic substance came from subsequent blood volume expansion experiments with equilibrated blood when a natriuresis was obtained from a kidney that was denervated and perfused at controlled pressure [2,3].

Subsequently urinary extracts were prepared [4]. Two natriuretic factors were obtained. One caused a natriuresis of rapid onset and duration and the other a delayed natriuresis with a prolonged action. Atrial natriuretic peptide induces a natriuresis of relatively rapid onset and of short duration. Nevertheless though plasma atrial natriuretic peptide rises with acute volume expansion to levels which are known to be natriuretic there is still some doubt whether the acute natriuresis which follows acute volume expansion with intravenous saline is due only to, or even predominantly to, the effect of increase in atrial natriuretic peptide. Recently Sosa et al [5] have observed in the dog that the natriuretic effect of atrial natriuretic peptide can be abolished by lowering the renal perfusion pressure to around 95mmHg [1]. On the other hand we showed some years ago that the natriuretic effect of a saline infusion to a dog (in contrast to a dehydrated rat) cannot be abolished by lowering the arterial pressure below 90mmHg. Furthermore Lever [personal communication] has recently demonstrated that an infusion of saline usually causes a natriuresis much more quickly than giving atrial natriuretic peptide intravenously.

To add to the confusion there is the observation of Hirth and her colleagues that an antibody raised against atrial natriuretic peptide abolishes the natriuresis of a volume expansion induced by 20ml of blood, or saline, given in two minutes to a rat [6]. This is an enormous and very rapid volume expansion which it is difficult to compare with the more moderate volume expansion procedures which are usually used. Yet it is a fascinating observation which certainly diminishes the importance of the so-called physical factors in the natriuresis of acute volume expansion. But it also seems to exclude the participation of any other hormonal natriuretic mechanism. It will be interesting to see what happens next for there *are* certainly other natriuretic substances in the plasma which control urinary sodium excretion in response to changes of volume.

The presence of a delayed action long-acting natriuretic substance in the plasma was first demonstrated in plasma extracts by Verress et al [7] and subsequently by Knock [8] in whole plasma. In Knock's experiment an increase in the blood volume of the rat was induced by an infusion of equilibrated blood. This caused a brisk natriuresis which was maximal at 60 minutes. At this time 2ml of blood was removed from the equilibrating reservoir. It was spun and the resultant 1ml of plasma was injected intravenously into a 300g dehydrated anaesthetized rat which did not receive any other intravenous fluid. There was a gradual rise in sodium excretion which became significant after one hour and was still rising at the end of the second hour. It was concluded that blood volume expansion appears to give rise to a potent natriuretic substance in the plasma, which has a delayed and prolonged effect. This substance cannot be the atrial natriuretic peptide. Little is known about the nature of this long-acting natriuretic substance. There is some evidence that it may be due to a small molecule of about 1500 daltons [7] bound to a large one of about 30,000 daltons [9].

Interwoven between these experiments there were others which demonstrated that acute blood volume expansion with equilibrated blood [10] or saline [11], or a high sodium intake [12,13] endowed the plasma not only with natriuretic properties but also with an increased capacity to inhibit sodium transport and Na/K-ATPase activity. This was demonstrated by studying the effect of whole blood or plasma or extracts of plasma on fragments of renal tubules, sections of kidneys, anuran membranes, erythrocytes and leucocytes and more recently cultures of smooth muscle [4].

For some years it was generally assumed that the natriuretic capacity of the plasma following acute volume expansion, or an increase in sodium intake, was due to a change in the concentration of the same substance as that which was responsible for the inhibition of Na/K-ATPase. This conclusion was fostered not only because it seemed reasonable, but also because initial fractionation procedures showed that the natriuretic activity appeared in the same fraction as the sodium transport, or Na/K-ATPase inhibiting activity. The assumption that the natriuretic and sodium transport inhibiting activities were due to the same substance was so deeply ingrained that, in some refereed papers, the authors were allowed to state that the natriuretic activity of their extract was assayed on the short circuit current of the frog skin or the toad bladder. When atrial natriuretic peptides appeared, therefore, it was something of a surprise to find that they do not inhibit Na/K-ATPase [14,15].

The hunt for the relevant circulating Na/K-ATPase inhibitor has been pursued for about 15 years. It is beset by many hazards. One principal cause of confusion is that the plasma contains numerous Na/K-ATPase inhibitors. Some have yet to be identified while others such as cholesterol, ascorbic acid, fatty acids and steroids are well recognized inhibitors of Na/K-ATPase. A recent finding of interest is that the plasma concentration of certain fatty acids rises with volume expansion [16] or a high salt diet [17] and that some fatty acids are natriuretic. It is not clear at the moment, however, whether the rise in plasma concentration of the potentially natriuretic fatty acids is within the natriuretic range.

The search continues. There is a general agreement that other substances than fatty acids are also involved. We are also agreed that we are not all pursuing the same substance. This is not surprising for the various workers in the field do not share the same aims, and our methods of detection differ. For these reasons I think it is best if I confine myself to our own work. For the past few years, we have used two cytochemical techniques to detect a substance which we consider may be relevant. One is a direct semi-quantitative assay which measures Na/K-ATPase activity in the proximal tubule of fresh guinea pig kidney [18]. An inhibition of Na/K-ATPase in an intact cell is associated with stimulation of glucose-6-phosphate dehydrogenase (G6PD) we have also measured G6PD activity at the same location [19]. This second cytochemical procedure has enabled us to validate a quantitative assay for a circulating cytochemically detectable stimulator of G6PD after two minutes of exposure in the plasma, hypothalamus and urine [20] which is an index of their capacity to inhibit Na/K-ATPase at four to six minutes. These two assays have a certain degree of selectivity. Though they cross react with ouabain they do not do so with any other known plasma substance so far tested, including several others which are known to inhibit purified preparations of Na/K-ATPase, such as vanadate, linoleic acid, lysophosphatidyl choline and dehydroepiandrosterone [20,21], some of which are known to be natriuretic.

Many organs have been examined in order to try and find the source of the substance responsible for the plasma Na/K-ATPase inhibiting activity. The only tissue which has yielded extracts of high activity is the hypothalamus. The time course of the effect of the hypothalamic extract is the same as that of plasma and the dose response is parallel.

The active substance in both the hypothalamus and the plasma has a molecular weight below 500 daltons, is not destroyed by heating in 6N HCl at 105°C for 18 hours or by several proteolytic enzymes, but it is destroyed by treatment with NaOH and ashing at 600°C, and on extraction the activity appears in the same fraction on silica gel electrophoresis [21]. Using these cytochemical techniques we have shown that: 1) a high sodium intake in man and the rat increases the plasma's concentration of the cytochemically detectable inhibitor of Na/K-ATPase [12]; 2) the hypothalamus is the only site in the rat which contains high concentrations of the inhibitor [20], and 3) the content of the inhibitor in the hypothalamus rises substantially when the rat is placed on a high sodium diet [22]. The plasma concentration of the cytochemically detectable Na/K-ATPase inhibitor is raised in essential hypertension [23] in the Okamoto spontaneously hypertensive rat (SHR) [24] and in the Milan hypertensive rat [25]. In the latter the plasma level rises before the rise in arterial pressure. It is also greatly raised in the plasma of the reduced renal mass hypertensive rat on a high sodium diet [unpublished observation]. And we have observed that the hypothalamus of the SHR rat has extremely high concentrations of activity, much greater than in a normal rat on a high sodium intake [24]. Thus in the normal rat the cytochemically detectable Na/K-ATPase inhibiting/G6PD stimulating activity in the plasma and hypothalamus is increased by a high sodium intake. Similarly in the SHR rat the Na/K-ATPase inhibiting/G6PD stimulating activity is increased in both the plasma *and* the hypothalamus. These additional similarities and the relative selectivity of these assays increase the likelihood that the cytochemically assayable Na/K-ATPase inhibiting/G6PD stimulating activity in the plasma and the hypothalamus is due to the same substance. We do not yet know what class of compound it is but we are pretty confident that it is not a peptide or a fatty acid. We have very recently obtained sufficient amounts of highly purified hypothalamic extract to enable us to infuse it intravenously into a whole 300g rat for one hour. Preliminary experiments show that this causes a sustained increase in blood pressure of about 10mmHg and a substantial natriuresis. If these initial observations are confirmed it looks as if the cytochemically assayable Na/K-ATPase inhibitor in the hypothalamus, which we consider is probably the same substance as that which is present in the plasma, both of which are influenced by sodium intake, is natriuretic and can raise the arterial pressure. In addition, Baylis et al [26] have found that our hypothalamic extract has another biological activity. It interferes with the effect of vasopressin on the thick ascending limb of the collecting duct. Their initial observation was that arginine vasopressin at a dilution of 10 to 10 produced a cytochemically detectable stimulation of Na/K-ATPase in the thick ascending limb of the rat kidney at 10 minutes, an effect which could be blocked by the addition of an antiserum against arginine vasopressin. Only medullary

ATPase activity appeared to be responsive to arginine vasopressin, no changes in proximal or distal convoluted tubular ATPase activity were observed [27].

This made it possible to validate a cytochemical technique with which to assay plasma vasopressin [28] with a rectolinear dose response curve between concentrations of 0.01 to 10fmol/L. The cytochemical assay correlated well with radioimmunoassays when vasopressin was added to plasma, and when the plasma level of vasopressin was altered by changes in hydration. Subsequently, however, Baylis, Pippard and Burd [29] observed that when plasma AVP was raised by an intravenous infusion of approximately 500ml of hypertonic saline (850mmol/L) to a 70kg man in two hours the expected rise in plasma radio-immunoassayable AVP was not accompanied by any change in plasma AVP as measured by the cytochemical technique [30]. Addition of synthetic AVP to plasma obtained after hypertonic saline infusion also failed to stimulate Na/K-ATPase activity. This suggested that the inability of AVP to stimulate Na/K-ATPase was due to the plasma having acquired a Na/K-ATPase inhibiting capacity as a result of the considerable volume expansion associated with the infusion of hypertonic saline.

The ability of AVP to stimulate thick ascending limb Na/K-ATPase was then tested when mixed with our hypothalamic extract. Though the extract can be shown to inhibit proximal tubule Na/K-ATPase after four to six minutes of exposure it has no effect on the thick ascending limb at the 10 minutes exposure used in the AVP assay. Nevertheless, when the thick ascending limb was exposed for 10 minutes to both AVP and the hypothalamic extract the ability of AVP to stimulate Na/K-ATPase was inhibited.

Now to melanocyte stimulating hormone (MSH). MSH peptides, including MSH have been shown to possess natriuretic properties for about 15 years [31]. The possibility that γMSH resides in the N terminal portion of the ACTH/B endorphine precursor molecule pro-opiomelanocortin. Instead of using some form of volume expansion as their model, Humphreys and his colleagues have studied the brief natriuresis which follows 30 to 60 minutes after acute unilateral nephrectomy [33]. They have performed a series of logical experiments which suggest, in that setting, that MSH may be a natriuretic hormone.

Their initial observations established that acute post-nephrectomy natriuresis was a reflex involving the renal nerves not only of the kidney that is removed, but also of the kidney that remains suggesting that both afferent and efferent renal nerves are involved in the reflex [34]. They then deduced that the reflex involved the central nervous opoid pathways for naloxone perfused into the cerebral ventricles abolished the reflex [35]. Furthermore, the reflex was not seen in hypophysectomized animals [36]. More recently they have developed a radioimmunoassay for γMSH [37] and have shown that: 1) after acute unilateral nephrectomy the plasma level of γMSH rises from about 40fmol/ml to 80fmol/ml; 2) there is a significant correlation between the rise in plasma γMSH and the urinary sodium excretion; 3) the natriuresis is blocked in rats treated with serum from animals immunized against γMSH, and 4) the administration of γMSH into the renal artery at a rate which should raise the renal plasma concentration of γMSH within the physiological range causes a natriuresis [unpublished observations].

Lin and colleagues conclude that acute unilateral nephrectomy triggers the release of γMSH, presumably from the anterior pituitary, into the circulation [36,37]. It is likely that the natriuresis is due to inhibition of tubular reabsorption of sodium for it is established that post-nephrectomy natriuresis occurs without an increase in glomerular filtration rate or renal plasma flow.

In conclusion, concepts about the control of body fluid volume, and its relation to hypertension are undergoing a major revolution. In this field the identification of the atrial natriuretic peptides and the recognition of their importance in the natriuresis of volume expansion has some points of resemblance with the fall of the Bastille. Things will never be the same again. It will be interesting to see what happens next.

References

1 de Wardener HE, Mills IH, Clapham WF, Hayter CJ. Studies on the efferent mechanism of the sodium diuresis which follows the administration of intravenous saline in the dog. *Clin Sci 1961; 21:* 249–258

2 Bahlman JS, McDonald J, Ventom MG, de Wardener HE. The effect on urinary sodium excretion of blood volume expansion without changing the composition of the blood in the dog. *Clin Sci 1967; 32:* 403–413

3 Kaloyanides GJ, Azer M. Evidence for a humoral mechanism in volume expansion natriuresis. *J Clin Invest 1971; 50:* 1603–1612

4 de Wardener HE, Clarkson EM. Concept of natriuretic hormone. *Physiol Rev 1985; 65:* 659–745

5 Sosa RE, Volpe M, Marion DN et al. Relationship between renal haemodynamics and natriuretic effects of atrial natriuretic factor. *Am J Physiol 1986; 250:* F520–F524

6 Hirth C, Stasch J-P, Kazda S et al. Blockade of the response to volume expansion by monoclonal antibodies against natriuretic peptide. *Klin Wochenschr 1987; 65 (Suppt VIII):* 87–91

7 Veress AT, Milojevic S, Sonnenberg H. Characterisation of the natriuretic activity in the plasma of hypervolaemic rats. *Clin Sci 1980; 59:* 183–189

8 Knock CA. Further evidence in vivo for a circulating antinatriuretic substance after expanding the blood volume in rats. *Clin Sci 1980; 59:* 423–433

9 Pearce JW, Sonnenberg H, Veress AT, Ackerman U. Evidence for a humoral factor modifying the renal response to blood volume expansion. *Can J Physiol Pharmacol 1969; 47:* 377–386

10 Clarkson EM, Talner LB, de Wardener HE. The effect of plasma from blood volume expanded dogs on sodium, potassium and PAH transport of renal tubule fragments. *Clin Sci 1970; 38:* 617–627

11 Buckalew VM, Martinez J, Green WS. The effect of dialysates and ultrafiltrates of plasma of saline-loaded dogs on toad bladder sodium transport. *J Clin Invest 1970; 49:* 926–935

12 de Wardener HE, Clarkson EM, Bitensky L et al. Effect of sodium intake on ability of human plasma to inhibit Na-K-adenosine triphosphatase in vitro. *Lancet 1981; i:* 411–412

13 Poston L, Wilkinson S, Sewell RB, Williams R. Sodium transport during the natriuresis of volume expansion in a study using peripheral blood leucocytes. *Clin Sci 1982; 63:* 243–249

14 Pollock DM, Mullins MM, Banks RO. Failure of atrial myocardial extract to inhibit renal Na-K-ATPase. *Renal Physiol 1983; 6:* 295–299

15 Thibault G, Garcia R, Cantin M, Genest J. Atrial natriuretic factor. Characterisation and partial purification. *Hypertension 1983 (Suppt I):* 175–180

16 Tamura M, Kuwano H, Kinoshita T, Inagami I. Identification of linoleic and oleic acids as endogenous Na,K-ATPase inhibits from acute volume expanded dog plasma. *J Biol Chem 1985; 260:* 9672–9677

17 Wauquier I, Pernollet M-G, Delva P et al. High sodium diet and circulating digitalis-like compound in the rat. *J Hypertension 1986; 4:* 463–469

18 Chayen J, Frost GI, Dodds RA et al. The use of hidden metalcapture reagent for the measurement of a Na-K-ATPase activity in a new concept of cytochemistry. *Histochem 1981; 71:* 533–541

19 Dikstein S. Stimulability, adenosine triphosphatases and their control by cellular redox processes. *Naturwissenschaften 1971; 58:* 439–443

20 Fenton S, Clarkson EM, MacGregor GA et al. An assay of the capacity of biological fluids to stimulate renal glucose-6-phosphate dehydrogenase activity in vitro as a marker of their ability to inhibit sodium potassium-dependent-adenosine triphosphatase activity. *J Endocrinol 1982; 94:* 99–110

21 Millett JA, Holland SM, Alaghband-Zadeh J, de Wardener HE. Extraction and characterization of a cytochemically assayable Na/K-ATPase inhibitor/glucose-6-phosphate dehydrogenase stimulator in the hypothalamus and plasma of man and the rat. *J Endocrinol 1987; 112:* 299–303

22 Alaghband-Zadeh J, Fenton S, Hancock K. Evidence that the hypothalamus may be a source of a circulating Na-K-ATPase inhibitor. *J Endocrinol 1983; 98:* 221–226

23 MacGregor GA, Fenton S, Alaghband-Zadeh J et al. An increase in a circulating inhibitor of Na,K-dependent ATPase: a possible link between salt intake and the development of essential hypertension. *Clin Sci 1981; 61:* S17–S20

24 Millett JA, Holland SM, Alaghband-Zadeh J, de Wardener HE. Na-K-ATPase-inhibiting and glucose-6-phosphate dehydrogenase-stimulating activity of plasma and hypothalamus of the Okamoto spontaneously hypertensive rat. *J Endocrinol 1986; 108:* 69–73

25 Holland SM, Millett J, Alaghband-Zadeh J et al. Cytochemically assayable Na-K-ATPase inhibition by Milan hypertensive rat plasma. *Hypertension 1987; 9:* 498–503

26 Baylis PH, Pitchfork J, Chayen J, Bitensky L. A cytochemical bioassay for arginine vasopressin: preliminary studies. *J Immunol 1980; 1:* 399–411

27 Pippard C, Baylis PH. The stimulation of Na-K-ATPase activity in the medulla of the rat kidney by (arginine) vasopressin and its analogues. *Clin Sci 1984; 66:* 561–567

28 Baylis PH, Pippard C, Gill GV, Burd J. Development of a cytochemical assay for plasma vasopressin: application to studies in water loading in man. *Clin Endocrinol 1986; 24:* 383–393

29 Baylis PH, Pippard C, Burd JM. Interference in the cytochemical assay of plasma vasopressin by a circulating factor induced by salt loading in man. *J Endocrinol 1986; 111:* 495–499

30 Pippard C, Baylis PH. Rat hypothalamic extract inhibits vasopressin-stimulated Na-K-ATPase activity in the rat renal medulla. *Cell Biochem Func 1986; 4:* 25–29

31 Orias R, McCann SM. Natriuresis induced by alpha and beta melanocyte stimulating hormone (MSH) in rats. *Endocrinol 1972; 90:* 700–706

32 Gruber KA, Klein MC, Hutchins PM et al. Natriuretic and hypertensive activities reside in a fragment of ACTH. *Hypertension 1984; 6:* 468–474

33 Humphreys MH, Ayus JC. Role of haemodynamic changes in the increased cation excretion after acute unilateral nephrectomy in the anaesthetised dog. *J Clin Invest 1978; 61:* 590–596

34 Ribstein J, Humphreys MH. Renal nerves and cation secretion after acute reduction in renal functioning mass of the rat. *Am J Physiol 1984; 246:* F260–F265

35 Lin S-Y, Humphreys MH. Centrally administered naloxone blocks reflex natriuresis after acute unilateral nephrectomy. *Am J Physiol 1985; 249:* F390–F395

36 Lin S-Y, Wiedeman E, Humphreys MH. Role of the pituitary in reflex natriuresis following acute unilateral nephrectomy. *Am J Physiol 1985; 249:* F282–F290

37 Lin S-Y, Chaves C, Weideman E, Humphreys MH. Evidence that an immunoreactive γ-MSH-like material (IR-γMSH) participates in reflex natriuresis following acute unilateral nephrectomy (AUN) in the rat. *Clin Research 1986; 34 (Abstract):* 481A

REGULATION OF INNER MEDULLARY COLLECTING DUCT SODIUM TRANSPORT BY ATRIAL NATRIURETIC PEPTIDE

M L Zeidel

Harvard Medical School, Boston, Massachusetts, USA

Atrial natriuretic peptide markedly enhances renal excretion of sodium and water, reduces aldosterone and renin secretion, and suppresses ADII release [1–5]. These actions permit atrial natriuretic peptide to decrease extracellular volume and lower blood pressure.

Despite the fact that atrial natriuretic peptide provokes dramatic increases in renal salt and water excretion in all species tested, the renal mechanisms of action of this peptide remain unclear. However, recent work has revealed two major nephron sites at which atrial natriuretic peptide enhances sodium excretion, the glomerulus and the inner medullary collecting duct.

In most, but not all studies, atrial natriuretic peptide or atrial extract simultaneously increased glomerular filtration rate and sodium excretion [2,3,6–8]. In addition, glomeruli are rich in atrial natriuretic peptide receptors and respond to atrial natriuretic peptides with striking elevations of cGMP [9–12], suggesting a rôle for the glomerulus in the stimulation of natriuresis by atrial natriuretic peptide in vivo. While not excluding effects of atrial natriuretic peptide on more distal segments, these observations have led several authors to conclude that enhanced glomerular filtration is the major renal mechanism of action of atrial natriuretic peptide [2,6,7]. The glomerulus cannot be the only direct site of action of atrial natriuretic peptide, because several studies in multiple species in vivo and in vitro have found that atrial natriuretic peptide can increase sodium excretion without measurably altering glomerular filtration rate [13–19].

Effects of atrial natriuretic peptide on net sodium reabsorption in the inner medullary collecting duct

The inner medullary collecting duct (IMCD) reabsorbs under normal conditions approximately 2% of the glomerular filtrate [20,21]. Although little is known about transport mechanisms in the IMCD, this segment reabsorbs sodium, secretes hydrogen ions and adds urea to the urine [21–30]. Micropuncture,

peptide inhibits sodium entry into IMCD cells, we have measured the accumulation of $^{22}Na^+$ by IMCD cells in the presence and absence of atrial natriuretic peptide or amiloride. In three similar experiments, atrial natriuretic peptide inhibited sodium uptake by 27.0±4.2%, 28.2±1.4%, and 29.4±7.2%, at one, three and five minutes respectively. Inhibition by amiloride at these three time points was 41.5±2.2%, 42.5±4.4% and 47.0±5.4%. Preliminary studies indicate that IMCD cell sodium uptake is sensitive to amiloride, but not to frusemide, bumetanide, or thiazide. Thus, sodium entry in rabbit IMCD cells appears to be mediated by Na/H exchange, electrogenic sodium channels, or both, and not by Na/K/Cl cotransport processes. Measurements of intracellular pH and membrane potential have provided evidence for both Na/H exchange and electrogenic sodium entry mechanisms in IMCD cells; atrial natriuretic peptide appears to inhibit sodium entry via the electrogenic pathway. We have also shown that atrial natriuretic peptide inhibits apical sodium entry by an amiloride-sensitive process in primary cultures of IMCD cells grown on filter bottom supports [41]. Our results with IMCD cells are entirely consistent with those obtained by Cantiello et al in cultures of the renal epithelial cell line, $LLCPK_1$ [47]. In these cells, atrial natriuretic peptide inhibits apical sodium entry via an electrogenic channel.

Thus, atrial natriuretic peptide inhibits sodium entry in IMCD cells via an amiloride-sensitive mechanism, probably an electrogenic sodium channel. This inhibition of sodium entry may contribute, in part to the natriuretic effect of atrial natriuretic peptide in the IMCD.

Mechanisms by which atrial natriuretic peptide regulates inner medullary collecting duct sodium handling-atrial natriuretic peptide receptors

We have begun to characterize specific, highly selective receptors for atrial natriuretic peptide on the surface of IMCD cells. Previous studies have demonstrated specific atrial natriuretic peptide binding sites in rat inner medulla in situ [48–50]. These binding sites have been localized in rat microdissected IMCD segments, and in suspensions enriched in IMCD [45,50]. Atrial natriuretic peptide radioligand binding data in a variety of cell types best fit single site models with a Kd in the 10^{-10}M range [10,11,51–54]. Photoaffinity labelling and the use of crosslinking agents have allowed molecular characterization of the atrial natriuretic peptide receptor from aorta, lung and adrenal [54–56]. Specific covalent labelling occurs in peptides of two sizes, 60,000–70,000, and 130,000 daltons. In rat lung endothelial cells, a receptor of 130,000 daltons appears to be tightly linked to particulate guanylate cyclase [57]. Adaptation of atrial natriuretic peptide receptor density but not Kd in response to atrial natriuretic levels has been shown in cultured aortic smooth muscle cells and in isolated glomeruli [10,11,53].

Using equilibrium binding techniques, we have recently begun to characterize IMCD atrial natriuretic peptide receptors [40]. At 22°C, binding of ^{125}I-ANP_{1-28}

to IMCD cells reached apparent equilibrium at 60–90 minutes and remained stable for three hours. Abrupt lowering of extracellular pH to 5.0 caused rapid release of the ligand, indicating a surface binding site. Rebinding experiments revealed preservation of >90% of initial specific activity of ligand bound to the cells as well as free in solution. Binding was saturable with increasing concentrations of radioligand; Scatchard plots were linear (R values averaged 0.97), suggesting a single class of binding sites, or two or more classes of similar affinity. Equilibrium dissociation constants from three such plots averaged 66±3pM, and the number of binding sites per cell, R_O, averaged 3567±222. The apparent dissociation constant agrees well with similar values obtained in vascular smooth muscle and glomeruli; the receptor density is in the range commonly observed for peptide hormones, and represents one-quarter the density of atrial natriuretic peptide receptors reported on mesangial cells.

Studies of the effect of increasing concentration of unlabelled ANP_{1-28} and analogues on binding of radioligand to IMCD cells (competitive binding inhibition) best fit a single site model with Kd of 130pM using ligand analysis, in good agreement with the saturation data. Subtle alterations in peptide structure resulted in striking changes in apparent affinity. Deletion of amino terminal residues (ANP_{4-28} and ANP_{5-28}) did not alter significantly the competition curve. Removal of carboxy terminal residues (ANP_{5-25}), however, resulted in a striking loss in ability to inhibit radioligand binding. Disruption of the disulfide bridge (ANP_{13-28}) abolished binding activity. Similarly, unrelated peptides, such as bradykinin, angiotensin II, and vasopressin exhibited no competitive binding activity.

In preliminary experiments, we have labelled covalently atrial natriuretic peptide receptors with ^{125}I-ANP and analysed the labelling patterns by polyacrylamide gel electrophoresis. Two bands, of molecular weights 130,000 daltons and 76,000 daltons are specifically labelled. The larger molecular weight band has been shown in other cell types to be tightly linked to particulate guanylate cyclase.

Mechanisms by which atrial natriuretic peptide regulates inner medullary collecting duct sodium handling – rôle of cGMP in mediating cellular response to atrial natriuretic peptide

In several atrial natriuretic peptide-responsive tissues, evidence is accumulating that cGMP mediates the actions of these peptides. In vascular smooth muscle, atrial natriuretic peptide elevates cGMP levels prior to inducing vasorelaxation. Atrial natriuretic peptide also stimulates directly particulate guanylate cyclase and cGMP-dependent protein kinase. Finally BrcGMP duplicates the vasorelaxant effects of atrial peptides [58–61]. In teleost intestine, both BrcGMP and atrial natriuretic peptide inhibit Na^+/Cl^- cotransport [62]. In $LLCKP_1$ cells, atrial natriuretic peptide elevates cGMP levels and BrcGMP reproduces the inhibitory effect of atrial natriuretic peptide on sodium entry [47]. In rat lung, atrial natriuretic peptide receptors and guanylate cyclase activity appear to reside in the same macromolecular complex [57].

Because cGMP appears to mediate the actions of atrial natriuretic peptide in a variety of cell types, we examined the rôle of cyclic nucleotides, particularly cGMP in inhibition of IMCD oxygen consumption by atrial natriuretic peptide [39]. We first determined whether analogues of cGMP or cAMP can mimic the inhibitory effect of $hANP_{4-28}$ on IMCD oxygen consumption. BrcGMP (1mM) inhibited oxygen consumption in these cells by 23.5±1.2%. The inhibition exhibited nucleotide specificity, in that only the cGMP analogue altered O_2 consumption; dibutyryl cAMP was without effect on IMCD cells. Like atrial natriuretic peptide, response to BrcGMP was observed only in IMCD cells and not in outer medullary collecting duct cells.

We examined the mechanism of action of BrcGMP and found it duplicates exactly the interaction of hANP with ouabain, amphotericin, and amiloride. We also found that this cGMP analogue did not give additive inhibition with atrial natriuretic peptide. Thus, like atrial natriuretic peptide, BrcGMP appears to inhibit sodium entry in IMCD cells.

If cGMP mediates the actions of atrial natriuretic peptide in IMCD cells, then atrial peptides would be expected to increase intracellular levels of cGMP. We therefore examined the effects of atrial natriuretic peptide on cyclic nucleotide levels in IMCD cells. Basal levels of cGMP were 0.314±0.058pmol/mg protein in IMCD cells (n=16) and 0.666±0.066pmol/mg protein in outer medullary collecting duct cells (n=4). These levels were similar to those obtained in rat glomeruli and whole kidney [33]. Atrial natriuretic peptide (10^{-8}M) stimulated cGMP accumulation 10-fold in IMCD cells in the absence of inhibition of phosphodiesterase. The peptide had little effect on cGMP levels in outer medullary collecting duct cells and did not alter cAMP levels in IMCD cells. These results are similar to those obtained in dog and rabbit IMCD suspensions, and in microdissected rat IMCD.

Following exposure of the cells to 10^{-8}M $hANP_{4-28}$ cellular cGMP levels rose within 10–30 seconds of exposure, reaching maximal levels at two minutes. The inhibition of oxygen consumption observed with hANP began two to four minutes after addition of peptide and reached a maximal value at five to seven minutes. Thus, the elevations of cellular cGMP levels observed with hANP occurred prior to inhibition of oxygen consumption. In all subsequent measurements of cGMP levels, two minute incubations were used.

We next examined the effect of increasing concentrations of $hANP_{4-28}$ and analogues on accumulation of cGMP. These peptides gave the same order of potency for stimulation of cGMP accumulation as for inhibition of oxygen consumption.

A characteristic of cyclic nucleotide-mediated responses to peptide hormones is enhanced effects of submaximal hormone levels in the presence of phosphodiesterase inhibition [63]. Using isobutyl methyl xanthine (IBMX), we determined the effects of phosphodiesterase inhibition on stimulation of cGMP accumulation and inhibition of oxygen consumption by submaximal levels ($<10^{-8}$ M) of $hANP_{4-28}$. IBMX (0.1mM) doubled IMCD cGMP levels, while 10^{-9} M $hANP_{4-28}$ alone gave a three to fourfold elevation. The same level of hANP in the presence of IBMX raised cGMP levels six to sevenfold. In addition to augmenting cGMP accumulation in response to atrial natriuretic peptide, IBMX markedly potentiated the degree of inhibition in oxygen consumption observed with 10^{-9} M hANP. The fact that IBMX potentiates both accumulation of cGAMP and inhibition of oxygen consumption in response to submaximal levels of hANP provides further evidence that cGMP mediates the effect of atrial natriuretic peptide on IMCD cells.

In thoracic aorta, elevation of cGMP levels by exposure to atrial natriuretic peptide or to nitroprusside results in vasorelaxation [60]. Recent studies in this and other tissues have shown that atrial natriuretic peptide stimulates particulate guanylate cyclase, while nitroprusside acts on the soluble form of this enzyme [64]. We therefore exposed IMCD and outer medullary collecting duct cells to nitroprusside and measured cGMP and response of oxygen consumption. Nitroprusside concentrations of 10^{-6} M or higher increased cGMP levels in both IMCD and outer medullary collecting duct cells. By contrast, oxygen consumption was inhibited only in IMCD cells by nitroprusside. These results agree with those described above in that BrcGMP inhibited oxygen consumption only in IMCD cells. Furthermore, these results suggest that stimulation of soluble IMCD guanylate cyclase can mimic the action of atrial natriuretic peptide.

To determine whether atrial natriuretic peptide elevates IMCD cGMP levels by stimulating guanylate cyclase or by inhibiting phosphodiesterase, we have measured guanylate cyclase in homogenates and particulate fractions freshly prepared from IMCD cells. Preliminary results indicate that atrial natriuretic peptide stimulates guanylate cyclase activity up to 10-fold in particulate fractions of IMCD cells. We plan to characterize more fully this guanylate cyclase response and to measure the response of phosphodiesterase to atrial natriuretic peptide as well.

It is clear that freshly prepared suspensions of IMCD cells provide an excellent experimental model for examining the mechanisms of atrial natriuretic peptide action in epithelial cells. Cells can be prepared rapidly and inexpensively and in sufficient quantity for biochemical studies. In addition, the results of tracer sodium uptakes and of ouabain-sensitive oxygen consumption can be directly correlated with biochemical events in the same cell preparations. We have shown that atrial natriuretic peptide inhibits oxygen consumption in IMCD cells. The inhibition exhibited selectivity for cell type and for peptide structure and occurred at peptide levels similar to those described in other atrial natriuretic peptide-responsive cells types. Atrial natriuretic peptide reduced oxygen consumption by impeding sodium entry, via sodium channels or Na/H exchange.

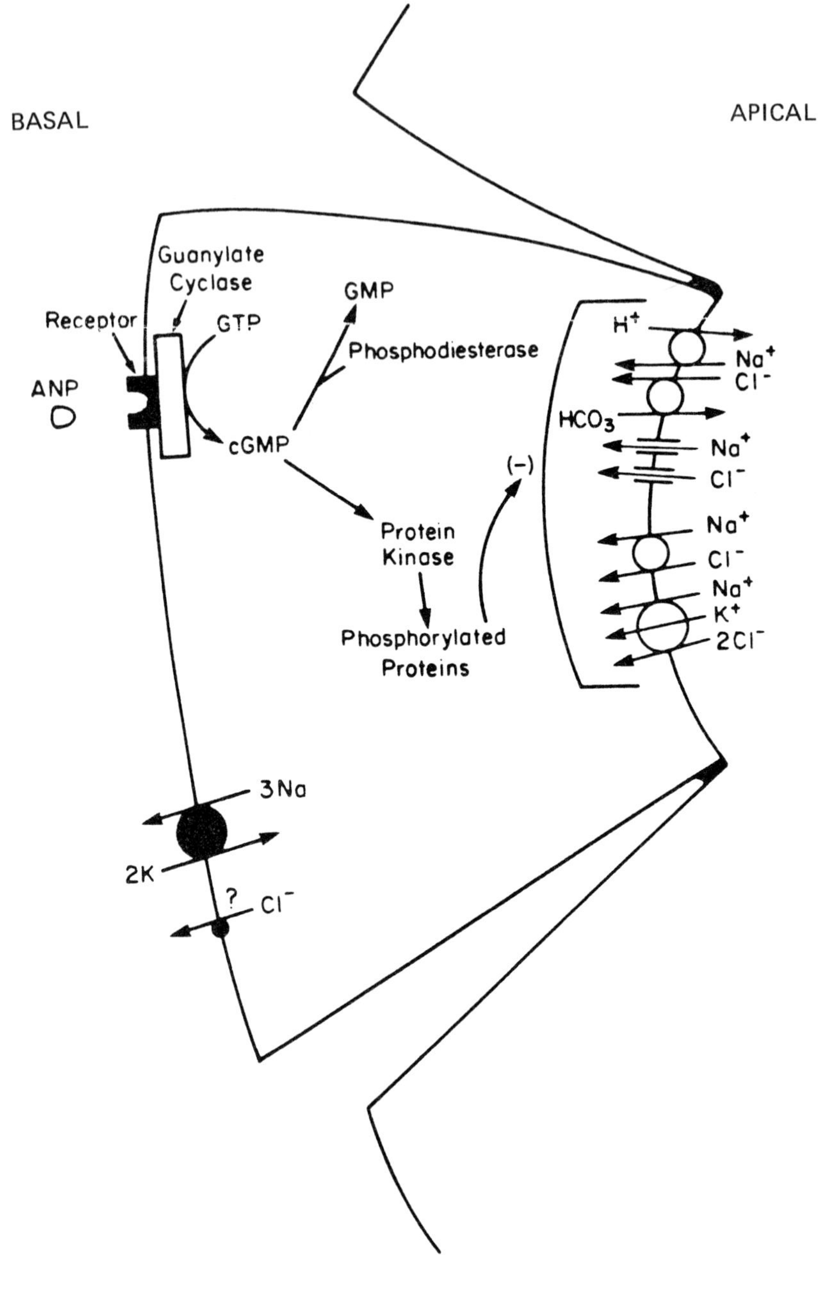

Figure 1. Model of regulation of IMCD sodium transport by atrial natriuretic peptide. See text for details

This impression was confirmed by our demonstration that atrial natriuretic peptide and amiloride inhibit isotopic sodium uptake by IMCD cells in fresh suspensions or in confluent epithelial sheets of these cells in primary culture. We have characterized specific, selective receptors for atrial natriuretic peptide on the surface of IMCD cells and have begun to explore their structure. We have provided strong evidence that cGMP mediates the response of IMCD cells to atrial natriuretic peptide. BrcGMP duplicated the effects of atrial natriuretic peptide in IMCD cells. The response exhibited cell type and nucleotide specificity. Atrial natriuretic peptide elevated IMCD cGMP with the appropriate time course and potency order of atrial natriuretic peptide peptides. Inhibition of phosphodiesterase enhanced both cGMP accumulation and inhibition of oxygen consumption in response to submaximal levels of hANP. Finally, nitroprusside elevated cGMP in both IMCD and outer medullary collecting duct cells, but inhibited oxygen consumption only in IMCD cells. These results indicate that raising cGMP by any mechanism leads to inhibition of oxygen consumption.

The results described in this review allow us to construct the model for the regulation of IMCD sodium transport by atrial natriuretic peptide depicted in Figure 1: atrial natriuretic peptide binds to specific receptors located on the basolateral surface of IMCD cells. Binding of atrial natriuretic peptide stimulates a guanylate cyclase which may be tightly coupled to the receptor. Stimulation of guanylate cyclase raises intracellular cGMP levels. The increase of cytosolic cGMP leads to an inhibition of sodium entry across the luminal membrane of the cell, thus inhibiting net sodium reabsorption. The possible pathways inhibited are shown in the figure. Our current data support best a sodium channel effect. Cyclic GMP may regulate sodium transport by any of several mechanisms, including direct binding to the transport protein [62] or stimulation of specific cGMP-dependent protein kinases. Over the next several years we plan to test directly several features of this model.

References

1 Ballermann BJ, Brenner BM. Biologically active atrial peptides. *J Clin Invest 1985; 76:* 2041–2048

2 Maack T, Marion DN, Camargo MJ et al. Effects of auriculin (atrial natriuretic factor) on blood pressure, renal function, and the renin-aldosterone system in dogs. *Am J Med 1984; 77:* 1069–1075

3 Burnett JC Jr, Granger JP, Opgenorth T. Effects of synthetic atrial natriuretic factor on renal function and renin release. *Am J Physiol 1984; 247:* F863–F866

4 Garcia R, Thibault G, Cantin M, Genest J. Effect of a purified atrial natriuretic factor on rat and rabbit vascular strips and vascular beds. *Am J Physiol 1984; 247:* R34–R39

5 Kudo T, Baird A. Inhibition of aldosterone production in the adrenal glumerulosa by atrial natriuretic factor. *Nature 1984; 312:* 756–757

6 Huang CL, Lewicki J, Johnson LK, Cogan MG. Renal mechanism of action of rat atrial natriuretic factor. *J Clin Invest 1985; 75:* 769–773

7 Cogan MG. Atrial natriuretic factor can increase renal solute excretion primarily by raising glomerular filtration. *Am J Physiol 1986; 251:* F710–F714

8 Camargo MJ, Kleinert HD, Atlas SA et al. Ca-dependent hemodynamic and natriuretic effects of atrial extract in isolated rat kidney. *Am J Physiol 1984; 247:* F447–F456

9 Ballermann BJ, Hoover RL, Karnovsky MJ, Brenner BM. Physiologic regulation of atrial natriuretic peptide receptors in rat renal glomeruli. *J Clin Invest 1985; 76:* 2049–2056

10 Ballermann BJ, Bloch KD, Seidman JG, Brenner BM. Atrial natriuretic peptide transcription, secretion, and glomerular receptor activity during mineralocorticoid escape in the rat. *J Clin Invest 1986; 78:* 840–843

11 Tremblay J, Gerzer R, Vinay P et al. The increase of cGMP by atrial natriuretic factor correlates with the distribution of particulate guanylate cyclase. *Febs Lett 1985; 181:* 17–22

12 Stokes TJ, McConkey CL, Martin KJ. Atriopeptin III increases cGMP in glomeruli but not proximal tubules of dog kidney. *Am J Physiol 1986; 251:* F456–F460

13 Briggs JP, Steipe B, Schubert G, Schnermann J. Micropuncture studies of the renal effects of atrial natriuretic substance. *Pfluegers Arch 1982; 395:* 271–276

14 Murray RD, Itoh S, Inagami T et al. Effects of synthetic atrial natriuretic factor in the isolated perfused rat kidney. *Am J Physiol 1985; 249:* F603–F609

15 Baines AD, deBold AJ, Sonnenberg H. Natriuretic effect of atrial extract on isolated perfused rat kidney. *Can J Physiol Pharmacol 1983; 61:* 1462–1466

16 Pollock DM, Banks RO. Effect of atrial extract on renal function in the rat. *Clin Sci 1983; 65:* 47–55

17 Seymour AA et al. Renal and systemic effects of synthetic atrial natriuretic factor. *Life Sci 1985; 36:* 33–44

18 Yukimura T, Ito K, Takenaga T et al. Renal effects of a synthetic human atrial natriuretic polypeptide in anesthetized dogs. *Eur J Pharmacol 1984; 103:* 353–366

19 Biollaz J et al. Synthetic human atrial natriuretic peptide: renal site of the natriuretic effect on normal volunteers. *Clin Res 1986; 34:* 590A

20 Jamison RL, Sonnenberg H, Stein JH. Questions and replies: role of the collecting tubule in fluid, sodium, and potassium balance. *Am J Physiol 1979; 237:* F247–F261

21 Diezi J, Michoud P, Aceves J, Giebisch G. Micropuncture study of electrolyte transport across papillary collecting duct of the rat. *Am J Physiol 1973; 224:* 623–634

22 Ullrich KJ, Papavassiliou F. Sodium reabsorption in the papillary collecting duct of rats. Effect of adrenalectomy, low Na+ diet, acetazolamide, HCO-3-free solutions and of amiloride. *Pfluegers Arch 1979; 379:* 49–52

23 Moran T, Ray C. The permeability of collecting ducts to 22 Na+ and 36Cl- in rat isolated papillae. *Clin Exp Pharmacol Physiol 1982; 9:* 657–663

24 Ullrich KJ, Papavassiliou F. Bicarbonate reabsorption in the papillary collecting duct of rats. *Pfluegers Arch 1981; 389:* 271–275

25 Graber ML, Bengele HH, Schwartz JH, Alexander EA. pH and PCO2 profiles of the rat inner medullary collecting duct. *Am J Physiol 1981; 241:* F659–F668

26 Graber ML, Bengele HH, Mroz E et al. Acute metabolic acidosis augments collecting duct acidification rate in the rat. *Am J Physiol 1981; 241:* F669–F676

27 Laski ME, Kurtzman NA. Characterization of acidification in the cortical and medullary collecting tubule of the rabbit. *J Clin Invest 1983; 72:* 2050–2059

28 Sonnenberg H, Wilson DR. Urea handling by the medullary collecting duct of the rat kidney during hydropenia and urea infusion. *Pfluegers Arch 1981; 390:* 131–137

29 Sonnenberg H, Wilson DR. Urea handling by the distal tubule and collecting duct of the rat during urea – saline, isotonic saline, or urea diuresis. *Can J Physiol Pharmacol 1982; 60:* 128–133

30 Rocha AS, Kudo LH. Water, urea, sodium, chloride, and potassium transport in the in vitro isolated perfused papillary collecting duct. *Kidney Int 1982; 22:* 485–491

31 Stanton B. Cellular conductive properties of rat inner medullary collecting duct (IMCD): effects of vasopressin. *Abstracts Xth Int Congress Nephrology*. London. 1987: 580

32 Grupp C, Kinne-Saffran E, Stokes JB, Kinne R. Evidence for a furosemide-sensitive Na-K-Cl cotransport system in rat papillary collecting duct cells. *Abstracts Xth Int Congress Nephrology*. London. 1987: 570

33 Kudo LH, Rocha AS. Chloride and sodium secretion by rat papillary collecting duct (PCD). *Abstracts Xth Int Congress Nephrology.* London. 1987: 574

34 Sonnenberg H, Cupples WA, de Bold AJ, Veress AT. Intrarenal localization of the natriuretic effect of cardiac atrial extract. *Can J Physiol Pharmacol 1982; 60:* 1149–1152

35 Sonnenberg H, Honrath U, Chong CK, Wilson DR. Atrial natriuretic factor inhibits sodium transport in medullary collecting duct. *Am J Physiol 1986; 250:* F963–F966

36 Fried TA, Osgood RW, Stein JH. The effect of synthetic atrial natriuretic peptide on chloride handling in the rat. *Abstracts First World Congress Biologically Active Atrial Peptides.* 1986: 117A

37 Van de Stolpe A, Jamison RL. Effect of atrial natriuretic peptide on Na reabsorption in the rat collecting tubule. *Kidney Int 1987; 31:* 290A

38 Zeidel ML, Seifter JL, Lear S et al. Atrial peptides inhibit oxygen consumption in kidney medullary collecting duct cells. *Am J Physiol 1986; 251:* F379–F383

39 Zeidel ML, Silva P, Brenner BM, Seifter J. cGMP mediates effects of atrial peptides on medullary collecting duct cells. *Am J Physiol 1987; 241:* F551–F559

40 Gunning M, Ballermann BJ, Silva P, Zeidel ML. Characterization of specific atrial natriuretic peptide receptors in rabbit inner medullary collecting duct cells. *Kidney Int 1987; 31:* 271A

41 Zeidel ML, Seifter JL, Brenner BM, Silva P. Atrial peptides inhibit Na^+ entry-dependent oxygen consumption in rabbit inner medullary collecting duct cells. *Trans Am Assoc Phys 1986; 49:* 258–265

42 Kaissling B, Kriz W. Structural analysis of the rabbit kidney. *Adv Anat Embryol Cell Biol 1976; 56:* 1–121

43 Zeidel ML, Silva P, Seifter JL. Intracellular pH regulation and proton transport by rabbit renal medullary collecting duct cells: role of plasma membrane proton adenosine triphosphatase. *J Clin Invest 1986; 77:* 113–120

44 Manillier C, Vinay P, Lalonde L et al. ANF does not inhibit respiration by nephron segments of dog and rat in vitro. *Kidney Int 1986; 29:* 340A

45 Nonoguchi H, Knepper MA, Manganiello VC. Effect of atrial natriuretic factor on cGMP and cAMP accumulation in renal tubule suspensions and isolated nephron segments. *Clin Res 1986; 34:* 604A

46 Harris SI, Balaban RS, Barrett L, Mandel LJ. Mitochondrial respiratory capacity and Na^+ and K^+ dependent adenosine triphosphatase-mediated ion transport in the intact renal cell. *J Biol Chem 1981; 256:* 10319–10328

47 Cantiello HF, Ausiello DA. Atrial natriuretic factor and cGMP inhibit amiloride-sensitive Na^+ transport in the cultured renal epithelial cell line, LLC-PK1. *Biochem Biophys Res Comm 1986; 134:* 852–860

48 Murphy KMM, McLaughlin L, Michener ML, Needleman P. Autoradiographic localization of atriopeptin III receptors in rat kidney. *Eur J Pharmacol 1985; 111:* 291–292

49 Healy DP, Fanestil DD. Localization of atrial natriuretic peptide binding sites within the rat kidney. *Am J Physiol 1986; 250:* F573–F578

50 Kosecki C, Hayashi Y, Torikai S et al. Localization of binding sites for rat atrial natriuretic polypeptide in rat kidney. *Am J Physiol 1986; 250:* F210–F216

51 Schiffrin EL, Chartier L, Thibault G et al. Vascular and adrenal receptors for atrial natriuretic factor in the rat. *Circ Res 1985; 56:* 801–807

52 Inui K, Saito H, Matsukawa Y et al. Specific binding activities and cyclic GMP responses by atrial natriuretic polypeptide in kidney epithelial cell line (IIC-PI1). *Biochem Biophys Res Comm 1985; 132:* 253–260

53 Hirata Y, Tomita M, Takada S, Yoshimi H. Vascular receptor binding activities and cyclic GMP responses by synthetic human and rat atrial natriuretic peptides (ANP) and receptor down-regulation by ANP. *Biochem Biophys Res Comm 1985; 128:* 538–546

54 Napier MA et al. Specific membrane receptors for atrial natriuretic factor in renal and vascular tissues. *Proc Natl Acad Sci USA 1984; 81:* 5946–5950

55 Vandlen RL, Arcuri KE, Napier MA. Identification of a receptor for atrial natriuretic factor and rabbit aorta membranes by affinity cross-linking. *J Biol Chem 1985; 260:* 10889–10892
56 Andresen JW, Kuno T, Kamisaki Y et al. Atrial natriuretic factor receptor heterogeneity in rat tissues. *Fed Proc 1986; 45:* 680A
57 Kuno T, Andresen J, Kamisaki Y et al. Copurification of an atrial natriuretic factor receptor and particulate guanylate cyclase from rat lung. *J Biol Chem 1986; 261:* 5817–5823
58 Ohlstein EH, Berkowitz BA. Cyclic guanosine monophosphate mediates vascular relaxation induced by atrial natriuretic factor. *Hypertension 1985; 7:* 306–310
59 Waldman SA, Rapoport RM, Murad F. Atrial natriuretic factor selectively activates particulate guanylate cyclase and elevates cyclic GMP in rat tissues. *J Biol Chem 1984; 259:* 14332–14334
60 Fiscus RR, Rapoport RM, Waldman SA, Murad F. Atriopeptin II elevates cyclic GMP, activates cyclic GMP-dependent protein kinase and causes relaxation in rat thoracic aorta. *Biochem Biophys Acta 1985; 846:* 179–184
61 Winquist RJ, Faison EP, Waldman SA et al. Atrial natriuretic factor elicits an endothelium-independent relaxation and activates particulate guanylate cyclase in vascular smooth muscle. *Proc Natl Acad Sci USA 1984; 81:* 7661–7664
62 O'Grady SM, Field M, Nash NT, Rao MC. Atrial natriuretic factor inhibits Na-K-Cl cotransport in teleost intestine. *Am J Physiol 1985; 249:* C531–C534
63 Robison GA, Butcher RW, Sutherland EW. *Cyclic AMP.* New York: Academic Press. 1971

FUNCTIONS OF THE PROXIMAL TUBULE

PATCH CLAMP ANALYSIS OF IONIC CHANNELS IN RENAL PROXIMAL TUBULES

H Gögelein, *R Greger

*Max-Planck-Institut für Biophysik, Frankfurt/Main, *Lehrstuhl II Physiologisches Institut der Universität Freiburg, FRG*

Introduction

The ionic conductances of the luminal and contraluminal cell membranes of renal proximal tubules are dominated by potassium permeabilities [1]. Potassium ions are actively transported into the cell by the basolateral Na/K-ATPase in exchange for sodium ions. It is generally accepted that the basolateral potassium conductance allows potassium ions to recycle from cytosol to blood. As a consequence, a cell potential (inside negative) is generated. The rôle of the luminal potassium permeability is not completely understood. It may be involved in potassium secretion. In fact, in proximal straight tubules net secretion of potassium ions has been observed [2], so luminal potassium conductance could be responsible for the potassium exit across the luminal membrane. On the other hand, in proximal convoluted tubules net reabsorption of potassium takes place [3]. As the intracellular potassium concentration is above its electrochemical equilibrium [4], potassium ions may leak from the cell into the tubular lumen and will consequently diminish potassium reabsorption. The potassium flux across the luminal membrane also enhances the hyperpolarization of the cytosol. The negativity of the cell interior and the low intracellular sodium activity [5] create a large electrochemical gradient for sodium uptake across the luminal membrane. It is well established that most of the reabsorbed sodium in the proximal tubule is taken up across the luminal membrane by coupled transport mechanisms, such as (Na^+/H^+) countertransport and various cotransport systems with sodium coupled to substrate [6]. In other epithelia, such as frog skin, urinary bladder or renal distal tubules sodium entry across the apical membrane occurs mainly via amiloride sensitive channels. Measurements of membrane voltage in renal proximal tubules do not provide evidence for a sodium conductance in the luminal membrane [1]. However, transepithelial sodium flux can be partially inhibited by amiloride [7], and this inhibitory effect is more pronounced in rats fed a sodium deficient diet than in controls.

These experiments could be explained by the existence of amiloride sensitive sodium channels in the luminal membrane. In addition, large sodium permeabilities in brush-border membrane vesicle have been observed by several investigators, although inhibitory effects of amiloride in vesicle studies have not been reported thus far [8].

Until recently it has not been possible to demonstrate the existence of ionic channels in renal tubules since, unlike other epithelia [9], it was not possible to apply fluctuation analysis to tubular structures. Only when methods were developed to apply the patch clamp technique to renal tubules could the existence of ionic channels be verified.

One way to gain access to renal cell membranes with a patch pipette is to use cultured cells. It has been possible to record sodium selective channels in the apical membrane of a cell line derived from toad kidney (A6 cells) [10] as well as in cells originating from pig kidney ($LLC\text{-}PK_1$) [11]. Sodium selective channels were also observed when vesicles derived from A6 cells were fused with a planar lipid bilayer [12]. Potassium selective channels were recorded in cultured cells derived from rabbit medullary thick ascending limbs [13] as well as from rabbit cortical collecting duct [14]. Recently, methods were developed to provide access to tubule cell membranes in vitro. One way is to start from dissected tubular segments and to open the tubule with sharpened needles, thus allowing access to the luminal membrane of cortical collecting ducts. This technique demonstrated potassium [15] as well as sodium selective channels [16,17]. Luminal membranes of Necturus proximal and Amphiuma early distal tubules were similarly investigated and potassium channels were observed [18]. In isolated tubules it is also possible to remove manually the connective tissue and basement membrane in order to reach the basolateral membrane. Hunter et al [18] found potassium selective channels using this method in Necturus proximal tubules.

We developed a slightly different method in order to apply the patch clamp method to renal proximal tubules. Tubule segments were isolated according to the method of Burg et al [19], cannulated and perfused with a modified perfusion system [20]. In contrast to conventional methods of isolated perfused tubules, the distal end of the tubule lay free on the bottom of the perfusion chamber. At the open end of the tubule, it was possible either to insert a patch pipette into the tubule lumen and to attach it to the brush-border membrane, or to bring the patch pipette into contact with the lateral membrane [21]. This technique has the advantage that the tubule remains structurally intact. Moreover, the tubule lumen is perfused so that the experimental conditions are similar to those under which micropuncture techniques have been performed. With this technique we observed potassium selective channels both in the apical and basolateral cell membrane [21–23]. To our surprise we recorded sodium selective channels in the luminal membrane [24] and a non-selective channel in the basolateral membrane [25]. Recently, potassium selective channels have been observed in lateral membranes of non-perfused tubules [26] and in isolated proximal tubular cells [27].

Results and discussion

Potassium channels in the basolateral membrane

In this first series of experiments tubule segments were bathed and perfused with physiological saline and the patch pipette was filled with a medium that resembled extracellular fluid (NaCl solution, Table I). In the absence of ionic channels we recorded in cell-attached basolateral membranes a potential of -63 ± 5mV (n=10)

TABLE I. Composition of solutions. Concentrations in mmol/L

Abbreviation	Na^+	K^+	Ca^{2+}	Mg^{2+}	Cl^-	Hepes	D-glucose	Acetate	NTA	EGTA
NaCl	143	4.7	1.3	1	144	10	5	3	0	0
KCl-10^{-3} Ca^{2+}	0	145	1	1	144	10	0	0	0	0
KCl-10^{-4} Ca^{2+}	0	145	0.1	1	142	10	0	0	0	0
KCl-10^{-6} Ca^{2+}	0	145	9.1×10^{-3}	1.5	142	10	0	0	1	0
KCl-Ca^{2+}free	0	145	0	1	137	10	0	0	0	5

NTA=nitrilotriacetic acid; EGTA=ethylene-bis(oxy-ethylenenitrile)tetraacetic acid

which is similar to the potential recorded with microelectrodes [28–30]. Figure 1 demonstrates a typical experiment, performed with NaCl solution in both the pipette and in the bath. At a clamp voltage of 0mV (lowest trace) the cell potential is present across the membrane patch, but single channel currents could not be resolved because background noise was too high. Applying positive clamp potentials, corresponding to depolarization of the membrane patch, elicited single channel responses, opening in the upward direction, and single channel amplitude increased with positive clamp voltage. These positive currents can be explained by potassium movement out of the cell and into the pipette. In one experiment both cell-attached and cell-excised modes were used to study the potassium selectivity of the channel. The current-voltage relationship of the channel was fitted by the Goldman-Hodgkin-Katz (GHK) current equation (dotted line in lower left panel of Figure 1). In order to fit the data adequately we assumed that the channels were selective for potassium ions, that intracellular potassium activity was 80mmol/L [4] and that the membrane potential was -60mV [28–30]. Extrapolation of the curve obtained by fitting the GHK equation to the data (dotted line in Figure 1) crosses the voltage axis at about -20mV. The slight negative value of the zero current potential indicates that intracellular potassium ions are above their electrochemical equilibrium. This fact is in agreement with data obtained by direct determination of intracellular potassium activity [4,31]. Mean values (±SEM) of the permeability coefficient P_K, the single channel slope conductance $g(V\infty)$, and the single channel conductance

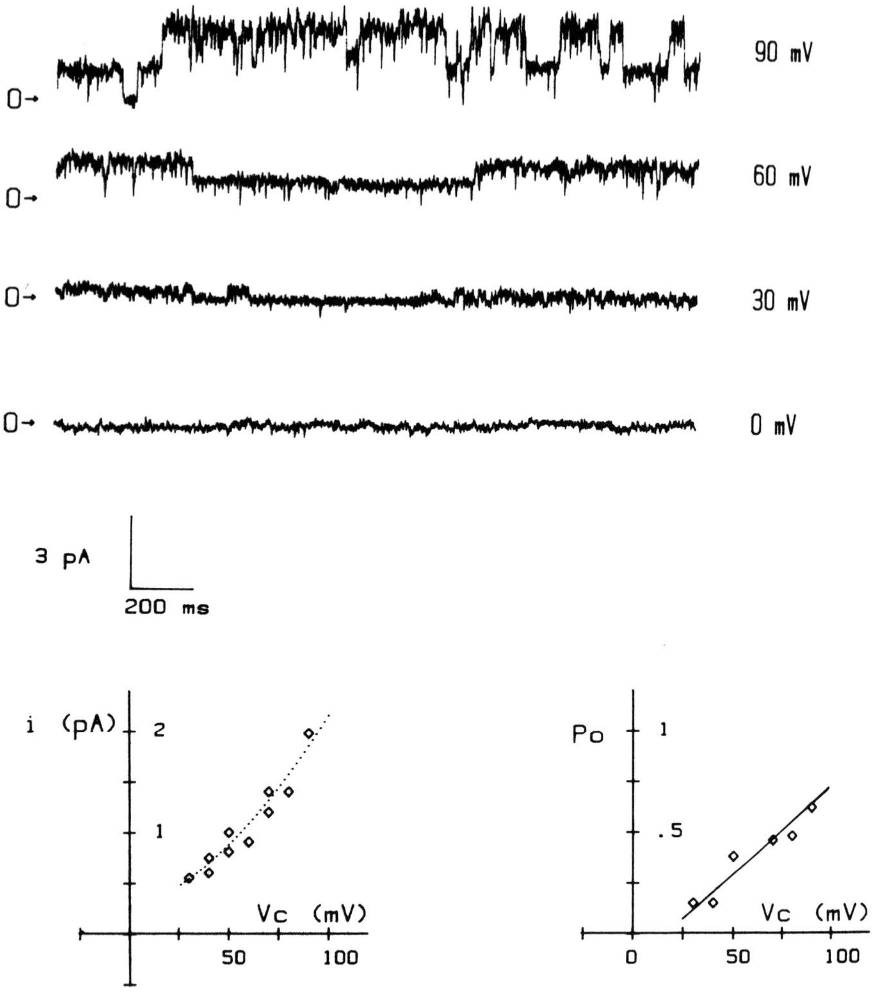

Figure 1. Outward directed (from cell into pipette) single potassium channel currents in a cell-attached patch of basolateral membrane. Pipette and bath contain NaCl Ringer solution. 0→ denotes the current level when channels are closed. The voltage given at the right side of the records denotes the clamp potential present between patch pipette and bath. The sign of the potential refers to the bath with respect to the pipette. Lower left panel: current-voltage relation. The single channel current of one current level is plotted as a function of the clamp voltage (Vc). The dotted line is obtained by fitting the Goldman-Hodgkin-Katz (GHK) current equation to the data. Lower right panel: the open-state probability (Po) of one channel is plotted as a function of the clamp potential

TABLE II. Permeability coefficients and single channel conductances of K^+ channels in the basolateral membrane of rabbit straight proximal tubule cells

	Cell-attached				Cell-excised			
	Pipette NaCl Bath NaCl		Pipette $KCl-10^{-3}\ Ca^{2+}$ Bath NaCl		Pipette NaCl Bath $KCl-10^{-6}\ Ca^{2+}$		Pipette $KCl-10^{-3}\ Ca^{2+}$ Bath NaCl	
P_K (cm^3/s)	$(0.17 \pm 0.04) \cdot 10^{-12}$	(4)			$(0.10 \pm 0.01) \cdot 10^{-12}$	(8)	$(0.12 \pm 0.01) \cdot 10^{-12}$	(6)
$g(V_{bl})$ (pS)	12 ± 3	(4)			7 ± 1	(8)	8 ± 1	(6)
$g(V_\infty)$ (pS)	50 ± 12	(4)	46 ± 3 and 36 ± 3	(9) (11)	40 ± 4	(8)	45 ± 5	(6)

The permeability coefficients (P_K) were obtained by least square fits of the current-voltage curves to the Goldman-Hodgkin-Katz current equation. $g(V_{bl})$ are the single channel conductances at the physiological membrane potential and $g(V_\infty)$ are the single channel slope conductances at infinite potential (linear range of the current-voltage curves). The values for $g(V_\infty)$ in cell attached mode with KCl in the pipette and NaCl in the bath were obtained by linear regression analysis of data at negative clamp potentials (cf text). The numbers in brackets are the numbers of experiments at 0mV clamp potential $g(B_{bl})$ (corresponding to the membrane potential of about −60mV) from four experiments are presented in Table II.

Close inspection of the single channel current recordings in Figure 1 reveals that with increasing positive clamp potentials superposition of two current amplitudes of equal magnitude occurs more frequently. Evaluation of the open-state probability of one channel demonstrates an increase of single channel activity with increasing depolarizing potentials (lower right panel of Figure 1). This indicates that the channel is voltage sensitive. Whether this voltage dependence is relevant for the regulation of basolateral potassium conductance under physiological conditions remains uncertain, since we are unable to resolve the channel current above noise in the potential range of 0±20mV, which corresponds to ±20mV deviation of the resting membrane voltage. After detecting potassium channels in membrane patches of intact cells, we investigated these channels in cell-excised patches, where the cytosolic membrane face is oriented towards the bath (inside out patches). Figure 2 demonstrates single channel current recordings of a representative experiment. The pipette was filled with NaCl solution, whereas the bath contained KCl-10^{-6} Ca^{2+} solution (Table I). Channel currents were positive, indicating potassium movement from the bath into the pipette. The amplitude of single channel currents decreased at negative and increased at positive clamp potentials. The i/V curve depicted in the lower left part of Figure 2 was fitted by the GHK equation. Mean values of the parameters obtained in this way are similar to those obtained in cell-attached patches (Table II). The kinetic appearance of the channels is also very similar to that observed in cell-attached experiments: channel openings appeared in bursts and exhibited fast flickering. We may assume, therefore, that we were observing the same type of channel in cell-attached and in cell-excised patches.

The lower right part of Figure 2 illustrates the dependence of the open-state probability (Po) of a single channel on the clamp potential. The curve shows that channel activity increased with positive (depolarizing) membrane potentials, as was the case in cell-attached patches (Figure 1). A similar voltage dependence was recently reported for inward directed potassium channels in the basolateral membrane of rabbit convoluted tubules [32]. In contrast, however, Hunter et al [18] observed a decrease of channel open probability with depolarizing potentials in Necturus proximal tubule, when the pipette contain KCl and the bath NaCl solution. It is unclear whether these differences are due to experimental or species differences.

In order to characterize these potassium channels more closely, movement of potassium into the cell was also studied using a pipette filled with KCl-10^{-3} Ca^{2+} solution (Table I). Figure 3a presents typical single channel current recordings, obtained with a cell-attached patch, with the tubule perfused and bathed in NaCl solution. In this figure, at 0mV clamp potential, downward single channel amplitude decreased with positive clamp voltage and disappeared into the baseline noise at about 50mV. With further increasing clamp potential

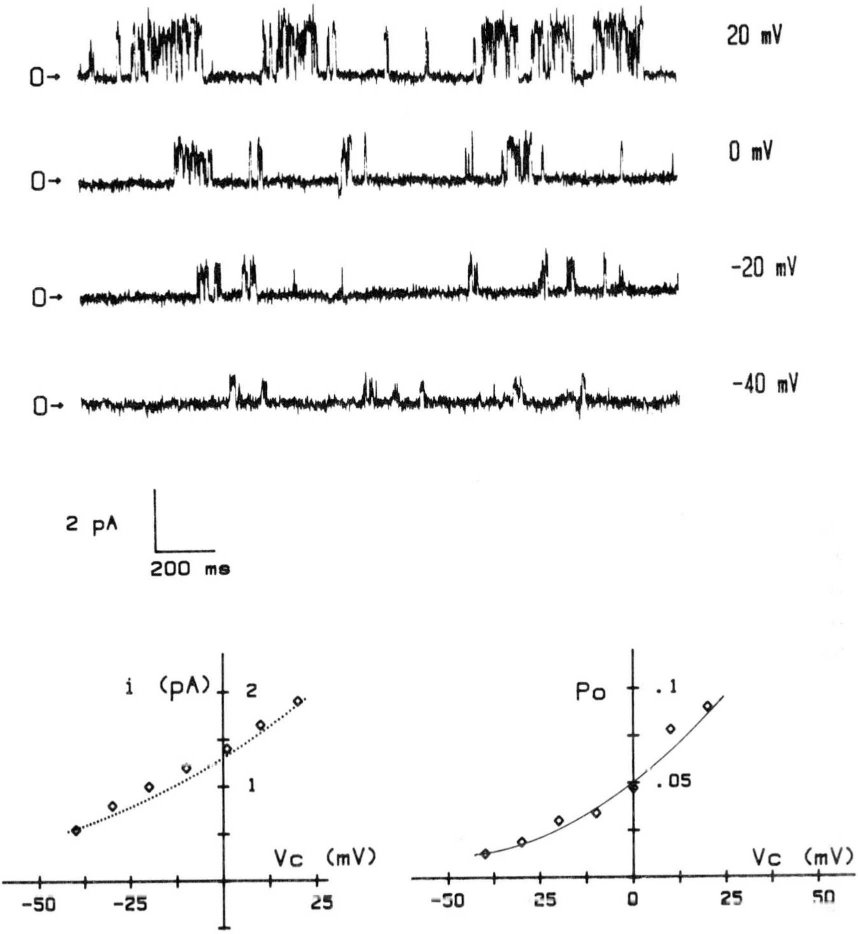

Figure 2. Outward directed (from bath into pipette) single potassium channel currents in a cell-excised basolateral membrane. The pipette contains NaCl, the bath KCl–10^{-6} Ca^{2+} solution (Table I). The data points of the i/V curve (lower left panel) are fitted to the GHK equation (dotted line). Lower right panel: open-state probability as a function of the clamp potential. The curve is fitted by eye (solid line)

upward channel currents, indicating movement of potassium ions into the pipette, were observed. The i/V curve on the right part of Figure 3a was non-linear indicating inward rectification of this potassium channel. However, unlike channels in the rectal gland [33], those in proximal straight tubules allow movement of potassium ions in both directions. The mean single channel conductance was calculated by linear regression of data points recorded with negative clamp voltages and is denoted as g/V∞) (see Table II). The interpolated reversal potential was 59±6mV (n=9).

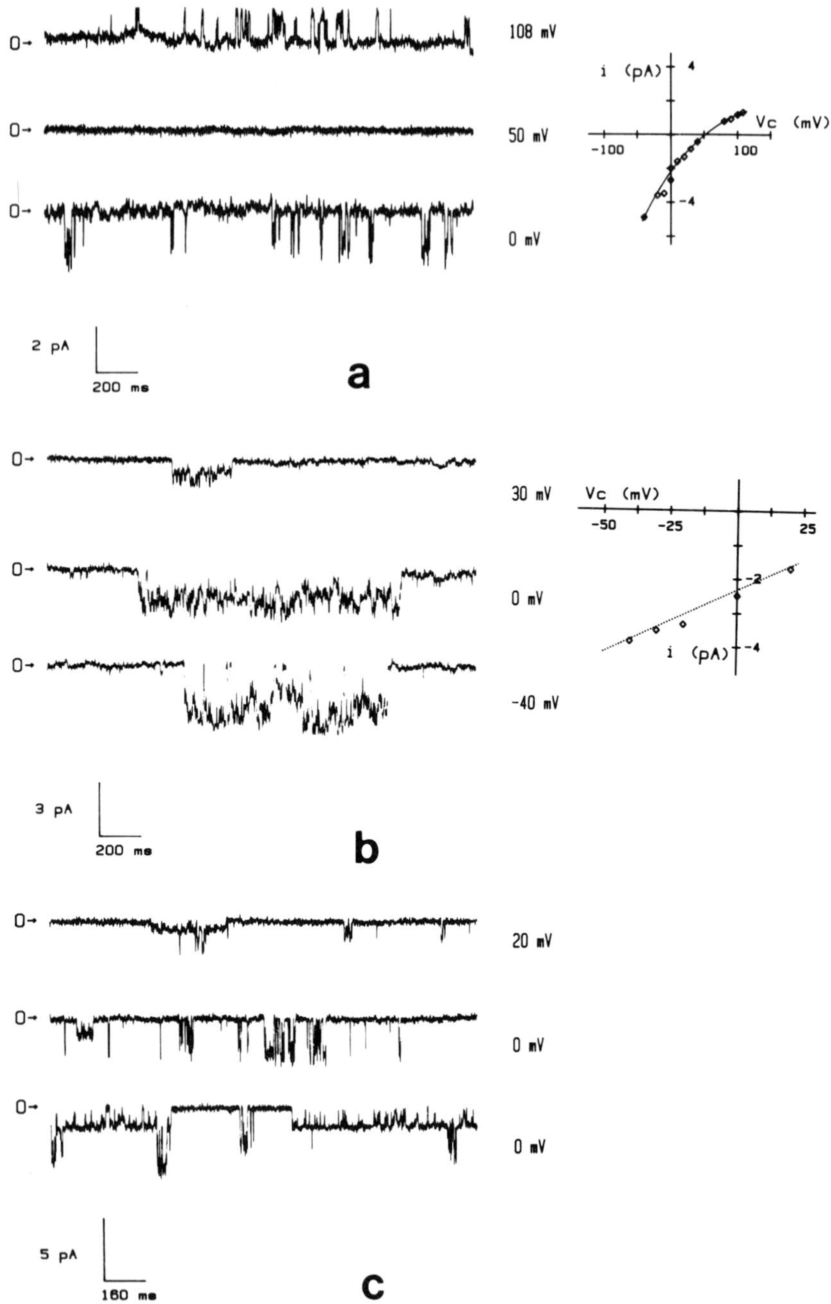

Figure 3. Inward directed potassium channels in a cell-attached basolateral membrane. The pipette contains KCl–10^{-3} Ca^{2+}, the bath NaCl solution (Table I). Two types of channels are observed. In (a) the channel with higher conductance (g=46 pS) is shown. The i/V curve, plotted on the right part of (a) is fitted by eye. In (b) the channel with lower conductance (g=36 pS) is shown. The corresponding i/V curve (right part of b) is fitted by linear regression. (c) shows an original record of an experiment where both channel types are present in one membrane patch

In addition to this potassium channel, we frequently observed a second type of inwardly directed potassium current, as shown in Figure 3b. The channels responsible have a somewhat lower single channel slope conductance (36 pS, Table II), and stay in the open-state for a longer period than the first type of potassium channel, making it easy to differentiate the two channels. The extrapolated zero current potential of 62±4mV (n=11) is very similar to that recorded for the larger conductance potassium channel (cf above), demonstrating that the lower conductance channel is mainly permeable to potassium ions. In a few cases, we observed both types of channels in the same membrane patch (see Figure 3c).

Inwardly directed potassium currents were also recorded in cell-excised patches (Figure 4) when the pipette was filled with KCl- 10^{-3} Ca^{2+} and the bath contained NaCl solution (Table I). Two channels with equal amplitude are present in this membrane patch. The i/V relation, depicted in the lower part of Figure 4, was fitted by the GHK equation. Mean values of single channel parameters are given in Table II. The kinetic appearance and magnitude of the single channel conductance demonstrate that this channel corresponds to the higher conductance channel, described in Figure 3a.

Further experiments were performed on the first type of potassium channel, i.e. the one with the shorter opening time and the higher conductance. It has been shown that barium ions inhibit potassium conductance of the basolateral cell membrane of proximal tubules [1,28,31]. In the first type of potassium channel in cell-excised membrane patches, single channel open probability was considerably reduced by barium ions (Figure 5a). In contrast, addition of 20mmol/L of tetraethylammonium (TEA^+) ions to the bathing solution reduced the single channel current amplitude (Figure 5a). Both effects were reversible. Similar results were recently observed in the dogfish rectal gland [34].

It is generally assumed that intracellular Ca^{2+} ions play a rôle in the regulation of basolateral potassium channels of transporting epithelia [35,36]. In cell-excised patches with NaCl in the pipette and KCl- 10^{-6} Ca^{2+} in the bath, outward potassium currents were recorded at 0mV clamp voltage. Replacing the bathing solution by KCl-Ca^{2+} free solution (Table I) did not change single channel open probability (Figure 5b). In one experiment where outward potassium currents were observed in a cell-attached patch, the Ca^{2+} ionophore A23187 (10^{-5}M) was added to the bath in order to increase intracellular Ca^{2+} activity; there were no changes in single channel open probability (data not shown). Detregger et al [39] have shown that addition of A23187 did not alter basolateral membrane potentials in isolated perfused rabbit tubules. Potassium channels in dogfish rectal gland [34] in Necturus proximal tubules [18] and in collapsed rabbit proximal tubules [26] showed no dependence on intracellular calcium ions.

We conclude that basolateral potassium channels of proximal tubule cells unlike those in pancreatic [37] or lacrimal gland cells [38] are not regulated by intracellular Ca^{2+} ions.

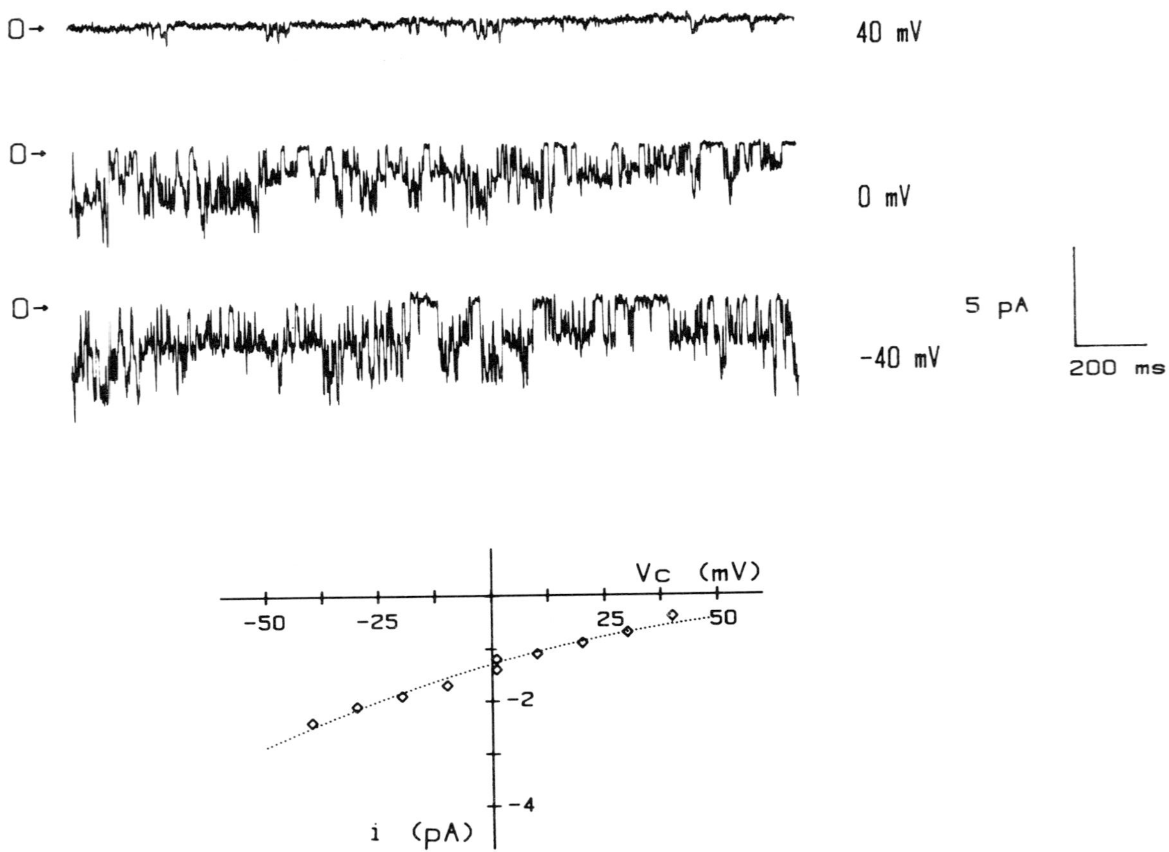

Figure 4. Inward directed single potassium channel currents in a cell-excised basolateral membrane. The pipette contains KCl–10^{-3} Ca^{2+}, the bath NaCl Ringer solution. The i/V curve (lower panel) is fitted to the data using the GHK equation

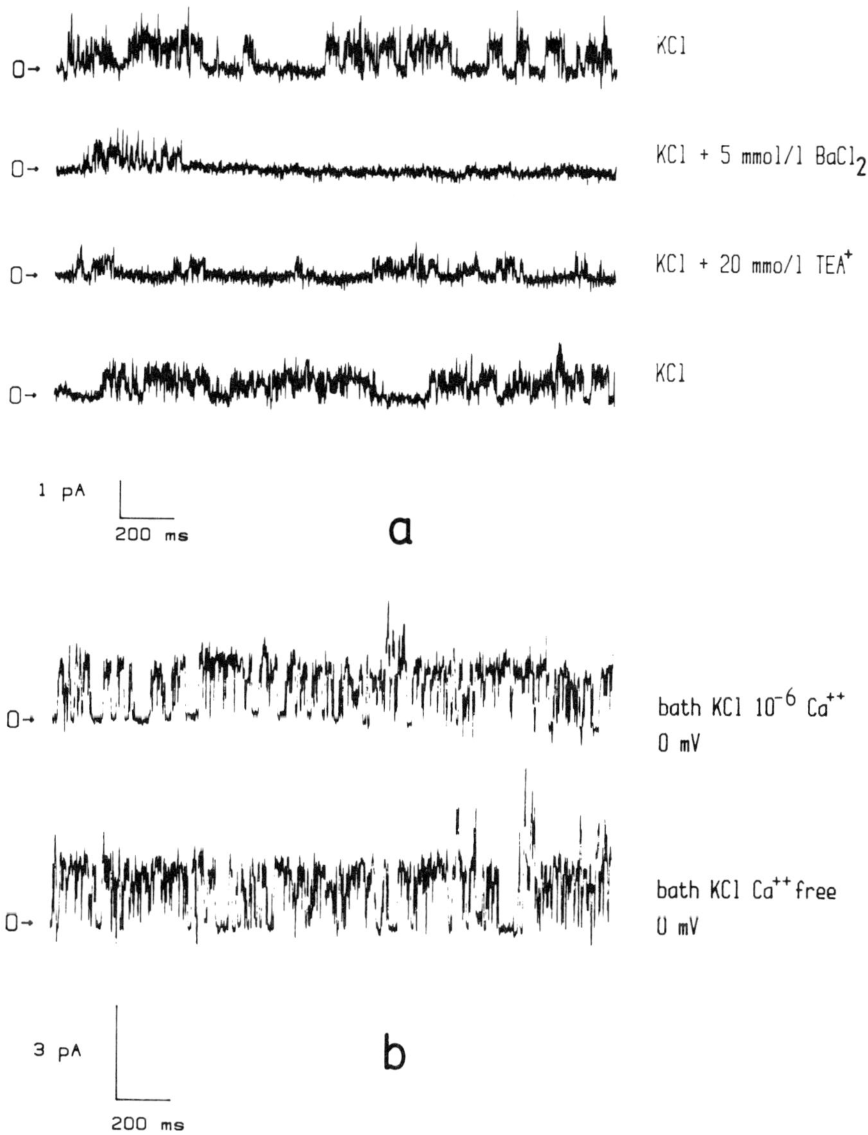

Figure 5. (a) Effects of barium and tetraethylammonium (TEA^+) ions on outward directed single potassium channels in the basolateral membrane of a cell-excised patch. The blocking effect of TEA^+ ions is reversible (last trace), as is the case for barium ions (not shown).
(b) Omission of bath calcium ions in a cell-excised basolateral membrane patch. Note there is no change in open probability of the channel

Figure 6. Non-selective channels in a cell-excised basolateral membrane patch. Pipette and bath contain NaCl Ringer solution.

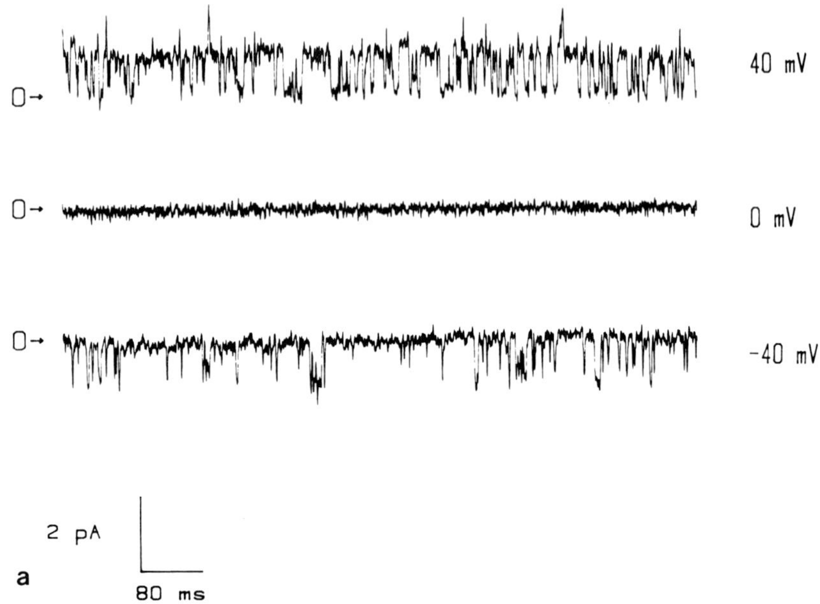

a

(a) Shows single channel current recordings of a representative experiment

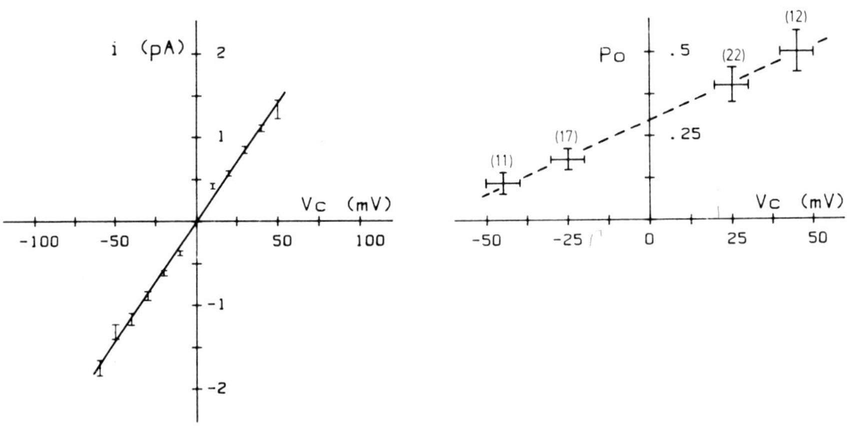

b

(b) Mean values (± SEM) of single currents (left part) and of the open-state probabilities (right part) are plotted as functions of the clamp potential. Both curves are fitted by linear regression. The numbers in parentheses denote the number of experiments

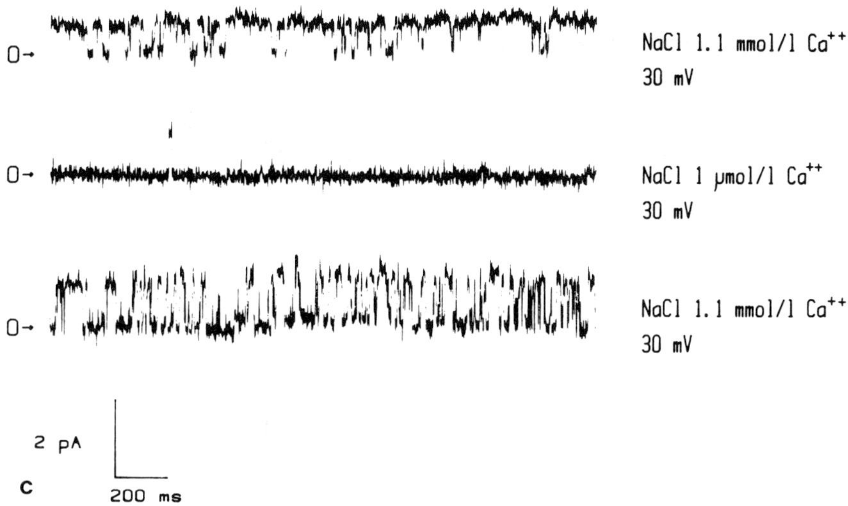

(c) The effect of lowering bath calcium concentration from 1.1mmol/L to 1μmol/L. The single channel current is almost completely inhibited (second trace). This effect is reversible (last trace)

Non-selective channel in the basolateral membrane
After excision of membrane patches another type of channel with a single channel conductance of 29±1 pS (n=28) was frequently observed. The channel was equally permeable to sodium and potassium ions [25] and its open-state probability increased markedly with positive clamp potentials (Figures 6a and 6b). Changing bath NaCl concentration from 145mmol/L to 70mmol/L shifted the i/V curve by 2.9±2.4mV (n=5) to the left (data not shown). According to the Nernst equation this yields a permeability ratio of sodium to chloride of 1.8±0.5. Decreasing bath (cytosolic) calcium concentration from 1.1mmol/L to 10^{-6} mol/L and lower inhibited the single channel activity completely and reversibly (Figure 6c). The inactivation of the channel at calcium concentrations above intracellular calcium activity [40], explains the apparent absence of the channel in cell-attached patches. The physiological significance of this non-selective channel is as yet unclear. A cation channel, which is inhibited by 10^{-6} mol/L calcium on the cytosolic side, has also been reported in a rat insulinoma cell line [41].

Luminal potassium channel
In luminal cell membranes, potassium channels were mainly recorded in cell-attached patches with KCl-10^{-3} Ca^{2+} in the pipette and NaCl as bathing medium. Figure 7 shows a typical experiment. The kinetic appearance of the luminal potassium channels is very similar to that of the basolateral potassium channels. Open-time distributions can be fitted by a single exponential, yielding

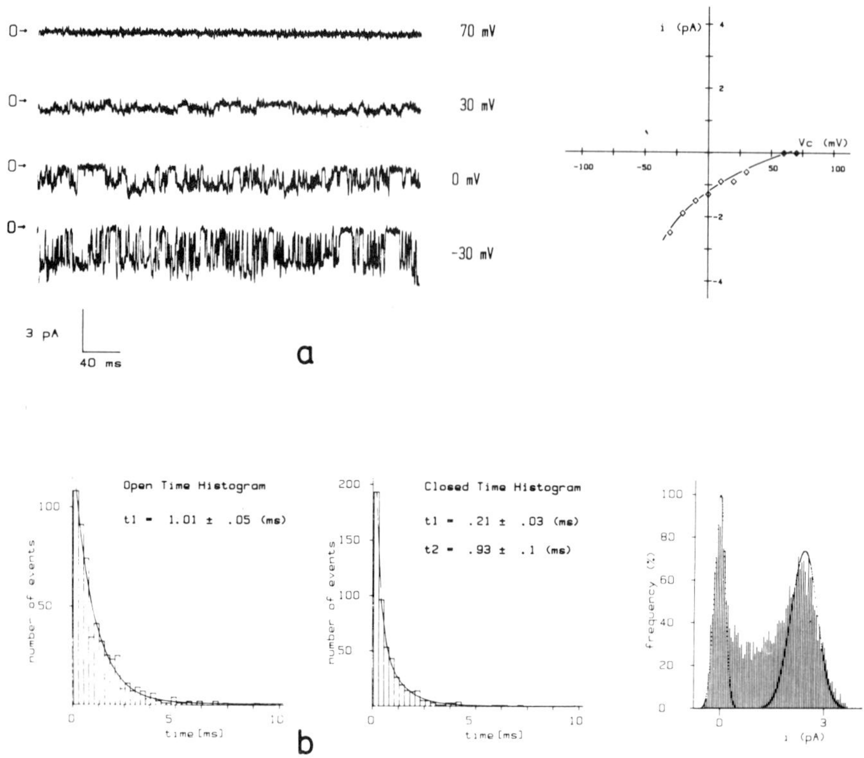

Figure 7. Inward directed potassium channels in a cell-attached patch of the luminal membrane. The pipette contains KCl–10^{-3} Ca^{2+}, the bath NaCl Ringer solution. The i/V curve (right panel of a) was fitted by eye. In (b), open- and closed-time distributions are shown. The clamp potential is −30mV. The data are low-pass filtered with 1kHz (−3 dB point of 4 pole Bessel filter) and are sampled at 0.2ms intervals. The open-time histogram is fitted by a single exponential, and the closed-times by two exponential functions. The time constants obtained in this way are given on the figures. The right panel of (b) depicts a current-amplitude histogram recorded at a clamp potential of −30mV. The dotted lines are obtained by fitting Gaussian curves to the peaks

a time-constant of about 1ms, whereas the closed-time histogram could be fitted by two exponentials, the first time-constant was about 0.2ms and the second about 1ms (lower part of Figure 7). These values are comparable to those obtained for basolateral potassium channels [23]. The i/V relation (right part of Figure 7) reveals inward rectification. The single channel slope conductance, calculated from data points at negative clamp voltages, was 33±3 pS (n=6). This value is somewhat lower than the single channel conductance of apical potassium channels of Necturus proximal tubules (about 50 pS) [18].

The current-amplitude histogram, depicted in the right lower part of Figure 7, reveals two peaks, which were fitted by Gaussian curves (dotted lines). The left peak represents the baseline (level at closed channels) and the right peak the open channel. The events between both peaks are due to fast transitions to the closed state (flickering). Because of the high frequency of flickering we cannot discriminate between incomplete closing and opening events, caused by low-pass filtering, and possible substates of this channel.

The luminal sodium channel

In addition to the potassium channel described above, we also observed a sodium selective channel in the luminal cell membrane. In cell-attached patches, with NaCl solution in both the pipette and bath, we recorded negative channel currents whose amplitude decreased with increasing positive clamp voltage (Figure 8a). The i/V curves could be adequately fitted by the GHK equation, assuming an intracellular sodium activity of about 17mmol/L and a luminal membrane potential of about −70mV. The single channel conductance in the linear range was 16 pS, and at 0mV potential was 14 pS (Table III). The kinetic

TABLE III. Permeability coefficient and single channel conductances of sodium channels in the luminal membrane of rabbit straight proximal tubule cells

	Cell-attached		Cell-excised			
	Pipette NaCl Bath NaCl		Pipette NaCl Bath NaCl		Pipette NaCl Bath KCl–10^{-4} Ca^{2+}	
P_{Na} (cm^3/s)	$(4.1\pm0.2)\cdot10^{-14}$	(10)	$(2.5\pm0.4)\cdot10^{-14}$	(9)	$(4.8\pm0.2)\cdot10^{-14}$	(8)
$g(V_{lu})$ (pS)	14±1	(10)			15±1	(8)
$g(V_{\infty})$ (pS)	16±1	(10)	10±1	(9)	18±1	(8)

P_{Na} is the permeability coefficient, $g(V_{lu})$ is the single channel conductance at the cell resting potential and $g(V_{\infty})$ is the single channel slope conductance

behaviour of the sodium channels was distinct from that of potassium channels since sodium channels do not exhibit flickering. In cell-excised patches, with NaCl in the pipette and KCl-10^{-4} Ca^{2+} solution (Table I) in the bath, the channel behaved as in cell-attached patches (Figure 8b). The i/V curve could be fitted by the GHK equation, assuming negligible permeability for potassium ions, as shown in Figure 8b (right side). The single channel conductance was comparable to that obtained in cell-attached membrane patches (Table III). However, with NaCl on both sides, the permeability coefficient single channel conductance were somewhat smaller than those recorded with KCl on the cytoplasmic side (Table III). The reason for this difference in single channel slope conductance is as yet unexplained.

The channel could be blocked by amiloride applied to the cytoplasmic side

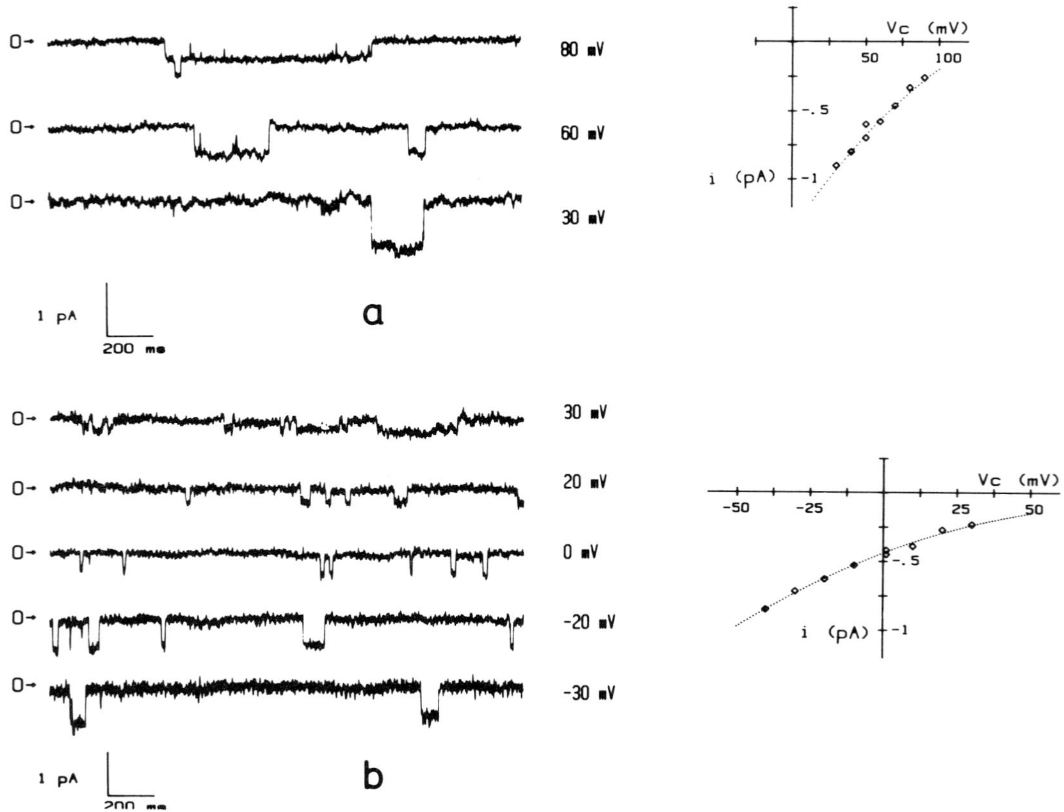

Figure 8. Inward directed single sodium channel currents in the luminal membrane. (a) An experiment performed with a cell-attached patch is shown. Pipette and bath contain NaCl Ringer solutions. The i/V curve (right panel) is fitted using the GHK equation.
(b) Shows single sodium channel currents in a cell-excised experiment, where the pipette is filled with NaCl and the bath with KCl–10^{-4} Ca^{2+} solution (Table I). The i/V curve (right panel) is fitted using the GHK equation

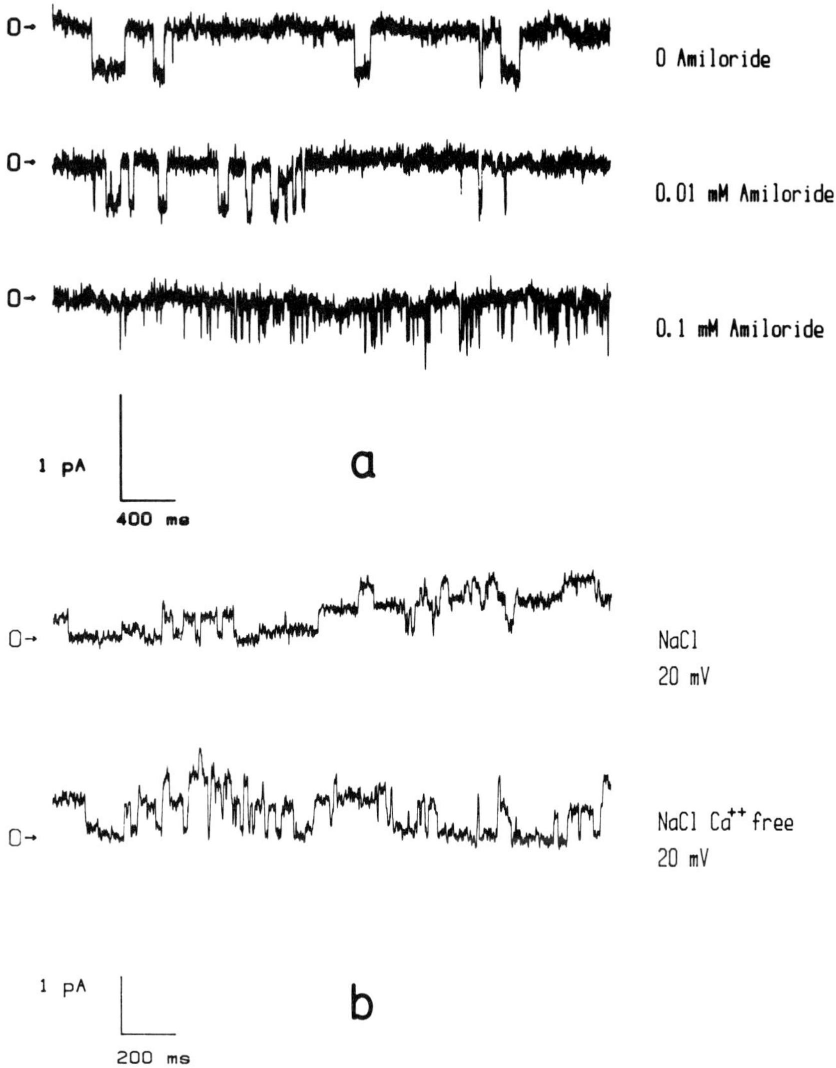

Figure 9. (a) Effects of amiloride on single sodium channel currents in a cell-excised patch of the luminal membrane. Amiloride was added to the bath (cytosolic side).
(b) Omission of bath calcium ions in a cell excised luminal membrane patch. The pipette contains KCl–10^{-3} Ca^{2+}, the bath NaCl Ringer solution

(Figure 9a). Administration of 0.01mmol/L and of 0.1mmol/L amiloride, decreased the channel open time in a dose dependent manner; with 1mmol/L amiloride the channel was completely inhibited [24]. The blocking effects were reversible. Omission of bath calcium ions (cytosolic side) did not affect single channel open-state probability of sodium channels in cell-excised patches (Figure 9b). It is therefore likely that the luminal sodium channel is not directly dependent on calcium ions.

Single sodium channels have also been recorded in a cultured cell line derived from toad kidney (A6) [10] and in cortical collecting ducts of rat kidney [16]. In the latter tissue, the channel was not dependent on calcium ions in cell-free membrane patches, but seemed to be inhibited by elevation of cytosolic calcium in cell-attached patches [39].

Conclusion

The application of the patch clamp technique to renal proximal tubules is in its infancy and many observations are as yet unexplained. Already, however, it has revealed something of the nature of the channel types that make up membrane conductances described in experiments with microelectrodes [1]. It is also feasible to investigate the mechanisms which regulate membrane conductances and, possibly, the factors responsible for the communication between luminal and basolateral transport processes. We provide evidence that intracellular calcium ions do not regulate the basolateral potassium conductance nor do they affect directly luminal sodium channels. The physiological significance of the sodium channel is unclear. Since most of the reabsorbed sodium crosses the luminal cell membrane by coupled transport systems [1], the channel mechanism probably plays only a minor rôle for total sodium transport.

Thus far, anion selective channels have not been detected in renal proximal tubules. It is not clear whether the non-selective channel in the basolateral membrane is involved in anion exit from the cell across the basolateral membrane. Anion selective channels might not be detected if anion exit across the basolateral membrane occurs through channels with a single channel conductance smaller than 5 pS; this could not be resolved by our method. Alternatively, it is possible that anion transport is mediated solely by coupled transport processes, which cannot be detected by the patch clamp technique.

Acknowledgment

We are grateful to Professor Dr K J Ullrich for his great interest in this work and for valuable discussion.

References

1 Frömter E. Viewing the kidney through microelectrodes. *Am J Physiol 1984; 247:* F695–F705

2 Schafer JA, Work J. Transport properties of the Pars Recta. In Robinson RR, ed. *Nephrology*. New York: Springer Verlag. 1984: 186–195

3 Giebisch G. Renal potassium transport. In Giebisch G, Tosteson DC, Ussing HH, eds. *Membrane Transport in Biology, Volume IVA.* New York: Springer Verlag. 1979: 215–298

4 Edelman A, Curci S, Samarzija I, Frömter E. Determination of intracellular K^+ activity in rat kidney proximal tubular cells. *Pfluegers Arch 1978; 378:* 37–45

5 Yoshitomi K, Frömter E. How big is the electrochemical potential difference of Na^+ across rat renal proximal tubular cell membranes in vivo? *Pfluegers Arch 1985; 405:* S121–S126

6 Ullrich KJ, Frömter E, Murer H. Principien des epithelialen Transportes in Niere und Darm. *Klin Wochenschr 1979; 57:* 977–991

7 Ullrich KJ, Cassola AC, Papavassiliou F et al. Induction by low Na^+ diet of amiloride-sensitive Na^+ transport in the proximal convolution of the rat kidney. *Pfluegers Arch 1982; 403:* R39

8 Elgavish GA, Elgavish A. Evidence from ^{23}Na NMR studies for the existence of sodium-channels in the brush border membrane of the renal proximal tubule. *Biochem Biophys Res Commun 1985; 128:* 746–753

9 Van Driessche W, Zeiske W. Ionic channels in epithelial cell membranes. *Physiol Rev 1985; 65:* 833–903

10 Hamilton KL, Eaton DC. Single-channel recordings from amiloride-sensitive epithelial sodium channel. *Am J Physiol 1985; 249:* C200–C207

11 Moran A, Moran N. Amiloride-sensitive channels in LLC-PK_1 apical membranes. *Fed Proc 1984; 43:* 447

12 Sariban-Sohraby S, Latorre R, Burg M et al. Amiloride-sensitive epithelial Na^+ channels reconstituted into planar lipid bilayer membranes. *Nature 1984; 308:* 80–82

13 Guggino SE, Suarez-Isla BA, Guggino WB, Sacktor B. Forskolin and antidiuretic hormone stimulate a Ca^{2+}-activated K^+ channel in cultured kidney cells. *Am J Physiol 1985; 249:* F448–F455

14 Gitter AH, Beyenbach KW, Christine CW et al. High-conductance K^+ channel in apical membranes of principal cells cultured from rabbit renal cortical collecting duct anlagen. *Pfluegers Arch 1987; 408:* 282–290

15 Hunter M, Lopes AG, Boulpaep EL, Giebisch GH. Single channel recordings of calcium-activated potassium channels in the apical membranes of rabbit cortical collecting tubules. *Proc Natl Acad Sci USA 1984; 81:* 4237–4239

16 Palmer LG, Frindt G. Amiloride-sensitive Na channels from the apical membrane of the rat cortical collecting tubule. *Proc Natl Acad Sci USA 1986; 83:* 2767–2770

17 Helman SI, Koeppen BM, Beyenbach KW, Baxendale LM. Patch clamp studies of apical membranes of renal cortical collecting ducts. *Pfluegers Arch 1985; 405:* S71–S76

18 Hunter M, Kawahara K, Giebisch G. Potassium channels along the nephron. *Fed Proc 1986; 45:* 2723–2726

19 Burg MB. Perfusion of isolated renal tubules. *Yale J Biol Med 1972; 45:* 321–326

20 Greger R, Hampel W. A modified system for in vitro perfusion of isolated renal tubules. *Pfluegers Arch 1981; 189:* 175–176

21 Gögelein H, Greger R. Single channel recordings from basolateral and apical membranes of renal proximal tubules. *Pfluegers Arch 1984; 401:* 424–426

22 Greger R, Gögelein H. Role of K^+ conductive pathways in the nephron. *Kidney Int 1987; 31:* 1055–1064

23 Gögelein H, Greger R. Properties of single K^+ channels in the basolateral membrane of rabbit proximal straight tubules. *Pfluegers Arch:* in press

24 Gögelein H, Greger R. Na^+ selective channels in the apical membrane of rabbit late proximal tubules (pars recta). *Pfluegers Arch 1986; 406:* 198–203

25 Gögelein H, Greger R. A voltage-dependent ionic channel in the basolateral membrane of late proximal tubules of the rabbit kidney. *Pfluegers Arch 1986; 407:* S142–S148

26 Parent L, Cardinal J, Sauve R. Single channel analysis of a K^+-inward rectifier channel in the basolateral membrane of the collapsed rabbit proximal convoluted tubule. *Proc Int Physiol Sci 1986; 16:* 346

27 Rufer L, Su-Tsai SM, von Riotte A, Chan YL. Single ionic channel recordings from isolated proximal cells of the rat kidney. *Clin Res 1986; 34:* 1006A

28 Bello-Reuss E. Electrical properties of the basolateral membrane of the straight portion of the rabbit proximal renal tubule. *J Physiol 1982; 326:* 49–63

29 Biagi B, Kubota T, Sohtell M, Giebisch G. Intracellular potentials in rabbit proximal tubules perfused in vitro. *Am J Physiol 1981; 240:* F200–F210

30 Defregger M, Voelkl H, Paulmichl M, Lang F. Effects of A23187, verapamil, and quinidine on electrical properties of Madin-Canine-Kidney and mouse straight proximal tubule cells. *J Clin Chem Clin Biochem 1986; 24:* 686–687

31 Biagi B, Sohtell M, Giebisch G. Intracellular potassium activity in the rabbit proximal straight tubule. *Am J Physiol 1981; 241:* F677–F686

32 Parent L, Lapointe JY, Sauve R. Kinetic characterization of a K channel at the basolateral membrane of the proximal convoluted tubule (PCT): a single channel study. *Kidney Int 1987; 31:* 440

33 Greger R, Gögelein H, Schlatter E. Potassium channels in the basolateral membrane of the rectal gland of the dogfish (Squalus acanthias). *Pfluegers Arch 1987; 409:* 100–106

34 Gögelein H, Greger R, Schlatter E. Potassium channels in the basolateral membrane of the rectal gland of Squalus Acanthias. Regulation and inhibitors. *Pfluegers Arch 1987; 409:* 107–113

35 Schultz SG. Homocellular regulatory mechanisms in sodium-transporting epithelia: avoidance of extinction by 'flush-through'. *Am J Physiol 1981; 241:* F579–F590

36 Taylor A, Windhager EE. Cytosolic calcium and its role in the regulation of transepithelial ion and water transport. In Seldin DW, Giebisch G, eds. *The Kidney. Physiology and Pathophysiology.* New York: Raven Press. 1985: 1297–1322

37 Petersen OH, Maruyama Y. Calcium-activated potassium channels and their role in secretion. *Nature 1984; 307:* 693–696

38 Marty A, Tan YP, Trautmann A. Three types of calcium-dependent channel in rat lacrimal glands. *J Physiol 1984; 357:* 293–325

39 Palmer L, Frindt G. Epithelial sodium channels: characterization by using the patch-clamp technique. *Fed Proc 1986; 45:* 2708–2712

40 Lee CO, Taylor A, Windhager EE. Cytosolic calcium ion activity in epithelial cells of Necturus kidney. *Nature 1980; 287:* 859–861

41 Ashford MLJ, Hales CN, Sturgess NC. A calcium-activated non-selective cation channel in a rat insulinoma cell line. *J Physiol 1986; 380:* 23P

MECHANISM OF CHLORIDE TRANSPORT ACROSS THE MAMMALIAN PROXIMAL TUBULE

G Giebisch, L Schild, *R Green

Yale University School of Medicine, New Haven, Connecticut, USA,
**University of Manchester, Manchester, United Kingdom*

Knowledge of the mechanism of chloride transport across the epithelium of the proximal tubule has advanced significantly. Whereas for a long time it has been held that chloride ions move passively with sodium ions – the mendicant position of chloride – more recent studies provide evidence for several characteristic chloride transport mechanisms in parallel, and a new model of chloride transport has evolved. It includes active transcellular and passive intercellular pathways and several lines of evidence strongly support the view that chloride reabsorption across the proximal tubule is critically linked to both sodium and hydrogen ion transport.

Active and passive components of transepithelial chloride movement

The mechanisms by which chloride is transported across the proximal tubule can be described phenomenologically [1] by:

$$J_s = P_s(\Delta C_s + \Psi \cdot \bar{C}_s \cdot zF/RT) + \bar{C}_s J_v (1 - \sigma_s) + J_{act}$$

where J_s is the net solute flux, C_s and ΔC_s are the mean concentrations and differences in concentration of solute, respectively, J_v is the rate of fluid reabsorption, σ is the reflection coefficient, P_s is the solute permeability, Ψ is the transepithelial potential difference, J_{act} is solute movement due to active transport, and z, F, R and T have their usual meanings. According to this approach, chloride movement can be divided into an electrodiffusive term, a solute drag term and an active term. In the following, we shall analyse evidence supporting the participation of each of these processes in transepithelial chloride movement across the mammalian proximal tubule.

Diffusion of chloride across the proximal tubule

The view that chloride ions move passively across the epithelium of the proximal tubule is based on two experimental observations. First, the proximal tubule has a high chloride permeability – particularly the intercellular shunt pathway [1,2] – and a favourable electrochemical potential gradient for passive translocation of chloride ions from the lumen to the peritubular fluid. Secondly, chloride movement across the proximal tubule is subject to modulation by passive driving forces: changes in the transepithelial chloride gradient or the transepithelial electrical potential difference, significantly affect chloride translocation across the proximal tubule [3–9].

Figures 1 and 2 provide data supporting the importance of passive transport mechanisms in transepithelial chloride movement across proximal tubules. Figure 1 summarizes the results of three series of in vivo microperfusion studies in rats in which the luminal perfusion fluid consisted essentially of an isosmotic chloride solution mimicking 'late' proximal tubule fluid [4]. Transepithelial fluid movement was monitored by measuring the concentration changes of inulin. The peritubular perfusion fluid was either a bicarbonate Ringer solution ('complete') or was similar to the perfusion fluid (chloride replaced bicarbonate). Finally, active transport could be abolished by deletion of potassium from the peritubular perfusion fluid. The left section of Figure 1 demonstrates the effects

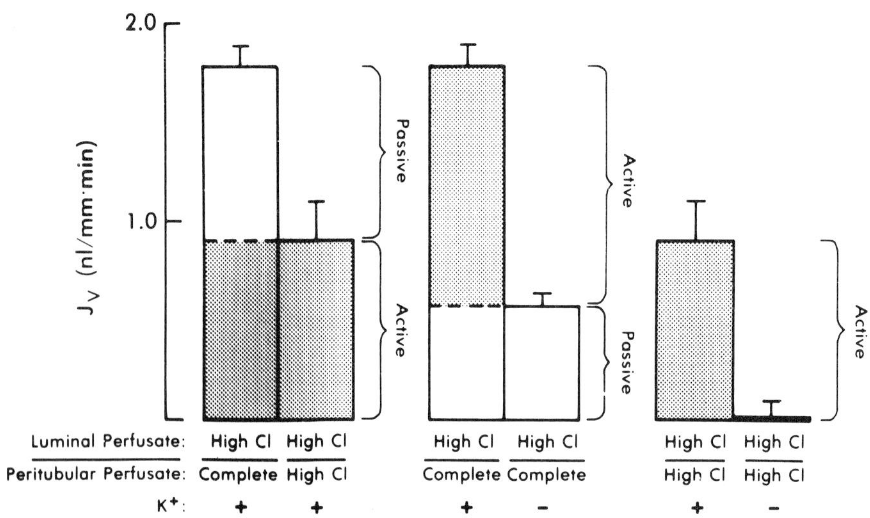

Figure 1. Summary of luminal and peritubular perfusion studies in which the effects of transepithelial chloride gradients and inhibition of active transport on fluid transport (J_V) were studied. Note that abolition of the transepithelial chloride gradients inhibits a significant fraction of proximal chloride reabsorption, that inhibition of active transport (deletion of potassium from the peritubular perfusion fluid) also inhibits a fraction of chloride reabsorption but leaves intact a component of passive chloride movement. The latter is suppressed in the absence of both active transport and a favourable electrochemical potential difference (high chloride in both luminal and peritubular perfusion fluid). From [4]

of abolishing the transepithelial chloride concentration gradient. This manoeuvre results in a significant reduction of transepithelial fluid and chloride movement, presumably that fraction of transepithelial chloride reabsorption due to the chloride concentration gradient. In the middle section of Figure 1 we note that a significant fraction of fluid and chloride reabsorption persists after active transport had been abolished by deletion of potassium from the peritubular perfusion fluid. As shown on the right of Figure 1, it is only in the absence of a transepithelial chloride concentration gradient that inhibition of active transport completely suppresses chloride reabsorption. These experiments fully support previous studies in which the important rôle of the concentration gradient in chloride reabsorption has been established [1,5–10].

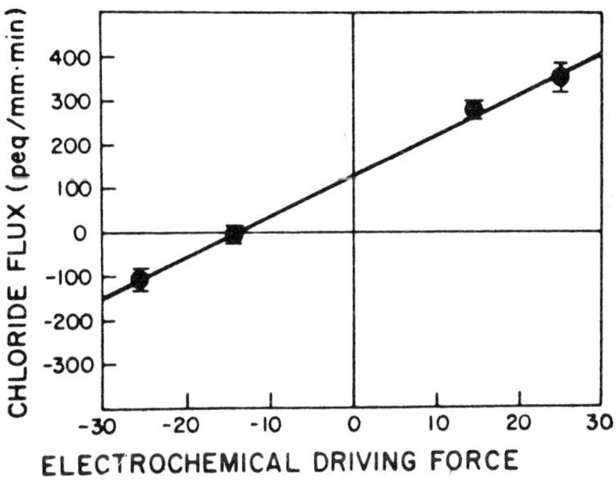

Figure 2. Summary of perfusion experiments in which the effects of changing the luminal chloride concentration on chloride movement was examined. Transepithelial electrical potentials and luminal chloride concentrations were measured to assess the transepithelial electrochemical driving force. Note that a significant amount of chloride continues to be reabsorbed in the absence of a measurable transepithelial electrochemical potential difference. From [3]

Figure 2 summarizes results of luminal and peritubular perfusion experiments in which the effects of changing electrochemical driving forces upon chloride movement is further analysed [3]. Two points deserve mention. First, it is apparent that chloride movement depends critically upon the electrochemical driving force, supporting the notion that a significant component of transepithelial chloride transport occurs by electrodiffusion. A second point concerns the observation that chloride transport continues in the absence of an apparent external driving force. We conclude from this that a significant component of chloride reabsorption occurs by active transport (see below).

Movement of chloride by solvent drag

Much conflicting evidence has been presented about solvent drag and its contribution to chloride reabsorption. This is critically dependent, in a phenomenological sense, on the reflection coefficient σ. In rabbit proximal tubules two groups of workers [11–13] have been unable to link chloride transport with fluid movement and have denied that solvent drag plays a significant rôle. By inference this means that σ must be 1 or very close. Analysis of some of their data [e.g. 11] shows, however, that if $\sigma = 0.6$ and an increased reabsorptive flux of 1.2nl · mm^{-1} · min^{-1} occurred with an average concentration of chloride of 120mmol · $litre^{-1}$, the amount of chloride transported by solvent drag would be expected to be about 58pmol · mm^{-1} · min^{-1}. For a perfusion rate of 20nl · min^{-1}, some 2400pmol · min^{-1} are perfused so that 58pmol · min^{-1} represents only a 2.5% change in the amount of chloride collected – an amount which is virtually undetectable with current methodology.

In rat proximal convoluted tubules perfused in vivo, there is much evidence that chloride reabsorption *is* linked to total fluid flux [1,14–16]. In recent experiments [16] we have perfused tubules and capillaries with cyanide containing solutions which inhibit active transport. The precise composition of the fluid was (in mmol · $litre^{-1}$): NaCl, 148; KCl, 5; $CaCl_2$, 1; NaCN, 2; with tracer amounts of ^{3}H-methoxyinulin as a volume marker. The tubular perfusion rate was 30nl · min^{-1}. As predicted, there was no significant net fluid reabsorption (-0.05±0.19nl · mm^{-1} · min^{-1}) or net chloride absorption (-43±37pmol · mm^{-1} · min^{-1}). When the peritubular perfusate was made hypertonic with either 25mM sodium chloride or with 40mM L-glucose there was an induced water flux and an associated chloride flux (see Table I).

TABLE I

Peritubular hypertonic agent	No. of tubules	Fluid flux (nl·mm^{-1}·min^{-1})	Net chloride flux (pmol·mm^{-1}·min^{-1})	Chloride flux due to solvent drag (pmol·mm^{-1}·min^{-1})
None	(48)	−0.05±0.19	−43±37	−3
25mM Sodium chloride	(27)	2.14±0.20	143±59	147
40mM L-glucose	(16)	2.91±0.37	172±68	186

When L-glucose was the osmotic agent there was a rise in chloride concentration in the tubular fluid which might have contributed to chloride reabsorption by diffusion, but no such objection can be raised when sodium chloride is the osmotic agent because the gradient for chloride movement is directed from the capillaries into the tubule. There seems, therefore, to be an undeniable link between water flux and chloride movement in rat proximal tubules.

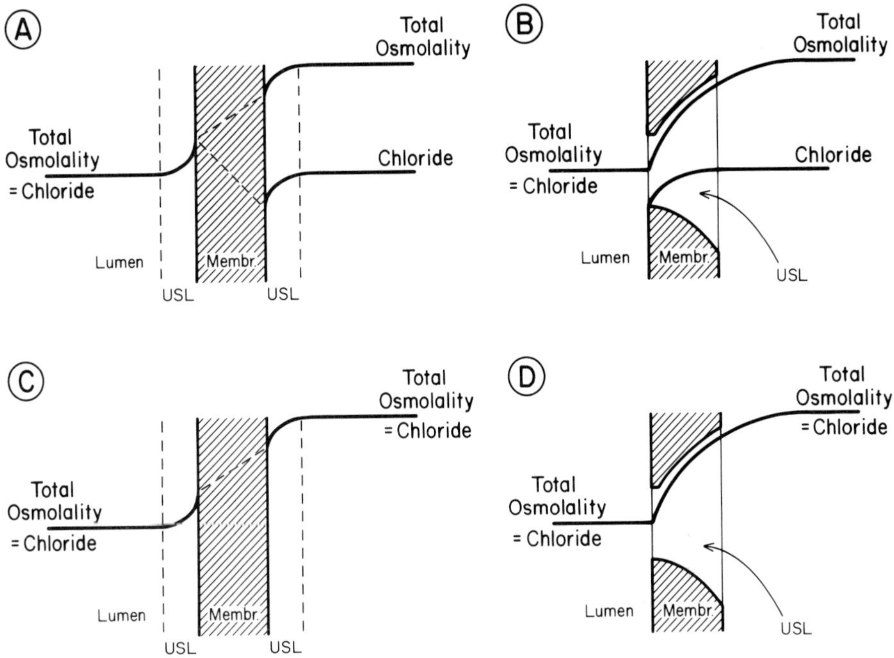

Figure 3. Effects of unstirred layer (USL) on gradients across membrane. A or B where L-glucose is the hypertonic driving agent, C or D where sodium chloride is the driving agent. In A and C the membrane is assumed to be homogenous with a USL *on either side*; in B and D the USL is depicted as in the interspace, with no USL on the luminal side of the membrane

It has been customary to describe this work of link as 'solvent drag' but a number of factors need to be considered before this can be truly defined as the frictional interactions between solute and solvent particles. One technical complication is the presence of unstirred layers. When volume reabsorption proceeds in response to an osmotic gradient, solute polarization occurs [17]. This could be either at the interface between the fluid and epithelium or, if all fluid passes through an intercellular compartment, within that compartment (see Figure 3). While such considerations might be applied to the experiments in which L-glucose was the hypertonic agent – where the water movement driven by L-glucose will create an apparent gradient down which chloride could move (Figures 3A and 3B), they cannot apply to the experiments with sodium chloride since, if there exists a gradient to cause water flow, that same gradient must oppose chloride reabsorption (Figures 3C and 3D). Calculation has shown that because of the diameter of the tubules, the unstirred layer is not, in any case, likely to have a major effect [18].

Setting aside technical considerations, it is possible to determine whether there are direct frictional forces between solute and solvent molecules. It can be shown [19] that:

$$\sigma = 1 - \frac{\omega \bar{V}_s}{L_p} - \frac{K f_{sw}}{\phi_w (f_{sw} + f_{sm})}$$

where ω is the diffusive salt permeability and $= P_s/RT$, L_p is the hydraulic water permeability and is equal to $P_f \bar{V}_w/RT$, $\bar{V}_s$ is the partial molar volume of solute, $\bar{V}_w$ is the partial molar volume of water, f_{sw} is the friction between solute and water, f_{sm} the friction between solute and the membrane , ϕ_w the overall cross-sectional area accessible to water, and K is the average solute distribution coefficient.

There are few relevant measurements of f_{sw}, f_{sm} and K, but in general if solute and solvent traverse the membrane by different routes, frictional interaction is 0 so that

$$\sigma = 1 - \frac{\omega \bar{V}_s}{L_p} .$$

Conversely if

$$\sigma < 1 - \frac{\omega \bar{V}_s}{L_p} ,$$

then some frictional interaction must occur, i.e. there is true solvent drag. From our recent data, we can show that $\sigma_{NaCl} = 0.59$, $P_f = 1030 \mu m \cdot sec^{-1}$ and $P_{NaCl} = 1.7 \mu m \cdot sec^{-1}$ (calculated for $P_{Na} = 1.3 \mu m \cdot sec^{-1}$ and $P_{Cl} = 2.2 \mu m \cdot sec^{-1}$, as $P_{NaCl} = 2\, P_{Na} \cdot P_{Cl}/(P_{Na} + P_{Cl})$ [16,20] and $\bar{V}_s$ for NaCl at 160mM $= 17 cm^3 \cdot mol^{-1}$ [21].

$1 - \frac{\omega V_s}{L_p}$ can be shown to be equivalent to $1 - \frac{P_s \bar{V}_s}{P_f \bar{V}_w}$ and this is equivalent to $1 - \left(\frac{1.7}{1030} \times \frac{17}{18}\right) = 0.998$. The difference between 0.998 and 0.59 is so large and significant that there must be an interaction between water and salt transport. We therefore conclude that at least some of the water and chloride ions follow the same route and that solvent drag *is* a significant mechanism for chloride transport. It says nothing, however, about what that common route is.

Transcellular mechanisms of chloride transport

The persistence of a significant component of transepithelial reabsorptive chloride movement in the absence of either a chemical or electrical potential gradient has led to an investigation of possible mechanisms by which *transcellular* chloride movement could occur. Possible transport routes of such modes of chloride reabsorption are schematically summarized in Figure 4 [22]. Chloride movement between cells has already been discussed when *passive* chloride

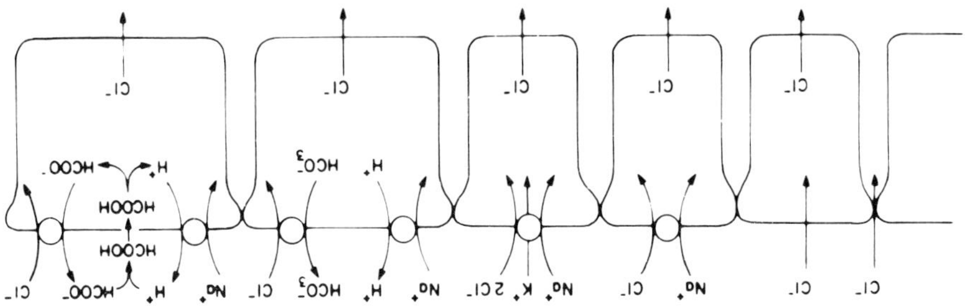

Figure 4. Possible mechanisms of chloride transport across the epithelium of the proximal tubule. Specific exit mechanisms of chloride across the basolateral cell membrane are not considered. From [22]

transport by electrodiffusion was considered. In contrast, chloride movement through cells must involve an active apical transport step in view of the insufficient electrochemical driving force that operates at this site [23]. Since no evidence supports the view of primary active chloride transport in the apical brush border membrane of proximal tubule cells, several types of secondary, active chloride transport have been considered [22]. These include direct, carrier-mediated linkage between sodium and chloride movement [24,25], coupling of chloride transport to sodium and potassium [26], and coupled exchange mechanisms of chloride for bicarbonate (or OH) [27,28], or of chloride for other anions of cellular origin, both coupled to the exchange of sodium for hydrogen ions [29].

Based on evidence obtained first by Karniski and Aronson in brush border vesicles of rabbit proximal tubules, a new model of transcellular chloride transport has emerged [30]. As shown in Figure 5, it involves several components. First, an anion exchanger in the apical cell membrane that binds both formate and chloride ions. Second, a potent sodium/hydrogen exchanger that prevents both cell and luminal pH changes and, third, a highly effective apical pathway

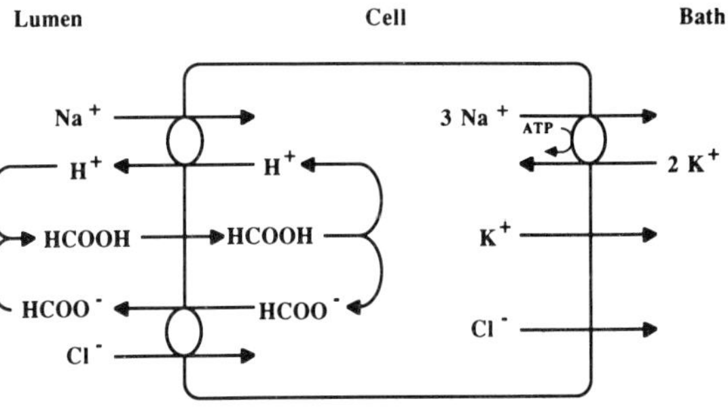

Figure 5. Proximal cell model demonstrating the rôle of formate in mediating electroneutral sodium chloride entry across the apical cell membrane. From [32]

for the diffusion of non-ionized formic acid. This allows for extensive recycling of formate from lumen to cell, necessary for operation of this transport mechanism in view of the much larger amount of chloride reabsorbed than that of formate secreted [30].

Evidence based on intracellular pH measurements has confirmed the presence of a chloride/base exchange mechanism involving formate [31]. When care is taken to block basolateral bicarbonate exit by stilbene inhibitors to amplify apical membrane effects on cell pH, addition of chloride leads to cell acidification, an effect significantly stimulated by formate. In parallel with sodium/hydrogen exchange, such anion exchange mechanisms are thus involved in active, transcellular chloride movement. Chloride/bicarbonate or chloride/OH exchange appears to play only a minor rôle in mediating net transcellular chloride movement, although this problem is not fully resolved [27,28,31].

The physiological rôle of chloride/formate exchange on fluid and chloride transport has been directly evaluated in perfusion studies of isolated rabbit proximal tubules [22,32]. These experiments were carried out using two types of luminal perfusion fluids. One solution mimicked 'late' proximal tubule fluid containing 3mM bicarbonate and 142mM chloride and having a pH of 6.5, another contained 25mM bicarbonate and had a pH of 7.4. Figure 6 summarizes the results of a study in which the effects of formate in the bath and the lumen on net fluid movement were tested [22,32]. It can be seen that addition of submillimolar amounts of formate, 0.25 and 0.5mM respectively, stimulated fluid movement across straight segments of proximal tubules. These effects on

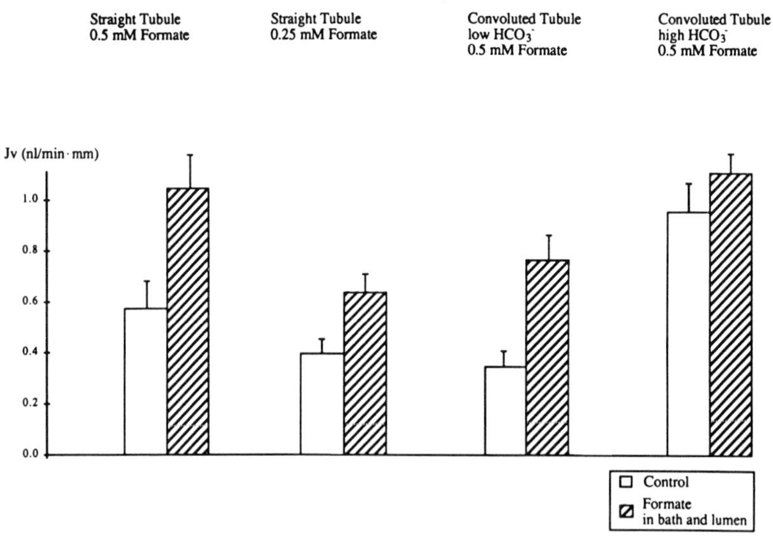

Figure 6. Summary of flux studies in isolated, perfused proximal tubules of the rabbit kidney. Shown is the effect of formate in the bath and lumen on water transport. Straight tubules were perfused with solutions simulating late proximal tubule fluid. Convoluted tubules were perfused with symmetrical solutions. From [22]

net transepithelial fluid movement indicate significant stimulation of chloride transport as well since chloride was the main anion in the perfusion fluid. The transport stimulation by formate was reversible, occurred without any changes in the transepithelial potential difference and could be blocked by SITS ((4,4′)-diisothiocyano-(2,2′)-disulfonic-stilbene). It should be noted that the addition of acetate or propionate in similar concentrations did not stimulate fluid and chloride transport.

Inspection of Figure 6 also shows that transport stimulation in the proximal convoluted tubule by formate depends on the bicarbonate content of the perfusion solution [22,32]. When proximal convoluted tubules were perfused with symmetrical high chloride/low bicarbonate solutions, transport was stimulated. However, no transport stimulation occurred when symmetrical low chloride/high bicarbonate solutions were used. This behaviour may be due to the different pH of the perfusion solutions. It can be shown that the solution with low buffer content (high chloride/low bicarbonate) is effectively acidified during perfusion, whereas a solution containing low chloride/high bicarbonate is less acidified [32]. In the latter situation, non-ionic back-diffusion of formic acid into the cell may occur at a low enough rate to compromise the chloride/formate exchange mechanisms.

These experiments suggest a rôle for formate/chloride exchange for the entry mechanism of chloride into proximal tubule cells. The mechanisms controlling formate metabolism, formate entry across the basolateral cell membrane and the control of apical formate/chloride exchange are presently poorly understood and need further investigation.

Chloride transport across the basolateral cell membrane

Three mechanisms are presently considered to facilitate chloride exit across the basolateral cell membrane: electrodiffusion of chloride through channels that allow the penetration by chloride ions [33], cotransport of chloride with potassium [34,35], and anion exchange mechanisms, mostly chloride/bicarbonate exchange [36–38]. A component of the latter exchange process has been shown to be dependent on extracellular sodium [38]. An unresolved problem of transcellular chloride transport in the proximal tubule concerns the relative magnitude and physiological importance of these parallel chloride exit steps and their rôle in the regulation of chloride reabsorption.

Acknowledgment

Work in the author's laboratory was supported by NIH grant AM 17433.

References

1 Frömter EE, Rumrich G, Ullrich KJ. Phenomenological description of Na, Cl and HCO_3 absorption from proximal tubules in the rat kidney. *Pfluegers Arch 1973; 343:* 189–220

2 Boulpaep EL. Electrophysiology of the kidney. In Giebisch G, Tosteson DC, Ussing HH, eds. *Membrane Transport in Biology, Vol IVA.* Berlin: Springer. 1979: 97–144

3 Alpern RJ, Howlin KJ, Preisig P. Active and passive components of chloride transport in the rat proximal convoluted tubule. *J Clin Invest 1985; 76:* 1360–1366

4 Chantrelle BN, Cogan MG, Rector FC Jr. Active and passive components of NaCl absorption in the proximal convoluted tubule of the rat kidney. *Min Electrolyte Metab 1985; 11:* 290–214

5 Giebisch G, Green R. Anion-driven fluid movement across proximal tubular epithelium. In *Alfred Benzon Symposium 15. Water Transport Across Epithelia.* Copenhagen: Munksgaard. 1980: 376–392

6 Green R, Giebisch G. Ionic requirements of proximal tubular sodium transport. II. Hydrogen ion. *Am J Physiol 1975; 229:* 1216–1226

7 Green R, Bishop JHV, Giebisch G. Ionic requirements of proximal tubular sodium transport. III. Selective luminal anion substitution. *Am J Physiol 1979; 236:* F268–F277

8 Green R, Giebisch G. Ionic requirements of proximal tubular sodium transport. I. Bicarbonate and chloride. *Am J Physiol 1975; 229:* 1205–1215

9 Green R, Moriarty RJ, Giebisch G. Ionic requirements of proximal tubular sodium transport. IV. Flow dependence of fluid transport. *Kidney Int 1981; 20:* 580–587

10 Frömter E. Solute transport across epithelia: what can we learn from micropuncture studies on kidney tubules? *J Physiol 1976; 228:* 1–31

11 Corman B, DiStephano A. Does water drag solute through kidney proximal tubule? *Pfluegers Arch 1983; 397:* 35–41

12 Jacobson HR, Kokko JP, Seldin DW, Holmberg C. Lack of solvent drag of NaCl and $NaHCO_3$ in rabbit proximal tubules. *Am J Physiol 1982; 243:* F342–F348

13 Hierholzer K, Kawamura SS, Seldin DW et al. Reflection coefficients of various substrates across superficial and juxtamedullary proximal convoluted segments of rabbit nephrons. *Min Electrolyte Metab 1980; 3:* 172–180

14 Bomsztyk K, Wright FS. Dependence of ion fluxes on fluid transport by rat proximal tubule. *Am J Physiol 1986; 250:* F680–F689

15 Andreoli TE, Schafer JA, Troutman SL, Watkins ML. Solvent drag component of Cl flux in superficial proximal straight tubule: evidence for a paracellular component of isotonic fluid absorption. *Am J Physiol 1979; 237:* F445–F462

16 Green R, Giebisch G. Reflection coefficients and fluid movement in rat proximal tubule. I. Absence of active transport. *Am J Physiol:* submitted for publication

17 House CR. *Water Transport in Cells and Tissues.* London: Edward Arnold. 1974: 104–114 and 141–143

18 Berry CA. Water permeability and pathways in the proximal tubule. *Am J Physiol 1983; 245:* F299–F294

19 Kedem O, Katchalsky A. A physical interpretation of the phenomenological coefficients of membrane permeability. *J Gen Physiol 1961; 45:* 143–179

20 Kedem O, Leaf A. The relation between salt and ionic transport coefficients. *J Gen Physiol 1966; 49:* 655–662

21 Gucker FT. The apparent molal heat capacity, volume and compressibility of electrolytes. *Chemical Reviews 1933; 13:* 111–130

22 Schild L, Giebisch G, Karniski L, Aronson PS. Chloride transport in the mammalian proximal tubule. *Pfluegers Arch 1986; 407:* S156–S159

23 Cassola AC, Mollenhauer M, Frömter E. The intracellular chloride activity of rat kidney proximal tubular cells. *Pfluegers Arch 1983; 399:* 259–265

24 Kimura G, Spring KR. Luminal Na^+ entry into Necturus proximal tubule cells. *Am J Physiol 1979; 236:* F295–F301

25 Oberleithner H, Greger R, Neuman S et al. Omission of luminal potassium reduces cellular chloride in early distal tubule of amphiuma kidney. *Pfluegers Arch 1983; 398:* 18–22

26 Greger R, Schlatter E. Presence of luminal K^+: a prerequisite for active NaCl transport in the cortical thick ascending limb of Henle's loop of rabbit kidney. *Pfluegers Arch 1981; 392:* 92–94

27 Warnock DG, Yee VJ. Chloride uptake by brush-border membrane vesicles isolated from rabbit renal cortex: coupling to proton gradients and K^+ diffusion potentials. *J Clin Invest 1981; 67:* 103–115

28 Seifter JL, Knickelbein R, Aronson PS. Absence of Cl-OH exchange and NaCl cotransport in rabbit renal microvillus membrane vesicles. *Am J Physiol 1984; 247:* F753–F759

29 Mahnensmith RL, Aronson PS. The plasma membrane sodium-hydrogen exchanger and its role in physiological and pathophysiological processes. *Circ Res 1984; 57:* 773–788

30 Karniski LP, Aronson PS. Chloride/formate exchange with formic acid recycling: mechanism of active chloride transport across epithelial membranes. *Proc Natl Acad Sci USA 1985; 82:* 6362–6365

31 Alpern RJ. Apical membrane Cl/base exchange in the rat proximal convoluted tubule. *J Clin Invest 1987; 79:* 1026–1030

32 Schild L, Giebisch G, Karniski LP, Aronson PS. Effect of formate on volume reabsorption in the rabbit proximal tubule. *J Clin Invest 1987; 79:* 32–38

33 Gögelein H, Greger R. A voltage-dependent ionic channel in the basolateral membrane of the late proximal tubule of the rabbit kidney. *Pfluegers Arch 1986; 407:* S142–S148

34 Eveloff J, Warnock DG. KCl cotransport systems in renal basolateral membrane vesicles. *Kidney Int 1987; 31:* 432

35 Gullans SR, Avison MJ, Ogino T et al. Furosemide-sensitive K^+ efflux induced by glucose in the rabbit proximal tubule. *Kidney Int 1986; 29:* 396

36 Alpern RJ, Chambers M, Basolateral membrane Cl/HCO_3 exchange in the rat proximal convoluted tubule. Na-dependent and independent modes. *J Gen Physiol 1987; 89:* 581–598

37 Alpern RJ. Mechanism of basolateral membrane $H^+/OH^-/HCO_3^-$ transport in the rat proximal convoluted tubule: a sodium-coupled electrogenic process. *J Gen Physiol 1985; 86:* 613–636

38 Guggino W, London R, Boulpaep EL, Giebisch G. Chloride transport across the basolateral cell membrane of the Necturus proximal tubule. Dependence on bicarbonate and sodium. *J Membrane Biol 1983, 71.* 227–240

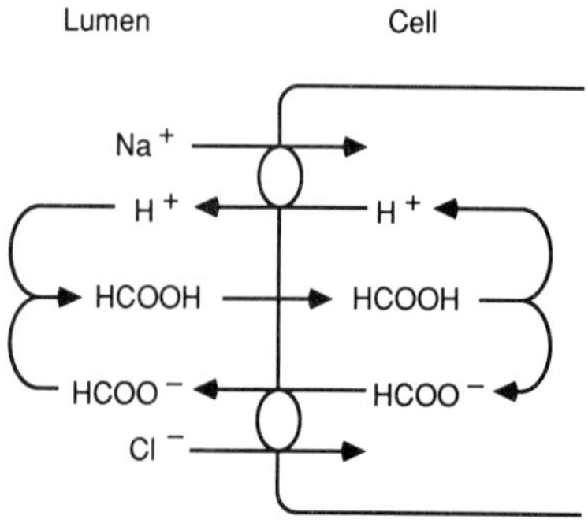

Figure 1. Schematic model of chloride uptake via chloride-formate exchange across the luminal membrane of the proximal tubule cell

uphill accumulation in renal microvillus vesicles was stimulated when a pH gradient (inside-alkaline) was imposed on the presence of a physiological concentration of formate (i.e. 0.2mM), but not when the same pH gradient was imposed in the absence of formate [6]. To the extent that active proton secretion across the luminal membrane occurs by a sodium-coupled mechanism such as sodium/proton exchange, as is largely the case in the proximal tubule, the net effect is equivalent to an electroneutral sodium-coupled chloride transport process (Figure 1). This process is driven by the inward sodium gradient that is present across the luminal membrane due to the primary active extrusion of sodium across the basolateral membrane via the Na/K-ATPase. In collaboration with Schild and Giebisch [9], we found that addition of physiological concentrations of formate to the bath and lumen of isolated, perfused proximal tubules from the rabbit markedly stimulated the rate of NaCl absorption. This finding strongly supports the concept that chloride-formate exchange is a major mechanism for transcellular chloride reabsorption in the intact proximal tubule under physiological conditions.

Chloride-oxalate exchange

Imposing a 10:1 outwardly directed oxalate gradient significantly stimulated the rate of chloride uptake into rabbit renal microvillus membrane vesicles, suggesting the presence of chloride-oxalate exchange [10]. This was confirmed by the finding that imposing a 10:1 outward chloride gradient markedly enhanced the rate of oxalate uptake and induced the transient uphill accumulation of oxalate above equilibrium. A 10:1 outwardly directed gradient of formate also stimulated uphill oxalate uptake, indicating the presence of formate-oxalate exchange [10]. Our initial hypothesis was that the processes of chloride-formate exchange, chloride-oxalate exchange and formate-oxalate exchange represented different modes of a single anion exchanger. Indeed, for each of several inhibitors and substrates, the dose response curve for inhibition of chloride-oxalate exchange was identical to that for inhibition of formate-oxalate exchange, suggesting that these two processes are modes of a single transport system [10]. However, chloride-formate exchange was less sensitive to inhibition by DIDS and was more sensitive to azide and frusemide than were the processes of chloride-oxalate exchange and formate-oxalate exchange [10]. Moreover, concentrations of oxalate that saturated the processes of chloride-oxalate exchange and formate-oxalate exchange caused only very modest inhibition of chloride-formate exchange. Studies utilizing potassium gradients in the presence of potassium ionophore valinomycin to vary the transmembrane electrical potential difference indicated that chloride-formate exchange is electroneutral, whereas the processes of chloride-oxalate exchange and formate-oxalate exchange are electrogenic in a manner consistent with exchange of one monovalent anion for divalent oxalate [10].

We therefore concluded that the major fraction of chloride-formate exchange occurs by an anion exchange pathway separate from that mediating chloride-oxalate exchange and formate-oxalate exchange [10]. According to this view, one transporter, the chloride-formate exchanger, accepts chloride and formate as substrates, has little or no affinity for oxalate, is more sensitive to inhibition by frusemide and azide than by DIDS, and is electroneutral. A second transporter, the chloride (formate)-oxalate exchanger, also accepts chloride and formate as substrates, but has high affinity for oxalate, is highly sensitive to inhibition by DIDS, less sensitive to inhibition by azide and frusemide, and is electrogenic.

Recently, we have observed hydroxyl-oxalate exchange in rabbit renal microvillus membrane vesicles [Kuo and Aronson, unpublished observations]. This process was found to be electrogenic, inhibited by chloride, and highly sensitive to inhibition by DIDS. These properties of the hydroxyl-oxalate exchange process indicate that it likely occurs as a mode of the chloride (formate)-oxalate exchanger. We have been unable to demonstrate appreciable chloride/hydroxyl exchange or chloride-formate exchange via the chloride (formate)-oxalate exchanger, suggesting that this system mediates exchange of monovalent anions for one another poorly if at all. Thus, this pathway appears to function principally in modes involving the exchange of monovalent anions for oxalate.

For chloride-oxalate exchange to play an important rôle in mediating active transcellular chloride reabsorption in the proximal tubule, a mechanism for recycling oxalate from lumen-to-cell would be necessary. There is evidence that oxalate shares the $2Na^+$-$SO_4^=$ cotransport system present in the luminal membrane [11], but we have found only minimal sodium gradient-stimulated oxalate uptake in rabbit renal microvillus vesicles [unpublished observations]. However, formate-oxalate exchange and hydroxyl-oxalate exchange are appreciable transport processes in these membrane vesicles, as discussed above. Thus, as shown in Figure 2, chloride-oxalate exchange with recycling of oxalate into the

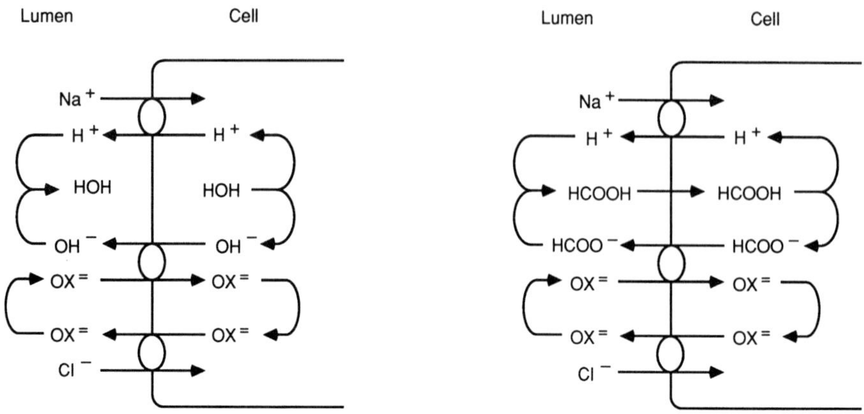

Figure 2. Schematic models of chloride uptake via chloride-oxalate exchange across the luminal membrane of the proximal tubule cell

cell by hydroxyl-oxalate exchange or by formate-oxalate exchange is a possible mechanism for mediating active uptake of chloride across the luminal membrane of the proximal tubule cell. Because cell-to-lumen gradients of hydroxyl and formate result from active proton secretion that takes place largely via sodium/proton exchange, any chloride transport occuring via chloride-oxalate exchange would be indirectly sodium-coupled, as illustrated in Figure 2.

Summary and conclusion

We have described at least two pathways by which active chloride uptake across the luminal membrane of the proximal tubule cell can occur by anion exchange. One pathway mediates the exchange of chloride for formate. Studies on the intact proximal tubule indicate that chloride-formate exchange may be a major mechanism for chloride transport under physiological conditions. The second pathway mediates the exchange of chloride for oxalate. To date, there is no evidence indicating whether this process may also contribute significantly to transtubular chloride transport.

It is interesting to speculate about the possible physiological utility of reabsorbing chloride in exchange for an organic anion, such as formate or oxalate. In effect, the organic anion, by recycling via a pH-coupled process, serves as a coupling factor to allow proton-coupled chloride transport across the luminal membrane. In parallel with sodium/proton exchange, this results in net NaCl entry. What is the physiological advantage of carrying out NaCl reabsorption in the proximal tubule by such a roundabout mechanism rather than by a more direct mechanism such as sodium/chloride cotransport? Is it possible that the local concentration of formate or oxalate is regulated in order to modulate proximal tubule NaCl reabsorption? Even in the absence of added formate or oxalate, a component of active, transcellular chloride reabsorption has been observed in the proximal tubule. Does this reflect the presence of additional pathways for chloride transport across the luminal membrane, or is endogenous production of formate or oxalate by proximal tubule cells sufficient to maintain a modest rate of chloride transport even in the absence of exogenously added organic anions? Answering these questions will require examining the metabolic production and/or disposal of formate and oxalate in proximal tubule cells, and measuring the concentration of formate and oxalate in luminal fluid, in peritubular blood and in proximal tubule cells as a function of manoeuvres known to alter proximal tubule NaCl reabsorption.

References

1 Giebisch G, Aronson PS. The proximal nephron. In Andreoli TE, Hoffman JF, Fanestil DD, Schultz SG, eds. *Physiology of Membrane Disorders, 2nd Edition.* New York: Plenum Medical Book Co. 1986: 669–700

2 Schild L, Giebisch G, Karniski L, Aronson PS. Chloride transport in the mammalian proximal tubule. *Pfluegers Arch 1986; 407 (Suppt 2):* S156–S159

3 Seifter JL, Knickelbein R, Aronson PS. Absence of Cl-OH exchange and Na-Cl cotransport in rabbit renal microvillus membrane vesicles. *Am J Physiol 1984; 247:* F753–F759

4 Warnock DG, Yee VJ. Chloride uptake by brush border membrane vesicles isolated from rabbit renal cortex. Coupling to proton gradients and K^+ diffusion potentials. *J Clin Invest 1981; 67:* 103–115

5 Shiuan D, Weinstein SW. Evidence for electroneutral chloride transport in rabbit renal cortical brush border membrane vesicles. *Am J Physiol 1984; 247:* F837–F847

6 Karniski LP, Aronson PS. Chloride/formate exchange with formic acid recycling: a mechanism of active chloride transport across epithelial membranes. *Proc Natl Acad Sci USA 1985; 82:* 6362 6365

7 Ives HE, Chen P-Y, Verkman AS. Mechanism of coupling between Cl^- and OH^- transport in renal brush-border membranes. *Biochim Biophys Acta 1986; 863:* 91–100

8 Walter A, Gutknecht J. Monocarboxylic acid permeation through lipid bilayer membranes. *J Membrane Biol 1984; 77:* 255–264

9 Schild L, Giebisch G, Karniski LP, Aronson PS. Effect of formate on volume reabsorption in the rabbit proximal tubule. *J Clin Invest 1987; 79:* 32–38

10 Karniski LP, Aronson PS. Anion exchange pathways for Cl^- transport in rabbit renal microvillus membranes. *Am J Physiol 1987: 253:* in press

11 Bästlein C, Burckhardt G. Sensitivity of rat renal luminal and contraluminal sulfate transport systems to DIDS. *Am J Physiol 1986; 250:* F226–F234

MECHANISMS OF NaCl TRANSPORT IN MAMMALIAN PROXIMAL TUBULE

F C Rector Jr, Christine A Berry

Cardiovascular Research Institute, University of California, San Francisco, California, USA

Introduction

The proximal tubule reabsorbs approximately 100% of the organic solutes, 90% of the $NaHCO_3$, and 50–60% of the NaCl and water filtered at the glomerulus. In the mammalian kidney there is considerable axial heterogeneity. The first millimetre of the proximal convoluted tubule reabsorbs bicarbonate and organic solutes at much faster rates than does the later portion [1], as a consequence the concentration of chloride in late portions of proximal convoluted tubule is higher than in plasma. The mechanisms for transepithelial reabsorption of chloride are different in early and late portions of the proximal tubule [2].

In the early proximal convoluted tubule sodium-coupled glucose and amino acid transport generate a lumen negative potential difference which drives the reabsorption of chloride passively through the highly permeable paracellular shunt pathway. In the late proximal convoluted tubule the high luminal concentration of chloride provides two possible driving forces for passive NaCl reabsorption: convection and diffusion. In 1966 Rector and associates [3] proposed that the reflection coefficient for NaCl in the proximal convoluted tubule was lower than that of $NaHCO_3$ and glucose, and as a consequence the reabsorption of $NaHCO_3$ and glucose would generate an effective osmotic force that promotes the reabsorption of water with some entrained NaCl. This solvent drag of NaCl requires that the reflection coefficient for NaCl be less than that for $NaHCO_3$ and organic solutes such as glucose and aminoacids. However, evidence suggesting a low NaCl reflection coefficient in the proximal convoluted tubule has been unconvincing. Direct studies in the isolated perfused proximal convoluted tubule from rabbits have failed to demonstrate any significant convective transport of NaCl coupled to osmotic water movement [4]. In contrast, the high luminal chloride concentration has been shown to promote diffusive NaCl reabsorption. Chloride diffusion is driven by the high luminal chemical concentration of chloride and sodium diffusion is driven by the lumen positive potential difference generated by the difference between lumen and bath chloride and bicarbonate concentrations in a chloride permselective membrane. Convective transport may be more important in the rat than the rabbit.

Evidence for active transcellular electroneutral NaCl transport

Passive NaCl reabsorption in the proximal tubule only accounts for a small percentage of proximal NaCl reabsorption. Studies in both the rat and rabbit proximal convoluted tubule have demonstrated that the passive reabsorption of NaCl accounts for only 20 to 50% of the total NaCl absorption from the late proximal tubule, while 50 to 80% appears to be reabsorbed actively via a transcellular route. The most convincing studies concerning the relative rates of passive and active NaCl transport are those of Baum and Berry [5]. They found that the rabbit proximal convoluted tubule, when perfused with a high chloride solution resembling late proximal fluid and bathed in a plasma-like solution, had a lumen-positive chloride diffusion potential difference and absorbed fluid at a rate of $0.56 nl \cdot mm^{-1} \cdot min^{-1}$. When the chloride concentration gradient was obliterated by changing the bath to a high chloride solution, the potential difference fell to zero and fluid absorption was reduced 20% to $0.45 nl \cdot mm^{-1} \cdot min^{-1}$. Thus, the rate of NaCl absorption was 80% of normal in the absence of any external electrochemical gradients for NaCl absorption; therefore, there must be some form of a transcellular, active NaCl transport process. The potential difference of zero suggests that the transport process is electroneutral. This conclusion was confirmed by additional experiments in which the tubules were perfused with high chloride perfusate and bathed in plasma-like solution in the absence and presence of ouabain in the bathing solution. Ouabain reduced the absorptive rate by 84% from 0.51 to $0.08 nl \cdot mm^{-1} \cdot min^{-1}$, but had no effect on the lumen-positive potential difference, which was +2.4mV and +2.5mV in the absence and presence of ouabain in the bathing solution. Ouabain reduced the absorptive rate by 84% from 0.51 to $0.08 nl \cdot mm^{-1} \cdot min^{-1}$, but had no effect on fluid was about 20% passive, while the remaining 80% was active, transcellular and electroneutral. Studies in the rat proximal tubule studied in vivo have also shown that NaCl reabsorption is active [6], transcellular [7], and electroneutral [8].

Apical membrane transport processes

The precise mechanisms involved in this process of electroneutral NaCl transport have not yet been defined completely. In this discussion we will first address the possible mechanisms by which sodium and chloride might enter the cell across the apical membrane, and thereafter consider the mechanisms by which chloride might exit the cell across the basolateral membrane. Although the overall process is electroneutral, parallel and equivalent electrogenic processes could be involved in either the apical or basolateral membranes, or both. A conductive chloride pathway has been observed in vesicles made from renal brush borders, but not in those made from basolateral membrane [9–11]. Electrophysiological studies on intact proximal convoluted tubules have failed to find any significant sodium or chloride ion conductances in either apical or basolateral membranes, however, [12] so parallel electrogenic sodium and chloride transport is highly unlikely. A second possibility is that there is directly coupled sodium:chloride electroneutral cotransport in the apical membrane. Studies on renal brush border membrane vesicles, however, have failed to demonstrate any direct coupling between chloride and sodium or potassium [9,11], so this also is an unlikely possibility. Most of the current evidence suggests that sodium and chloride are moved across the apical membrane of the proximal convoluted tubule by the action of two parallel ion exchangers: Na/H exchange and Cl/base exchange. The Na/H antiporter in brush border membrane vesicles was first demonstrated by Murer, Hopfer and Kinne [13], and has been extensively characterized by Aronson and others [14]. The various mechanisms involved in anion transport in renal brush border membrane vesicles have been discussed in the preceding chapter.

Preisig et al [15] have recently quantified the rôle of the Na/H antiporter in NaCl reabsorption in the rat proximal convoluted tubule, microperfused in vivo, by measuring net NaCl absorption in the presence and absence of varying amounts of amiloride in the luminal fluid. In these studies we evaluated Na/H antiporter activity by measuring the change in cell pH in response to a rapid change in luminal sodium concentration. In the absence of luminal amiloride Na/H antiporter activity was designated 100% and the inhibition caused by 1 and 4mM amiloride measured. The effect of the same doses of amiloride on total NaCl absorption was also measured and the fraction of total NaCl mediated by the antiporter was calculated. Under these conditions in the rat proximal convoluted tubule approximately 50% of NaCl absorption is passive and 50% is active and virtually all of the active component of NaCl absorption was mediated by Na/H exchange. Baum [16] has performed similar studies in the rabbit proximal convoluted tubule and has found that 1mM amiloride inhibits active NaCl absorption by 50%. (Note that this figure was not corrected for the corresponding percentage inhibition of the Na/H antiporter.) Thus, the evidence suggests that the Na/H antiporter plays a major (50–100%) rôle in the active transcellular absorption of NaCl in both the rat and rabbit proximal convoluted tubule.

Evidence has been presented in the two preceding chapters that sodium chloride is transported across the apical cell membrane by Cl/formate exchange acting in parallel with the Na/H antiporter.

Basolateral cell membrane transport processes

To complete the process of vectorial transport of NaCl from lumen to blood, sodium and chloride which enter the cell across the apical membrane must exit the cell across the basolateral membrane. The sodium, at least in part, will be transported out of the cell by the basolateral Na/K-ATPase pump system. The mechanism by which the chloride leaves the cell is poorly understood. Although the electrochemical gradient is favourable for passive diffusion of chloride out of the cell, there is no evidence from either electrophysiological or vesicle studies for the existence of simple chloride conductive pathways in the basolateral membrane. Any anion current crossing the basolateral membrane would depolarize this membrane to a potential difference below the potassium equilibrium potential difference. Kuwahara, Rector and Berry [17] have found that in proximal convoluted tubule perfused and bathed with symmetrical high chloride solutions inhibition of anion currents by the disulphonic stilbene SITS in the bath caused hyperpolarization of the basolateral membrane, establishing the existence of anion current under these conditions. However, baseline basolateral membrane potential difference and the SITS-dependent anion current were completely independent of the presence or absence of chloride. Thus, there appears to be no Cl-dependent anion current crossing the basolateral membrane during electroneutral NaCl transport. Other studies by Berry and her associates have shown that chloride transport is in fact insensitive to the basolateral membrane potential difference. They found that depolarization of the basolateral potential difference by addition of Ba^{++} to the bathing solution inhibited net $NaHCO_3$ absorption by 50% [18], but had no significant effect on net NaCl absorption [5]. Thus, chloride exit across the basolateral membrane must be predominantly by an electroneutral process which is indifferent to basolateral membrane potential difference.

Baum and Berry [5] suggested that the mechanism for electroneutral chloride exit across the basolateral membrane might be via a coupled K/Cl cotransport, driven by the potassium concentration gradient between cell and bathing solution. The fraction of basolateral chloride transport which could occur by this mechanism depends on the Na/K-ATPase coupling ratio. If the coupling ratio is 3Na:2K, then only two-thirds of the chloride transport could occur via electroneutral K/Cl cotransport, while the remaining one-third would have to exit via an electrogenic pathway. Only if the Na/K-ATPase coupling ratio were 1Na:1K could *all* basolateral chloride transport be via K/Cl cotransport. Efforts to demonstrate K/Cl cotransport in renal basolateral membrane vesicles have resulted in conflicting results. Eveloff and Warnock [19] have shown Cl-dependent ^{86}Rb uptake in basolateral membrane vesicles, but neither Grassl et al [20] nor Chen and Verkman [21] have been able to demonstrate any potassium-dependence of chloride uptake using ^{36}Cl and the new chloride-sensitive dye, SPQ, respectively. The reason for these discrepant results is still unresolved.

Other mechanisms for electroneutral chloride transport in the basolateral membrane have been identified. $Cl/OH/HCO_3$ exchange has been found in the intact rat proximal convoluted tubule by Alpern and Chambers [23] and in basolateral membrane vesicles of rabbit kidney by Chen and Verkman [21]. This transport system, however, cannot play an important rôle in net chloride absorption, since the orientation of the chloride and bicarbonate concentration gradients would result in chloride entry into rather than exit from the cell. A potentially more important transport system, originally described by Guggino et al [22] in *Necturus* proximal tubule and later found by Alpern and Chambers [23] in the intact rat proximal convoluted tubule and by Chen and Verkman in the rabbit basolateral membrane vesicles [21], is Na:2HCO_3/Cl countertransport. This transporter, which is electroneutral, would move Na–2HCO_3 into the cell in exchange for chloride. Although this transporter in itself is electroneutral, the Na:2HCO_3 which enters the cell would have to recycle out of the cell via the electrogenic Na:3HCO_3 cotransport system. Thus, in the steady state the net movement of chloride out of the cell by the interaction of these two transport systems would be electrogenic and should be dependent on the basolateral membrane potential difference. The failure of Ba^{++}, which depolarizes the basolateral potential difference, to inhibit NaCl absorption to the same extent as $NaHCO_3$ absorption, argues against an Na:2HCO_3/Cl countertransporter being responsible for *all* of basolateral chloride transport. However, this system operating in conjunction with an electroneutral K/Cl cotransport could reconcile the difficulties posed by a 3:2 coupling ratio of the Na/K-ATPase pump. Although the current crossing the basolateral membrane would be equal to one-third the net chloride flux it might be too small to see using electrophysiological techniques or to measure using the volume marker inulin as an index of chloride transport following addition of Ba^{++} to the bathing fluid.

Summary

To summarize, we have described the evidence for net active transcellular NaCl transport in the mammalian proximal tubule. This transport process does not generate a transepithelial potential difference and therefore appears to be electroneutral. At the luminal membrane sodium and chloride are probably transported by the Na/H antiporter and by a Cl/base and Cl/formate antiporter, respectively. Chloride movement across the basolateral membrane is poorly understood. There appears to be little if any simple conductive chloride transport from cell to peritubular fluid. In addition, net NaCl absorption does not appear to be sensitive to the basolateral membrane potential difference, suggesting that chloride exit is probably not associated with any combination of current-carrying transport processes. On the other hand, there is only contradictory evidence for the presence of an electroneutral KCl symport mechanism for chloride efflux. More studies are needed to address the mechanisms of chloride transport across the basolateral cell membrane during active, electroneutral, transcellular NaCl reabsorption in the mammalian proximal tubule.

References

1 Liu F-Y, Cogan MG. Axial heterogeneity in the rat proximal convoluted tubule. I. Bicarbonate, chloride and water transport. *Am J Physiol 1984 (Renal Fluid Electrolyte Physiol 16)*: F816–F821

2 Rector FC. Sodium, bicarbonate, and chloride absorption by the proximal tubule. *Am J Physiol 1983; 244 (Renal Fluid Electrolyte Physiol 13):* F461–F471

3 Rector FC, Martinez-Maldonado M, Brunner FP, Seldin DW. Evidence for passive reabsorption of NaCl in proximal tubule of rat kidney. *J Clin Invest 1966:* 1060

4 Jacobson HR, Kokko JP, Seldin DW, Holmberg C. Lack of solvent drag of NaCl and $NaHCO_3$ in rabbit proximal tubules. *Am J Physiol 1982; 243 (Renal Fluid and Electrolyte Physiol 12):* F342–F348

5 Baum M, Berry CA. Evidence for neutral transcellular NaCl transport and neutral basolateral chloride exit in the rabbit proximal convoluted tubule. *J Clin Invest 1984; 74:* 205–211

6 Chantrelle BM, Cogan MG, Rector FC. Active and passive components of NaCl absorption in the proximal convoluted tubule of the rat kidney. *Min and Elect Metab 1985; 11:* 209–214

7 Alpern RJ, Howlin KJ, Preisig PA. Active and passive components of chloride transport in the rat proximal convoluted tubule. *J Clin Invest 1985; 76:* 1360–1366

8 Howlin KJ, Alpern RJ, Berry CA, Rector FC. Evidence for electroneural sodium chloride transport in rat proximal convoluted tubule. *Am J Physiol 1986; 250 (Renal Fluid Electrolyte Physiol 19):* F644–F648

9 Seifter J, Knickelbein R, Aronson PS. Absence of Cl/OH exchange and NaCl cotransport in rabbit renal microvillus membrane vesicles. *Am J Physiol 1984; 247 (Renal Fluid Electrolyte Physiol 16):* F753–F759

10 Warnock DG, Yee VJ. Chloride uptake by brush-border membrane vesicles: coupling to proton gradients and K^+ diffusion potentials. *J Clin Invest 1981; 67:* 103–115

11 Chen PY, Illsley NP, Verkman AS. Renal brush border chloride transport mechanisms characterized using a fluorescent indicator. *Am J Physiol:* in press

12 Cardinal J, Lapointe JY, Laprade R. Luminal and peritubular ionic substitutions and intracellular potential of the rabbit proximal convoluted tubule. *Am J Physiol 1984; 247 (Renal Fluid Electrolyte Physiol 16):* F352–F364

13 Murer H, Hopfer U, Kinne R. Sodium/proton antiport in brush-border membrane vesicles isolated from rat small intestine and kidney. *Biochem J 1976; 154:* 597–604

14 Aronson PS. Mechanisms of active H^+ secretion in the proximal tubule. *Am J Physiol 1983; 245:* F647–F659

15 Preisig PA, Ives HE, Cragoe EJ et al. Na^+/H^+ exchange mediates most, but not all of apical membrane proton secretion in the rat proximal tubule. *J Clin Invest:* in press

16 Baum M. Evidence that parallel Na-H and Cl-HCO_3 (OH) antiporters transport NaCl in the proximal tubule. *Am J Physiol 1987; 252 (Renal Fluid Electrolyte Physiol 21):* F338–F345

17 Kuwahara M, Rector FC, Berry CA. Basolateral anion current during transcellular electroneutral sodium chloride transport in rabbit proximal convoluted tubules. *Am J Physiol:* submitted

18 Sasaki S, Berry CA. Mechanism of bicarbonate exit across basolateral membrane of the rabbit proximal convoluted tubule. *Am J Physiol 1984; 246 (Renal Fluid Electrolyte Physiol 15):* F889–F896

19 Eveloff J, Warnock DG. KCl transport systems in renal basolateral membrane (BLM) vesicles. *Kidney Int 1987; 31:* 432

20 Grassl SM, Holohan PD, Ross CR. Cl/HCO_3 exchange in rat renal cortical basolateral membrane vesicles (BLMV). *Kidney Int 1987; 31:* 409

21 Chen PY, Verkman AS. Chloride transport pathways in basolateral vesicles isolated from rabbit proximal tubule. *Biophysics J:* submitted

22 Guggino WB, London R, Boulpaep EL, Giebisch G. Chloride transport across the basolateral cell membrane of the *Necturus* proximal tubule: dependence on bicarbonate and sodium. *J Membr Biol 1983; 71:* 227–240

23 Alpern RJ, Chambers M. Basolateral membrane Cl/HCO_3 exchange in the rat proximal convoluted tubule: Na-dependent and independent modes. *J Gen Physiol:* in press

BICARBONATE TRANSPORT MECHANISMS ACROSS PERITUBULAR CELL MEMBRANE OF PROXIMAL CONVOLUTED TUBULE

R J Alpern, Patricia A Preisig

University of Texas Health Science Center at Dallas, Southwestern Medical School, Dallas, Texas, USA

The proximal tubule reabsorbs large amounts of bicarbonate. This process is mediated by the active secretion of protons across the apical membrane. Base generated in the cell must then exit across the basolateral membrane. In this paper we will discuss recent evidence from our laboratory relating to the mechanisms by which hydroxyl and bicarbonate cross the basolateral membrane.

Burckhardt, Sato and Frömter [1] first demonstrated that rapid changes in peritubular bicarbonate concentration cause rapid changes in the potential difference of cells in the rat proximal tubule, consistent with a basolateral membrane pathway for bicarbonate movement. This was initially assumed to be a simple bicarbonate conductance. Boron and Boulpaep [2] confirmed the presence of a basolateral membrane bicarbonate conductance in the salamander (Ambystoma) proximal tubule, and in addition, found that lowering peritubular sodium caused cell depolarization. This change in potential difference was in the opposite direction expected for a sodium conductance and was interpreted as a sodium-coupled bicarbonate conductance (the transporter carried one sodium ion and at least two bicarbonate ions in a similar direction). The first suggestion that such a transporter could be present in the mammalian proximal tubule was raised by Biagi and Sohtell [3] who found that lowering peritubular sodium concentration caused a paradoxical spike depolarization in rabbit proximal tubules perfused in vitro.

We approached the mechanism of basolateral membrane bicarbonate movement using the fluorescent measurement of cell pH in the in vivo microperfused rat proximal tubule. With this technique, the kidney of a rat is exposed using a flank incision [4]. Methods were developed which allow measurement of cell pH during perfusion of lumen and capillary with separate solutions [5]. Cell pH is measured using the pH-sensitive fluorescent dye, 2′7′-biscarboxyethyl-5,6-carboxyfluorescein (BCECF) [5]. The lumen of the tubule to be studied is perfused with the acetyoxymethyl derivative of BCECF which is lipid soluble and able to penetrate into the cells. Cytoplasmic esterases then cleave off the acetyoxymethyl groups forming a compound with four to five negative charges, which is trapped within the cell. Fluorescence is measured using an epifluorescence microscope at two excitation wavelengths, 500nm and 450nm, with emission at 530nm. Excitation at 450nm is pH-independent while excitation at 500nm is pH-dependent. Ratioing these values gives a result which is independent of dye concentration or changes in the optical pathway, but is dependent on intracellular pH. The dyes have been calibrated intracellularly by measuring fluorescence after cell pH has been set with the ionophore nigericin [5,6]. Results are shown in Figure 1.

Figure 2 shows a typical tracing during a change in luminal and peritubular pH (bicarbonate concentration). Tracings representing measurement with 450nm

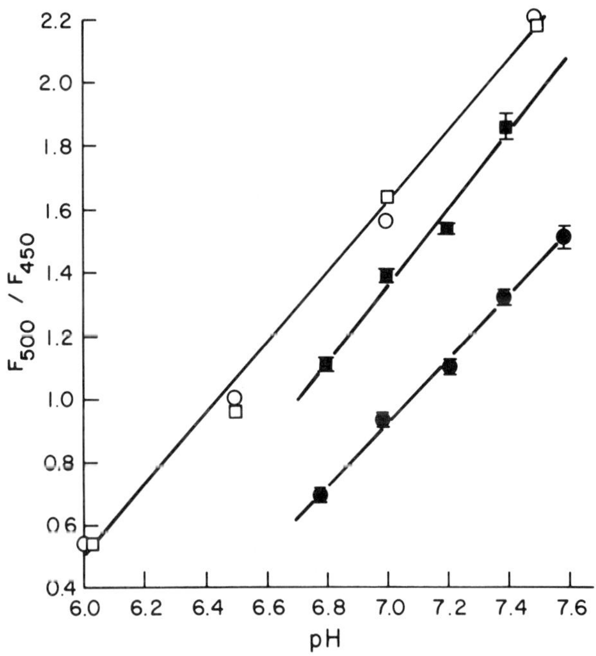

Figure 1. Dye calibration by epifluorescent microscopy. Open symbols represent calibration of acidic form of BCECF in solutions of set pH. Closed symbols represent calibration of BCECF loaded into proximal tubule cells, using the Nigericin method [5]. Squares represent studies performed with BCECF from Research Development Corp (Toronto, Canada), whilst circles represent studies performed with BCECF from Molecular Probes (Junction City, OR). It can be seen that the acidic forms of the compound from the two suppliers behaved similarly. However, the acetoxymethyl forms, when loaded into cells, give different calibrations. When results from each of the dyes is corrected for their respective calibration, similar values for intracellular pH result. Borrowed with permission from [6]

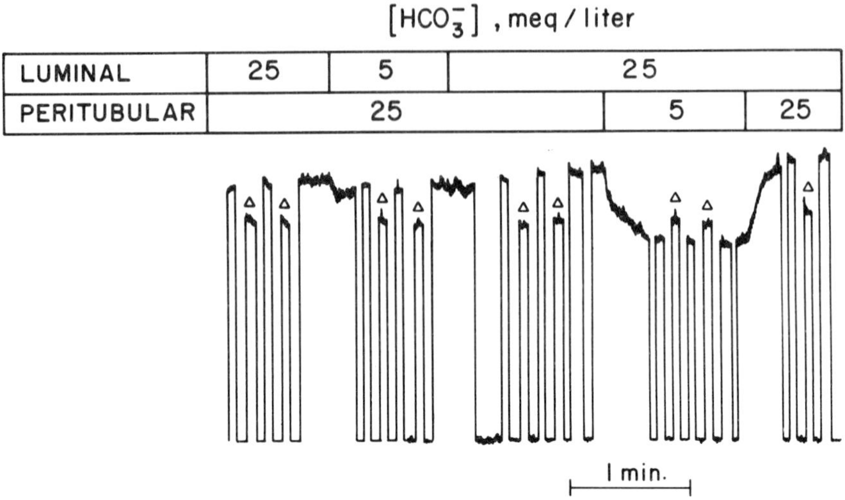

Figure 2. A typical study showing the effect of luminal and peritubular bicarbonate concentration on cell pH. Lumens and capillaries were perfused with CO_2-containing solutions with either 25 (pH 7.32) or 5 (pH 6.63) mEq/litre bicarbonate. Intensity of fluorescence in arbitrary units is indicated by the height of the bars. Measurements with 450nm excitation, the pH-insensitive wavelength, are indicated by triangles over the bars. All other measurements are with 500nm excitation, the pH-sensitive wavelength. Borrowed with permission from [7]

excitation are denoted by triangles. All other tracings represent measurements with 500nm excitation (the pH-sensitive wavelength). It can be seen that upon luminal acidification (0.7pH units), there is a small cell acidification, whereas a similar change in peritubular pH causes a large cell acidification denoted by large changes in 500nm fluorescence. Results in six tubules showed that acidifying the lumen by 0.7pH units caused the cell to acidify by 0.08pH units, whilst a similar change in peritubular pH caused the cell to acidify by 0.32pH units [7]. Thus, the basolateral membrane transport mechanisms appear to control cell pH to a greater extent than apical membrane transporters.

As mentioned above, bicarbonate movement across the basolateral membrane is believed to occur across a conductive pathway. As such it might be expected that changes in cell potential difference would lead to changes in cell pH. In order to test this, we examined the effect of increasing peritubular capillary potassium concentration from 5 to 50mEq/litre. Because the basolateral membrane contains a large potassium conductance, this manoeuvre is expected to cause cell depolarization [8,9]. The results are shown in Figure 3 (left). Increasing peritubular potassium from 5 to 50mEq/litre caused cell pH to increase from 7.12±0.03 to 7.30±0.04 ($p<0.01$) [5]. This effect was reversible upon lowering the potassium concentration back to 5mEq/litre.

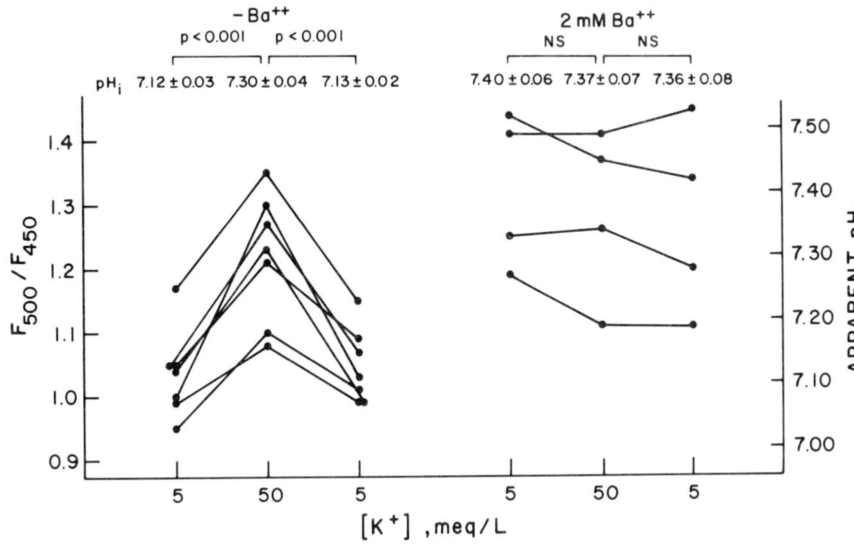

Figure 3. Effect of cell depolarization on cell pH. Capillaries were perfused with solutions containing either 5 or 50mEq/litre potassium. On the left, experiments were performed in the absence of barium, whilst on the right, 2mM barium was added to all solutions. Ratio of 500/450nm fluorescence is shown on the left ordinate whilst the calculated pHi is shown on the right ordinate. Borrowed with permission from [5]

These pH changes are consistent with a bicarbonate conductive pathway. However, these results are also consistent with cotransport of potassium and bicarbonate. We, therefore, next examined the effect of 2mM barium on this interaction. Barium blocks the potassium conductance and prevents any effect of changing peritubular potassium concentration on cell potential difference [8,9]. As can be seen in the right side of Figure 3, barium blocked the effect by changing capillary potassium concentration on cell pH [5]. In addition, barium, which in itself depolarizes the cell, caused cell alkalinization. These results thus suggest the existence of a potential-sensitive bicarbonate pathway.

We next examined whether there was a sodium-coupled pathway on the basolateral membrane. Peritubular sodium concentration was lowered from 147 to 25mEq/litre by substitution with either choline or tetramethylammonium. As can be seen in Figure 4, in both cases lowering peritubular sodium caused a cell acidification [5], consistent with cotransport of sodium and bicarbonate, as in the salamander proximal tubule [2].

These results, however, are also consistent with two other possible explanations. First, there could be an amiloride-sensitive Na/H antiporter. Second, these results could be explained by parallel sodium and bicarbonate conductances. The next studies addressed these possibilities. First, we examined whether amiloride inhibited the effect of sodium on cell pH. Because amiloride competes

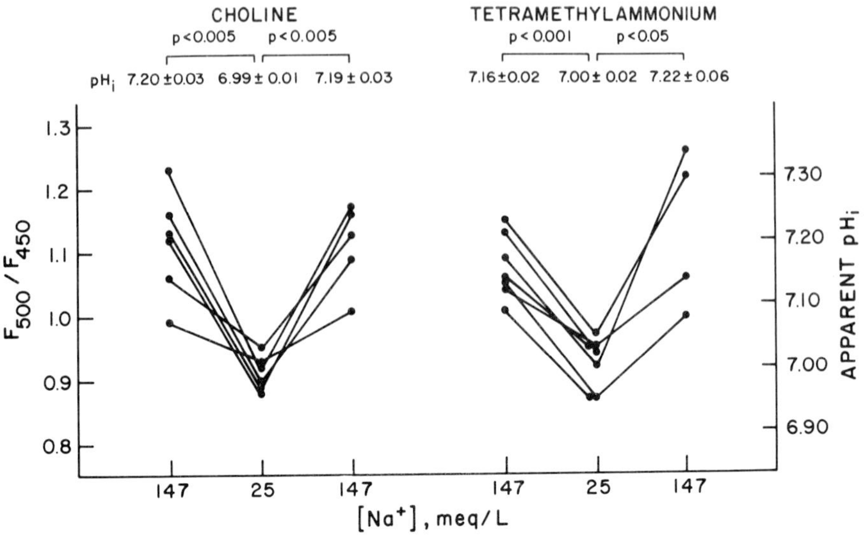

Figure 4. Effect of peritubular sodium on cell pH. Capillaries were perfused with solutions containing either 147 or 25mEq/litre sodium. On the left choline replaced sodium, and on the right tetramethylammonium replaced sodium. The ratio of 500/450nm fluorescence is shown on the left ordinate and the calculated pHi on the right ordinate. Borrowed with permission from [5]

with sodium, we used low sodium concentrations for these studies. When peritubular sodium concentration was lowered from 50mEq/litre to 0mEq/litre, cell pH decreased by 0.18pH units at an initial rate of 1.4±0.2pH units/min. Both the magnitude of the pH change and the initial rate of pH change were unaffected by 1mM amiloride [5].

We next examined the effect of SITS (4-acetamido-4′-isothiocyanostilbene-2,2′-disulfonate). SITS is an inhibitor of anion transporters, which Boron and Boulpaep found inhibited the sodium bicarbonate cotransporter in the salamander proximal tubule [2]. We found that SITS completely blocked the effect of either peritubular pH changes or peritubular sodium changes on cell pH [5]. These results are consistent with sodium bicarbonate cotransport, but are also consistent with a sodium conductance in parallel with a SITS-sensitive bicarbonate conductance.

To examine this question further, we next studied the effect of sodium removal on basolateral membrane bicarbonate permeability. If the only effect of sodium is to provide a conductance in parallel to the bicarbonate conductance, sodium removal should have no effect on the bicarbonate permeability of the basolateral membrane. We thus examined the rate of cell pH change in response to lowering peritubular bicarbonate concentration from 25 to 5mEq/litre in the presence and absence of luminal and peritubular sodium. In the presence of sodium, cells acidified at an initial rate of 2.4±0.3pH units/min. In the absence of luminal and peritubular sodium, cells acidified at a rate of only 0.2±0.1pH units/min ($p<0.001$) [5]. Thus, removal of sodium from lumen and peritubular capillary decreased the apparent permeability of the basolateral membrane to H^+/HCO_3^- by more than 90%. These results therefore suggest that the interaction between sodium and bicarbonate is related to cotransport on a SITS-sensitive anion transporter.

We next raised the question as to whether the potential difference-sensitive pathway was the sodium/bicarbonate transporter. If so, then removal of sodium from lumen and peritubular capillary should inhibit the effect of changing peritubular potassium concentration on cell pH. Siebens and Boron [10] have found in the salamander proximal tubule that increases in peritubular potassium concentration still caused a cell depolarization in the absence of sodium. We found, however, that total removal of luminal and peritubular sodium completely inhibited the effect of peritubular potassium concentration on cell pH [5]. Thus, it appears that the potential-sensitive pathway is the sodium/bicarbonate cotransporter. These results suggest that the sodium/bicarbonate cotransporter has a bicarbonate to sodium stoichiometry greater than one, and is thus electrogenic. This is consistent with the electrophysiological results of Burckhardt et al [1], Boron and Boulpaep [2], and Biagi and Sohtell [3].

To test if the sodium/bicarbonate cotransporter is also coupled to chloride, we examined the effect of chloride removal from luminal and capillary solutions on the response of cell pH to lowering peritubular sodium concentration. As noted above, lowering peritubular sodium concentration from 147 to 25mEq/litre in the presence of chloride caused a cell acidification of 0.20±0.03pH units [5]. In the absence of a luminal and peritubular chloride the similar manoeuvre caused a similar cell acidification of 0.21±0.01pH unit (NS) [6]. Thus, the majority of sodium/bicarbonate cotransport across the basolateral membrane is independent of chloride.

Next, we examined whether this transporter actually transported bicarbonate or hydroxyl. Because of difficulties controlling the CO_2 tension in the renal cortex, these studies were performed in the rabbit proximal convoluted tubule perfused in vitro. Initial studies demonstrated the presence of a SITS-sensitive basolateral membrane sodium/base cotransporter, similar to that found in the rat proximal tubule in vivo [11]. To examine whether this transporter actually carried hydroxyl or bicarbonate, we studied the effect of removing all exogenous CO_2 and bicarbonate from the perfusate. In this setting, sodium/base cotransport was still present, although at one-third of the control rate [11]. In the absence of exogenous CO_2/bicarbonate, changing peritubular pH or sodium concentration caused a cell pH change which was inhibited by SITS and not affected by amiloride [11]. In addition, sodium removal in this setting inhibited the apparent H^+/OH^- permeability [11]. Whereas these studies suggested that the transporter was indeed a sodium/hydroxyl cotransporter, an alternative explanation was that the transporter carried bicarbonate, and that metabolic CO_2 production was sufficiently high to supply the needed bicarbonate.

To explore this possibility, two sets of studies were performed. First, we examined whether the sodium/base cotransporter was dependent on the presence of carbonic anyhydrase. In theory, if the transporter actually was a sodium/hydroxyl cotransporter, carbonic anyhydrase should not be required for an effect on cell pH. To examine this, the effect of a peritubular pH or sodium concentration change in the absence of exogenous CO_2 was examined in the absence and in the presence of acetazolamide. In both of these sets of studies acetazolamide inhibited greater than 90% of the base flux [11]. These results suggest that the transporter is actually transporting sodium/bicarbonate. However, an alternative explanation is that the transporter is directly inhibited by acetazolamide.

A second approach was to examine the effect of metabolic inhibition in this setting. In theory, if the transporter is a sodium/bicarbonate cotransporter functioning on metabolically produced CO_2/bicarbonate then inhibition of metabolism should inhibit the transporter. To examine this, we studied the effect of lowering peritubular sodium in the absence of exogenous CO_2 in the absence and then in the presence of cyanide. Two millimolar bath cyanide completely inhibited the effect of changing bath sodium on cell pH in this setting [11]. In addition, cyanide had no effect on the transporter when studied in the presence of exogenous CO_2, thus ruling out a direct effect on the transporter [11]. These studies suggest that the transporter is a sodium/bicarbonate cotransporter which can function in the absence of exogenous CO_2/bicarbonate by utilizing metabolically produced CO_2/bicarbonate.

Thus, the above studies demonstrate in the intact renal tubule a basolateral membrane, sodium-coupled, chloride-independent, electrogenic bicarbonate transport mechanism. This transport mechanism is the major basolateral membrane bicarbonate transport mechanism. However, when working with whole cells, there is always the danger of regulatory mechanisms affecting the results. We, therefore, wanted to confirm the presence of this transporter in isolated basolateral membranes.

^{22}Na uptake into isolated basolateral membrane vesicles was studied in the the absence and presence of bicarbonate with a potassium gradient (out greater than in). The results are shown in Figure 5. It can be seen that addition of bicarbonate to the vesicles doubled the rate of ^{22}Na uptake [12]. SITS addition had no effect on the rate of sodium uptake in the absence of bicarbonate, but completely inhibited the stimulation by bicarbonate [12]. Addition of valinomycin in the presence of the imposed potassium gradients should lead to an interior positive potential difference, which would be expected to slow the rate of sodium uptake through a sodium conductance. It can be seen in Figure 5 that valinomycin had no effect on sodium uptake in the absence of bicarbonate and actually accelerated sodium uptake in the presence of bicarbonate, consistent

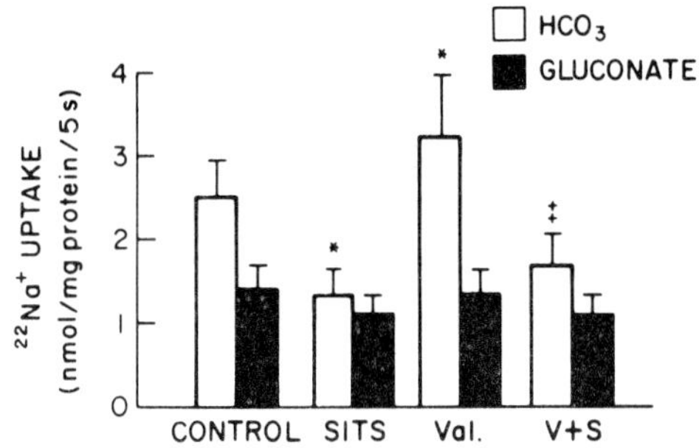

Figure 5. ^{22}Na uptake in basolateral membrane vesicles in the presence of bicarbonate (open bars), and in the absence of bicarbonate (presence of gluconate) (solid bars). Borrowed with permission from [12]

with sodium moving in an anion transporter [12]. SITS inhibited the stimulatory effect of valinomycin. These studies, therefore, are most consistent with a sodium/bicarbonate cotransport mechanism which carries negative charge and is SITS sensitive. This is similar to the conclusions of the tubule studies.

Other investigators have also obtained results consistent with electrogenic sodium/bicarbonate cotransport of the basolateral membrane. Yoshitomi et al [13] and Sasaki et al [14] used intracellular pH and sodium microelectrodes in perfused rat and rabbit tubules, respectively. Lowering peritubular sodium lowered cell pH, and lowering peritubular pH lowered cell sodium. Grassl and Aronson [15] used basolateral membrane vesicles from rabbit renal cortex and obtained results consistent with sodium/bicarbonate cotransport. In addition, the results of Yoshitomi et al [13] and Soleimani et al [16] suggest a stiochiometry for this transporter of one sodium to three bicarbonate ions.

We next examined whether the basolateral membrane contained any chloride-coupled base transport mechanisms. Tubules were perfused in the absence of luminal and peritubular chloride, and the effect of peritubular chloride addition on cell pH was examined. Addition of peritubular chloride caused cells to acidify rapidly from pH 7.34±0.04 to 7.21±0.04 ($p<0.001$), an effect which was reversible on chloride removal [6]. As these cells do not possess a chloride conductance [9,17–19], the results suggest chloride/bicarbonate exchange. In addition, peritubular SITS inhibited the effect of chloride addition on cell pH [6]. Guggino et al [20] have identified a sodium bicarbonate/chloride exchanger on the basolateral membrane of the salamander (Necturus) proximal tubule. This transporter is believed to function by allowing sodium bicarbonate to enter the cell in exchange for chloride. It would thus provide a mechanism by which chloride could exit across the basolateral membrane. To examine if our apparent chloride/bicarbonate exchanger was actually coupled to sodium, we examined the effect of sodium removal on chloride/bicarbonate exchange. In the absence of luminal and peritubular sodium, addition of chloride to the peritubular capillary caused only a 0.04pH unit acidification [6]. Thus, approximately three-quarters of apparent chloride/bicarbonate exchange is dependent on the presence of sodium and may indeed be coupled to it. The remaining fraction may represent simple chloride/bicarbonate exchange.

These studies demonstrate the presence of basolateral membrane chloride/bicarbonate exchange, most of which is dependent upon sodium and possibly coupled to it. Vesicle studies by Grassl et al [21] have previously reported the presence of chloride/bicarbonate exchange in rabbit basolateral membranes. In addition, Grassl et al [22] have recently reported in rat basolateral membranes that chloride gradients can modify the bicarbonate-dependent transport of sodium in a manner consistent with sodium bicarbonate/chloride exchange. It is important to emphasize at this point that these chloride-coupled transporters may be related to chloride transport but are unlikely to be quantitatively important in bicarbonate absorption. Studies have found that whilst greater than 90% of basolateral membrane bicarbonate permeability is dependent on the presence of sodium [5,13,14], only 30% of basolateral membrane bicarbonate permeability is dependent on the presence of chloride [14 and unpublished observations]. In addition, Burg and Green [23] and Sasaki and Berry [24] found that total chloride removal from lumen and peritubular solutions did not modify the rate of bicarbonate absorption.

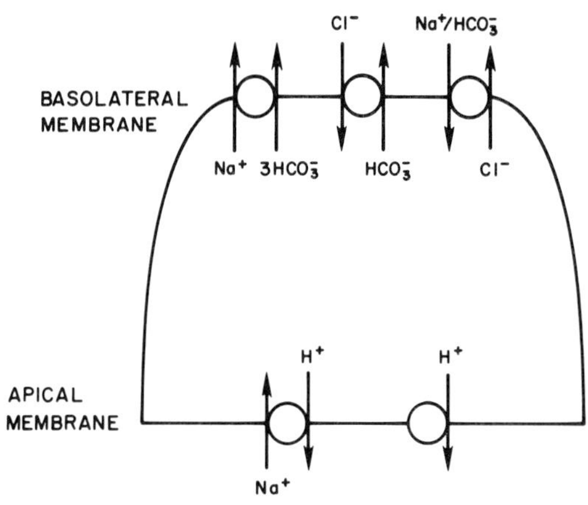

Figure 6. Cell model for proximal tubular acidification

In summary, these studies demonstrate the presence of three transport mechanisms on the basolateral membrane (Figure 6). The first is an electrogenic sodium-coupled chloride-independent bicarbonate transport mechanism. This is the major pathway for basolateral membrane bicarbonate transport and appears to function as a sodium bicarbonate cotransporter. In parallel with this are two chloride-coupled transporters. One is sodium-dependent and may be similar to the sodium-coupled transporter described by Guggino et al [20] (i.e. $Na(HCO_3)_2$/ Cl exchanger). If so, it could provide a mechanism for chloride efflux from the cell. The third transporter, a simple Cl/HCO_3 exchanger, is quantitatively of minor importance and its rôle is unclear. It could not function as a chloride efflux mechanism but rather would function as a bicarbonate efflux mechanism, or may be involved in cell pH regulation.

Acknowledgment

The studies detailed herein were supported in part by NIH grants DK27045, DK38875 and DK01229.

References

1 Burckhardt B-Ch, Sato K, Frömter E. Electrophysiological analysis of bicarbonate permeation across the peritubular cell membrane of rat kidney proximal tubule. I. Basic observations. *Pfluegers Arch 1984; 401:* 34–42

2 Boron WF, Boulpaep EL. Intracellular pH regulation in the renal proximal tubule of the salamander. Basolateral HCO_3^- transport. *J Gen Physiol 1983; 81:* 53–94

3 Biagi BA, Sohtell M. Electrophysiology of basolateral bicarbonate transport in the rabbit proximal tubule. *Am J Physiol 1986; 19:* F267–F272

4 Alpern RJ. Bicarbonate-water interactions in the rat proximal convoluted tubule. An effect of volume flux on active proton secretion. *J Gen Physiol 1984; 84:* 753–770

5 Alpern RJ. Mechanism of basolateral membrane $H^+/OH^-/HCO_3^-$ transport in the rat proximal convoluted tubule. A sodium-coupled electrogenic process. *J Gen Physiol 1985; 86:* 613–636

6 Alpern RJ, Chambers M. Basolateral membrane Cl/HCO_3 exchange in the rat proximal convoluted tubule. Na-dependent and -independent modes. *J Gen Physiol 1987; 89:* 581–598

7 Alpern RJ, Chambers M. Cell pH in the rat proximal convoluted tubule. Regulation by luminal and peritubular pH and sodium concentration. *J Clin Invest 1986; 78:* 502–510

8 Biagi B, Kubota T, Sohtell M, Giebisch G. Intracellular potentials in rabbit proximal tubules perfused in vitro. *Am J Physiol 1981; 9:* F200–F210

9 Burckhardt B-Ch, Cassola AC, Frömter E. Electrophysiological analysis of bicarbonate permeation across the peritubular cell membrane of rat kidney proximal tubule. II. Exclusion of HCO_3^--effects on other ion permeabilities and of coupled electroneutral HCO_3^--transport. *Pfluegers Arch 1984; 401:* 43–51

10 Siebens AW, Boron WF. Intracellular alkalinization induced by depolarization in ambystoma proximal tubules. *Kidney Int 1985; 27 (Abstract):* 288

11 Krapf R, Alpern RJ, Rector FC Jr, Berry CA. Basolateral membrane Na/base cotransport is dependent on CO_2/HCO_3^- in the proximal convoluted tubule. Submitted for publication

12 Akiba T, Alpern RJ, Eveloff J et al. Electrogenic sodium/bicarbonate cotransport in rabbit renal cortical basolateral membrane vesicles. *J Clin Invest 1986; 78:* 1472–1478

13 Yoshitomi K, Burckhardt B-Ch, Frömter E. Rheogenic sodium-bicarbonate cotransport in the peritubular cell membrane of rat renal proximal tubule. *Pfluegers Arch 1985; 405:* 360–366

14 Sasaki S, Shiigai T, Yoshiyama N, Takeuchi J. Mechanism of bicarbonate exit across basolateral membrane of rabbit proximal straight tubule. *Am J Physiol 1987; 21:* F11–F18

15 Grassl SM, Aronson PS. Na^+/HCO_3^- co-transport in basolateral membrane vesicles isolated from rabbit renal cortex. *J Biol Chem 1986; 19:* 8778–8783

16 Soleimani M, Grassl SM, Aronson PS. Stiochiometry of Na^+-HCO_3^- cotransport in basolateral membrane vesicles isolated from rabbit renal cortex. *J Clin Invest 1987; 79:* 1276–1280

17 Cassola AC, Mollenhauer M, Frömter E. The intracellular chloride activity of rat kidney proximal tubular cells. *Pfluegers Arch 1983; 399:* 259–265
18 Guggino WB, Boulpaep EL, Giebisch G. Electrical properties of chloride transport across the *Necturus* proximal tubule. *J Membr Biol 1982; 65:* 185–196
19 Shindo T, Spring KR. Chloride movement across the basolateral membrane of proximal tubule cells. *J Membr Biol 1981; 58:* 35–42
20 Guggino WB, London R, Boulpaep EL, Giebisch G. Chloride transport across the basolateral cell membrane of the *Necturus* proximal tubule: dependence on bicarbonate and sodium. *J Membr Biol 1983; 71:* 226–240
21 Grassl SM, Karniski LP, Aronson PS. Cl-HCO_3 exchange in rabbit renal cortical basolateral membrane vesicles (BLMV). *Kidney Int 1985; 27 (Abstract):* 282
22 Grassl SM, Holohan PD, Ross CR. HCO_3^- transport in basolateral membrane vesicles isolated from rat renal cortex. *J Biol Chem 1987; 262:* 2682–2687
23 Burg M, Green N. Bicarbonate transport by isolated perfused rabbit proximal convoluted tubules. *Am J Physiol 1977; 2:* F307–F314
24 Sasaki S, Berry CA. Mechanism of bicarbonate exit across basolateral membrane of the rabbit proximal convoluted tubule. *Am J Physiol 1984; 15:* F889–F896

INTRACELLULAR pH REGULATION IN THE S3 SEGMENT OF THE RABBIT PROXIMAL TUBULE

W F Boron, N L Nakhoul

Yale University School of Medicine, New Haven, Connecticut, USA

One of the major functions of the proximal tubule is the reabsorption of bicarbonate. The consensus is that bicarbonate reabsorption is not brought about by direct transport out of the tubular lumen, but rather by the secretion of proton into the lumen by Na-H exchange. The secreted H^+ combines with the luminal bicarbonate to form H_2CO_3, which in turn dissociates to form H_2O and CO_2. The latter then diffuses from the lumen. This H^+ secretion and titration of luminal bicarbonate is only half of the process of bicarbonate reabsorption. The second half is the movement of bicarbonate from the proximal tubule cell across the basolateral membrane. The net effect is thus the disappearance of bicarbonate from the luminal fluid, and its reappearance in the basolateral fluid.

Although the above picture, the one presented in textbooks, is correct in its most general features, recent work indicates that acid-base transport in the proximal tubule is actually much more complex. Work on brush-border membrane vesicles [1] has shown the presence of a formate-chloride exchanger, which in combination with the non-ionic diffusion of formic acid, could participate in the recycling of formate across the luminal membrane and the net reabsorption of hydrochloric acid. Indeed, work on isolated perfused S3 segments of the rabbit proximal tubule has shown that a component of chloride reabsorption is dependent upon formate [2], and fluorescence measurements of pH_i in microperfused rat proximal tubules indicates that formate-chloride exchange can have a small effect on the steady-state pH_i [3].

Over the past three years, our group has been using an optical technique to study pH_i regulation in the isolated perfused S3 segment of the rabbit proximal tubule. Our approach has been to load proximal tubule cells with the pH-sensitive dye dimethylcarboxyfluorescein, and then measure the intracellular absorbance spectrum of this dye by passing a 10μm diameter beam of light through the tubule. The transmitted light, which has passed through from two to six cells, is focused on a diffraction grating, which breaks the white light up

Acknowledgments

This work was supported by NIH grants RO1-DK30344 and KO4-DK01022.

References

1 Karniski LP, Aronson PS. Chloride/formate exchange with formic acid recycling: a mechanism of active chloride transport across epithelial membranes. *Proc Natl Acad Sci USA 1985; 82:* 6362–6375

2 Schild L, Giebisch G, Karniski L, Aronson PS. Chloride transport in the mammalian proximal tubule. *Pfluegers Arch 1086; 407:* S156–S159

3 Alpern RJ. Apical membrane Cl/base exchange in the rat proximal convoluted tubule (PCT). *Kidney Int 1987; 31:* 428

4 Thomas JA, Buchsbaum RN, Zimniak A, Racker E. Intracellular pH measurements in Ehrlich ascites tumor cells utilizing spectroscopic probes generated in situ. *Biochem 1979; 81:* 2210–2218

5 Boron WF, De Weer P. Intracellular pH transients in squid giant axons caused by CO_2, NH_3 and metabolic inhibitors. *J Gen Physiol 1976; 67:* 91–112

6 Chaillet JR, Boron WF. Intracellular pH regulation in rabbit proximal tubules studied with a pH-sensitive dye. *Kidney Int 1984; 25:* 273

7 Murer H, Hopfer U, Kinne R. Sodium/proton antiport in brush-border-membrane vesicles isolated from rat small intestine and kidney. *Biochem J 1976; 154:* 597–604

8 Kinsella JL, Aronson PS. Properties of the Na^+-H^+ exchanger in renal microvillus membrane vesicles. *Am J Physiol 1980; 238:* F461–F469

9 Kinsella JL, Aronson PS. Amiloride inhibition of the Na^+-H^+ exchanger in renal microvillus. *Am J Physiol 1981; 241:* F374–F379

10 Siebens AW, Boron WF. Effect of electroneutral luminal and basolateral lactate transport on intracellular pH in salamander proximal tubules. *J Gen Physiol 1987:* in press

11 Chan YL, Giebisch G. Relationship between sodium and bicarbonate transport in the rat proximal convoluted tubule. *Am J Physiol 1981; 240:* F222–F230

MOLECULAR IDENTIFICATION OF THE PROXIMAL TUBULAR Na^+/H^+ EXCHANGER

G Burckhardt, T Friedrich

Max-Planck-Institut für Biophysik, Frankfurt Main, FRG

Properties and localization of the proximal tubular Na^+/H^+ exchanger

A considerable portion of salt and water reabsorption in the mammalian proximal tubule is due to the operation of an antiporter which is located in the luminal ('brush border') membrane of proximal tubule cells and exchanges intracellular protons (H^+) for luminal sodium (Na^+) ions [1]. The existence of this Na^+/H^+ exchanger (antiporter) had first been demonstrated by Murer et al in experiments with vesicles isolated from rat kidney cortex and small intestine [2]. Since that time the antiporter has been intensively investigated in the intact kidney as well as in studies with isolated membrane vesicles. The characteristics of the Na^+/H^+ exchanger are in brief [1–4]:

- Electroneutral exchange of cations (1:1 exchange).
- Affinity for H^+>>lithium>ammonium≥Na^+, but not for potassium, rubidium, caesium.
- Highest translocation rates when loaded with Na^+, and lowest with lithium.
- Competitive inhibition by amiloride and its analogues.
- Activation by protonation of a modifier site at intracellular pH<7.0.
- Modulation by acid/base status and hormones.

Highest activities of the Na^+/H^+ exchanger were found in outer cortical brush border membrane vesicles which presumably originate from proximal convoluted tubules. Outer medullary brush border membrane vesicles corresponding to proximal straight tubules exhibited lower activities [5] which is in agreement with a decline of proton secretion along the proximal tubule. Within the proximal tubule cells the Na^+/H^+ exchanger shows a highly asymmetric distribution since it is found only in the luminal membrane. This has been demonstrated with membrane vesicles isolated separately from the luminal and contraluminal cell membrane [6].

In parentheses it should be mentioned that Na^+/H^+ exchangers have been found in a great variety of epithelial and non-epithelial cells. The antiporters serve important physiological functions as for instance the maintenance of intracellular pH and cellular volume. Furthermore Na^+/H^+ exchangers are involved in the onset of cell division and differentiation [4,7]. At present it is not known whether all these functions are governed by a single type of Na^+/H^+ exchanger or whether a family of antiporters exists. This question can only be solved when the Na^+/H^+ exchangers from different cells have been identified and isolated.

Strategies for molecular identification

Although the renal Na^+/H^+ exchanger plays an important rôle in fluid reabsorption, it was not until recently that experiments were begun to identify the membrane proteins involved in the exchange process. In general, the biochemical identification of a protein involved in transmembrane substrate transport involves several consecutive steps which are summarized as follows:

- Application of substrate or inhibitor derivatives that can bind covalently to the transporter: a) derivatives with chemically reactive groups; b) derivatives with photolabile groups.
- Application of side group-specific reagents.
- Proof of covalent binding by demonstration of an irreversible inhibition of the transport process.
- Proof of modification at the substrate binding site by demonstration of substrate protection.
- Application of radioactively labelled derivatives or side group-specific reagents. Separation of labelled proteins according to their molecular weight.
- Proof of specific labelling by demonstration of substrate protection.

Since natural substrates interact reversibly with their transport system they do not remain attached to the transporter protein during its isolation. It is, therefore, necessary to design substrate or inhibitor derivatives which react covalently with the transporter. The covalent binding can occur between a chemically reactive group of the substrate derivative and a side group within the substrate binding site of the transporter (affinity labelling). Alternatively, substrate or inhibitor derivatives can carry a photolabile group which is split off during irradiation. Thereby, highly reactive radicals are generated which can insert into the carrier protein independently of the presence of specific side groups (photoaffinity labelling). Whenever substrates or inhibitors are appropriately modified the transport system will recognize them as natural substrates and handle them with high affinity. Thus, affinity and photoaffinity labelling are the most specific techniques to modify a transport system.

Where substrate or inhibitor derivatives are not available, a side group-specific reagent can be used to modify the transporter. However, a side group-specific reagent usually modifies several membrane proteins carrying the same side groups making this approach less specific as compared to affinity and photoaffinity labelling. Irrespective of the technique applied, a covalent modification of the transport system at the substrate binding site causes an irreversible inhibition of the transport process. This inhibition is attenuated when substrate derivatives or side group reagents are offered together with an excess of the natural substrate due to a competition for a common binding site (subtrate protection).

After having demonstrated irreversible inhibition and substrate protection, and thus modification of the transporter at or close to the substrate binding site, radioactive derivatives can be used to label the respective membrane proteins and to detect them after separation, e.g. by sodium dodecylsulphate (SDS) polyacrylamide gel electrophoresis. Using these guidelines we shall now describe the modification and identification of the rat renal Na^+/H^+ exchanger.

Photoaffinity labelling of the Na^+/H^+ exchanger

The organic cation amiloride (for structural formula see Figure 1) inhibits the Na^+/H^+ exchanger by competing with Na^+ for a common binding site [8]. We observed a half-maximal inhibition of the rat renal Na^+/H^+ exchanger at 43μM which is in excellent agreement with a K_i of 50μM reported for the rabbit renal Na^+/H^+ exchanger [8]. Since amiloride interacts reversibly with the antiporter,

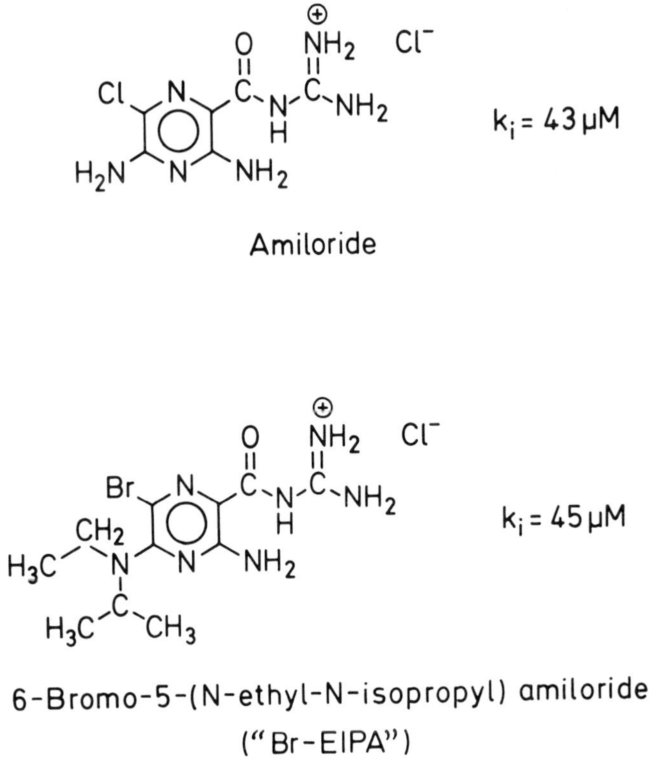

Figure 1. Inhibitors of the rat renal Na^+/H^+ exchanger

this drug cannot be used to identify the membrane protein involved in Na^+/H^+ exchange. Therefore, we replaced the chlorine at position 6 of the pyrazine ring by a bromine and, in addition, the amino group at position 5 by the hydrophobic N-ethyl-N-isopropyl group. Details of the synthetic procedure are given elsewhere [9]. The introduction of a bromine renders the molecule sensitive to irradiation [10]. The hydrophobic substitution at position 5 serves to retain a high affinity of the bromine derivative to the Na^+/H^+ exchanger: indeed, the K_i of 6-bromo-5-(N-ethyl-N-isopropyl) amiloride (Br-EIPA) is similar to that of the parent compound amiloride (see Figure 1).

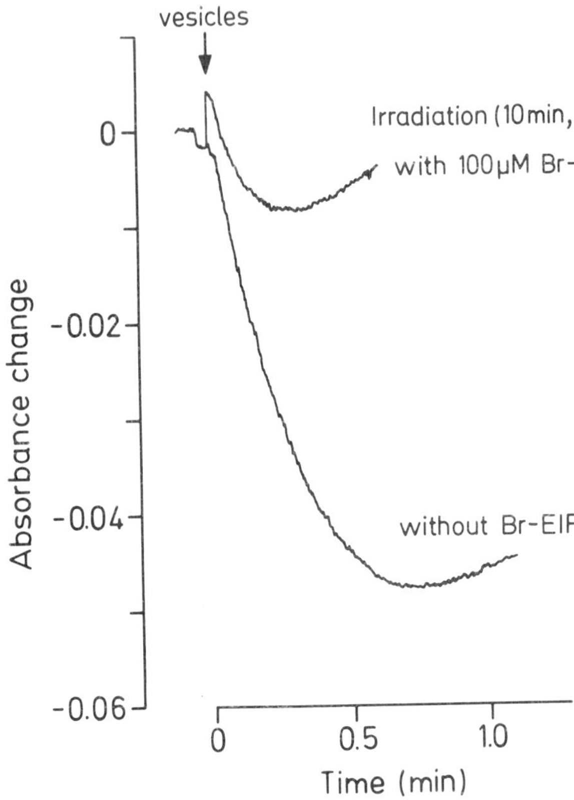

Figure 2. Irreversible inhibition of rat renal Na^+/H^+ exchanger by photoaffinity labelling with 6-bromo-5-(N-ethyl-N-isopropyl) amiloride (Br-EIPA). Brush border membrane vesicles were irradiated at 350nm for 10 minutes in buffers containing 100mM tetramethylammonium chloride, 50mM KCl, 5mM HEPES/Tris, pH 7.0, and 0 or 0.1mM Br-EIPA. After irradiation the vesicles were washed in the dark in Br-EIPA-free buffer containing 100mM NaCl, 50mM KCl, 5mM HEPES/Tris, pH 7.0. These Na^+-loaded vesicles were then added to a buffer containing 100mM tetramethylammonium chloride, 50mM KCl, 5mM HEPES/Tris, pH 7.0, 2.5μM valinomycin, and 6μM acridine orange. The figure shows the absorbance decrease of acridine orange as a function of time

To investigate the effect of Br-EIPA on the Na^+/H^+ exchanger we have irradiated rat renal brush border membrane vesicles in the presence or absence of 0.1mM Br-EIPA. Thereafter the vesicles were thoroughly washed, loaded with Na^+ and suspended in a Na^+-free buffer which contained the pH indicator acridine orange. Since Na^+ efflux out of the vesicles is coupled to H^+ entry via the antiporter, an intravesicular acidification occurs which can be visualized by a time-dependent absorbance decrease of acridine orange (Figure 2). Figure 2 clearly shows that the initial rate and maximal degree of intravesicular acidification are severely decreased in vesicles that have been irradiated in the presence of Br-EIPA suggesting that photoproducts of Br-EIPA have modified and irreversibly inhibited the Na^+/H^+ exchanger. This modification must have taken place at or close to the cation binding site because Na^+ and lithium (Li^+) present together with Br-EIPA during the irradiation protected the Na^+/H^+ exchanger from the irreversible inhibition [9].

Since Br-EIPA fulfilled the criteria for a suitable photoaffinity label we next applied [^{14}C]-labelled Br-EIPA to detect the membrane proteins possibly involved in Na^+/H^+ exchange. To this end brush border membrane vesicles from rat kidney cortex were irradiated with [^{14}C] Br-EIPA in the absence of Na^+ (control) or in the presence of Na^+ (substrate protection). Thereafter, vesicles were washed and membrane proteins were separated by SDS polyacrylamide gel electrophoresis. The distribution of incorporated ^{14}C along the gel is found in a band with an apparent molecular weight of 65,000 (Figure 3). As the labelling of this band is decreased by Na^+ (compare lower with upper panel in Figure 3) we conclude that a protein with an apparent molecular weight of 65,000 is involved in Na^+/H^+ exchange. This conclusion is supported by the absence of a Na^+-protectable [^{14}C] Br-EIPA-labelled band in basolateral membranes which do not contain a Na^+/H^+ exchanger [6,9].

Affinity labelling of the rat renal Na^+/H^+ exchanger

As outlined above, side group-specific reagents provide an alternative approach for the biochemical identification of a transporter protein. So far, three different classes of side group-specific reagents have been tested as possible irreversible inhibitors of renal Na^+/H^+ exchange: sulfhydryl-group reagents, histidyl-group reagents and carboxyl group reagents. The sulfhydryl group reagent N′-ethylmaleimide (NEM) inhibited the rabbit renal Na^+/H^+ exchanger [11] and the antiporter present in thymic lymphocytes [12]. Since Na^+ and amiloride did not protect the exchanger from irreversible inhibition, NEM most probably did not bind to the cation site. The histidyl-group reagent diethylpyrocarbonate (DEPC) inhibited the rabbit renal Na^+/H^+ exchanger [13] and the antiporter present in the human placenta [14]. Amiloride and protons afforded protection suggesting that histidines are involved in the binding and translocation of protons [13]. Finally, the carboxyl group reagents N-ethoxycarbonyl-2-ethoxy-1,2-dihydroquinoline (EEDQ) and N,N′-dicyclohexylcarbodiimide (DCCD)

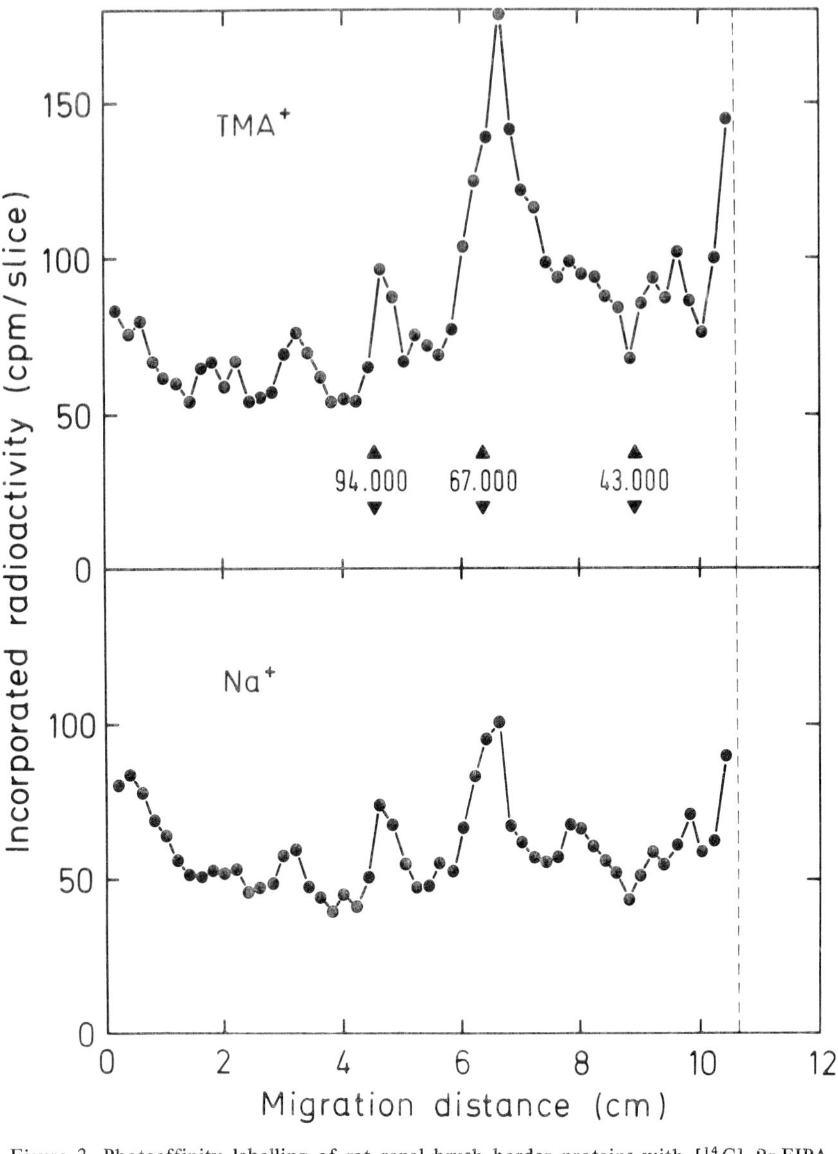

Figure 3. Photoaffinity labelling of rat renal brush border proteins with [^{14}C] Br-EIPA. Vesicles were irradiated for 10 minutes in the presence of 0.1mM [^{14}C] Br-EIPA and 100mM tetramethylammonium chloride (top panel) or 100mM NaCl (bottom panel). In addition the buffers contained 50mM KCl, 5mM HEPES/Tris, pH 7.0. After washing in [^{14}C] Br-EIPA-free buffers the membrane proteins were separated by SDS polyacrylamide gel electrophoresis. The gel was then cut into 2mm slices and the incorporated radioactivity was determined in each slice by liquid scintillation techniques. The ordinate shows the migration distance of the proteins from the top of the gel, the ordinate the incorporated radioactivity. Arrow heads indicate the position of molecular weight marker proteins run in parallel gel tracks. The figure is taken from [9]

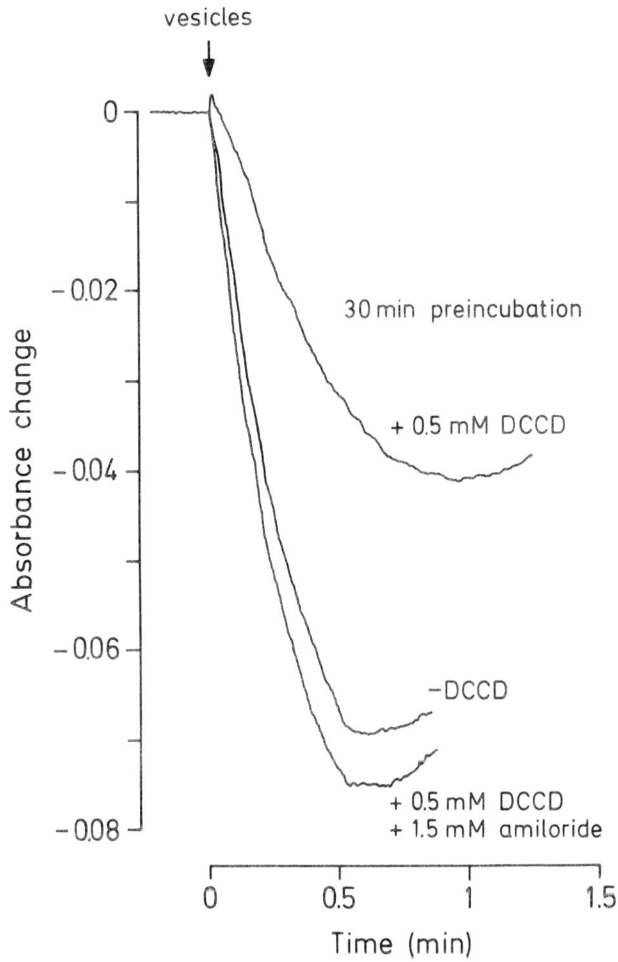

Figure 4. Irreversible inhibition of Na^+/H^+ exchange by N,N′-dicyclohexylcarbodiimide (DCCD) and protection by amiloride. Rat renal brush border membrane vesicles were pretreated for 30 minutes without or with 0.5mM DCCD in buffers containing 100mM tetramethylammonium chloride, 50mM KCl, 5mM HEPES/Tris, pH 7.0, without or with 1.5mM amiloride as indicated. Thereafter the vesicles were washed in DCCD-free buffers and tested for Na^+/H^+ exchanger activity as described in the legend to Figure 2

were shown to cause irreversible inhibition of proximal tubular Na^+/H^+ exchangers [9,11,15–17]. Figure 4 shows an experiment with rat renal brush border membrane vesicles that had been pretreated with 0.5mM DCCD (controls: no DCCD) for 30 minutes. Following washing and loading with Na^+, intravesicular acidification as visualized by the absorbance decrease of acridine orange is slower in DCCD-treated vesicles as compared to controls. Vesicles pretreated with DCCD in the presence of amiloride show no inhibition of

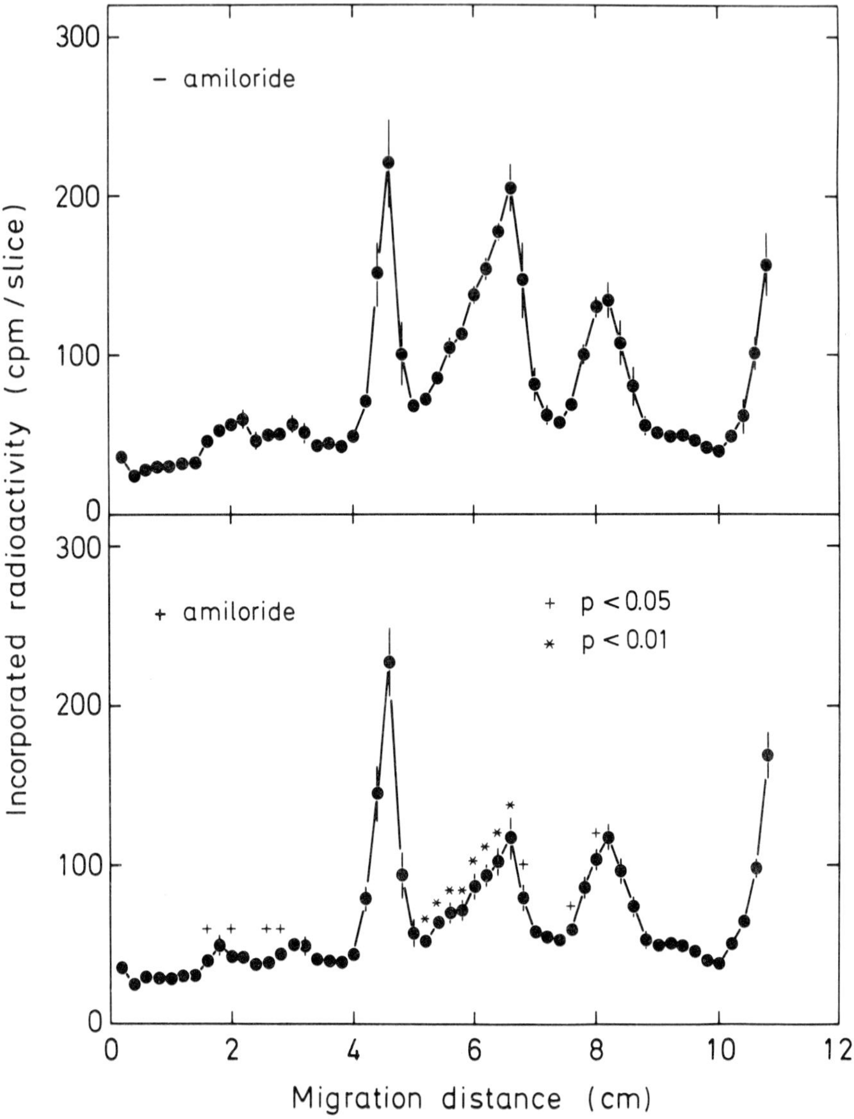

Figure 5. Labelling of rat renal brush border membrane vesicles with [^{14}C] DCCD and protection by amiloride. Brush border membrane vesicles were incubated for 30 minutes with 2.3nmol [^{14}C] DCCD/mg protein in buffers containing 100mM tetramethylammonium Cl, 50mM KCl, 5mM HEPES/Tris, pH 7.0, without (top panel) or with 1mM amiloride (bottom panel). Thereafter, the vesicles were spun down and left without supernatant for three hours on ice. The pellets were then prepared for gel electrophoresis as previously described [9]. Four gels were run in parallel for each condition, cut into 2mm slices and the radioactivity was determined. Each point shows the mean of these four determinations with standard errors if they exceed the symbol size. Statistical differences were calculated using Student's 't' test for unpaired data. The figure is taken from [9]

subsequently determined Na^+/H^+ exchange. In agreement with other studies [11,14,17] these data suggest that DCCD modifies a carboxyl group which is either directly involved in Na^+ and amiloride binding or is closely related to the substrate binding site. Therefore, DCCD is suited to label the membrane protein involved in Na^+/H^+ exchange.

Figure 5 shows the distribution of [^{14}C] DCCD-labelled membrane proteins along an SDS gel. For this experiment rat renal brush border membrane vesicles have been incubated with [^{14}C] DCCD in the absence (top panel) or presence of amiloride (bottom panel). [^{14}C] DCCD is mainly incorporated into three bands corresponding to the apparent molecular weights (from left to right) of 89,000, 65,000, and 51,000. A significant protection from labelling is observed with the MW 65,000 band. Since the activity of the Na^+/H^+ exchanger could also be protected by amiloride from inactivation by DCCD (c.f. Figure 4) it is likely that a protein within the MW 65,000 band is related to the antiporter. This conclusion is strongly supported by two lines of evidence. First, the amiloride-protectable [^{14}C] DCCD-labelled band is not present in basolateral membranes which lack the Na^+/H^+ exchanger [6,9]. Second, a band of similar molecular weight showed a Na^+-protectable [^{14}C] Br-EIPA incorporation (c.f. Figure 3). Thus, we believe that a membrane protein with apparent molecular weight of 65,000 is involved in Na^+/H^+ exchange in rat renal brush border membranes.

Specificity of N,N′-dicyclohexylcarbodiimide

As already outlined, group-specific reagents can interact with many membrane proteins carrying similar side groups. To test for the specificity of DCCD we have determined the effect of this carboxyl group reagent on a series of Na^+-coupled transport systems present in the brush border membrane. All tested transport systems, i.e. the Na^+-cotransporters for sugars, neutral, acidic and basic aminoacids, citric acid cycle intermediates and for sulphate were irreversibly inhibited by DCCD, although to a different extent [9]. Similar inhibitions were reported by Kinsella et al [17] for the Na^+-dependent phosphate transporter. The Na^+/substrate cotransport systems, however, differ in one important aspect from the Na^+/H^+ exchanger: amiloride afforded protection against inactivation by DCCD only for the Na^+/H^+ exchanger. Therefore, the amiloride-protectable [^{14}C] DCCD-binding protein described above cannot be related to any of the tested Na^+-dependent substrate transport systems. At present it is not known which of the other amiloride-insensitive [^{14}C] DCCD-labelled bands corresponds to one or more of the cotransport systems.

Differences between rat and rabbit renal Na^+/H^+ exchangers

Igarashi and Aronson [11] reported that a protein with an apparent molecular weight of 100,000 bound [^{14}C] DCCD and was protected by amiloride in rabbit renal brush border membrane vesicles. Their data which indicated a molecular weight of 100,000 for the Na^+/H^+ exchanger were clearly in disagreement with our findings (Figures 3 and 5 [9]) which suggested a molecular weight of 65,000 for the rat renal Na^+/H^+ exchanger. A possible explanation for this discrepancy was the presence of species differences. We therefore tested both, rat and rabbit renal brush border membrane vesicles under identical experimental conditions [18]. Both exchangers showed comparable affinities towards amiloride and amiloride analogues and both exchangers could be irreversibly inhibited by photoaffinity labelling with Br-EPIA. However, the rabbit renal Na^+/H^+ exchanger required higher DCCD concentrations than the rat renal antiporter to achieve a comparable degree of irreversible inhibition (Figure 6). This result

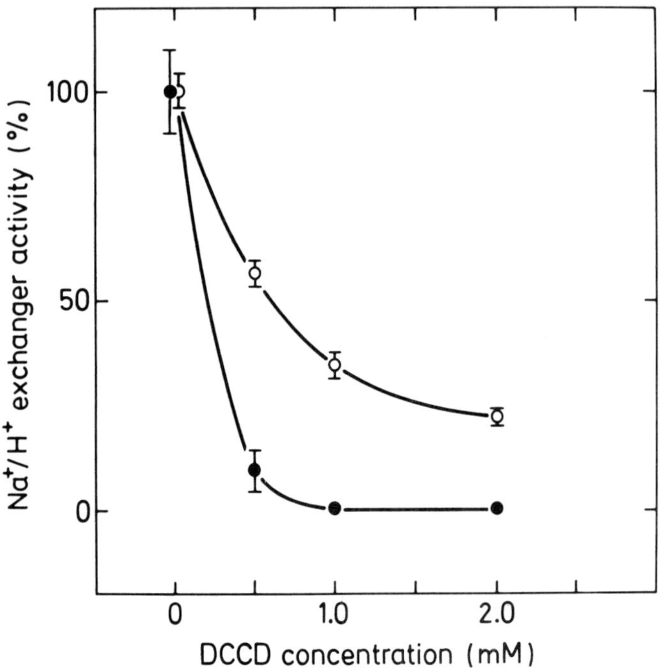

Figure 6. Different sensitivities towards DCCD of rat (•) and rabbit (○) renal Na^+/H^+ exchangers. Rat and rabbit renal brush border membrane vesicles were incubated for 30 minutes at room temperature in buffers containing the indicated DCCD concentrations and 100mM tetramethylammonium chloride, 50mM KCl, 5mM HEPES/Tris, pH 7.0. Na^+/H^+ exchanger activity was assayed after washing the vesicles in DCCD-free buffer and loading with Na^+ as described in the legend to Figure 2

suggests that the molecular structure of the cation binding site differs between both species. When we labelled rabbit renal brush border membrane vesicles with [^{14}C] DCCD and separated the membrane proteins by SDS polyacrylamide gel electrophoresis, we could not detect an amiloride-protectable [^{14}C] DCCD-labelled band with an apparent molecular weight of 65,000 [18]. Such a band is clearly visible under identical experimental conditions with rat renal brush border membrane vesicles (c.f. Figure 6) supporting the notion of species differences. Thus, it seems at present that in rat and rabbit renal brush border membranes different proteins are involved in Na^+/H^+ exchange.

Purification of the rat renal Na^+/H^+ exchanger

Future experiments are directed to isolate and purify from rat renal brush border membranes the protein with an apparent molecular weight of 65,000 which we think is involved in Na^+/H^+ exchange. Preliminary evidence suggests that an affinity column with amiloride as ligand can be used to highly enrich the M_r 65,000 protein from Triton X-100-solubilized brush border membranes. A further purification can be achieved by high pressure liquid chromatography. The purified protein can then be used to determine a partial aminoacid sequence and to raise antibodies against the renal Na^+/H^+ exchanger. The final proof of the identity of the M_r 65,000 protein with the Na^+/H^+ exchanger awaits the functional reconstitution of the purified protein in liposomes.

Acknowledgments

This work was supported by the Sonderforschungsbereich 169/A2.

References

1 Aronson PS. Mechanisms of active H^+ secretion in the proximal tubule. *Am J Physiol 1983; 245:* F647–F659

2 Murer H, Hopfer U, Kinne R. Sodium/proton antiport in brush border membrane vesicles from rat small intestine and kidney. *Biochem J 1976; 154:* 597–604

3 Aronson PS. Kinetic properties of the plasma membrane Na^+-H^+ exchanger. *Ann Rev Physiol 1985; 47:* 545–560

4 Seifter JL, Aronson PS. Properties and physiological role of the plasma membrane sodium-hydrogen exchanger. *J Clin Invest 1986; 78:* 859–864

5 Jacobson C, Kragh-Hansen U, Sheikh MI. Na^+-H^+ exchange in luminal-membrane vesicles from rabbit proximal convoluted and straight tubules in response to metabolic acidosis. *Biochem J 1986; 239:* 411–416

6 Sabolić I, Burckhardt G. Proton pathways in rat renal brush-border and basolateral membrane vesicles. *Biochim Biophys Acta 1983; 734:* 210–220

7 Grinstein S, Rothstein A. Mechanisms of regulation of the Na^+/H^+ exchanger. *J Membrane Biol 1986; 90:* 1–12

8 Kinsella JL, Aronson PS. Amiloride inhibition of the Na^+-H^+ exchanger in renal microvillus membrane vesicles. *Am J Physiol 1981; 241:* F374–F379

9 Friedrich T, Sablotni J, Burckhardt G. Identification of the renal Na^+/H^+ exchanger with N,N'-dicyclohexylcarbodiimide (DCCD) and amiloride analogues. *J Membrane Biol 1986; 94:* 253–266

10 Benos DJ, Mandel LJ. Irreversible inhibition of sodium entry sites in frog skin by a photosensitive amiloride analog. *Science 1978; 199:* 1205–1206

11 Igarashi P, Aronson PS. Covalent modification of the renal Na^+/H^+ exchanger by N,N'-dicyclohexylcarbodiimide. *J Biol Chem 1987; 262:* 860–868

12 Grinstein S, Cohen S, Rothstein A. Chemical modification of the Na^+-H^+ exchanger of thymic lymphocytes. Inhibition by N-ethylmaleimide. *Biochim Biophys Acta 1985; 812:* 213–222

13 Grillo FG, Aronson PS. Inactivation of the renal microvillus membrane Na^+-H^+ exchanger by histidine-specific reagents. *J Biol Chem 1986; 261:* 1120–1125

14 Ganapthy V, Balkovetz DF, Ganapathy ME et al. Evidence for histidyl and carboxy groups at the active site of human placental Na^+-H^+ exchanger. *Biochem J 1987; 245:* 473–477

15 Burnham C, Munzesheimer C, Rabon E, Sachs G. Ion pathways in renal brush border membranes. *Biochim Biophys Acta 1982; 685:* 260–272

16 Rocco VK, Cragoe EJ Jr, Warnock DG. N-ethoxycarbonyl-2-ethoxy-1,2-dihydroquinolone, amiloride analogues, and renal Na^+/H^+ antiporter. *Am J Physiol 1987; 252:* F517–F524

17 Kinsella JL, Sehrle J, Wilkins N, Sacktor B. Inhibition of Na^+-H^+ exchange by N,N'-dicyclohexylcarbodiimide in isolated rat renal brush border membrane vesicles. *J Biol Chem 1987; 262:* 7092–7097

19 Friedrich T, Sablotni J, Burckhardt G. Species differences between rat and rabbit renal Na^+/H^+ exchangers. *Biochem Biophys Res Commun 1987; 144:* 869–875

FUNCTIONS OF THE LOOP OF HENLE

FUNCTION OF THE THIN ASCENDING LIMB IN URINE CONCENTRATING MECHANISM

M Imai, K Yoshitomi, Y Kondo, J Taniguchi, C Koseki

National Cardiovascular Center Research Institute, Osaka, Japan

Introduction

The thin ascending limb of Henle's loop is assumed to play an important rôle in the generation of a steep osmotic gradient in the inner medulla as a major component of the countercurrent multiplication system [1,2]. An essential requirement for the countercurrent multiplier is that the ascending limb has a capability to generate hypotonic luminal fluid by selectively transporting solutes without a sizeable volumetric flux. The existence of active NaCl transport has been well established in the cortical ascending limb as well as medullary thick ascending limb [3,4]. Since these thick segments of Henle's loop have a low water permeability luminal fluid becomes hypotonic relative to ambient fluid. On the other hand there is controversy about whether active solute transport exists in the thin segment [1,2]. Technical difficulties in studying the function of the thin segments are the major sources for the disagreement.

In vitro microperfusion of isolated renal tubules [5] is a useful method of examining the transport properties of the thin ascending limb without complications from changes in haemodynamics. The purpose of this communication is to summarize the data on solute and water transport properties of the thin ascending limb, which have been mainly derived from in vitro microperfusion studies, and to discuss the rôle of the thin ascending limb in the operation of the countercurrent multiplication system in the renal inner medulla. Special attention will be focused on the mechanism of chloride transport across the thin ascending limb.

GENERAL TRANSPORT PROPERTIES OF THE THIN ASCENDING LIMB

Failure to demonstrate active solute transport

In vitro microperfusion studies revealed that the transmural voltage (V_T) across the thin ascending limb is zero when the composition of the perfusate is identical to that in the bathing fluid [6]. Under these circumstances the collected fluid to perfusate (CF/PF) ratios of osmolality, sodium, chloride and volume marker were not different from unity [6], indicating that there is no fluid movement, net NaCl or solute transport in the absence of driving forces. In hypertonic solution, no net solute transport was demonstrated. These observations favour the view that there is no active solute transport in the thin ascending limb.

However, one may argue that the failure to demonstrate active solute transport may be due to the lack of humoral factors which maintain active solute transport in vivo. Vasopressin is one such candidate, since it is known to stimulate NaCl transport in the medullary thick ascending limb [3,4]. Although Imai and Kusano [7] confirmed that there is vasopressin-sensitive adenylate cyclase in hamster thin ascending limb, the administration of arginine vasopressin did not increase V_T or chloride flux.

Permeabilities to water and solutes

The osmotic water permeability of the thin ascending limb was reported to be very low in various species including rabbits [6], rats and hamsters [8]. Diffusional permeability to water was also reported to be low in the rabbit thin ascending limb [6]. These findings are in accord with the observations by in vivo micropuncture studies [9,10] and in vitro microperfusion in papillary slices [11].

The thin ascending limb is highly permeable to sodium and to chloride, but less permeable to urea. These characteristics are common among rabbits, rats

TABLE I. Transport parameters of the thin ascending limb isolated from kidneys of rabbits, rats and hamsters

		Rabbits [6]	Rats [8]	Hamsters [8]
L_p	10^{-6} cm sec^{-1} atm^{-1} (10^{-7} cm^2 sec^{-1} atm^{-1})	0.93±0.61 (0.58±0.38)	1.80±1.44 (1.13±0.90)	2.11±1.30 (1.33±0.82)
P_{dw}	10^{-5} cm sec^{-1} (10^{-7} cm^2 sec^{-1})	45.3±5.4 (28.4±3.4)	ND	ND
P_{Na}	10^{-5} cm sec^{-1} (10^{-7} cm^2 sec^{-1})	25.5±1.8 (16.0±1.1)	79.6±3.6 (50.0±2.3)	87.6±7.3 (55.0±4.5)
P_{Cl}	10^{-5} cm sec^{-1} (10^{-7} cm^2 sec^{-1})	117.0±9.1 (73.5±5.7)	183.7±19.6 (115.4±5.8)	196.0±12.3 (123.1±7.7)
P_{urea}	10^{-5} cm sec^{-1} (10^{-7} cm^2 sec^{-1})	6.7±1.0 (4.2±0.6)	22.8±4.5 (14.3±2.8)	18.5+6.2 (11.6±3.9)
P_{Cl}/P_{Na}		8.81±0.16 [12]	2.17±0.15	2.35±0.14

Data in parentheses are converted to values expressed by unit tubular length assuming that tubular diameter is 20μm. All data are means ± SEM.
Abbreviations: L_p=hydraulic conductivity; P_{dw}=diffusional water permeability; P_{Cl}/P_{Na}= permeability ratio calculated from NaCl diffusion voltage; ND=not determined

and hamsters (Table I). It should be noted that chloride permeability is extraordinarily high. The permeability properties of the thin ascending limb are in favour of the view that dilution of the luminal fluid occurs by passive mechanisms.

MECHANISM OF CHLORIDE TRANSPORT

Evidence for facilitated transport

Since the apparent chloride permeability in the thin ascending limb is extremely high, it is possible that there is a special mechanism which accelerates chloride transport across this segment. Three lines of evidence support this hypothesis [13]. First, the unidirectional flux of ^{36}Cl from the lumen to bath exhibited a saturation kinetic when ambient chloride concentration was increased. Second, the chloride flux was competitively inhibited by bromide. Third, when Ussing's flux ratio analysis was performed at various transmural voltages generated by salt diffusion, the flux ratios for chloride clearly deviated from the line of identity which represents simple passive diffusion. These findings suggest that at least a part of chloride transport is mediated by a facilitated transport mechanism. On the other hand, sodium transport is mediated entirely by simple passive diffusion.

Effects of anion transport inhibitors

If chloride transport is mediated by a process involving transporters in membranes, there may be specific inhibitors. Kondo et al [14] addressed this issue by examing effects of stilbene disulfonates (SITS, DIDS), phloretin and frusemide on NaCl transport across the hamster thin ascending limb.

Stilbene disulfonates

When DIDS was added to the bath at 10^{-3}M, the lumen positive diffusion voltage which was generated upon reduction of NaCl concentration in the bath was reduced and the polarity of the voltage was reversed, indicating that the permeability to chloride was less than the permeability to sodium. This effect of DIDS was irreversible. The decrease in P_{Cl^-}/P_{Na^+} ratio can be explained by 1) a decrease in chloride permeability, 2) an increase in sodium permeability, 3) a combination of the two, 4) a decrease in both with a much greater fall preferential in chloride permeability, and 5) an increase in both with a much greater rise in sodium permeability. Therefore, we measured permeabilities for ^{36}Cl and ^{22}Na to obtain more direct information. Since there is no active solute transport in the thin ascending limb, the unidirectional flux coefficients measured in the absence of driving forces represent the passive permeability coefficients. The results summarized in Figure 1 clearly show that DIDS suppresses the chloride permeability without affecting the Na^+ permeability. SITS had a similar effect, but it was less potent.

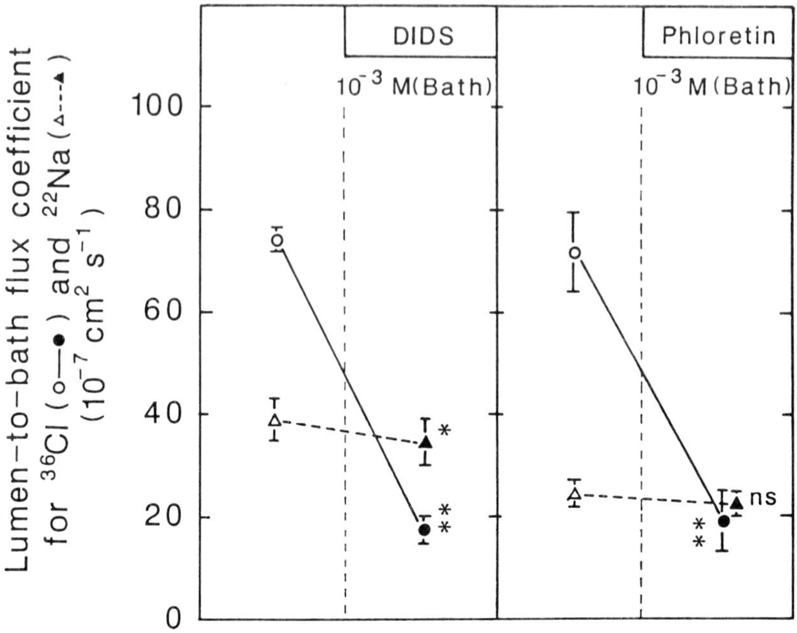

Figure 1. Effects of DIDS on ^{36}Cl and ^{22}Na flux coefficients in the hamster thin ascending limb. *$P<0.05$; **$P<0.01$ (paired samples). Figure is constructed from the data of Kondo et al [14]

Stilbene disulfonates are known to be inhibitors of the Cl^- HCO_3^- or Cl^-/Cl^- antiporter equated with band 3 protein in red blood cells [15]. The specificity of these agents on red blood cell membranes depends on the fact that the band 3 protein is almost the only protein exposed on the outside of the membranes that is modified by stilbene derivatives. In other cells stilbene derivatives bind to many other functional proteins and modify their functions, e.g. they also inhibit a Na^+:HCO_3^- symport [16–19] and chloride channels [20]. Thus, the inhibitory effect of stilbene disulfonates on chloride transport in the thin ascending limb does not necessarily mean that chloride is transported by Cl^-/HCO_3^- or Cl^-/Cl^- antiporters. It may rather mean that chloride transport in the thin ascending limb shares a common mechanism with other anion transport systems which are sensitive to stilbene disulfonate derivates.

Phloretin

Phloretin is also known to be an inhibitor of Cl^-/HCO_3^- or Cl^-/Cl^- antiporter of red blood cells [15]. Therefore, we tested whether phloretin also inhibits chloride transport in the hamster thin ascending limb [14]. Since chloride transport in the thin ascending limb is unaffected by removal of bicarbonate (vide infra), we used bicarbonate-free solutions. Phloretin added either to the bath or to the lumen caused a reversible reduction of the NaCl diffusion voltage generated by decreasing NaCl concentration in the bath, indicating again that phloretin reduced the P_{Cl}/P_{Na} ratio. We also confirmed this inhibitory effect of phloretin was specific to chloride permeability (Figure 1). Sodium flux was unchanged by phloretin.

Phloretin is known to be one of the inhibitors of the glucose-sodium cotransporter [21]. Phlorizin, another inhibitor of glucose-sodium cotransport, did not affect the P_{Cl^+}/P_{Na^+} ratio in the thin ascending limb however, so the inhibitory effect of phloretin on chloride transport is unlikely to be related to glucose-sodium transport. Phloretin is also known to inhibit urea transport in membranes of red blood cells [22], toad bladder [23] and collecting duct of mammalian kidneys [24]. Thus it is impossible to specify the mechanism of chloride transport in the thin ascending limb by the effect of phloretin.

Frusemide

Although frusemide is known to be an inhibitor of the Na^+-K^+-$2Cl^-$ cotransporter in various biological membranes [3], it also, at higher concentrations, inhibits chloride channels [25]. Frusemide (10^{-3}M) added to the bath reversibly reduced chloride permeability and the P_{Cl}/P_{Na} ratio [14]. However, when it was added to the lumen at this concentration, chloride transport was unchanged. Although these observations suggest that frusemide is more potent on the basolateral side than on the luminal side in inhibiting chloride transport, they do not identify the mechanism of chloride transport. The failure of frusemide to inhibit chloride transport from the lumen indicates that the mechanism of chloride transport is different from that in the thick ascending limb.

Effects of ion substitution

There are several mechanisms by which chloride transport across biological membranes is facilitated. They are classified into three categories: 1) antiport mechanisms, which include Cl^-/Cl^- or Cl^-/HCO_3^- exchange; 2) symport mechanisms, which include K^--Cl^- cotransport; and 3) channels through which chloride moves down its electrochemical gradient without being coupled to any other ion. In order to identify the mechanism of chloride transport in the thin ascending limb, we examined the effect of removal of bicarbonate, potassium and sodium on chloride flux. The results of these studies are summarized in Table II.

The elimination of bicarbonate did not decrease chloride flux, but rather increased it. Failure of bicarbonate elimination to suppress chloride flux indicates that the Cl^-/HCO_3^- exchanger is not responsible for chloride transport in the thin ascending limb, but it is difficult to explain why elimination of bicarbonate caused an *increase* in chloride flux.

When sodium was completely removed from bathing fluids chloride was

TABLE II. Effects of elimination of bicarbonate, sodium or potassium on lumen-to-bath ^{36}Cl flux coefficient

	Lumen-to-bath chloride flux coefficient ($10^{-7} cm^2 sec^{-1}$)
Control	75.9±7.1
Bicarbonate-free	101.7±10.5*
Control	119.2±6.9
Sodium-free	107.3±8.3
Control	111.9±7.2
Potassium-free + 5mM $BaCl_2$	115.9±12.7

In experimental periods, the indicated ions were eliminated from both perfusate and bathing fluid. *$P<0.05$. Data from [26]

unchanged, indicating that chloride transport is not coupled to sodium, excluding both Na^+-Cl^- and Na^+-K^+-$2Cl^-$ cotransport mechanisms. Further, when KCl of the artificial solution was replaced by $BaCl_2$, chloride flux was unchanged. This would exclude both K^+-Cl^- and Na^+-K^+-$2Cl^-$ cotransport mechanisms.

Possible existence of chloride channels

Based on these studies we can postulate, by exclusion, that chloride is transported across the thin ascending limb by a process of electrodiffusion most probably via chloride channels. Since sodium, potassium and bicarbonate are the major ions in body fluids, the absence of coupling of chloride transport with these ions strongly suggests that chloride is transported across the thin ascending limb without coupling to other ions. The effects of anion transport inhibitors are not inconsistent with the existence of chloride channels. A patch clamp study is necessary to draw a final conclusion.

ROUTE OF CHLORIDE TRANSPORT

Morphological studies have shown that epithelial cells of the thin ascending limb are closely opposed to neighbouring cells, with complicated interdigitations and shallow tight junctions [27]. These features are characteristic of leaky epithelia. Therefore, it is reasonable to assume that the paracellular shunt pathway may play an integral part for the high ion permeability of the thin ascending limb.

Based on observations in the rabbit thin ascending limb Imai and Kokko [28] suggested that the chloride flux of this segment consist of two components, one saturable, the other non-saturable. On the other hand, there is no saturable component for the sodium flux. It is possible that sodium is transported exclusively via the paracellular route, whereas chloride is transported by both a transcellular and a paracellular route. Although the permeability of the thin ascending limb to sodium is much less than that of chloride, the absolute value for sodium permeability is very high, much higher than in the proximal convoluted tubule, which is recognized as a leaky epithelium. So, although electrical resistances have yet to be measured, we are confident that the thin ascending limb can be classified as a leaky epithelium.

It is also reasonable to assume that the saturable component of chloride transport is associated with the transcellular route. This hypothesis is supported in part by the observations that anion transport inhibitors selectively inhibit chloride without affecting sodium transport. The observation that the NaCl diffusion voltage, which is a measure of the chloride permselectivity, was symmetrical whether NaCl was decreased in the lumen or in the bath seems to contradict this hypothesis, but it might be explained by assuming that there are chloride conductances in series in the luminal and basolateral cell membranes.

In order to substantiate this hypothesis, it is necessary to impale the epithelium of the thin ascending limb with microelectrodes. Because of the size of the cells in the thin ascending limb, this is extremely difficult. Recently, Yoshitomi et al [29] succeeded in impaling 18 cells of the hamster thin ascending limb. The basolateral membrane voltage (V_B) ranged from −14.0 to −40.0mV with a mean of −24.5±1.5mV (SEM). This voltage was not affected by 10^{-4}M ouabain on the basolateral side. When chloride concentration in the bathing fluid was abruptly reduced from 165 to 5mM, a sharp and transient positive deflection of V_B was observed. When chloride concentration in the bathing fluid was returned to 165mM again, a mirror-image negative deflection of V_B was observed. This observation suggests that there is a chloride conductance in the basolateral membrane and that the chloride concentration in the cell rapidly reaches a new equilibrium level. The peak of positive deflection was 49.1±2.7mV (n=18). This voltage was even greater than the transmural voltage (V_T) simultaneously observed (33.4+1.2mV) indicating that a considerable portion of the chloride conductance is attributable to the transcellular route.

It is worth emphasizing that the deflection of V_T was stable during the time the NaCl gradient was imposed, while the response of V_B was transient. Apical membrane voltage (V_A) can be predicted to remain altered during reduction of chloride concentration in the bath and from this pattern, we may deduce that chloride conductance in the apical membrane constitutes a rate-limiting step to transcellular chloride transport, i.e. the chloride conductance is less in the apical than in the basolateral membrane. In fact, when chloride concentration in the luminal fluid was suddenly reduced, a stable positive voltage deflection of V_A was observed amounting to −34.2±1.9mV (n=6), a value less than V_T (−31.8±2.2mV). Observations that anion transport inhibitors were more potent in the bath than in the lumen support this view.

Although biochemical studies have shown that vasopressin [7,30] and prostaglandins [31] stimulate adenylate cyclase activity in the thin ascending limb, the physiological significance of these hormones or autoacoids in the regulation of the function of the thin ascending limb is unknown. Since chloride channels are likely to be responsible for transcellular chloride transport across the thin ascending limb (vide supra), we here examined whether this chloride conductance is modulated by calcium or pH [26,32].

pH dependence of chloride transport

It is well known that many ion transporting systems including channels, antiporters and cotransporters consist of protein subunits. Ion transport mediated by these systems is influenced by the ambient pH. The titration curves of ion conductances vary depending on the aminoacids which play a critical rôle in the

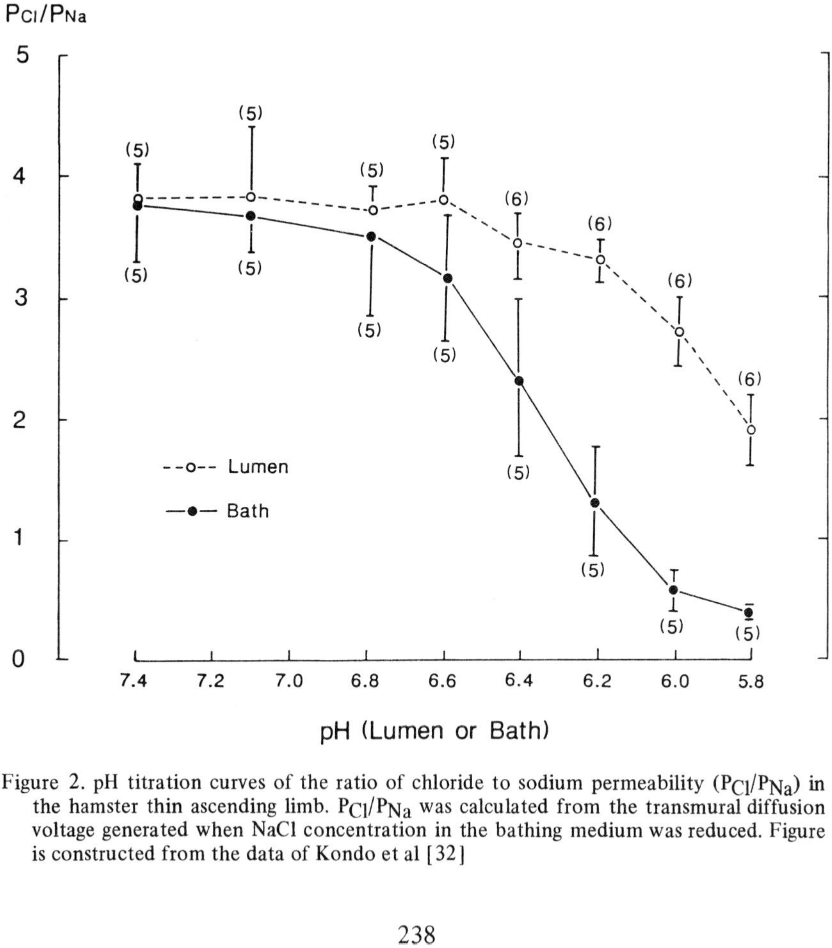

Figure 2. pH titration curves of the ratio of chloride to sodium permeability (P_{Cl}/P_{Na}) in the hamster thin ascending limb. P_{Cl}/P_{Na} was calculated from the transmural diffusion voltage generated when NaCl concentration in the bathing medium was reduced. Figure is constructed from the data of Kondo et al [32]

translocation of the ion in question. Kondo et al [32] demonstrated that chloride transport across the hamster thin ascending limb was inhibited by an acid pH which was more potent at the basolateral side than in the lumen (Figure 2). Analyses of pH titration curves revealed that pK values were 6.13 and 5.78 for the basolateral and the luminal side, respectively, but that the maximal inhibitory effect was identical on both sides. Hill's coefficients of these curves were close to 2, so it is reasonable to speculate that there are two proton binding sites for the modulation of the conductive chloride pathways. The alkalinization of the bathing fluid to pH 9.0 did not affect chloride conductance.

It is of interest to note that selective intracellular acidification by addition of o-nitrophenylacetate also inhibited the chloride conductance. This provides further evidence that chloride is transported at least in part by a transcellular route. At the present time, it is not known whether changes in intracellular pH have a physiological relevance in the regulation of chloride transport across the thin ascending limb.

Calcium dependence of chloride transport

In other biological membranes chloride channels are regulated by the ambient calcium concentration [33,34]. We have examined whether the chloride conductance

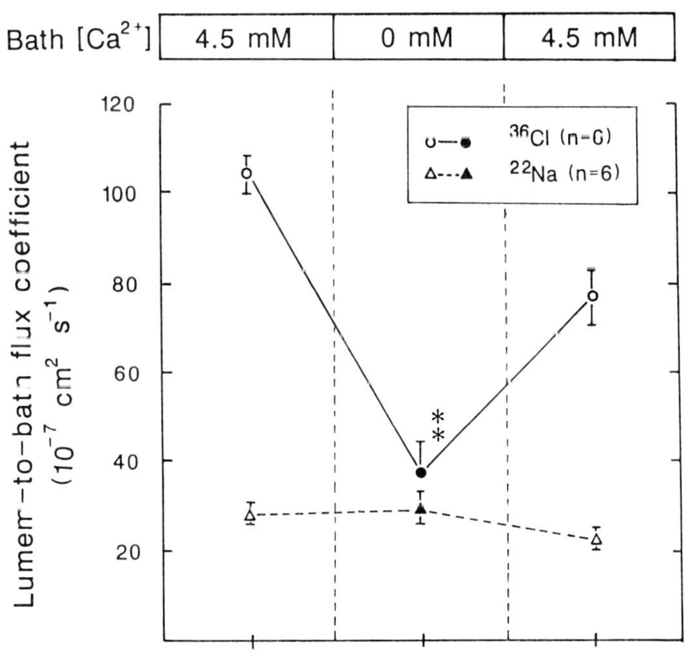

Figure 3. Effects of elimination of calcium from the bath on ^{36}Cl and ^{22}Na flux coefficients in the hamster thin ascending limb. **P<0.01. Figure is constructed from the data of Kondo et al [26]

in the thin ascending limb is regulated by calcium [26]. We found that reducing calcium concentration caused a decrease in chloride conductance.

As shown in Figure 3, the P_{Cl}/P_{Na} ratio calculated from the NaCl diffusion potential was reduced when the calcium concentration in the bath was nominally zero. The elimination of calcium from lumen fluid was without effect. Removal of calcium from the bath selectively inhibited the chloride flux coefficient from $104.6 \pm 3.4 \times 10^{-7}$ to $37.2 \pm 7.2 \times 10^{-7}$ $cm^2\ s^{-1}$ ($P<0.01$, n=6) with little increase in sodium flux coefficient (from $28.0 \pm 3.0 \times 10^{-7}$ to $29.3 \pm 3.1 \times 10^{-7}$; $P<0.05$, n=6). The observed slight increase in sodium flux coefficient may represent an increased leakiness of the tight junction which occurs with removal of calcium. The fact that the elimination of calcium caused a decrease rather than an increase in chloride flux coefficient accords with the view that the transcellular route is a major component of chloride transport and is regulated by calcium concentrations.

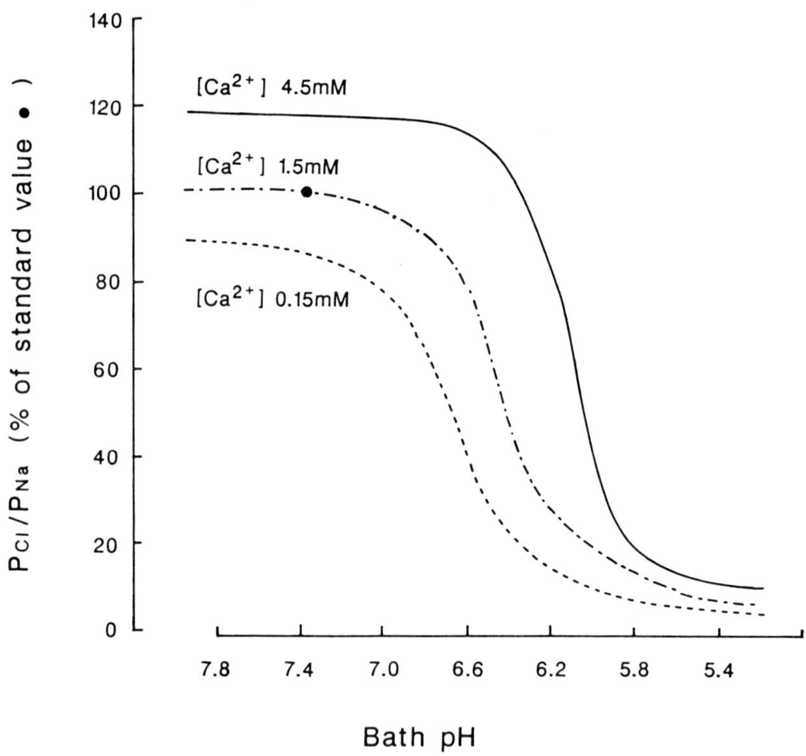

Figure 4. Interaction between effects of calcium and pH in modulating P_{Cl}/P_{Na} ratio in the hamster thin ascending limb. pH titration curves were measured at three calcium concentrations. The P_{Cl}/P_{Na} ratio was calculated from deflection of the transmural voltage generated when NaCl concentration in the bathing medium was reduced. Figure is constructed from the data of Kondo et al [26]

The modulatory effect of calcium on chloride transport may depend on changes in intracellular calcium concentration. In support of this view, we found that the acetyoxymethyl ester of quin 2, which is supposed to decrease intracellular calcium concentration by its chelating capability suppressed the chloride flux as well as the P_{Cl}/P_{Na} ratio.

Since chloride transport is also regulated by pH (vide supra), it is important to examine whether there are interactions between pH and calcium in the regulation of chloride transport across the thin ascending limb. Therefore, we performed titration studies of chloride conductance at three different calcium concentrations, 0.15, 1.5 and 4.5mM. We found increases in calcium concentration are associated with both increases in the transport maximum and decreases in the affinity to proton (Figure 4). Thus it is highly likely that calcium concentration modulates chloride transport by a mechanism or mechanisms distinct from the hydrion binding site.

Rôles of sulfhydryl groups

In order to examine whether sulfhydryl groups on the putative chloride transporter play an important rôle, we observed the effects of sulfhydryl reagents on chloride transport across the thin ascending limb [35]. As summarized in Figure 5, all the agents tested, including parachloromercuribenzene sulfonate (PCMBS), maleimide, and N-ethylmaleimide (NEM) decreased the P_{Cl}/P_{Na} ratio, as determined by NaCl diffusion potentials, as well as the ^{36}Cl flux. Kondo and

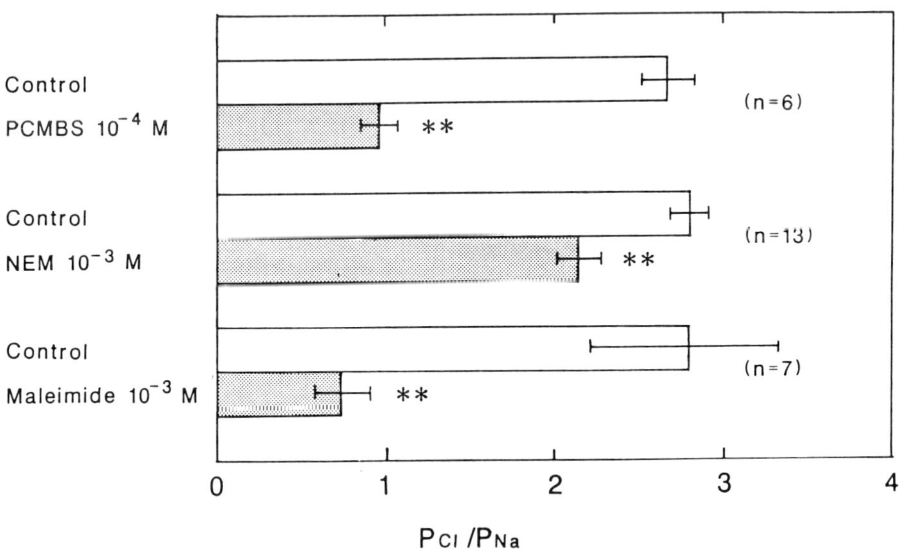

Figure 5. Effect of sulfhydryl reagents on the P_{Cl}/P_{Na} ratio in the hamster thin ascending limb. Figure is constructed from the data of Imai et al [34]

Imai [35] have reported that treatment of hamster thin ascending limb with glutaraldehyde preferentially inhibited halogen permselectivity. This could also be attributed to a modification of sulfhydryl groups. The inhibitory effects caused by the modification of sulfhydryl groups with these agents were irreversible but were prevented by pretreatment with dithiothreitol. NEM exhibited a unique stimulatory effect on chloride conductance of the thin ascending limb [35] when it was applied to the segment which had been pretreated with sulfhydryl reagents (Figure 6). The stimulatory effect was reversible and prevented or reversed by administration of dithiothreitol. Since NEM exhibited a dual action it is likely that there are at least two distinct sites with sulfhydryl groups which regulate chloride transport across the thin ascending limb. Dextran maleimide did not show any inhibitory effect on chloride conductance, so the inhibitory site may be located inside cells.

In order to clarify the relationship between these sites modified by sulfhydryl reagents and those regulated by proton or by calcium, we have examined combined effects of NEM and pH or those of NEM and calcium on the P_{Cl}/P_{Na}

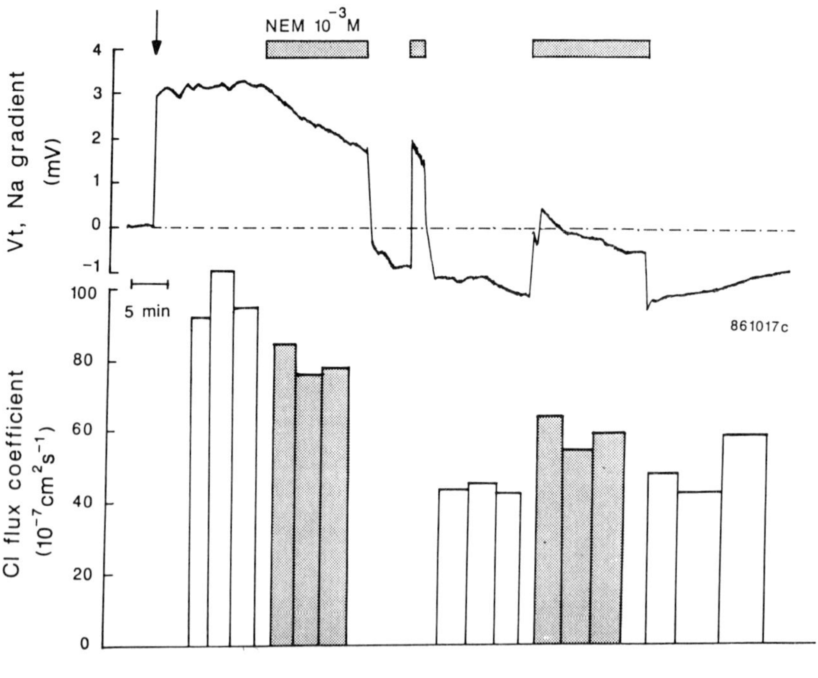

Figure 6. A representative study showing a dual action of NEM on diffusion voltage (V_T) and lumen-to-bath ^{36}Cl flux coefficient. The arrow indicates the time when NaCl concentration in the bath was reduced to approximately a half of that in the perfusate. In this particular experiment, the ^{36}Cl flux was measured in the presence of the transmural voltage. In the absence of the diffusion voltage, similar effects of NEM on the chloride flux were observed

ratio estimated by NaCl diffusion potential. While the P_{Cl}/P_{Na} was lowered by an initial administration of NEM, acidification of the bathing fluid to pH 5.8 further decreased the ratio. The stimulatory effect of a second administration of NEM on the parameter was markedly suppressed when the bathing fluid was made acidic to pH 5.8. These findings suggest that the sites regulated by protons are located distally to both stimulatory and inhibitory sulfhydryl sites.

On the other hand, after the NEM treatment, elimination of calcium from the bath caused a similar decrease in P_{Cl}/P_{Na} ratio as occurred before the NEM treatment. The stimulatory effect of NEM in the NEM treated segments was unchanged in the nominal absence of calcium in the bath. These observations suggest that the regulatory site controlled by calcium is distinct from the stimulatory as well as the inhibitory sites affected by sulfhydryl reagents.

In summary, the conductive chloride pathway across the thin ascending limb is regulated either by a stimulatory or by an inhibitory mechanism having sulfhydryl groups in critical positions. Protonation of the transporter may shut the pathway at a site distal to these dual regulatory systems, calcium may stimulate the chloride pathway by a separate mechanism.

ROLE OF THIN ASCENDING LIMB IN URINE CONCENTRATING MECHANISM

Although the conclusive evidence that there is no active NaCl transport in the thin ascending limb is still lacking, the demonstration of the highly efficient conductive chloride transport system in the thin ascending limb led us to conclude that active NaCl transport may not contribute significantly to net solute transport across this segment and hence to the countercurrent multiplication system in the inner medulla. In this regard, the passive equilibration models as proposed by Kokko and Rector [36] and Stephenson [37] are very attractive. However, these models require the existence at the hair-pin turn of large transmural concentration gradients for NaCl oriented from the lumen to peritubular region. Micropuncture studies and computer analyses have failed to support this hypothesis [1,2]. Since a considerable amount of urea enters the descending limb, urea must diffuse out of the thin ascending limb. Thus the dilution of the luminal fluid along the thin ascending limb should be established by diffusion of both NaCl and urea out of the tubule. Imai, Taniguchi and Tabei [2] proposed an alternative passive equilibration model for the countercurrent multiplication in the inner medulla. According to this model the single effect which provides osmotic work for multiplication comes from passive equilibration between three compartments: the thin ascending limb, the capillary networks and the papillary collecting duct. The essential features of the proposed single effect is depicted in Figure 7. If we assume that the reflection coefficient for urea in the papillary collecting duct is low and that the solutes in the luminal

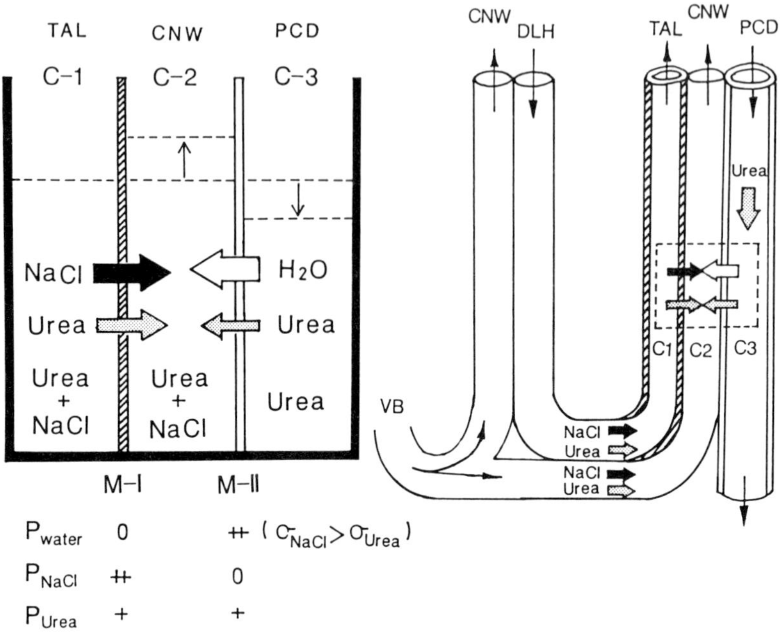

Figure 7. Three compartments–two solutes model (left) and assignment of each compartment to the structure of the inner medulla (right). C-1, C-2 and C-3 represent three compartments, where initial solute compositions are indicated at the bottom. Membrane I (M-I) is impermeable to water, highly permeable to NaCl and moderately permeable to urea. Membrane II (M-II) is highly permeable to water and moderately permeable to urea, but impermeable to NaCl. The reflection coefficients of membrane are higher for NaCl than for urea. CNW=capillary networks; DLH=descending limb of Henle; PCD= papillary collecting duct; TAL=thin ascending limb; VB=vascular bundle. From [2] with permission

fluid in the papillary collecting duct are mainly urea and NaCl, the effective osmolality in the latter compartment is higher than in the former even though nominal or cryoscopic osmolality is equal. Thus, this would become a primary driving force to induce water flux from the papillary collecting duct to the capillary networks. This could, in turn, dilute solute concentration in the capillary networks, generating concentration gradients favourable for diffusion of both NaCl and urea from the thin ascending limb to the capillary networks. Thus both NaCl and urea can diffuse out of the thin ascending limb and the luminal fluid in the thin ascending limb would be diluted. The net result of this system is concentration in the compartment of the papillary collecting duct and the dilution in the compartment of the thin ascending limb. It is conceivable that this single effect can be multiplied by an appropriate counterflow system.

Conclusion

Function of the thin ascending limb has been reviewed based on the data derived from in vitro microperfusion studies. The segment is characterized by impermeability to water, high permeability to NaCl and moderate permeability to urea. Chloride is transported mainly through a conductive transcellular pathway, which is sensitive to various anion transport inhibitors and regulated by ambient proton and calcium concentrations. The putative transporter may have two distinct sulfhydryl sites which operate either stimulatory or inhibitory regulation of chloride conductance. These characteristics are in accord with the passive model of the countercurrent multiplication system, which is based on the single effect among three compartments including the thin ascending limb, capillary networks and papillary collecting duct.

Acknowledgments

We wish to thank Mrs Yayoi Ueshima for her secretarial work in preparing this typescript. The works quoted in this review were supported in part by Research Grant for Cardiovascular Diseases (59-C8) from the Ministry of Health and Welfare of Japan and a grant from the Ministry of Education, Sciences and Culture of Japan (No 58480104).

References

1 Jamison RL, Kriz W. *Urinary Concentrating Mechanism: Structure and Function.* New York: Oxford University Press. 1982

2 Imai M, Taniguchi J, Tabei K. Function of thin loops of Henle. *Kidney Int 1987; 31:* 565–579

3 Greger R. Ion transport mechanisms in thick ascending limb of Henle's loop of mammalian nephron. *Physiol Rev 1985; 65:* 760–797

4 Hebert SC, Andreoli TE. Control of NaCl transport in the thick ascending limb. *Am J Physiol 1984; 246:* F745–F756

5 Burg MB, Grantham J, Abramow M, Orloff J. Preparation and study of fragments of single rabbit nephron. *Am J Physiol 1966; 210:* 1293–1298

6 Imai M, Kokko JP. Sodium, chloride, urea, and water transport in the thin ascending limb of Henle. Generation of osmotic gradients by passive diffusion of solutes. *J Clin Invest 1974; 53:* 393–402

7 Imai M, Kusano E. Effects of arginine vasopressin on the thin ascending limb of Henle's loop of hamsters. *Am J Physiol 1982; 243:* F167–F172

8 Imai M. Function of the thin ascending limb of Henle of rats and hamsters perfused in vitro. *Am J Physiol 1977; 232:* F201–F209

9 Marsh DJ. Solute and water flows in thin limb of Henle's loop in the hamster kidney. *Am J Physiol 1970; 218:* 824–831

10 Sakai F, Tadokoro M, Teraoka M. Experimentalle Untersuchungen über die Funktion des Nierenmarkes mit der Mikropunktionsmethode. *Tokyo J Med Sci 1971; 79:* 1–30

11 Morgan T, Berliner RW. Permeability of loop of Henle, vasa recta, and collecting duct to water, urea, and sodium. *Am J Physiol 1968; 215:* 108–115

12 Imai M, Kokko JP. Relative permeability of the thin ascending limb of Henle (tALH) to various ions. *6th Annual Meeting Am Soc Nephrol.* Washington DC 1973: 52 (Abstract)

13 Imai M, Kokko JP, Mechanism of sodium and chloride transport in the thin ascending limb of Henle. *J Clin Invest 1976; 58:* 1089–1097

14 Kondo Y, Yoshitomi K, Imai M. Effects of anion transport inhibitors and ion substitution on Cl^- transport in the thin ascending limb of Henle's loop. *Am J Physiol:* submitted

15 Wieth JO, Brahm J. Cellular anion transport. In Seldin DW, Giebish G, eds. *The Kidney. Physiology and Pathophysiology.* New York: Raven Press. 1985: 49–89

16 Alpern RJ, Mechanism of basolateral membrane $H^+/OH^-/HCO_3^-$ transport in the rat proximal convoluted tubule. A sodium-coupled electrogenic process. *J Gen Physiol 1985; 86:* 613–636

17 Boron WF, Boulpaep EL. Intracellular pH regulation in the renal proximal tubule of the salamander. Basolateral HCO_3^- transport. *J Gen Physiol 1983; 81:* 53–94

18 Yoshitomi K, Frömter E. Cell pH rat renal proximal tubule in vivo and the conductive nature of peritubular HCO_3^- (OH^-) exit. *Pfleugers Arch 1984; 402:* 300–305

19 Yoshitomi K, Burckhardt B-Ch, Frömter E. Rheogenic sodium-bicarbonate cotransport in the peritubular cell membrane of rat renal proximal tubule. *Pfleugers Arch 1985; 405:* 360–366

20 Nelson DJ, Tang JM, Palmer LG. Single-channel recordings of apical membrane chloride conductance in A6 epithelial cells. *J Membr Biol 1984; 80:* 81–89

21 Kinne R, Murer H, Kinne-Saffran E et al. Sugar transport by renal plasma membrane vesicles. Characterization of the systems in the brush-border microvilli and basal-lateral plasma membrane. *J Membr Biol 1975; 21:* 375–395

22 Macey RJ, Farmer REL. Inhibition of water and solute permeability in human red cells. *Biochem Biophys Acta 1970; 211:* 104–106

23 Levine S, Franki N, Hays RM. Effect of phloretin on water and solute movement in the toad bladder. *J Clin Invest 1973; 52:* 1435–1442

24 Kondo Y, Imai M. Effects of glutaraldehyde fixation on renal tubular function. I. Preservation of vasopressin-stimulated water and urea pathways in rat papillary collecting duct. *Pfleugers Arch 1987; 408:* 479–483

25 Evans MG, Marty A, Tan YP, Trautmann A. Blockage of Ca-activated Cl conductance by furosemide in rat lacrimal glands. *Pfleugers Arch 1986; 406:* 65–68

26 Kondo Y, Yoshitomi K, Imai M. Effects of Ca^{2+} on Cl^- transport in the thin ascending limb of Henle's loop. *Am J Physiol:* submitted

27 Schwartz MM, Venkatachalam MA. Structural differences in thin limbs of Henle: physiological implications. *Kidney Int 1974; 6:* 193–208

28 Imai M, Kokko JP. Mechanism of sodium and chloride transport in the thin ascending limb of Henle. *J Clin Invest 1976; 58:* 1089–1097

29 Yoshitomi K, Kondo Y, Imai M. Evidence for conductive Cl^- pathways across the cell membranes of the thin ascending limb of Henle's loop. *J Clin Invest:* submitted

30 Morel F. Sites of hormone action in the mammalian nephron. *Am J Physiol 1981; 240:* F159–F164

31 Torikai S, Kurokawa K. Effect of PGE_2 on the cell cyclic AMP content in the thin ascending limb of Henle of the rat. *Mineral Electrolyte Metab 1984; 10:* 21–25

32 Kondo Y, Yoshitomi K, Imai M. Effects of pH on Cl^- transport in the thin ascending limb of Henle's loop. *Am J Physiol:* submitted

33 Owen DG, Segal M, Barker JL. A Ca-dependent Cl^- conductance in cultured mouse spinal neurons. *Nature 1984; 311:* 567–570

34 Imai M, Kondo Y, Koseki C, Yoshitomi K. Dual actions of N-ethylmaleimide (NEM) on Cl^- transport across the thin ascending limb of Henle's loop (TAL). *Japan J Pharmacol 1987; 43 (Suppl):* 128P

35 Kondo Y, Imai M. Effect of glutaraldehyde on renal tubular function. II. Selective inhibition of Cl^- transport in the hamster thin ascending limb of Henle's loop. *Pfleugers Arch 1987; 408:* 484–490

36 Kokko JP, Rector FC Jr. Countercurrent multiplication system without active transport in renal inner medulla. *Kidney Int 1972; 2:* 214–223

37 Stephenson JL. Concentration of urine in a central Core model of the renal counterflow system. *Kidney Int 1972; 2:* 85–94

MULTIPLE HORMONAL CONTROL OF THE Na/K-ATPase ACTIVITY IN THE THICK ASCENDING LIMB

A Doucet

Laboratoire de Physiologie Cellulaire, Collège de France, Paris, France

Introduction

We have previously reported that adrenalectomy decreases Na/K-ATPase activity in the medullary thick ascending limb of Henle's loop of rabbit kidney, and that a single injection of dexamethasone (100μg/kg body weight) restores this activity up to normal level within three hours [1]. Unexpectedly, we also observed [2] that this stimulation of Na/K-ATPase activity is not paralleled by any increase

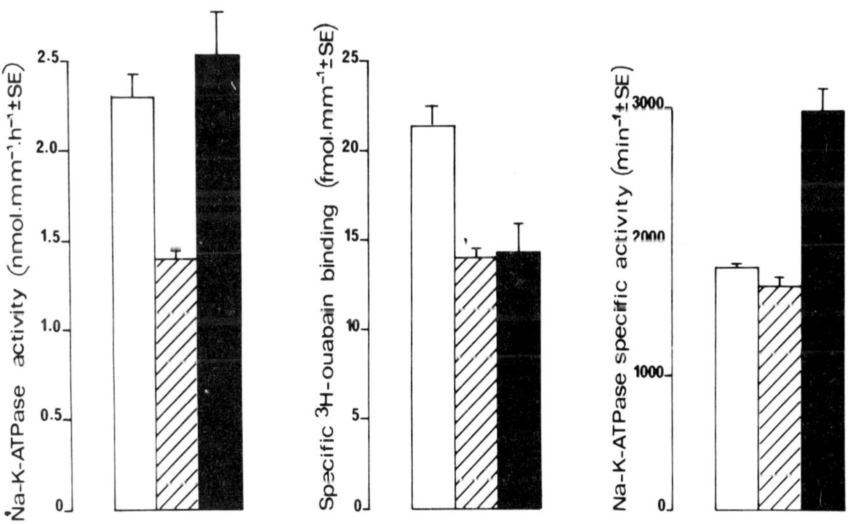

Figure 1. Na/K-ATPase activity and specific binding of ^{3}H-ouabain were determined in the medullary thick ascending limb from four normal rabbits (open bars), six rabbits adrenalectomized 5–7 days previously (hatched bars) and four adrenalectomized rabbits injected with dexamethasone (100μg/kg body weight) three hours before killing (black bars). The specific activity of Na/K-ATPase was calculated as the number of cycles (ATP split) per ouabain binding site and per minute

in the number of catalytic sites of the enzyme, as measured by the specific binding of ^{3}H-ouabain (Figure 1). Therefore, it was concluded that glucocorticoids enhances the V_{max} of pre-existing Na/K-ATPase units.

The recent development [3] of a procedure to maintain single segments of the medullary thick ascending limb under viable conditions allowed us to reproduce the action of glucocorticoids in vitro in the medullary thick ascending limb dissected from adrenalectomized rats. This protocol, which eliminates all possible interactions with other hormones and with hormonal effects originating elsewhere in the kidney or in the whole organism, allowed us to confirm that dexamethasone stimulates Na/K-ATPase in the medullary thick ascending limb of adrenalectomized rats and to demonstrate that this action is dependent on protein synthesis, as it is abolished by cycloheximide and actinomycin D (Figure 2). From these results, it was concluded that dexamethasone might induce the

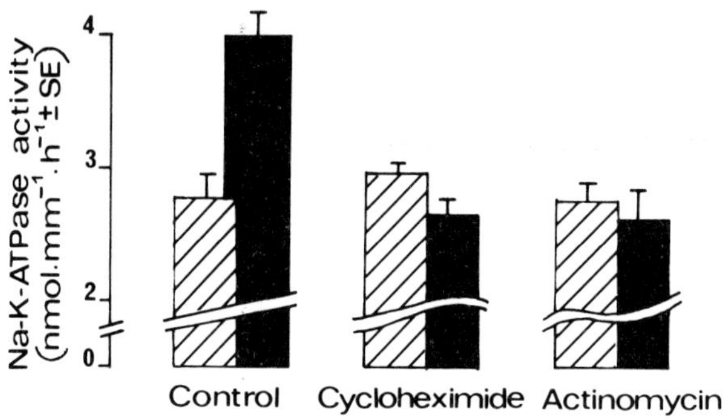

Figure 2. Inhibition of in vitro stimulatory action of dexamethasone on Na/K-ATPase in the medullary thick ascending limb by cycloheximide and actinomycin D. Tubules from the same adrenalectomized rat were incubated at 37°C for two hours in the absence (hatched bars) or in the presence of 10^{-8} M dexamethasone (black bars), under normal conditions (control) or in the presence of 10μM cycloheximide or 5μM actinomycin D. Neither cycloheximide nor actinomycin D had an action per se but both inhibited dexamethasone-induced stimulation of Na/K-ATPase activity. Note that Na/K-ATPase activity is higher in rat medullary thick ascending limb (compare with Figure 1)

synthesis of an activator of Na/K-ATPase (or repress the synthesis of an inhibitor of Na/K-ATPase). However, the precise nature of such a modulator remained unknown at that time.

At about the same time, Schwartzman and colleagues reported that cells derived from rabbit medullary thick ascending limb display a cytochrome P450-dependent monoxygenase system which metabolized arachidonic acid into two biologically active products, one of which inhibited the activity of Na/K-ATPase from canine heart microsomes [4]. Furthermore, these authors reported that the production of this inhibitor of Na/K-ATPase by medullary thick ascending limb-derived cells is enhanced by cyclic AMP-generating hormones such as arginine vasopressin and calcitonin [4].

Since glucocorticoids inhibit the release of arachidonic acid in several systems, including kidney cells, by blocking the activity of phospholipase A_2 through the synthesis of lipomodulin [5–8], we investigated whether the stimulatory action of dexamethasone on Na/K-ATPase activity in the medullary thick ascending limb could be due to the inhibition of the synthesis of the Na/K-ATPase inhibitor described by Schwartzman et al. For this purpose, experiments were carried out to determine:

1. Whether or not the inhibitor of Na/K-ATPase synthesized by a single micro-dissected medullary thick ascending limb segment in response to arginine vasopressin might inhibit Na/K-ATPase activity of that same segment.
2. The metabolic pathway responsible for the synthesis of this inhibitor;
3. Whether or not dexamethasone interferes with this pathway.

Experimental procedures used in this study were previously described and are only briefly summarized here. Segments of medullary thick ascending limb were micro-dissected under stereomicroscopic observation from collagenase-treated rat kidneys [9] and their length, which serves as reference for enzyme activities, was automatically determined by computerized image analysis [10]. Tubule segments were individually incubated at 37°C in an Eagle's MEM derived solution [3] for various times in the presence of the drugs and/or hormones to be tested. Thereafter, the segments were rinsed, permeabilized by exposure to a hypo-osmotic medium and by rapid freeze-thawing, and assayed for Na/K-ATPase activity [9].

Inhibition of Na/K-ATPase activity in rat medullary thick ascending limb by vasopressin

Results shown in Figure 3 indicate that incubation of medullary thick ascending limb micro-dissected from normal rats in the presence of 10^{-7}M vasopressin resulted in a marked inhibition of Na/K-ATPase activity (control: 3.74±0.21 $nmol \cdot mm^{-1} \cdot h^{-1} \cdot$ ±SE, arginine vasopressin : 2.28±0.11$nmol \cdot mm^{-1} \cdot h^{-1}$ ±SE, n=5, $p<0.001$). This inhibitory action of vasopressin was dose-dependent (apparent K_i~$2x10^{-8}$M) and reached a maximum within five minutes of incubation. Furthermore, this inhibition was probably mediated by cyclic AMP as it was mimicked either by calcitonin, another hormone stimulating adenylate-cyclase in the rat medullary thick ascending limb [11], or by dibutyryl-cyclic AMP.

These results are consistent with previous reports of Schwartzman et al [4] showing the existence of an arginine vasopressin-induced inhibitor of Na/K-ATPase in thick ascending limb cells and of Giesen et al [12] who demonstrated that forskolin inhibits Na/K-ATPase activity in rat kidney medulla. They also indicate that this inhibitor is of likely physiological relevance since it can alter Na/K-ATPase activity in the cells where it is produced in response to hormone stimulation. Finally, they suggest that the interaction between Na/K-ATPase

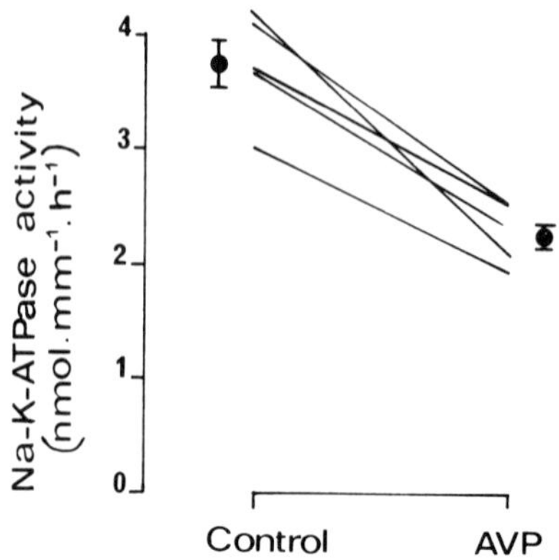

Figure 3. Inhibition by vasopressin of Na/K-ATPase in rat medullary thick ascending limb. Segments of medullary thick ascending limb were incubated at 37°C for 15 minutes in the absence (control) or presence of 10^{-7} M vasopressin (AVP) before Na/K-ATPase measurement. Lines join results obtained on same animals. Points are mean ± SE

and the inhibitor is only slowly reversible since inhibition is still observed after the permeabilization of tubular segments, a procedure carried out at 0–4°C but which lasts over 15 minutes.

The physiological significance of the inhibitory action of arginine vasopressin on Na/K-ATPase activity in rat medullary thick ascending limb is not yet clear. Indeed, it is now clearly admitted that NaCl reabsorption by the thick ascending limb of Henle's loop is an active process primarily energized by the peritubular Na/K-ATPase [13]. Thus, inhibition of Na/K-ATPase activity by cyclic AMP-generating hormones such as vasopressin or calcitonin would thwart the well-known stimulatory action of these hormones on NaCl reabsorption by the thick ascending limb [14–17]. It is possible, however, that partial inhibition of Na/K-ATPase activity by cyclic AMP may be part of a regulatory feedback mechanism.

Metabolic pathway involved in the inhibitory action of vasopressin on Na/K-ATPase activity

In order to evaluate whether or not the inhibitory action of vasopressin on Na/K-ATPase activity involves the metabolism of arachidonic acid through the monoxygenase pathway, we tested the effects of mepacrine, which inhibits phospholipase A_2, and of SKF525A, which inhibits the cytochrome P450-dependent monoxygenase.

Results given in Figure 4 indicate that both mepacrine and SKF525A completely abolished the inhibition of Na/K-ATPase induced by arginine vasopressin. Furthermore, incubation of the medullary thick ascending limb in the presence of 10^{-4} M arachidonic acid inhibited Na/K-ATPase activity to the same extent

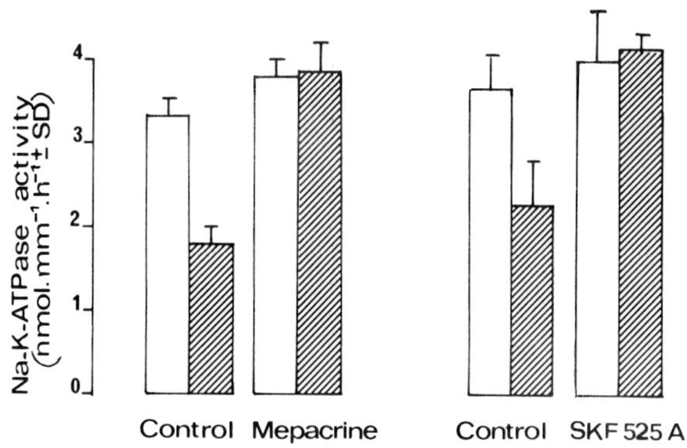

Figure 4. Suppression of the inhibitory action of arginine vasopression on Na/K-ATPase by mepacrine and SKF525A. Segments of medullary thick ascending limb were incubated at 37°C for 15 minutes in the presence (hatched bars) or absence (open bars) of 10^{-7} M AVP either under normal conditions (control) or in the presence of 10^{-5} M of the phospholipase A_2 inhibitor mepacrine or of 50μM of the cytochrome P450-monoxygenase inhibitor SKF525A. Both mepacrine and SKF525A abolished the inhibitory action of vasopressin

as did vasopressin. Finally, arachidonate-induced inhibition of Na/K-ATPase was abolished by SKF525A.

These results confirm that inhibition of Na/K-ATPase is due to the synthesis of an arachidonate metabolite through the monoxygenase pathway. They also indicate that arginine vasopressin acts prior to the generation of arachidonic acid, most likely at the level of phospholipase A_2.

Interaction between dexamethasone and vasopressin in the control of Na/K-ATPase

Next, we evaluated whether dexamethasone would block the inhibitory action of vasopressin. For this purpose, segments of medullary thick ascending limb were preincubated in the absence or presence of dexamethasone for 1.5 hours and then challenged with cyclic AMP. Results in Figure 5A clearly show that:

1. In the absence of dexamethasone, cyclic AMP induced the previously observed inhibition of Na/K-ATPase activity;
2. After dexamethasone pretreatment, cyclic AMP also inhibited Na/K-ATPase activity;
3. Pretreatment with dexamethasone increased Na/K-ATPase activity of medullary thick ascending limb segments which were not exposed to cyclic AMP.

In fact, as clearly shown in Figure 5B, dexamethasone did not increase Na/K-ATPase activity but rather prevented the time-dependent decrease observed when segments of medullary thick ascending limb were incubated over a three hour period in the absence of dexamethasone. This time-dependent decrease

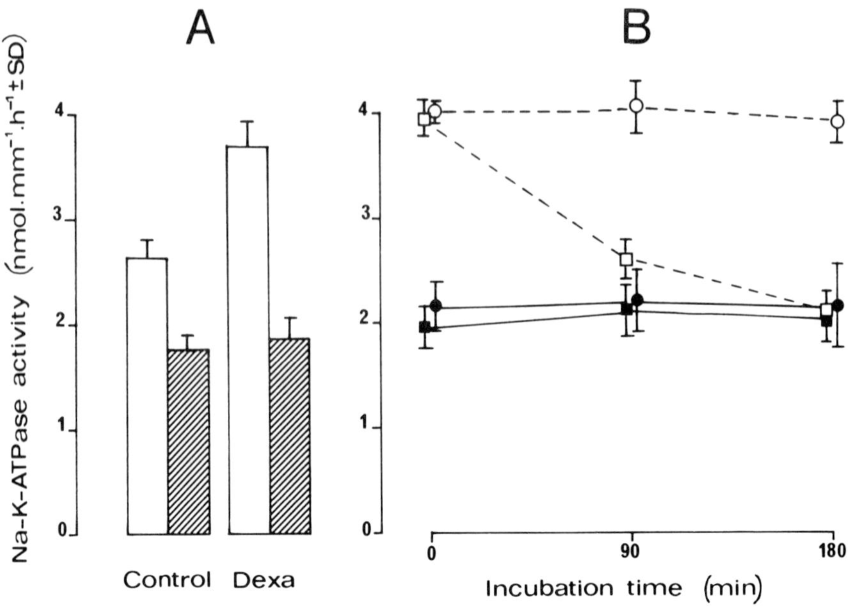

Figure 5. Interaction between vasopressin and dexamethasone in the control of Na/K-ATPase activity. A. Segments of medullary thick ascending limb were incubated at 37°C for 90 minutes in the absence (control) or presence of 10^{-8} M dexamethasone (Dexa) and, during the last five minutes of incubation, 10^{-4} M dibutyryl cyclic AMP was added (hatched bars) or not (open bars). B. The protocol was similar to that used in A but incubation time varied from 0 to 3 hours: without dexamethasone (□,■); with dexamethasone (○,●); without dibutyryl-cyclic AMP (□,○); with dibutyryl-cyclic AMP (■,●)

of Na/K-ATPase activity led, within three hours, to the same activity as that observed after inhibition by cyclic AMP.

Possible mechanism of action of cyclic AMP and dexamethasone

One of the best known actions of dexamethasone is to induce the synthesis of a protein (macrocortin or lipomodulin) which inhibits phospholipase A_2 [6–8]. If one admits that dexamethasone acts in this way on medullary thick ascending limb cells, the decrease of Na/K-ATPase observed after prolonged incubation in the absence of dexamethasone (see Figure 5B) is probably due to the disappearance of lipomodulin, and thus to the activation of arachidonate release and of the synthesis of Na/K-ATPase inhibitor.

The fact that disappearance of lipomodulin inhibits Na/K-ATPase activity to the same extent as cyclic AMP does (see Figure 5B), suggest that cyclic AMP might act through inactivation of lipomodulin. This hypothesis is supported by the observation that lipomodulin from rabbit neutrophils is phosphorylated by cyclic AMP-dependent protein kinase with a concomitant loss of its ability to inhibit phospholipase A_2 [18].

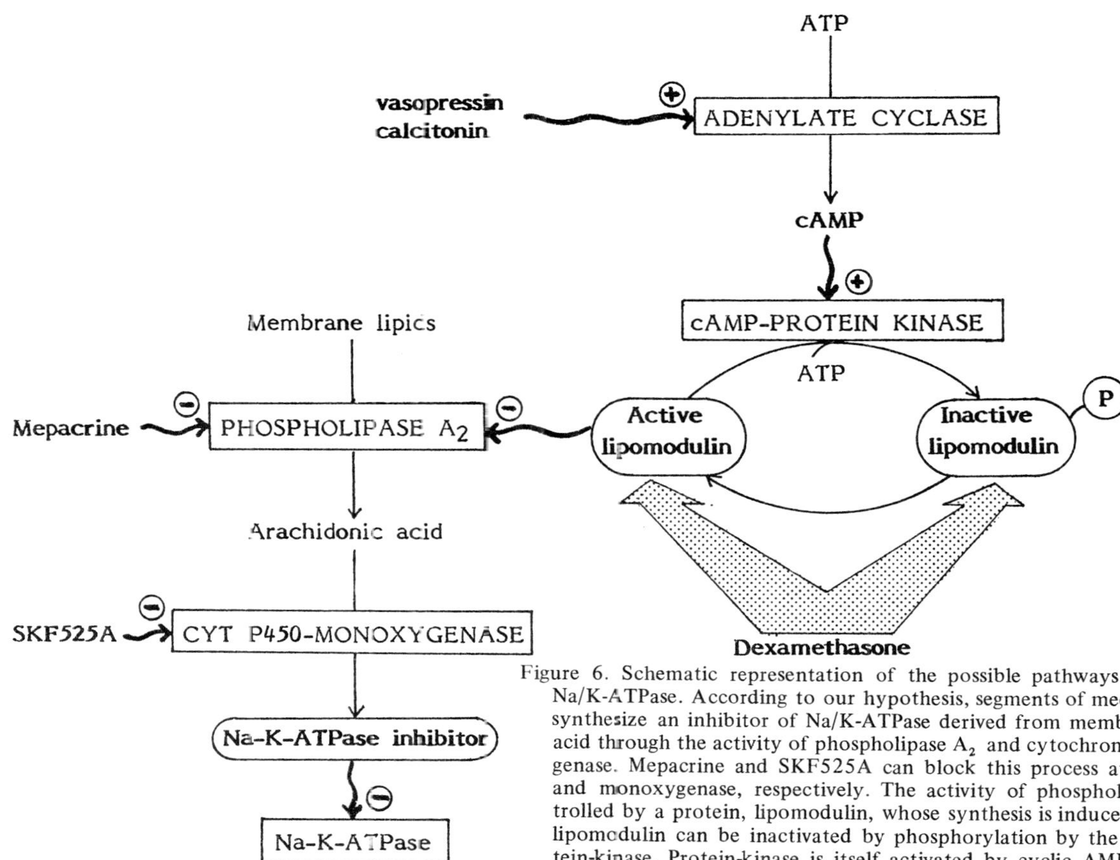

Figure 6. Schematic representation of the possible pathways involved in the control of Na/K-ATPase. According to our hypothesis, segments of medullary thick ascending limb synthesize an inhibitor of Na/K-ATPase derived from membrane lipids and arachidonic acid through the activity of phospholipase A_2 and cytochrome P450-dependent monoxygenase. Mepacrine and SKF525A can block this process at the level of phospholipase and monoxygenase, respectively. The activity of phospholipase A_2 is negatively controlled by a protein, lipomodulin, whose synthesis is induced by dexamethasone. Active lipomodulin can be inactivated by phosphorylation by the cyclic AMP-dependent protein-kinase. Protein-kinase is itself activated by cyclic AMP synthetized by adenylate-cyclase in response to stimulation by vasopressin or calcitonin. Inactive lipomodulin can probably be activated by dephosphorylation by a phosphatase

The postulated mechanism of control of Na/K-ATPase in medullary thick ascending limb cells is schematized in Figure 6.

Acknowledgments

This work was supported in part by a grant from the Centre National de la Recherche Scientifique to the Unité Associée 219. The author gratefully acknowledges Dr Fort and Dr Skidmore from Smith Kline and French Laboratories Ltd for kindly providing SKF525A.

References

1 El Mernissi G, Doucet A. Short term effects of aldosterone and dexamethasone on Na-K-ATPase along the rabbit nephron. *Pfluegers Arch 1983; 399:* 147–151
2 El Mernissi G, Doucet A. Specific activity of Na-K-ATPase after adrenalectomy and hormone replacement along the rabbit nephron. *Pfluegers Arch 1984; 402:* 258–263
3 Doucet A, Hus-Citharel A, Morel F. In vitro stimulation of Na-K-ATPase in rat thick ascending limb by dexamethasone. *Am J Physiol 1986; 251:* F851–F857
4 Schwartzman M, Ferreri NR, Carroll MA et al. Renal cytochrome P450-related arachidonate metabolite inhibits (Na^+ + K^+) ATPase. *Nature 1985; 314:* 620–622
5 Russo-Marie F, Paing M, Duval D. Involvement of glucocorticoid receptors in steroid-induced inhibition of prostaglandin secretion. *J Biol Chem 1979; 254:* 8498–8504
6 Flower RJ, Blackwell GJ. Anti-inflammatory steroids induce biosynthesis of a phospholipase A_2 inhibitor which prevents prostaglandin generation. *Nature 1979; 278:* 456–459
7 Hirata F, Schiffmann E, Venkatusabramanian K et al. A phospholipase A_2 inhibitory protein in rabbit neutrophils induced by glucocorticoids. *Proc Natl Acad Sci USA 1980; 77:* 2533–2536
8 Blackwell GJ, Carnuccio R, Di Rosa M et al. Macrocortin: a polypeptide causing the anti-phospholipase effect of glucocorticoids. *Nature 1980; 287:* 147–149
9 Doucet A, Katz AI, Morel F. Determination of Na-K-ATPase activity in single segments of the mammalian nephron. *Am J Physiol 1979; 237:* F105–F113
10 Khadouri C, Marsy S, Barlet-Bas C, Doucet A. Effect of adrenalectomy on NEM-sensitive ATPase along the rat nephron and on urinary acidification. *Am J Physiol:* in press
11 Morel F, Chabardès D, Imbert-Teboul M et al. Multiple hormonal control of adenylate cyclase in distal segments of the rat kidney. *Kidney Int 1982; 21:* S55–S62
12 Giesen EM, Grima M, Imbs JL et al. Forskolin inhibits ouabain-sensitive ATPase in the medulla of rat kidney. *IRCS Med Sci 1983; 11:* 957–968
13 Greger R. Ion transport mechanisms in thick ascending limb of Henle's loop of mammalian nephron. *Physiol Rev 1985; 65:* 760–797
14 Hall DA, Varney DM. Effect of vasopressin on electrical potential difference and chloride transport in mouse medullary thick ascending limb of Henle's loop. *J Clin Invest 1980; 66:* 792–802
15 Hebert SC, Culpepper RM, Andreoli TE. NaCl transport in mouse medullary thick ascending limb. I. Functional nephron heterogeneity and ADH-stimulated NaCl transport. *Am J Physiol 1981; 241:* F412–F431
16 Rouffignac C De, Corman B, Roinel N. Stimulation by antidiuretic hormone of electrolyte tubular reabsorption in rat kidney. *Am J Physiol 1983; 244:* F156–F164
17 Elalouf JM, Roinel N, Rouffignac C De. ADH-like effects of calcitonin on electrolyte transport by Henle's loop of rat kidney. *Am J Physiol 1984; 246:* F213–F220
18 Hirata F. The regulation of lipomodulin, a phospholipase inhibitory protein, in rabbit neutrophils by phosphorylation. *J Biol Chem 1981; 256:* 7730–7733

EFFECTS OF PEPTIDE HORMONES ON JUXTAMEDULLARY NEPHRON FUNCTION

C de Rouffignac, J M Elalouf

Service de Biologie Cellulaire, CEN Saclay, Gif-sur-Yvette, France

Introduction

The thick ascending limb of Henle is one of the major nephron segments participating in the mechanisms of urinary concentration and dilution. Its transport functions are regulated by several peptide hormones. However, the active hormones differ from one animal species to another [1]. In the rat, the medullary portion of the thick ascending limb of Henle is a target suite of antidiuretic hormone (ADH), calcitonin and glucagon, while the cortical portion responds not only to these three hormones but also to parathyroid hormone and β agonists.

In vivo studies carried out on hormone-deprived Brattleboro rats [2], i.e. in the absence of circulating ADH, parathyroid hormone, calcitonin and glucagon, have demonstrated that all four hormones elicit similar physiological effects on the thick ascending limb of Henle. They are all capable of stimulating magnesium, calcium and potassium transport [2–4], and all except parathormone [3] also stimulated sodium and chloride [2,4,5] in this nephron segment. The data obtained in vitro on isolated perfused segments, although extremely fragmentary, are in agreement with these observations [see ref 6].

This review examines the effects of each of these four hormones on the composition of the fluid delivered at the bend of the loop of Henle of the juxtamedullary nephrons and on the amplitude of the cortico-medullary concentration gradient. Two calcitonins were used, human and salmon.

In all the experiments considered here, in order to avoid undesirable interference with ADH, parathormone, calcitonins and glucagon, the effects of each of these four hormones were investigated in 'hormone deprived' rats. These were Brattleboro rats lacking endogenous ADH, acutely thyroparathyroidectomized to suppress parathormone and calcitonin and given somatostatin to inhibit glucagon secretion. Infusions of the hormone being investigated were given to achieve concentrations in the plasma close to those obtained during maximal stimulation of endogenous secretory processes ('physiological doses') and micropuncture experiments performed.

Effects of 'hormone deprivation'

The experiments [7–10] were carried out on relatively young rats, in which it is possible to perform micropunctures of the loop of Henle of juxtamedullary nephrons. Figure 1 shows that in hormone-deprived rats the ratio of the osmolality in tubular fluid to that of plasma (TF/P_{osm}) at the tip of Henle's loop of the longest nephron was no greater than 1.10–1.20. The corresponding osmolality of fluid at this level was thus about 350mOsm/kg, implying that the cortico-medullary concentration gradient is greatly reduced, though not totally abolished.

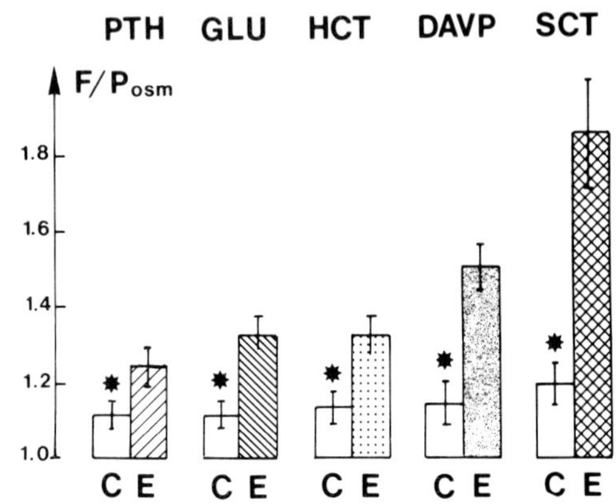

Figure 1. Tubular fluid-to-plasma concentration ratios of total solutes (F/P_{osm}) at the bend of the loop of Henle of juxtamedullary nephrons. Experiments were performed in hormone-deprived (C=control) rats or in hormone-deprived rats receiving (E=experimental) either parathyroid hormone (PTH), glucagon (GLU), human calcitonin (HCT), dDAVP or salmon calcitonin (SCT). Administration rates of the peptides were (per 100g body weight): PTH 5mU/min; GLU 5ng/min; HCT 1mU/min; dDAVP 20pg/min; SCT 2.5mU/min. Hormone-deprived rats were DI Brattleboro rats which were acutely thyro-parathyroidectomized and infused with somatostatin to inhibit glucagon secretion. * Significantly different from C, p at least <0.05. Each column represents the mean value obtained from five to six different animals. Data from refs 7–10

Suppression of the four hormones thus leads to a major disturbance of the function of the renal medulla. At this stage, it is of interest to note that in the least concentrated of the samples collected in the thin descending limb, just before the hairpin turn, the TF/P_{osm} was strictly equal to unity (0.99±0.02, n=10) but the ratio of tubular fluid sodium concentration to that in the ultra-filtrate (TF/UF_{Na}) was only 0.84±0.05 [8], a value significantly different from unity ($p<0.001$). This indicates that some sodium can be reabsorbed from the descending limb if, as is likely, the sodium concentration at the end of the proximal tubule was equal to that in plasma.

Physiological effects of individual peptide hormones

The single nephron glomerular filtration rate of the juxtamedullary nephrons did not vary significantly under the influence of any of the peptides except for

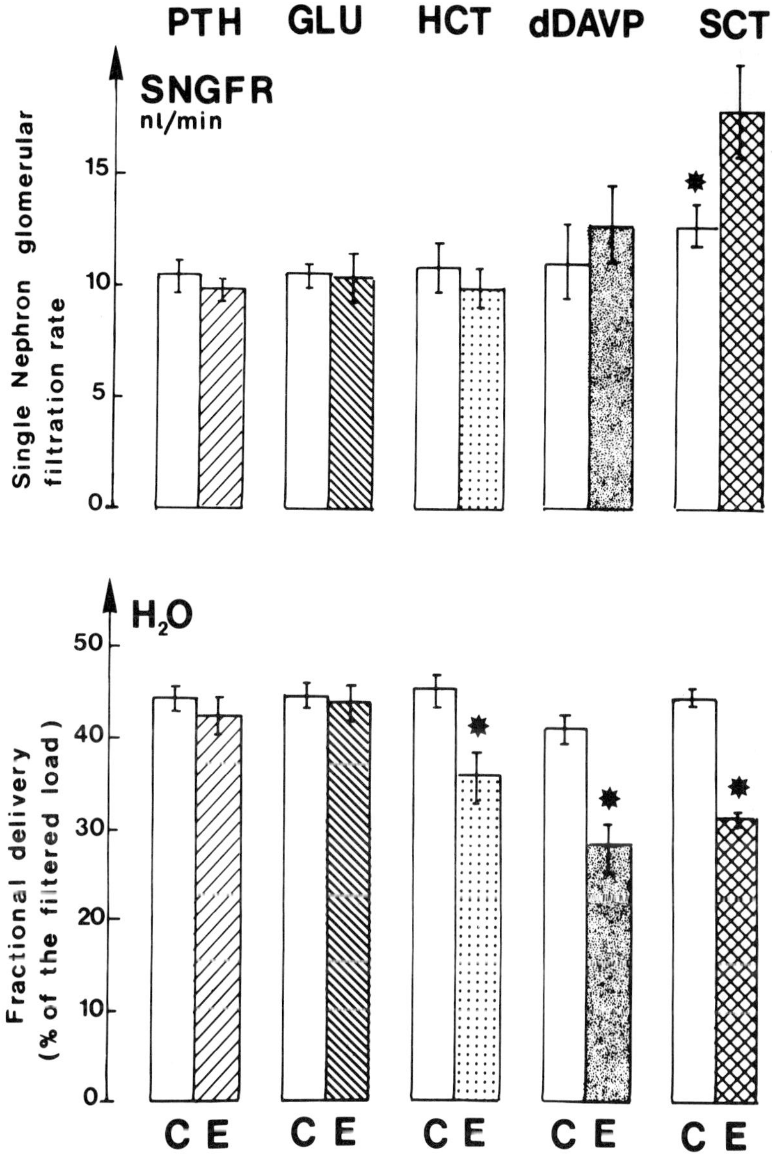

Figure 2. Single nephron filtration rate (SNGFR) of juxtamedullary nephrons (JM) and fractional delivery of water (as % of the SNGFR) at the tip of the loop of Henle of these nephrons. Experiments were performed in hormone-deprived (C) rats and in hormone-deprived rats receiving (E) either PTH, glucagon (GLU), human calcitonin (HCT), dDAVP or salmon calcitonin (SCT). Administration rates of the peptides were as indicated in Figure 1. * Significantly different from C, p at least <0.05. Each column represents the mean values obtained from five to six different animals. Data from refs 7–10

salmon calcitonin (Figure 2). Hence for parathormone, glucagon, human calcitonin and dDAVP, since the plasma electrolyte concentrations were virtually unaltered, any change in delivery to the tip of the loop of Henle must be a result of tubular action.

All peptides increased the osmolality of the fluid reaching the hairpin turn (Figure 1), thereby confirming that the washout of the cortico-medullary concentration gradient in hormone-deprived rats was due to hormonal depletion. Parathormone had the least effect. Neither glucagon nor human calcitonin alone were capable of completely restoring the cortico-medullary concentration gradient occurring in intact DI Brattleboro rats ($1.73 < TF/P_{osm} < 1.96$ [see 11]). This was obtained only with salmon calcitonin infused at 2.5mU/min/100g body weight (Figure 1). Surprisingly, the effect of dDAVP, although greater than that of glucagon or human calcitonin, was not so pronounced as that of salmon calcitonin.

The mechanism responsible for the increase of the tubular fluid osmolality at the hairpin turn was not the same for all the peptides. Glucagon [8] enhanced both the osmolality and the NaCl concentration of the tubular fluid, but left unchanged the absolute and fractional water delivery (Figure 2). Consequently, the NaCl fractional delivery was increased (Figure 3). The effects of glucagon, therefore, may be attributed entirely to net NaCl entry (secretion) in the tubular lumen. This conclusion was supported by a positive correlation between the sodium (or chloride) fractional delivery at the hairpin turn and the tubular fluid osmolality, indicating that the more concentrated this fluid the greater the amounts of NaCl delivered at the hairpin turn [8].

The effects of calcitonins [9,10] and dDAVP [7] were quite different. Unlike glucagon, calcitonins and dDAVP decreased the rate of fluid delivery to the tip of the loop of Henle (Figure 2). In addition, they did not increase the fractional deliveries of sodium and chloride; the small decrease was not statistically significant (Figure 3). It is known that ADH induces water removal along the descending limb by a mechanism involving urea. According to the theory of passive concentration in the inner medulla [12], ADH, thanks to its effect on the water permeability of the distal and collecting tubules, delivers to the collecting tubules in the inner medulla a fluid with a urea concentration sufficiently high for this solute to diffuse into the interstitium. The interstitial hyperosmolality thus created induces in turn an osmotic water removal along the descending limb [11,12] and increases the rate of urea entry in this segment [13]. Calcitonin, considered to produce the same physiological effects as ADH on the cortical collecting tubules of the rat [14], should thus bring about water removal along the descending limb by a process similar to that induced by ADH, although to a lesser degree since calcitonin has no action on the medullary collecting duct in this species.

The most probable explanation to account for the difference between the acute effects of glucagon, ADH and calcitonin is as follows: glucagon stimulates

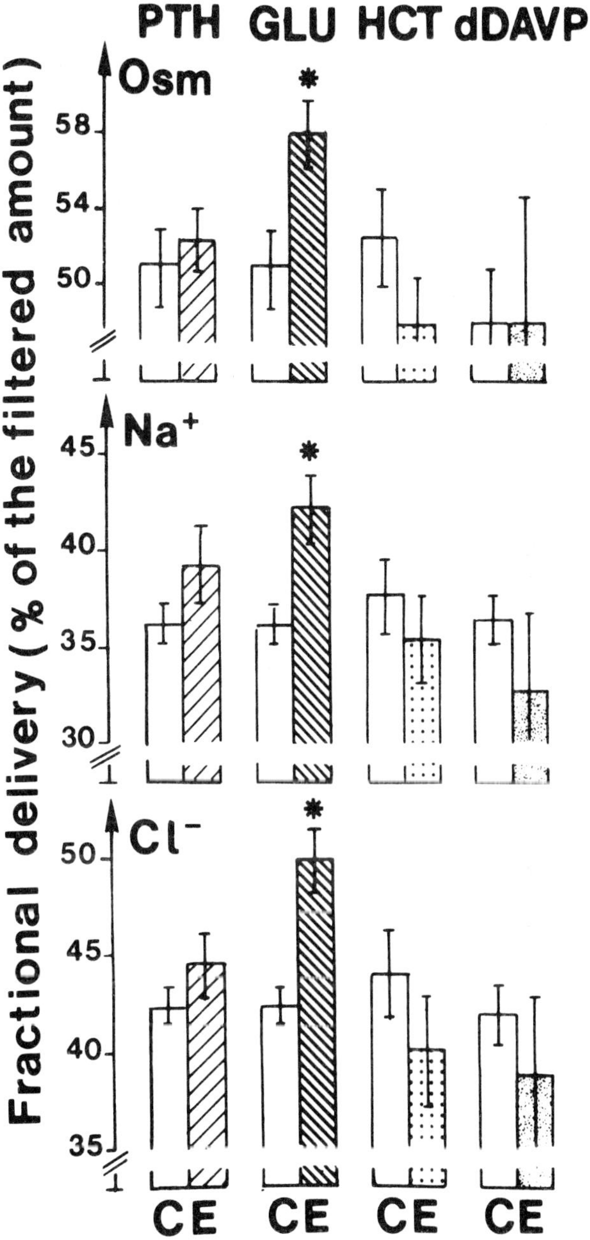

Figure 3. Fractional delivery of total solutes, sodium and chloride at the bend of the loop of Henle of juxtamedullary nephrons. Experiments were performed in hormone-deprived (C) rats and in hormone-deprived rats receiving (E) either PTH, glucagon (GLU), human calcitonin (HCT), dDAVP or salmon calcitonin (SCT). Administration rates of the peptides were as indicated in Figure 1. * Significantly different from C, p at least <0.05. Each column represents the mean value obtained from five to six different animals. Data from refs 7–19

NaCl transport in the thick ascending limb. The sodium chloride delivered to the interstitium would create a gradient favourable to its diffusion into the descending limb. NaCl would therefore undergo medullary recycling, as has already been proposed as part of the concentrating mechanism in a desert rodent, *Psammomys obesus* [15–17]. This recycling would be facilitated by the structure of the thin descending limb of juxtamedullary nephrons, the epithelium of which is much more permeable to sodium than is that of the thin descending limb of the superficial nephrons [18]. Nevertheless, if some sodium were later to escape from the descending limb, only a fraction of the salt thus added to the lumen by the recycling process would be present at the tip of the loop. Such an escape might occur if the transepithelial gradient of sodium concentration reversed somewhere along this segment, as the data obtained with hormone-deprived rats also suggest (see above): in these rats the TF/UF_{Na} was found to be 15% lower than unity at the bend of the loop [8].

Human calcitonin and dDAVP both induce water removal along the descending limb. We propose that this water removal increases the escape of NaCl at some point along the descending limb. This NaCl removal would counterbalance the upstream NaCl addition induced by hormone action, masking the hormonal stimulation of NaCl recycling. Data on calcium and magnesium support this view. Human calcitonin and dDAVP both reduced by 30% the delivery of magnesium and calcium at the hairpin turn [7,9] whereas parathormone and glucagon, which did not induce any water movement along the descending limb, had no effect on these deliveries [8]. Osmotic water withdrawal would therefore cause (for magnesium and calcium) or accentuate (for sodium and chloride) electrolyte reabsorption out of the descending limb. As shown below, the data obtained with diabetes insipidus (DI) Brattleboro rats which had been subjected to a long-term (three weeks) treatment with dDAVP fully confirm this interpretation. Before considering these data, the effects of chronic dDAVP treatment on superficial nephron function will be examined, since this treatment induces marked hypertrophy of the thick ascending limb [19].

Effects of long-term treatment with dDAVP on superficial nephron function

Long-term administration of ADH [20] or dDAVP [19] to DI Brattleboro rats is known to increase the renal concentrating ability more efficiently than acute infusion. This was confirmed in the present study, the osmolality of final urine reaching 1500 to 2500mOsm/kg in long-term treated rats [21]. After cessation of the treatment, the rats returned to water diuresis within four days. The animals were studied by micropuncture during maximal antidiuresis, i.e. when the treatment (dDAVP, 400ng/day, was given in a peanut oil emulsion) was continued right up to micropuncture experimentation, or during water diuresis, i.e. when the treatment was stopped four days before experiments. In both cases, throughout the period of micropuncture experiments, the animals were

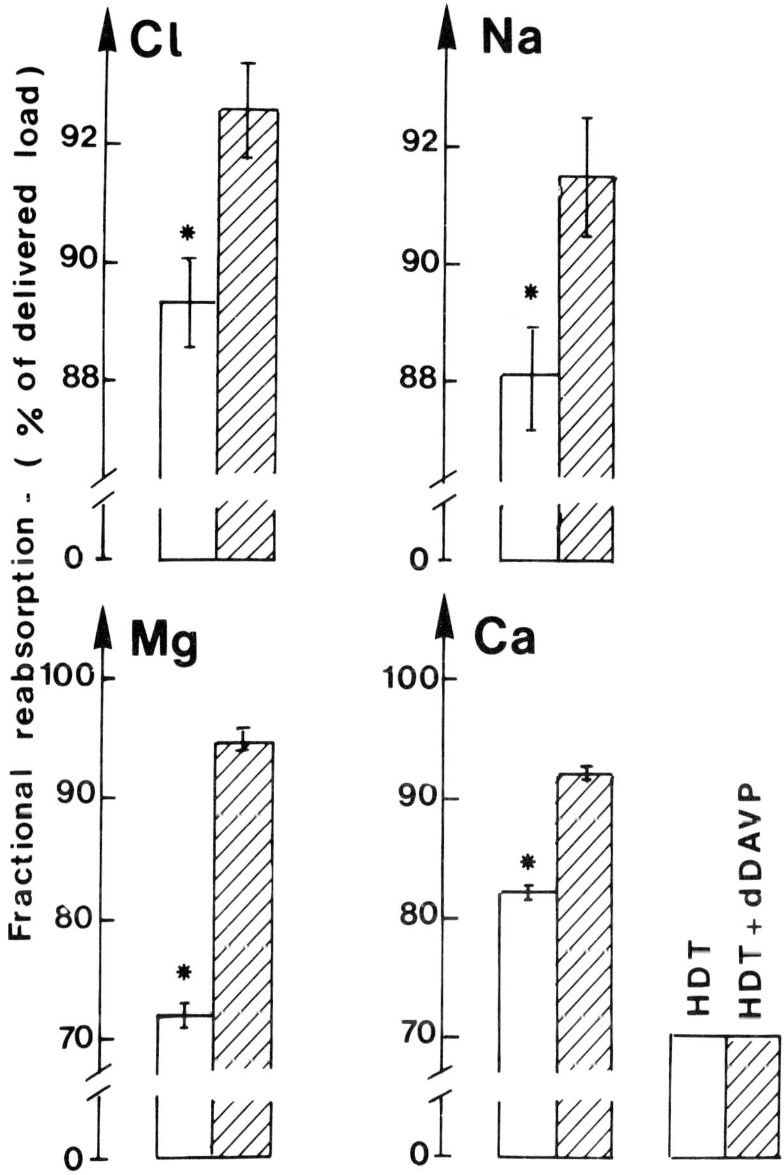

Figure 4. Chloride, sodium, magnesium and calcium fractional reabsorptions in the loop of Henle of superficial nephrons (reabsorbed amounts, as percent of delivered load). Experiments were performed in diabetes insipidus (DI) Brattleboro rats treated for three weeks with dDAVP (400, 500, 600ng/day during the first, second and third week respectively). The rats, acutely deprived of endogenous calcitonin, parathyroid hormone and glucagon (hormone-deprived rats), were examined either four days after cessation of dDAVP treatment (HDT, control diuretic rats) or when the treatment was continued until the micropuncture experiments, during which dDAVP was also given intravenously (20pg/min/100g body weight) (HDT + dDAVP experimental non-diuretic rats). Each column represents the mean value obtained from six different animals. * Significantly different from HDT+dDAVP rats. p at least <0.05. Data from ref 21

'hormone-deprived'. Non-diuretic rats were given dDAVP intravenously (20pg/min/100g body weight) during experiments, while the water-diuretic rats only received a hypotonic saline solution to compensate for water losses.

dDAVP administration during the micropuncture experiments changed neither the single nephron glomerular filtration rate nor the functional characteristics of the proximal convoluted tubule of the treated Brattleboro rats, but greatly affected tubular transport in the loop of Henle, as had already been observed in untreated Brattleboro rats given dDAVP acutely [2]. In the loop, it considerably enhanced fractional reabsorption (as % of the delivered load) of magnesium and calcium and, to a lesser extent, of sodium and chloride (Figure 4). Phosphate reabsorption was not affected. dDAVP had, therefore, the same effects on these treated rats as those already described in untreated animals. The effects in treated animals were not accompanied by any significant change in the filtered load of electrolytes, as in untreated rats, confirming the previous conclusion that dDAVP directly stimulates transport of magnesium, calcium, sodium and chloride in the loop of Henle, and hence in the thick ascending limb.

Effects of long-term treatment with dDAVP on juxtamedullary nephron function

Before considering the acute effect of the peptide in diabetes insipidus rats chronically treated with dDAVP, it is necessary to describe the consequences of the treatment itself on the function of the juxtamedullary nephron, i.e. in hormone-deprived (water diuretic) treated rats.

We have seen above that after hormone depletion, i.e. suppression of ADH, parathormone, calcitonin and glucagon, the cortico-medullary concentration gradient was almost completely dissipated. Removal of water along the descending limb was therefore minimal and fractional delivery of water at the hairpin turn ranged from 40 to 45% of the single nephron glomerular filtration rate (see Figure 2). In the hormone-deprived treated rats not infused with dDAVP during the experiments, the situation was identical and the fractional delivery of water fell in this range (Figure 5). With regard to electrolytes, the fractional delivery of calcium and magnesium at the hairpin turn was similar in hormone-deprived treated and untreated hormone-deprived rats. On the other hand, fractional delivery of sodium and chloride at the hairpin turn was significantly greater in the hormone-deprived treated controls than in hormone-deprived untreated rats (compare Figures 3 and 5). Besseghir et al [22] recently demonstrated that medullary thick ascending limbs of Henle in diabetes insipidus Brattleboro rats chronically treated with ADH expressed a higher transepithelial potential difference and chloride efflux, even in the absence of ADH in the bath, than do the medullary thick ascending limbs of Henle of diabetes insipidus untreated rats. This indicates that thick ascending limb hypertrophy consequent to chronic ADH administration is accompanied by an increase in NaCl transport by that segment. In the experiments in hormone-deprived rats presented

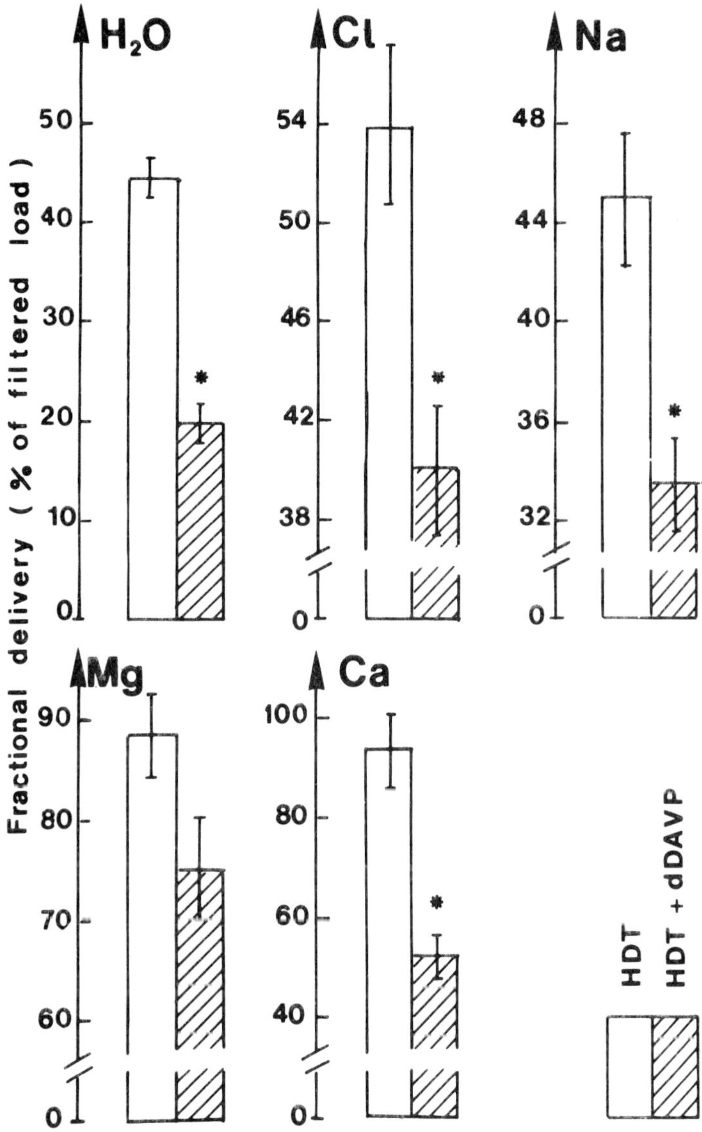

Figure 5. Water, chloride, sodium, magnesium and calcium fractional deliveries (as percent of filtered load) at the end of the loop of Henle of juxtamedullary nephrons. Experiments were performed in diabetes insipidus (DI) Brattleboro rats chronically treated with dDAVP (the amounts injected increased from 150ng/day during the first week of treatment to 360ng/day during the fifth week). The rats, acutely deprived of endogenous calcitonin, parathyroid hormone and glucagon (hormone-deprived rats) were examined either four days after cessation of dDAVP treatment (HDT, control diuretic rats) or when the treatment was continued until the micropuncture experiments, during which dDAVP was also given intravenously (20pg/min/100g body weight) (HDT+dDAVP experimental non-diuretic rats). Each column represents the mean value obtained from seven different animals. * Significantly different from HDT rats. p at least <0.05. Data from ref 21

above it was shown that glucagon, which stimulates NaCl transport in medullary thick ascending limb of Henle, increases sodium and chloride fractional delivery at the hairpin turn of juxtamedullary nephrons, without altering the water delivery. In addition, fractional delivery of sodium and chloride at the hairpin turn was in these rats, as in hormone-deprived treated control rats in the present study [21], significantly correlated to fluid osmolality. We concluded that glucagon enhances salt delivery at the tip of the loop by favouring net NaCl addition from the medullary thick ascending limb of Henle to the thin descending limb in the outer medulla. In hormone-deprived treated rats, the rise in NaCl delivery at the hairpin turn might, therefore, as in hormone-deprived rats given glucagon, also result from a medullary recycling process.

When dDAVP was given during the micropuncture experiments, fractional water delivery at the hairpin turn fell significantly (Figure 5), as consistently observed with low doses of this peptide [7] or with ADH [11]. This confirms that in the non-diuretic rat, water removal along the descending limb accounts for much of the increase in loop fluid osmolality. The increase in osmolality in the hormone-deprived treated and dDAVP treated rats was accounted for by increased water absorption, leaving fractional delivery of total solutes unchanged as compared with hormone-deprived treated rats (data not shown). On the other hand, fractional delivery of chloride, sodium and calcium was significantly lower in hormone-deprived treated and dDAVP than in hormone-deprived treated animals (Figure 5). A fractional delivery of total solutes similar in both groups therefore indicates that the decrease in the delivery of chloride and sodium was compensated by an increase in that of some other osmotically active solute. Urea is probably the chief candidate for this increase, since urea recycling is known to increase in the non-diuretic rat [13]. It was calculated that the non electrolyte solute concentration in the loop fluid in the present study was three times higher in non-diuretic than in diuretic rats.

Water removal along the descending limb probably increases the transepithelial NaCl concentration gradient between the descending limb lumen and the medullary interstitium. The reduction in the fractional delivery of chloride and sodium at the bend of the loop in the treated rats given dDAVP, might therefore be due to the enhancement of passive reabsorption along the descending limb. The positive correlation between the fractional delivery of sodium and osmolality at the hairpin turn observed in hormone-deprived treated rats was indeed completely abolished in hormone-deprived treated and dDAVP rats. That water removal along the descending limb might induce outward diffusion of electrolytes was first proposed to account for the decrease of calcium and magnesium fractional deliveries induced by calcitonin and dDAVP at the bend of the loop [7,9 and see above]. In the hormone-deprived treated and dDAVP rats, the fractional delivery of calcium to this site was also significantly decreased. The main findings from these studies on the effects of peptide hormones on the function of juxtamedullary nephrons are summarized in Figure 6.

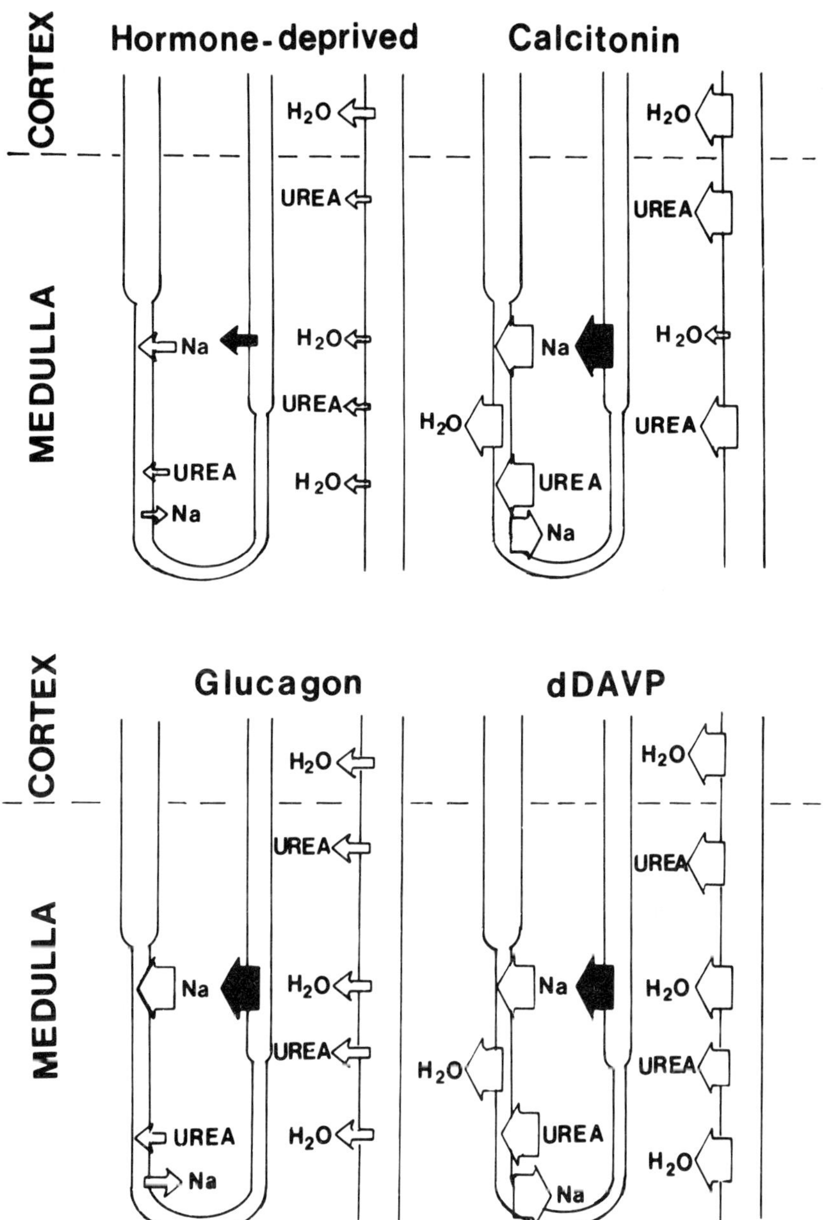

Figure 6. Effect of calcitonin, glucagon and dDAVP on the concentrating mechanism along the descending limb of juxtamedullary nephrons. This diagram is based on studies of the effects of the peptides in rats deprived of endogenous ADH, calcitonin, parathormone and glucagon, four hormones which stimulate the adenylate-cyclase activity of common target cells in the thick ascending limb. Administration rate of the peptides were as indicated in Figure 1. Black and white arrows refer to active and passive transport, respectively. Small arrows refer to unstimulated transport. Large arrows mean that the solute and water movements were increased by the peptides, either directly or indirectly. Data from refs 7–9, 21

On the basis of permeability properties measured in vitro, Imai et al modelled the transport of water and solutes along the descending limb of the long-looped nephrons of the hamster [18]. They concluded that in a simulated antidiuresis, the increase in loop fluid osmolality at the hairpin turn could be entirely accounted for by water removal. In their model, there was addition of urea, totally compensated by sodium output from the descending limb. This sodium reabsorption was due to diffusion and solvent drag. The authors also anticipated that an increase in the cortico-medullary urea concentration gradient would increase outward diffusion of sodium and that, conversely, a reduction in this gradient and an increase in the sodium gradient would reverse sodium absorption to net secretion. This mathematical determination of water and solute movements fully agrees with our finding that dDAVP reduces fractional delivery of chloride and sodium at the hairpin turn.

While the physiological significance of the hormonal effects on the NaCl medullary recycling is easy to understand (it contributes to the maintenance of the hyperosmolality of the medulla) such is not the case for the NaCl removal from the descending limb. It is possible that a NaCl escape from the descending limb in the inner medulla is a necessity for limiting the diluting effects on the interstitial osmolality of free water addition from both the medullary collecting ducts and the thin descending limbs. It is also relevant to note that, according to the 'central core' model, the mass balance equations indicate that, of several factors, net solute transport out of the descending limb should enhance the concentration gradient in the inner medulla, while pure medullary recycling of solutes should decrease it [23].

References

1 Morel F. Imbert-Teboul M, Chabardes D. Distribution of hormone-dependent adenylate cyclase in the nephron and its physiological significance. *Ann Rev Physiol 1981; 43:* 569–581

2 Rouffignac C de, Corman B, Roinel N. Stimulation by antidiuretic hormone of electrolyte tubular reabsorption in rat kidney. *Am J Physiol 1983; 244:* F156–F164

3 Bailly C, Roinel N, Amiel C. PTH-like glucagon stimulation of Ca and Mg reabsorption in Henle's loop of the rat. *Am J Physiol 1984; 246:* F205–F212

4 Elalouf JM, Roinel N, Rouffignac C de. ADH-like effects of calcitonin on electrolyte transports by Henle's loop of rat kidney. *Am J Physiol 1984; 246:* F213–F220

5 Elalouf JM, Chabane-Sari D, Roinel N, Rouffignac C de. ADH induces homologous desensitization in rat renal thick ascending limb cells. *Xth Int Congr Nephrol* (abstract)

6 Rouffignac C de, Elalouf JM, Roinel N. Phsyiological control of the urinary concentrating mechanism by peptide hormones. *Kidney Int 1987; 31:* 611–620

7 Elalouf JM, Roinel N, Rouffignac C de. Effects of dDAVP in rat juxtamedullary nephrons: stimulation of medullary K recycling. *Am J Physiol 1985; 249:* F292–F298

8 Elalouf JM, Roinel N, Rouffignac C de. Effects of glucagon and PTH on the loop of Henle of rat juxtamedullary nephrons. *Kidney Int 1986; 29:* 807–813

9 Elalouf JM, Roinel N, Rouffignac C de. Effects of human calcitonin on water and electrolyte movements in rat juxtamedullary nephrons. Inhibition of medullary K recycling. *Pfluegers Arch 1986; 406:* 502–508

10 Rouffignac C de, Elalouf JM. Effects of calcitonin on the renal concentrating mechanism. *Am J Physiol 1983; 245:* F506–F511

11 Jamison RL, Buerkert J, Lacy FB. A micropuncture study of Henle's thin loop in Brattleboro rats. *Am J Physiol 1973; 224:* 180–185

12 Kokko JP, Rector FC. Countercurrent multiplication system without active transport in inner medulla – a new model. *Kidney Int 1972; 2:* 214–223

13 Pennell JP, Lacy FB, Jamison RL. An *in vivo* study of the concentrating process in the descending limb of Henle's loop. *Kidney Int 1974; 5:* 337–347

14 Morel F, Chabardes D, Imbert-Teboul M et al. Multiple hormonal control of adenylate cyclase in distal segments of the rat kidney. *Kidney Int 1982; 21:* 55–62

15 Jamison RL, Roinel J, Rouffignac C de. Urinary concentrating mechanisms in the desert rodent *Psammomys obesus. Am J Physiol 1979; 236:* F448–F453

16 Rouffignac C de, Morel F. Micropuncture study of water, electrolyte and urea movements along the loops of Henle in *Psammomys. J Clin Invest 1969; 48:* 474–486

17 Rouffignac C de, Morel F, Moss N, Roinel N. Micropuncture study of water and electrolyte movements along the loop of Henle in Psammomys with special reference to magnesium, calcium and phosphorus. *Pfluegers Arch 1973; 344:* 309–326

18 Imai M, Taniguchi J, Tabei K. Function of thin loops of Henle. *Kidney Int 1987; 31:* 565–579

19 Bouby N, Bankir L, Trinh-Trang-Tan MM et al. Selective ADH-induced hypertrophy of the medullary thick ascending limb in Brattleboro rats. *Kidney Int 1985; 28:* 456–466

20 Harrington AR, Valtin H. Impaired urinary concentration after vasopressin and its gradual correction in hypothalamic diabetes insipidus. *J Clin Invest 1968; 47:* 502–510

21 Elalouf JM, Chabane-Sari D, Roinel N, Rouffignac C de. NaCl and Ca delivery at the bend of rat deep nephrons decreases during antidiuresis. *Am J Physiol 1987:* in press

22 Besseghir K, Trimble ME, Stoner L. Action of ADH on isolated medullary thick ascending limb of the Brattleboro rat. *Am J Physiol 1986; 251:* F272–F277

23 Stephenson J. Concentration of urine in a central core model of the renal counter flow system. *Kidney Int 1972; 2:* 85–94

REGULATION OF ELECTROLYTE TRANSPORT PROCESSES IN THE MEDULLARY THICK ASCENDING LIMB

D A Molony, W B Reeves, T E Andreoli

University of Texas Medical School, Houston, Texas, USA

Introduction

In this review, we summarize recent observations pertaining to the mechanism of active salt absorption by the thick ascending limb of Henle's loop, and how this process is modulated by antidiuretic hormone, prostaglandins and peritubular hypertonicity.

Mechanism of salt absorption

Early studies in isolated thick ascending limb segments demonstrated that chloride absorption occurs against both an electrical and chemical potential gradient, that is, chloride absorption is an energy requiring process [1,2]. It is now clear that chloride absorption in the thick ascending limb is an example of secondary active transport wherein the movement of chloride against its electrochemical gradient is coupled to the active transport of sodium. A model of the mechanism of salt absorption in the thick ascending limb is presented in Figure 1 [3]. Sodium, potassium and chloride enter the cell across the luminal membrane via an electroneutral, diuretic-sensitive cotransporter. In parallel with this cotransporter is a barium-sensitive potassium channel which allows potassium to recycle across the apical membrane, so that net potassium secretion is about 10% of net Cl^- absorption [4]. The activity of chloride in the cell is above its electrochemical equilibrium by virtue of its coupled entry with sodium. Dissipative chloride efflux, in turn, proceeds through chloride channels in the basolateral membrane. Sodium is pumped out actively across the basolateral membrane of the cell by the Na/K-ATPase pump, thereby maintaining a favourable gradient for further sodium entry across the apical membrane. Thus, active transcellular absorption of chloride is ultimately driven by the Na/K-ATPase pump.

An interesting feature of this model is that while chloride absorption is transcellular, a significant proportion of sodium absorption occurs via the paracellular pathway [3,4]. The electrogenic movement of chloride across the

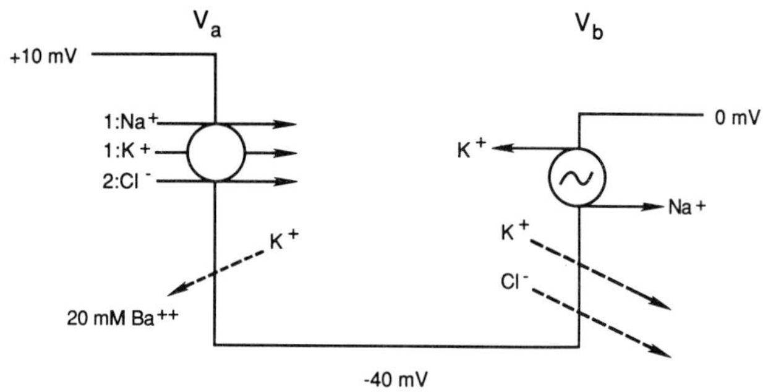

Figure 1. Electrical characteristics of the mouse medullary thick ascending limb cell. The apical membrane contains an electroneutral Na^+:K^+:$2Cl^-$ triporter in parallel with a barium inhibitable potassium channel. The basolateral membrane contains chloride and potassium channels and the Na/K-ATPase pump. The intracellular potential is −40mV, lumen positive [3]

basolateral cell membrane depolarizes this membrane relative to the apical membrane producing a lumen positive transepithelial electrical potential of 5–10mV [5]. This electrical potential provides the driving force for additional sodium absorption through the cation selective paracellular pathway. Approximately half of the net transepithelial sodium absorption occurs transcellularly, by way of the basolateral membrane Na/K-ATPase pump and the remaining sodium is absorbed through the paracellular pathway [3].

Regulation of NaCl absorption

Studies of thick ascending limb segments perfused in vitro have revealed it to be a heterogenous structure. For example, transport processes in the mouse medullary thick ascending limb are subject to modulation by a number of agents, including antidiuretic hormone (ADH), prostaglandins (PG), peritubular osmolality, glucagon and isoprenaline [6–8] while salt absorption in the cortical thick ascending limb is not affected by ADH or PGE_2, but is partially dependent upon carbon dioxide or bicarbonate [9]. The remainder of our remarks will focus specifically on the modulation of medullary thick limb function by ADH, prostaglandin and peritubular osmolality.

The ADH effect: features and mechanisms

It is well established, particularly for the medullary thick ascending limb of the mouse and rat, that ADH enhances adenylate cyclase activity [10], the net rate of NaCl absorption and the spontaneous transepithelial voltage (Table I) [6]. Coincident with the ADH-stimulation of net salt absorption, the transcellular electrical conductance is increased 30% and the apical and basolateral membranes depolarize by 6 and 11mV, respectively [4,5]. The transcellular conductance includes, at a minimum, apical membrane potassium channels and basolateral

TABLE I. Effects of ADH on NaCl transport in the mouse medullary thick ascending limb

	No ADH	ADH present
Spontaneous transepithelial voltage (mV)	5	11
Net rate of Cl^- absorption (pEq sec^{-1} cm^{-2})	2,600	10,800
Transepithelial conductance (mS cm^{-2})	100	120
Transcellular conductance (mS cm^{-2})	45	60
Basolateral membrane voltage (mV)	-49	-38

The data are from [4,6,11]

membrane chloride and potassium channels. The paracellular conductance, which accounts for roughly half of the total transepithelial conductance, is unaffected by ADH [4].

The ADH-induced increase in transcellular conductance is due primarily to an increase in basolateral chloride conductance [4,5,11,12]. This increase in the basolateral chloride conductance, in turn, could result either directly from an ADH effect on basolateral membrane permeability of chloride, or indirectly as a consequence of an ADH-dependent increase in apical membrane salt entry, which raises intracellular chloride activity and depolarizes the basolateral membrane voltage.

In order to differentiate between a primary and secondary effect of ADH on the basolateral membrane chloride conductance, we studied [11] the effect of ADH on transcellular conductance when both the cell chloride activity and basolateral membrane voltage were held constant by the luminal application of frusemide. As shown in Table II, in the presence of frusemide, ADH no longer increased transcellular conductance [11]. In other words, the increase in basal chloride conductance produced by ADH is due to a hormone-dependent increase in apical admittance for chloride, which increases intracellular chloride activity and, secondarily, increases basolateral membrane chloride conductance.

TABLE II. Effects of ADH and frusemide on the transcellular conductance

	Transcellular conductance (mS cm^{-2})		Difference
	No ADH	ADH Present	(mS cm^{-2})
No frusemide in lumen	44.5±5.6	58.9±8.9	14.3±5.5 ($p<0.02$)
Frusemide present in lumen	36.5±4.4	41.5±6.4	5.0±4.3 (NS)

The data are from [11]

Prostaglandin-ADH interactions

In mouse medullary thick ascending limb segments, prostaglandin E_2 inhibits the ADH-dependent components of the spontaneous transepithelial voltage and net salt absorption but does not alter these variables in the absence of ADH, nor in the ADH-unresponsive mouse cortical thick ascending limb [7]. This PGE_2

inhibition of transepithelial voltage and net salt absorption can be overcome by dibutyryl-cAMP, suggesting that PGE_2 interferes with ADH-dependent chloride absorption by inhibiting the rate of cAMP formation [7]. This view is supported by the observations of Torikai and Murokawa, who found that PGE_2 produced an inhibition of the ADH-stimulated rate of cAMP formation in isolated rat medullary thick ascending limb segments [13]. In addition, forskolin, a non-hormonal stimulator of the catalytic subunit of adenylate cyclase, stimulates transepithelial voltage even in the presence of PGE_2, whereas cholera toxin, which causes ADP ribosylation and activation of the stimulatory guanine regulatory subunit, N_S, fails to stimulate salt absorption in the presence of PGE_2 [14].

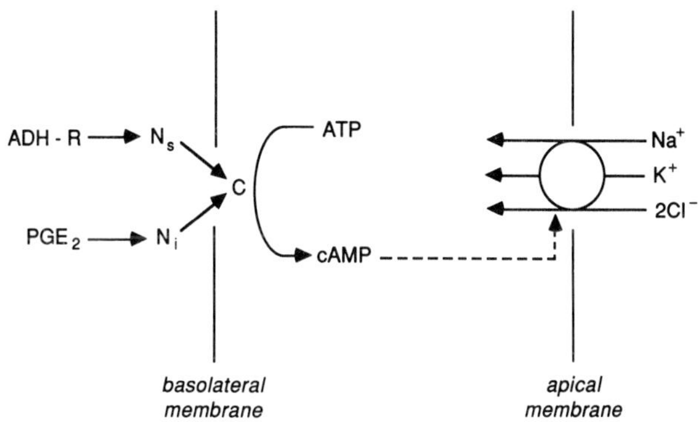

Figure 2. Modulation of medullary thick ascending limb transport by antidiuretic hormone (ADH) and the prostaglandin, PGE_2. ADH-receptor interaction results in the activation of the stimulatory guanine nucleotide subunit, N_S and the activation of the enzyme adenylate cyclase for the production of cyclic AMP (cAMP). cAMP acts as a second messenger signalling augmented apical salt admittance via the Na^+:K^+:$2Cl^-$ triporter. PGE_2 activates the N_i or inhibitory subunit, which, in turn, inhibits adenylate cyclase activity and ADH-stimulated generation of cAMP [14]

A scheme explaining how antidiuretic hormone and PGE_2 interact to modulate salt transport in the medullary thick ascending limb is shown in Figure 2. The adenylate cyclase complex in the basolateral membrane includes a stimulatory guanine nucleotide regulatory subunit, N_S, and an inhibitory guanine nucleotide regulatory subunit, N_i. ADH, when coupled to its receptor (R), activates N_S and thus increases the rate of cAMP formation. PGE_2, independently of hormone-receptor interactions, activates N_i and consequently suppresses the rate of cAMP formation. Thus, PGE_2 inhibits only the ADH-stimulated component of net salt absorption.

Modulation of medullary thick ascending limb function by peritubular osmolality

In contrast to the PGE_2 effect, increasing peritubular hypertonicity reversibly inhibits both the basal and ADH-stimulated rates of net salt absorption and the

TABLE III. The effects of peritubular hypertonicity on the spontaneous transepithelial voltage in the mouse medullary thick ascending limb in the presence of antidiuretic hormone

Experimental manoeuvre	ADH concentration (μU/ml)	Transepithelial voltage (mV)
Control	10	9.2±1.3
600mM bath urea	10	1.3±0.7
	250	0.7±0.8
600mM bath and perfusate urea	10	1.2±0.8
600mM bath mannitol	10	2.9±0.8
	250	2.8±0.8

The data are from [15]

spontaneous transepithelial voltage in the mouse medullary thick ascending limb [15]. Thus the addition of 600mM urea to peritubular solutions abolishes both net salt absorption, measured electrotitrametrically, and spontaneous transepithelial voltage in mouse medullary thick ascending limb segments studied in vitro [15]. The combined effect of different osmotic agents and of ADH on transepithelial voltage are shown in Table III. The inhibitory effects of increased peritubular osmolality could not be overcome with a 25-fold increase in bath ADH concentration (250μU/ml). These data are consistent with the view that peritubular hypertonicity suppresses salt absorption by a mechanism not involving the adenylate cyclase cascade.

In further contrast to the specific effects of PGE_2 and ADH on medullary but not cortical thick limbs, peritubular hypertonicity reversibly inhibits the spontaneous transport voltage in mouse cortical thick limbs as well as in rabbit medullary thick limbs studied in vitro [15]. Thus, specificity for this suppressive effect of peritubular hypertonicity on medullary thick ascending limb transport is the consequence in vivo of the location of the medullary thick ascending limb, in a hypertonic interstitial environment. In this context, it is relevant to examine the effects of various degrees of external hypertonicity on the transport properties of thick limb segments. A dose response curve for the inhibition of the transport voltage by peritubular hypertonicity in mouse thick ascending limb segments studied in vitro is shown in Figure 3. In both medullary and cortical thick limbs, there was a graded response to increasing peritubular osmolality with urea [16]. Thus, it is plausible to argue that in vivo, peritubular hypertonicity can modulate diluting segment function over a range of medullary interstitial osmolalities.

Mechanism for the urea effect

Our recent observations [16] indicate that peritubular urea hypertonicity also reduces the transcellular electrical conductance and hyperpolarizes the basolateral

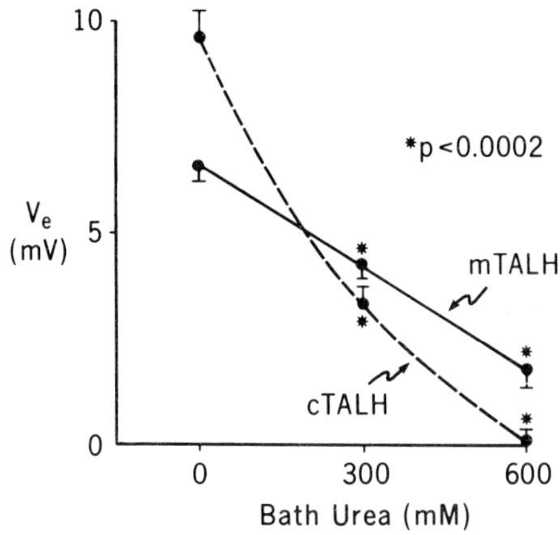

Figure 3. The effect of graded increases in bath urea (mM) and on the spontaneous transepithelial voltage, V_e (mV), in isolated perfused segments of mouse medullary thick ascending limbs (mTALH) and cortical thick ascending limbs (cTALH). V_e values at 300 and 600mM urea are significantly less than the control V_e values at zero bath urea [15]

membrane voltage by causing a direct blockade of basolateral membrane chloride conductance. Thus in vivo, peritubular hypertonicity may serve as an integral component of a negative feedback system designed to suppress metabolic work by the medullary thick ascending limb when urinary concentrating power has been made maximal by enrichment of medullary interstitial osmolality.

References

1 Burg MB, Green N. Function of the thick ascending limb of Henle's loop. *Am J Physiol 1973; 224:* 659–668

2 Rocha AS, Kokko JP. Sodium chloride and water transport in the medullary thick ascending limb of Henle. *J Clin Invest 1973; 52:* 612–623

3 Hebert SC, Andreoli TE. Control of NaCl transport in the thick ascending limb. *Am J Physiol 1984; 246:* F745–F756

4 Hebert SC, Friedman PA, Andreoli TE. The effects of antidiuretic hormone on cellular conductive pathways in mouse medullary thick ascending limbs of Henle. I. ADH increases transcellular conductance pathways. *J Memb Biol 1984; 80:* 201–219

5 Hebert SC, Andreoli TE. Effects of antidiuretic hormone on cellular conductive pathways in mouse medullary thick ascending limbs of Henle. II. Determinants of the ADH-mediated increases in transepithelial voltage and in net Cl^- absorption. *J Memb Biol 1984; 80:* 221–233

6 Hebert SC, Culpepper RM, Andreoli TE. NaCl transport in mouse thick ascending limbs. I. Functional nephron heterogeneity and ADH-stimulated NaCl cotransport. *Am J Physiol 1981; 241:* F412–F431

7 Culpepper RM, Andreoli TE. Interactions among prostaglandin E_2, antidiuretic hormone, and cyclic adenosine monophosphate in modulating Cl^- absorption in single mouse medullary thick ascending limbs of Henle. *J Clin Invest 1983; 71:* 1588–1601

8 Culpepper RM. Multiple regulators of adenylate cyclase (AC) in mouse medullary thick ascending limb (mTAL): significance for NaCl transport. *Clin Res 1984; 32:* 65A

9 Friedman PA, Andreoli TE. CO_2-stimulated NaCl absorption in the mouse renal cortical thick ascending limb of Henle. *J Gen Physiol 1982; 80:* 683–711

10 Morel F. Sites of hormone action in the mammalian nephron. *Am J Physiol 1981; 240:* F159–F164

11 Molony DA, Reeves WB, Hebert SC, Andreoli TE. ADH increases apical Na^+, K^+, $2Cl^-$ entry in mouse medullary thick ascending limbs of Henle. *Am J Physiol 1987; 252:* F177–F187

12 Schlatter E, Gregor R. cAMP increases the basolateral Cl^- conductance in the isolated perfused medullary thick ascending limb of Henle's loop of the mouse. *Pfluegers Arch 1985; 405:* 367–376

13 Torikai S, Kurokawa K. Effect of PGE_2 on vasopressin-dependent cell cAMP in isolated nephron segments. *Am J Physiol 1983; 245:* F58–F66

14 Culpepper RM, Andreoli TE. PGE_2, forskolin, and cholera toxin interactions in modulating NaCl transport in mouse mTALH. *Am J Physiol 1984; 247:* F784–F792

15 Hebert SC, Culpepper RM, Andreoli TE. NaCl transport in mouse medullary thick ascending limbs. III. Modulation of the ADH effect by peritubular osmolality. *Am J Physiol 1981; 241:* F443–F451

16 Molony DA, Andreoli TE. Peritubular hypertonicity reduces transcellular electrical conductance and hyperpolarizes basolateral membranes of isolated mouse medullary thick ascending limbs (mTALH). *Kidney Int 1987; 31:* 439

BICARBONATE AND CHLORIDE ABSORPTION IN HENLE'S LOOP AND THE ROLE OF PEPTIDE HORMONES

M Paillard, M Bichara, Odile Mercier, Francoise Leviel, M Delahousse, A Prigent

Université Paris VII, Hôpital Louis Mourier, Colombes, France

Little is known about the hormonal control of urinary acidification. Up to now, most studies have focused on the effects of steroid hormones but recent data from our laboratory suggest that peptide hormones may influence urinary acidification in the rat. Parathyroid hormone stimulates bicarbonate absorption in Henle's loop and enhances urinary acidification through increase in urinary phosphate concentration that stimulates proton secretion in the distal nephron [1,2]. Among other peptide hormones known to stimulate adenylate cyclase activity in the thick ascending limb of Henle and collecting system [3], antidiuretic hormone (ADH) has been recently shown to enhance, and glucagon to inhibit urinary acidification in the rat (data from our laboratory presented at this meeting). Finally other investigators have shown that cyclic AMP, the common intracellular second messenger for several peptide hormones, can affect the transepithelial hydrion and/or bicarbonate transport in the mammalian collecting system perfused in vitro [4,5].

These observations prompted us to study by free-flow micropuncture the effects of glucagon and ADH on the segmental handling of hydrion and/or bicarbonate in the superficial nephron of the rat. The peptide hormones, parathormone, glucagon, ADH, and thyrocalcitonin have been shown to stimulate the adenylate cyclase in the same tubular cells and to elicit similar biological effects on the thick ascending limb of Henle [6]. Thus we investigated the effects of glucagon and ADH in rats whose endogenous secretion of the four peptide hormones were suppressed or restrained. We used an acute peptide hormone-derived model. At variance with the model previously described [7], in which ADH secretion was chronically suppressed (Brattleboro rats), we chose to suppress acutely the four peptide hormone secretions in previously intact rats.

Methods

Paired micropuncture experiments were performed in acutely thyroparathyroidectomized rats that were plasma replete, as previously described [1]. The endogenous secretion of glucagon was reduced by an infusion of somatostatin ($0.7ng \cdot min^{-1} \cdot g^{-1}$ body wt), and the endogenous secretion of ADH by hypotonic volume expansion, using an infusion of 75mM NaCl to 7% of body weight in 60 minutes followed by a sustaining infusion at $0.3\mu l \cdot min^{-1} \cdot g^{-1}$ body weight during two hours of equilibration. The latter procedure was shown to reduce endogenous ADH secretion as evidenced by a dramatic fall in urinary osmolality and in urinary ADH excretion rate [8].

The renal and nephronal handling of hydrion and/or bicarbonate was studied twice in each rat, first during a 60 minute control period, and then during a 60 minute experimental period. In studies with glucagon, the experimental period started after glucagon (Novo Industrie, Bagswaerd, Denmark) was infused at $0.05ng \cdot min^{-1} \cdot g^{-1}$ body weight for 30 minutes. In ADH studies, the experimental period started after dDAVP (Ferring, Sweden) was infused at $0.2pg \cdot min^{-1} \cdot g^{-1}$ body weight for 30 minutes. Then, the 75mM NaCl infusion rate was diminished so that the rate of the infused solution balanced the reduced urinary flow rate.

Group I: Glucagon effects on Henle's loop and the whole kidney

This group comprised six Sprague Dawley rats. Superficial tubules were punctured first at early distal and then at end-proximal sites during the control period; fresh tubules were punctured during the experimental period.

Group II: Glucagon effects on the distal nephron

This group comprised seven Sprague Dawley rats. The proton secretion in the collecting system was assessed by measuring urine-minus-blood pCO_2 difference (U-B pCO_2) during bicarbonate loading as previously described [2], both during the control and experimental periods.

Group III: ADH effects on Henle's loop and whole kidney

This group comprised seven Sprague Dawley rats, and the same micropuncture protocol as described above was used.

Group IV: ADH effects on the distal nephron

This group comprised six rats. The U-B pCO_2 test during bicarbonate loading could not be used as an index of proton secretion in the distal nephron during dDAVP infusion, since the dramatic reduction in urinary flow rate increased the urinary osmolality, which is known to influence per se the generation and maintenance of U-B pCO_2. Thus we decided to assess directly the proton secretion in the superficial distal tubule in Wistar rats. This strain of rat was used because both the distal convoluted tubule (early distal) and the initial collecting tubule (late distal) are accessible to micropuncture [9].

Group V: Time control

This group comprised five Sprague Dawley rats. Tubular micropuncture of superficial nephrons was conducted as previously described from our laboratory

[1]. Methoxy-^{3}H inulin (New England Nuclear) was used to determine whole kidney glomerular filtration rate and single nephron glomerular filtration rate. Analytical procedures were performed as previously described from our laboratory [1]. Chloride and total CO_2 (tCO_2) were measured in tubule fluid samples by electrometric titration method of Ramsay et al and microcalorimetry respectively. Results are expressed by means ± SE. Statistical significance was assessed by the two-tailed paired or unpaired 't' test, as appropriate.

Results

Effects of glucagon and dDAVP on blood composition and urinary acidification

Mean arterial blood pressure and blood composition did not significantly vary between control and experimental periods in each group. Glucagon infusion inhibited urinary acidification, with an increase in urinary pH and bicarbonate excretion rate. The ammonium ion excretion rate did not vary and titratable acid excretion declined, with a reduction in net acid excretion (Table I). Infusion

TABLE I. Effect of glucagon and dDAVP on urinary acidification in acutely peptide hormone-deprived rats

	Urinary pH	Urinary excretion rates nmol/min			
		HCO_3^-	TA	NH_4^+	NA
Control	6.52±0.16	90±32	31±6	794±65	735±66
Glucagon	7.09±0.09	371±75	4±2	824±65	457±133
	P<0.01	P<0.02	P<0.05	NS	P<0.02
Control	6.90±0.1	189±54	22±7	840±53	731±77
dDAVP	5.92±0.09	2±0.5	41±7	653±44	692±47
	P<0.01	P<0.01	P<0.05	NS	NS

Values are means ± SE. Absolute rates were factored by kidney weight. TA=titratable acid; NA=net acid

of dDAVP stimulated urinary acidification, with a fall in urinary pH and disappearance of bicarbonate from the urine. Ammonium excretion did not change despite the reduction in urinary flow rate, and titratable acid excretion rate remained low (Table I). It should be noted that net acid excretion (calculated as ammonium + titratable acid - bicarbonate) did not change. In time control rats, the variables of urinary acidification remained unchanged.

Effects of glucagon and dDAVP in Henle's loop

Glucagon and dDAVP increased significantly the capability of the loop of Henle of superficial nephrons to absorb chloride, and decreased that for tCO_2. This is attested by an increase in the loop fractional absorption of chloride (which did not reach significance for glucagon), and a significant decrease for

TABLE II. Effects of glucagon and dDAVP on the Henle's loop handling of chloride and tCO_2 in acutely peptide hormone-deprived rats

	End proximal delivery		Henle's loop fractional absorption		Early distal TF/UF	
	Chloride	tCO_2	Chloride	tCO_2	Chloride	tCO_2
	pmol/min/g kidney wt					
Control	1,835±105	107±11	0.847±0.005	0.68±0.04	0.35±0.01	0.17±0.01
Glucagon	2,054±132	118±14	0.861±0.008	0.56±0.06	0.29±0.01	0.21±0.02
	NS	NS	P<0.01	P<0.02	P<0.01	P<0.05
Control	2,439±217	122±19	0.829±0.009	0.64±0.02	0.39±0.01	0.18±0.01
dDAVP	1,957±140	124±13	0.857±0.006	0.58±0.02	0.32±0.01	0.25±0.02
	NS	NS	P<0.02	P<0.05	P<0.01	P<0.05

Values are means ± SE. TF/UF=tubular fluid to ultrafiltrate concentration ratio

that of tCO_2 (Table II). As a consequence of these effects of glucagon and dDAVP, the tubular fluid-to-ultrafiltrate concentration ratio at the early distal site decreased for chloride, and increased for tCO_2 (Table II). It should be noted that the loads of chloride and tCO_2 delivered to the Henle's loop did not change (Table II) in the presence of glucagon or dDAVP. The unchanged end proximal delivery of chloride and bicarbonate in the presence of glucagon was not really unexpected due to the lack of increase in single nephron glomerular filtration rate. Indeed, the rats of the present study were plasma replete after completion of surgery and had a slight extracellular fluid volume expansion. In previous studies in which an increase in glomerular filtration rate was observed, the rats were probably hydropenic, since they exhibited a chronic diabetes insipidus and surgically induced plasma losses were not replaced [10]. It may be expected that hydropenic animals with elevated renal vascular resistance are much more responsive to the vasodilator effects of glucagon than plasma replete and slightly volume-expanded rats.

Effects of glucagon and dDAVP in the distal nephron

The effects of glucagon infusion in the distal nephron were assessed by measuring U-B pCO_2 during bicarbonate loading (urinary pH>7.6). U-B pCO_2 was about 15mmHg lower for any value of urinary bicarbonate concentration in the presence of glucagon than in its absence (P<0.001). The effects of dDAVP infusion in the distal nephron were assessed from micropuncture of the accessible distal tubules of superficial nephrons of Wistar rats. While the early distal tCO_2 delivery did not differ in this group (41±6 versus 47±7pmol/min), we observed tCO_2 secretion in the control period, −13±6pmol/min (significantly different from zero, P<0.05), which reversed to a tCO_2 absorption in the experimental period, +19±3pmol/min (significantly different from zero, P<0.05). This indicated clearly that antidiuretic hormone increased proton secretion or inhibited bicarbonate secretion in the distal tubule.

Discussion

The main original results of the present study in rats acutely deprived of four peptide hormones (parathormone, thyrocalcitonin, glucagon and antidiuretic hormone) are the following: 1) glucagon as well as antidiuretic hormone inhibits bicarbonate and stimulates chloride absorption in Henle's loop. The effect of antidiuretic hormone on chloride absorption in Henle's loop has previously been shown in thyroparathyroidectomized glucose-infused Brattleboro rats [7]; 2) glucagon inhibits and antidiuretic hormone stimulates proton secretion in the distal nephron; and 3) the whole kidney resulting effects are an inhibition of urinary acidification for glucagon and an enhancement for antidiuretic hormone.

Similar effects of glucagon and antidiuretic hormone in Henle's loop of superficial nephron are probably located in the thick ascending limb. First, glucagon and antidiuretic hormone have been shown to stimulate adenylate cyclase activity of the same cells in thick ascending limb [3]. Second, glucagon and antidiuretic hormone have been found to enhance chloride absorption in the rat or mouse medullary thick ascending limb perfused in vitro [11]. Third, it has been recently shown that a significant absorption of bicarbonate occurs in the rat cortical and medullary thick ascending limb perfused in vitro, probably via a Na:H exchange [12]. The mechanisms of action of glucagon and antidiuretic hormone on bicarbonate absorption were not addressed in the present study, and we can only propose a hypothesis. Antidiuretic hormone has been recently shown to increase the functional number of apical membrane Na^+-K^+-$2Cl^-$ cotransport units in the thick ascending limb [13]. The resultant increase in sodium entry and consequently cellular sodium concentration, might inhibit the Na:H exchange in the apical membrane, and thus reduce bicarbonate absorption. The possibility that glucagon's actions are mediated by similar mechanisms is much more speculative.

The opposing effects of glucagon and antidiuretic hormone on the proton secretion in the distal nephron are not unexpected. In contrast to the thick ascending limb of Henle, there are several types of cells in the distal nephron. Glucagon and antidiuretic hormone might stimulate adenylate cyclase activity of different target cells influencing proton secretion, i.e. proton and bicarbonate secreting intercalated cells, principal cells that absorb NaCl and secrete potassium and may indirectly influence proton secretion by modifying the transepithelial voltage. It should be noted that antidiuretic hormone enhances NaCl absorption in the distal tubule (probably in principal cells), while glucagon does not [14].

The physiological significance of the effects of antidiuretic hormone and glucagon on urinary acidification remains to be determined.

References

1 Bichara M, Mercier O, Paillard M, Leviel F. Effects of parathyroid hormone on urinary acidification. *Am J Physiol 1986; 251 (Renal Fluid Electrolyte Physiol 20):* F444–F453

2 Mercier O, Bichara M, Paillard M, Prigent A. Effects of parathyroid hormone and urinary phosphate on collecting duct hydrogen secretion. *Am J Physiol 1986; 251 (Renal Fluid Electrolyte Physiol 20):* F802–F809

3 Morel F. Sites of hormone action in the mammalian nephron. *Am J Physiol 1981; 240 (Renal Fluid Electrolyte Physiol 9):* F159–F164

4 Schuster VL. Cyclic adenosine monophosphate-stimulated bicarbonate secretion in rabbit cortical collecting tubules. *J Clin Invest 1985; 75:* 2056–2064

5 Hays S, Kokko JP, Jacobson HR. Hormonal regulation of proton secretion in rabbit medullary collecting duct. *J Clin Invest 1986; 78:* 1279–1286

6 Rouffignac C de, Elalouf JM, Roinel N. Physiological control of the urinary concentrating mechanism by peptide hormones. *Kidney Int 1987; 31:* 611–620

7 Rouffignac C de, Corman B, Roinel N. Stimulation by antidiuretic hormone of electrolyte tubular reabsorption in rat kidney. *Am J Physiol 1983; 244 (Renal Fluid Electrolyte Physiol 13):* F156–F164

8 Kauker ML, Crofton JT, Share L, Nasjletti A. Role of vasopressin in regulation of renal kinin excretion in Long-Evans and diabetes insipidus rats. *J Clin Invest 1984; 73:* 824–831

9 Woodhall PB, Tisher CC. Response of the distal tubule and cortical collecting duct to vasopressin in the rat. *J Clin Invest 1973; 52:* 3095–3108

10 Bailly C, Roinel N, Amiel C. PTH-like glucagon stimulation of Ca and Mg reabsorption in Henle's loop of the rat. *Am J Physiol 1984; 246 (Renal Fluid Electrolyte Physiol 15):* F205–F212

11 Hebert SC, Andreoli TE. Control of NaCl transport in the thick ascending limb. *Am J Physiol 1984; 246 (Renal Fluid Electrolyte Physiol 15):* F745–F756

12 Good DW. Sodium-dependent bicarbonate absorption by cortical thick ascending limb of rat kidney. *Am J Physiol 1985; 248 (Renal Fluid Electrolyte Physiol 17):* F821–F829

13 Hebert SC, Reeves WB, Molony DA, Adreoli TE. The medullary thick limb: function and modulation of the single-effect multiplier. *Kidney Int 1987; 31:* 580–588

14 Bailly C, Roinel N, Amiel C. Stimulation by glucagon and PTH of Ca and Mg reabsorption in the superficial distal tubule of the rat kidney. *Pfluegers Arch 1985; 403:* 28–34

FUNCTIONS OF THE COLLECTING DUCT

CORTICAL COLLECTING DUCT ANION TRANSPORT

V L Schuster

University of Iowa and Veterans Administration Medical Center, Iowa City, USA

The major anions transported by the mammalian cortical collecting duct are chloride and bicarbonate. Although there are several in vivo micropuncture studies in the rat 'distal tubule' dealing with anion transport in that species and because the 'distal tubule' contains more than one functionally distinct part of the nephron most of our understanding of *true* cortical collecting duct anion transport comes from rabbit in vitro microperfusion studies. Therefore, this discussion will be confined predominantly to data from the rabbit.

Bicarbonate absorption

The cortical collecting duct cells are capable of reabsorbing bicarbonate from the lumen, particularly if the animal has been acid-loaded in vivo [1,2]. Our understanding of the cellular mechanisms by which the cortical collecting duct reabsorbs bicarbonate ions derives in a large part from studies of acidification by the outer medullary collecting duct dissected from the inner stripe (OMCDi). In another later section of this symposium, Koeppen discusses the electrophysiology of the OMCDi segment. For purposes of understanding cortical collecting duct acidification mechanisms, suffice it to say here that OMCDi reabsorbs bicarbonate by electrogenically secreting protons (H^+) across the apical membrane via a H^+-ATPase [3]. Bicarbonate generated within the cell as a consequence of the proton pump exits the OMCDi cell via chloride/bicarbonate exchange process [4].

Investigation of this particular collecting duct anion exchanger, that is the basolateral chloride/bicarbonate exchanger, at the molecular level has provided the strongest evidence that acidification by the cortical collecting duct occurs by a mechanism very similar, if not identical, to that in OMCDi. We recently showed that a monoclonal antibody made to the membrane (anion-transporting) domain of the human erythrocyte chloride/bicarbonate exchange protein 'band 3' reacts immunocytochemically with the basolateral membrane of a subpopulation of rabbit cortical collecting duct and OMCDi cells [5]. These cells are the mitochondria-rich, or intercalated cells. Similar findings have been reported by Drenckhahn et al in the rat kidney [6]. In the rabbit, we found that the number of band 3-positive cells was much higher in OMCDi than in cortical collecting ducts, consistent with the higher bicarbonate reabsorptive rates in the former segment [5]. A similar proton-secreting, bicarbonate reabsorbing mitochondria-rich cell in the turtle bladder has been termed the alpha cell by Stetson and Steinmetz [7]. As shown in Figure 1, we have adapted this terminology to the acid-secreting rabbit intercalated cells as well.

The exact molecular nature of the alpha cell basolateral chloride/bicarbonate exchanger remains unclear. Is the protein identical to erythrocyte band 3 or is it only antigenically related? In the rat, Drenckhahn et al reported that the kidney membrane protein has a molecular weight of ~120kd when an antibody to whole red cell band 3 is used on immunoblots [6], i.e. its size is similar to that of rat erythrocyte band 3 (110kd). In similar experiments, we have found that we get different results vis-a-vis protein size depending upon the antibodies used in the immunoblotting (unpublished). In rabbit, mouse, and cow kidney membranes, a polyclonal antibody to the cytoplasmic (cytoskeletal-anchoring) domain of human erythrocyte band 3 does label a protein of a size similar to that of the erythrocyte protein, ~95kd. However, several monoclonals directed at the membrane domain of either human or rabbit erythrocyte band 3 consistently identify only a single, smaller protein of ~45kd. It seems unlikely that proteolysis could explain these findings given our experimental conditions. All of the antibodies identify the same group of OMCDi and cortical collecting duct cells on immunocytochemistry, and all label only the basolateral membrane. Thus at present it is not clear whether there are two (or possibly more) band 3-like basolateral membrane proteins of different sizes or if there is only one protein, nor is it clear whether the protein(s) is/are identical to the erythrocyte exchanger in both domains.

Bicarbonate secretion

Unlike OMCDi, the rabbit cortical collecting duct can secrete bicarbonate, particularly if the animal has been loaded with alkali in vivo [1]. Studies by Schwartz et al [8] first suggested that this bicarbonate secretion is mediated by an *apical* membrane chloride/bicarbonate exchanger in a subpopulation of cortical collecting duct cells. Using the pH-sensitive dye 6-carboxyfluorescein, these investigators showed that a group of cells exhibited acidification of cell pH when chloride ions were removed from the tissue bath. These results are most easily explained on the following schema: a chloride gradient into the cell across the apical membrane drives bicarbonate exit out of the cell across the same membrane by chloride/bicarbonate exchange. Schwartz et al noted that such cortical collecting duct cells bind peanut lectin at the apical membrane, an important point as will become evident shortly.

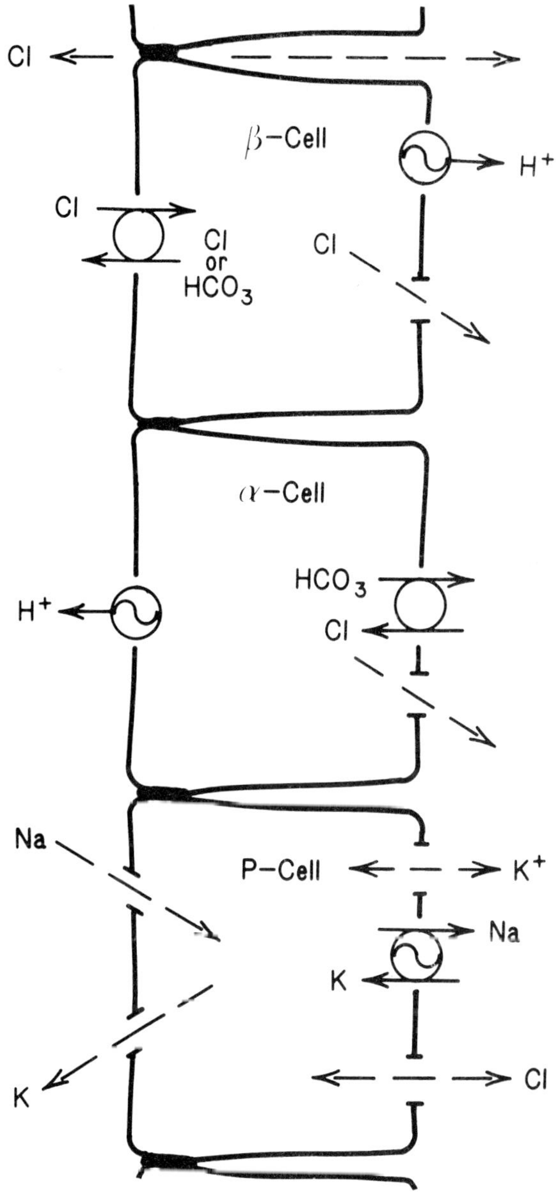

Figure 1. The three cell types identified to date in the rabbit cortical collecting duct. At the top is a beta-cell, or bicarbonate-secreting intercalated cell. The existence of the basolateral H^+-ATPase in rabbit cortical collecting duct is not yet proven. Flux data indicate that the apical exchanger can function in either a chloride/bicarbonate or chloride/chloride exchange mode. In the centre is an alpha-cell, or bicarbonate-absorbing intercalated cell. The cell is modelled after functional data on OMCDi and immunocytochemical data in both cortical collecting duct and OMCDi. At bottom is a principal cell containing apical membrane sodium and potassium conductances

Our laboratory recently examined the chloride dependence of cortical collecting duct bicarbonate secretion. Luminal chloride concentrations were varied and unidirectional bicarbonate secretory rates were then measured. As expected for a carrier-mediated chloride/bicarbonate exchanger, bicarbonate secretion varied as a function of mean luminal chloride concentration with saturation kinetics. The 'epithelial Km' for luminal chloride was about 4–11mM [9] and the V_{max} about 10pmol/mm/min. This rate of chloride/bicarbonate exchange should be noted for comparison later with the rate of chloride self-exchange (below). Further evidence for chloride/bicarbonate exchange has been provided by the experiments of Star et al [10], who showed that net chloride reabsorption varied linearly with bicarbonate secretion.

Our immunocytochemistry studies have suggested that the chloride/bicarbonate exchanger at the apical membrane responsible for chloride-dependent bicarbonate secretion [9] or cell acidification [8] is not the same as the basolateral exchanger responsible for bicarbonate reabsorption by alpha type intercalated cells. Not only does our monoclonal antibody to human erythrocyte band 3 fail to localize to the apical membrane of any cortical collecting duct cells [5] but, as mentioned above, several monoclonals raised recently to the membrane domain of rabbit erythrocyte band 3, as well as a polyclonal antibody to the cytoplasmic domain of human erythrocyte band 2, all immunolabel only the basolateral membrane of rabbit cortical collecting duct cells. With each antibody, the cells labelled are mitochondria-rich, or intercalated cells.

Studies using inhibitors of chloride/bicarbonate exchange, the disulfonic stilbenes, also suggest that the apical membrane chloride/bicarbonate exchanger is different from the basolateral exchanger: the latter is sensitive to stilbenes, whereas the former is not [4,9].

In keeping with the notion that the exchangers are different, it should be noted that we have identified two populations of rabbit cortical collecting duct intercalated cells based on cytochemistry. The alpha cells, as discussed earlier, immunolabel with antibodies to band 3 at the basolateral membrane; these cells do not bind peanut lectin at the apical cell membrane. Another group of cortical collecting duct intercalated cells does bind peanut lectin at the apical membrane but has no band 3 staining. This latter group almost certainly represents the cells responsible for bicarbonate secretion: the distribution of these cells axially along the collecting duct parallels bicarbonate secretory fluxes [5], and the cells noted by Schwartz et al to contain an apical chloride/bicarbonate exchanger bound peanut lectin at the apical membrane [8]. By analogy with the turtle bladder nomenclature, we have termed putative bicarbonate-secreting cells the beta type intercalated cells (Figure 1).

Bicarbonate secretion by cortical collecting ducts is stimulated by cyclic AMP. In testing the two first-messengers known to stimulate cortical collecting duct adenylate cyclase [11], we found that isoprenaline, but not vasopressin stimulated bicarbonate secretion [2]. Because isoprenaline has no effect on cortical collecting duct sodium transport, a principal cell function [12,13], it seems likely that beta-adrenergic receptors are coupled to adenylate cyclase in intercalated cells, especially intercalated cells of the beta type, whereas vasopressin receptors seem most likely coupled to adenylate cyclase in principal cells. This hypothesis remains to be directly tested in separated cortical collecting duct cell populations, however.

Chloride absorption by anion exchange

The cortical collecting duct can absorb chloride against an electrochemical gradient, as first demonstrated by Hanley et al [14]. It seems most likely that this active transport of chloride is mediated by the same chloride/bicarbonate exchange system discussed above for lectin-positive, bicarbonate-secreting, beta type intercalated cells, i.e. by a luminal exchanger. We have measured the lumen-to-bath flux of ^{36}Cl in bicarbonate/carbon dioxide-free and bicarbonate/carbon dioxide-containing solutions and have found that bath (basolateral) bicarbonate/carbon dioxide stimulates the ^{36}Cl flux [15], consistent with chloride absorption via chloride/bicarbonate exchange. Why postulate such an exchanger at the apical membrane? That is, why not model the beta type intercalated cell with a conductive apical chloride entry step and a basolateral chloride/bicarbonate exchanger? Such a cell would certainly demonstrate an increased lumen-to-bath ^{36}Cl flux upon imposing a bath-to-lumen bicarbonate gradient. There are several reasons for modelling this cell as shown in Figure 1. First, Sansom et al [16] have electrophysiologically studied a subpopulation of cortical collecting duct cells differing from principal cells. The cells described are undoubtedly intercalated cells and, given the fact that no conductive pathways for any ions were found at the apical membrane of these cells, chloride tracer entry across the apical membrane would have to occur via an electroneutral pathway. Second, the same investigators showed that these minority cells do have a basolateral chloride conductance [16], suggesting that chloride exit from the cells across that membrane is conductive. Furthermore, as discussed below, our ability to block ^{36}Cl flux by basolateral addition of chloride channel blockers also supports a conductive step at that membrane. Thus, the model of the beta cell shown in Figure 1 appears to be the more likely.

Chloride self-exchange

Related to chloride absorption via chloride/bicarbonate exchange is the interesting phenomenon of chloride self-exchange. Self-exchange occurs when an ion exchange protein transfers one of the same ion species in each of two opposite directions; that is, no net transport occurs. Self-exchange appears to be a general feature of ion hetero-exchangers. For example, the brush-border sodium/hydrogen exchanger can function in a sodium/sodium exchange mode [17], and the erythrocyte band 3 protein can function in a chloride self-exchange mode [18]. Although teleologically futile, self-exchange costs the cell nothing energetically and may represent a necessary structural constraint on such exchangers, i.e. one has to accept a certain degree of self-exchange in order to achieve some hetero-exchange.

Self-exchange can only be appreciated using isotopes so that, for example, one chloride ion can be distinguished from another. Self-exchange has several features. First, the ion tracer flux is much larger than can be accounted for by the measured electrical conductive pathways, i.e. most of the tracer movement is electroneutral. Second, if one monitors unidirectional tracer flux from a cis to a trans compartment (across a cell membrane), removal of non-tracer ion from the trans compartment will eliminate tracer movement from cis to trans. Third, a large unidirectional tracer flux is found to be accompanied by no measurable net flux.

All three of these features have been observed for chloride transport by the rabbit cortical collecting duct. Stoner et al first showed that the calculated partial ionic conductance for chloride, derived from the lumen-to-bath chloride tracer flux, was several times larger than the total measured transepithelial conductance [19]. In other words, the epithelium did not have a high enough electrical conductance to allow for the chloride tracer flux. We have confirmed this observation many times in our laboratory. In an extensive series of additional experiments we defined conditions that produced chloride self-exchange: bicarbonate/carbon dioxide-free solutions minimized chloride/bicarbonate exchange, and amiloride added to the perfusate clamped the transepithelial voltage near zero [20]. Under these conditions we demonstrated two more features of self exchange: 1) a substantial lumen-to-bath ^{36}Cl tracer flux was associated with no measurable net chloride flux, and 2) substitution of gluconate for chloride in the basolateral solution substantially lowered the lumen-to-bath ^{36}Cl flux [20]. In fact, varying the basolateral chloride concentration altered the lumen-to-bath ^{36}Cl flux with saturation kinetics [9]. The latter of these two properties allows us to operationally define the magnitude of chloride self-exchange: self-exchange is that lumen-to-bath ^{36}Cl flux which is inhibited by bath (trans) chloride removal. We presume that the remainder of the ^{36}Cl flux occurs by diffusion, presumably via the paracellular pathway.

Having established the presence of chloride self-exchange, we next studied several aspects in more detail. We found that the overall process of chloride self-exchange was inhibited when blockers of chloride channels, such as anthracene-9-carboxylate and diphenylamine carboxylate were added to the basolateral solutions [21]. This suggested that chloride tracer movement across the basolateral membrane occurred via a conductive pathway. Because the overall process of ion self-exchange across an epithelium requires only that there be an ion exchanger at one of the two cell membranes (the ion transfer step at the series membrane can occur via any mechanism, including conductive), these experiments with chloride channel blockers suggested that the cell be modelled with an apical anion exchanger in series with a basolateral chloride conductance.

Such a cell model for chloride self-exchange is similar to that of the beta intercalated cell described above for chloride/bicarbonate exchange. Indeed, as we continued to investigate chloride self-exchange we found that it has many properties in common with bicarbonate secretion via chloride/bicarbonate exchange. Both processes are stimulated by cyclic AMP, share the same 'first messenger' (isoprenaline), are insensitive to 0.1mM DIDS, are stimulated by alkali-loading and inhibited by acid-loading the animal, are inhibited by acetazolamide, are unaffected by ouabain, and are sensitive to exogenous bicarbonate/carbon dioxide [9,10,12,15,20].

For these reasons it seems likely that chloride self-exchange and chloride/bicarbonate exchange (bicarbonate secretion) represent alternative modes of operation of the same anion exchanger. In this regard, it is of interest to consider estimates of turnover rates for such an exchanger in the chloride/bicarbonate versus chloride/chloride exchange modes. Under experimental conditions optimal for chloride/bicarbonate exchange (lumen-to-bath chloride gradient and bath-to-lumen bicarbonate gradient) we found a 'V_{max}' for chloride/bicarbonate exchange of about 10pmol/mm/min [9]. In contrast, the 'V_{max}' for chloride self-exchange varies from 50 to 400pmol/mm/min [20, and unpublished observations]. Thus, assuming that both processes occur on the same anion exchange protein, these data suggest that the exchanger 'turns over' 5–40 times as often in the chloride self-exchange mode as in the chloride/bicarbonate exchange mode. It should be emphasized that these relative turnover rates may only apply to the experimental conditions used, and may be quite different in vivo where luminal chloride concentrations are not over 100mM and luminal bicarbonate concentrations may be higher than zero. Nonetheless it appears that chloride self-exchange represents a major mode of action of the anion exchanger.

Another interesting feature of chloride/bicarbonate versus chloride/chloride exchange emerges from studies on the effect of acute bicarbonate/carbon dioxide addition on the lumen-to-bath ^{36}Cl flux. In one set of experiments we used chloride-free basolateral solutions and simultaneously measured the bath-to-lumen bicarbonate secretory rate, the lumen-to-bath ^{36}Cl flux, and the transepithelial conductance (with principal cell cellular conductances blocked by luminal amiloride and barium). In this way we were able to eliminate chloride self-exchange and could assess conductive chloride absorption via diffusion as well as chloride absorption via electroneutral chloride/bicarbonate exchange. Under these conditions we found that acute isohydric replacement of HEPES-buffered solutions with bicarbonate/carbon dioxide-buffered solutions stimulated chloride absorption via chloride/bicarbonate exchange by about 5–10pmol/mm/min [9]. This manoeuvre also increased chloride absorption via a conductive (diffusive) pathway by about 10pmol/mm/min. These experiments were also done with chloride present in the basolateral solution, so that much of the (now larger) lumen-to-bath ^{36}Cl flux occurred via chloride self-exchange. Under these conditions, acute replacement of basolateral HEPES by bicarbonate/carbon dioxide solutions caused a total increase in the lumen-to-bath ^{36}Cl flux of about 35–100pmol/mm/min [15, and unpublished]. Assuming that the presence of chloride in the basolateral solution in this second set of experiments did not alter the effect of bicarbonate/carbon dioxide on chloride diffusion or chloride/bicarbonate exchange (as determined previously in the absence of bath chloride), then it would appear, by adding up the various fluxes, that bicarbonate/carbon dioxide stimulates chloride self-exchange by 25–80pmol/mm/min. Recent experiments using carbon dioxide pulses in HEPES solutions without bicarbonate added have shown a similar stimulation of chloride self-exchange (unpublished). Because bicarbonate is generated whenever carbon dioxide is added to a solution (including cytoplasm), it is not possible to determine at present whether the bicarbonate ion per se, or perhaps an accompanying change in cell pH represents the intracellular signal stimulating chloride self-exchange. Preliminary experiments aimed at altering cell pH with potassium-nigericin in the absence of carbon dioxide (and thus bicarbonate) indicate that there is a direct correlation between predicted cell pH and the lumen-to-bath ^{36}Cl flux [unpublished]. Complete elucidation of the intracellular modifers of chloride self-exchange will require measurement of cell pH; these studies are currently in progress. Nonetheless, the data to date strongly suggest that the apical membrane chloride/bicarbonate or chloride/chloride exchanger is modulated by one or more intracellular signals such as bicarbonate or hydrogen concentration. Such modulation may play a rôle in altering the stoichiometry of chloride/bicarbonate versus chloride/chloride exchange, or may affect the absolute turnover rate of the exchanger without changing the stoichiometry. These and other possibilities will require further investigation.

The issue of polarity reversal

Because the rabbit cortical collecting duct can either secrete or reabsorb bicarbonate, and because the models of alpha and beta intercalated cells are 'mirror images', at least in terms of chloride/bicarbonate exchangers and proton pumps (see Figure 1), the question arises as to whether alpha and beta type intercalated cells might be interchangeable manifestations of a common pluri-potent intercalated cell. Indeed, data from Schwartz et al [8] have suggested that beta intercalated cells can convert into alpha intercalated cells upon acid-loading the animal. This conclusion is based upon defining alpha cells functionally as those that endocytose macromolecules from the lumen (presumably as part of an endo-exo-cytosis process characteristic of H^+ ATPases), and upon defining beta cells as those that bind peanut lectin at the apical cell membrane. Upon acid-loading, the number of endocytosing cells increased by the same amount as the decrease in lectin-binding cells, suggesting that there had been a one-for-one shift in the distribution of the two cell types. These authors concluded from these results that acid-loading had induced the beta cell to convert into an alpha cell [8].

As discussed above, several lines of evidence raise questions about the notion of such 'polarity reversal'. First, no antibody to band 3 in any species applied to kidney from any species or to turtle bladder has yet been reported in the literature or observed by us to immunolabel the apical membrane of mitochondria-rich cells [5,6,22, unpublished observations]. This accumulating evidence with antibodies against multiple different epitopes of band 3 argues that the beta cell apical chloride/bicarbonate exchanger is not identical with alpha cell basolateral chloride/bicarbonate exchanger. Second, as discussed above the apical versus basolateral anion exchange processes appear to have different sensitivities to disulfonic stilbenes.

Third, we recently used the principle of chloride self-exchange to ask whether alpha intercalated cells can convert to beta cells upon being stimulated by metabolic alkalosis. Because the OMCDi segment represents essentially a pure population of alpha-type cells, we studied OMCDi. We found that OMCDi from normal rabbits demonstrated no evidence for transepithelial chloride self-exchange or chloride/bicarbonate exchange [23]. We previously presented evidence for the existence of a basolateral chloride/bicarbonate exchanger in alpha cells. Because, as discussed above, self-exchange across a two-membrane epithelium only requires one anion exchanger in series with some ion transport step, the absence of transepithelial chloride self-exchange in OMCDi indicates that there must be no route for ^{36}Cl movement across the apical membrane of OMCDi alpha cells. If there were, transepithelial ^{36}Cl flux should have been altered by basolateral bicarbonate or chloride removal. Because the lumen-to-bath ^{36}Cl flux is such a sensitive indicator of an apical anion exchanger, these negative results in OMCDi from normal rabbits strongly suggest the absence of an apical anion exchanger in OMCDi alpha cells.

We then produced metabolic alkalosis in rabbits by treatment with frusemide, desoxycorticosterone, and drinking water containing bicarbonate ions. We reasoned that such an alkalosis, as opposed to merely alkali loading, might constitute a signal strong enough to induce an apical chloride/bicarbonate exchanger in alpha cells, i.e. polarity reversal. This was not observed [23] as judged by ^{36}Cl fluxes. OMCDi from these alkalotic rabbits showed no evidence for induction of either chloride self-exchange or chloride/bicarbonate exchange. Additionally, immunocytochemical studies showed no band 3 labellings at the apical membrane of any intercalated cells.

These results can be interpreted in several ways. It may be that our stimulus was insufficient to induce polarity reversal. Alternatively, it may be that alpha cells cannot convert into beta cells, or that OMCDi alpha cells are not the same as cortical collecting duct alpha cells. The interpretation most in line with our stilbene inhibitor and immunocytochemistry data, however, is that intercalated cells do not reverse their polarity. If so, the bicarbonate secretion versus bicarbonate absorption by the cortical collecting duct in response to metabolic perturbations could occur by differential stimulation and suppression of function of each of two different cell types whose polarity is fixed [5]. The proof of the presence or absence of polarity reversal will require application of more sophisticated tools of cell biology such as in situ hybridization using cDNA probes for band 3. If no mRNA for band 3 were to ever appear in bicarbonate-secreting intercalated cells, it would seem very unlikely that the apical chloride/bicarbonate exchanger functionally identified in such cells represents some post-translationally modified, immunologically-unreactive version of band 3. Such studies are currently underway in the author's laboratory.

Summary

In conclusion, the rabbit cortical collecting duct absorbs or secretes bicarbonate via two types of intercalated cells termed alpha and beta respectively. Both cells contain chloride/bicarbonate exchangers, though several lines of evidence suggest that the exchangers are distinct proteins. The beta cell chloride/bicarbonate exchanger serves to reabsorb chloride from the lumen into the cell, whereupon it exits into the blood via a chloride channel. The beta cell chloride/bicarbonate exchanger can also function in a chloride self-exchange mode, and is controlled acutely by bicarbonate/carbon dioxide and cyclic AMP and chronically by acid-base conditions in vivo. Future investigations will be directed at describing the function and control of these anion exchangers at the molecular level.

Acknowledgments

Work in the author's laboratory was supported by NIH grants DK 01343 and DK 25231, and by the American Heart and Veterans Administration.

References

1 McKinney TD, Burg MB. Bicarbonate transport by rabbit cortical collecting tubules. Effect of acid and alkali load in vivo on transport in vitro. *J Clin Invest 1977; 60:* 766–768

2 Schuster VL. Cyclic adenosine monophosphate-stimulated bicarbonate secretion in rabbit cortical collecting tubules. *J Clin Invest 1985; 75:* 2056–2064

3 Steinmetz PR. Cellular organization of urinary acidification. *Am J Physiol 1986; 251 (Renal Fluid Electrolyte Physiol 20):* F173–F187

4 Stone DK, Seldin DW, Kokko JP, Jacobson HR. Anion dependence of medullary collecting duct acidification. *J Clin Invest 1983; 71:* 1505–1508

5 Schuster VL, Bonsib SM, Jennings ML. Two types of collecting duct mitochondria-rich (intercalated) cells: lectin and band 3 cytochemistry. *Am J Physiol 1986; 251 (Cell Physiol 20):* C347–C355

6 Drenckhahn D, Schluter K, Allen DP, Bennett V. Colocalization of band 3 with ankyrin and spectrin at the basal membrane of intercalated cells in the rat kidney. *Science Wash DC 1985; 230:* 1287–1289

7 Stetson DL, Steinmetz PR. α and β types of carbonic anhydrase-rich cells in turtle bladder. *Am J Physiol 1985; 249 (Renal Fluid Electrolyte Physiol 18):* F553–F565

8 Schwartz GJ, Barasch J, Al-Awqati Q. Plasticity of functional epithelial polarity. *Nature 1985; 318:* 368–371

9 Schuster VL. Cyclic adenosine monophosphate-stimulated anion transport in rabbit cortical collecting duct. Kinetics, stoichiometry, and conductive pathways. *J Clin Invest 1986; 78:* 1621–1630

10 Star RA, Burg MB, Knepper MA. Bicarbonate secretion and chloride absorption by rabbit cortical collecting ducts. Role of chloride/bicarbonate exchange. *J Clin Invest 1985; 76:* 1123–1130

11 Morel F, Chabardes D. Functional segmentation of the nephron. In Seldin DW, Giebisch G, eds. *The Kidney: Physiology and Pathophysiology.* New York: Raven Press. 1985: 519–530

12 Schuster VL, Stokes JB. Cl transport by the cortical and outer medullary collecting duct. *Am J Physiol 1987: 253 (Renal Fluid Electrolyte Physiol 22):* in press

13 Iino Y, Troy JL, Brenner BM. Effects of catecholamines on electrolyte transport in cortical collecting tubule. *J Membr Biol 1981; 61:* 67–73

14 Hanley MJ, Kokko JP, Gross JB, Jacobson HR. Electrophysiologic study of the cortical collecting tubule of the rabbit. *Kidney Int 1980; 17:* 74–81

15 Tago K, Schuster VL, Stokes JB. Stimulation of chloride transport by HCO_3-CO_2 in rabbit cortical collecting tubule. *Am J Physiol 1986; 251 (Renal Fluid Electrolyte Physiol 20):* F49–F56

16 Sansom S, Muto S, Giebisch G. Microelectrode assessment of conductive properties of 'minority cells' of the rabbit cortical collecting duct (Abstract). *Federation Proc 1986; 45:* 541

17 Kinsiella JL, Aronson PS. Interaction of NH_4 and Li with the renal microvillus membrane Na-H exchanger. *Am J Physiol 1981; 24 (Cell Physiol 10):* C220–C226

18 Lowe AG, Lambert A. Chloride-bicarbonate exchange and related transport processes. *Biochim Biophys Acta 1983; 694:* 353–374

19 Stoner LC, Burg MB, Orloff J. Ion transport in cortical collecting tubule; effect of amiloride. *Am J Physiol 1974; 227:* 453–459

20 Tago K, Schuster VL, Stokes JB. Regulation of Cl self exchange by cAMP in cortical collecting tubule. *Am J Physiol 1986; 251 (Renal Fluid Electrolyte Physiol 20):* F40–F48

21 Tago K, Warden DW, Schuster VL, Stokes JB. Effects of inhibitors of Cl conductance on Cl self-exchange in rabbit cortical collecting tubule. *Am J Physiol 1986; 251 (Renal Fluid Electrolyte Physiol 20):* F1007–F1009

22 Drenckhahn D, Oelmann M, Schaaf P et al. Band 3 is the basolateral anion exchanger of dark epithelial cells of turtle urinary bladder. *Am J Physiol 1987; 252 (Cell Physiol 21):* C570–C574

23 Hayashi M, Schuster VL, Stokes JB. Chloride transport by rabbit medullary collecting tubule: contrasts with the cortical segment (Abstract). *Federation Proc 1987; 46:* 1285

CORTICAL COLLECTING DUCT CATION TRANSPORT

E Schlatter, J A Schafer*

Albert-Ludwigs-Universität, Physiologisches Institut, Freiburg, FRG
**Nephrology Research and Training Center, University of Alabama at Birmingham, Birmingham, Alabama, USA*

The cortical collecting duct of the mammalian kidney is an important site for the regulation of the excretion of cations such as sodium and potassium. The reabsorption of sodium and secretion of potassium is stimulated by hormones such as mineralocorticoids [1–4] and antidiuretic hormone [3–6]. Aldosterone increases both sodium and potassium transport in the rabbit and the rat, the two species studied most. In the rabbit the effect of antidiuretic hormone (ADH) on sodium reabsorption is transient [7] and no effect of ADH on potassium secretion has been found [8]. In the rat, however, the stimulatory effect of ADH on sodium and potassium transport is sustained over several hours. The enhancement of sodium and potassium transport in the cortical collecting duct of the rat by ADH is much greater when the animals are pretreated with the synthetic aldosterone analogue desoxycorticosterone (DOC) for several days.

This article will summarize the recent evidence regarding the mechanisms involved in cation transport in the cortical portion of the collecting duct and its possible regulation. Ion flux studies and electrophysiological measurements in the isolated perfused cortical collecting tubule will be discussed. Special emphasis will be placed on tubules from DOC-treated rats, because sodium and potassium transport rates are high and maximally stimulated under these conditions.

Fluxes of sodium and potassium

Table I summarizes the net sodium, potassium and rubidium transport rates, obtained from sodium and potassium chemical determinations and unidirectional isotopic fluxes, and transepithelial voltages for tubules from normal and DOC-treated rats [3–6]. The table also shows the stimulatory effect of ADH in the two groups of animals. In tubules dissected from normal animals there is no significant net absorption of sodium or secretion of potassium either measured as net potassium fluxes or unidirectional rubidium fluxes; in addition the transepithelial potential is only slightly lumen negative, indicating a very low active transport activity under these conditions. Addition of ADH to the bathing

TABLE I. Effects of desoxycorticosterone (DOC) and antidiuretic hormone (ADH) on net transport of sodium, potassium and rubidium (J_{Na}, J_K, J_{Rb}) and on transepithelial voltage (PD_{te}) in the rat cortical collecting tubule

	net J_{Na}	net J_K	net J_{Rb}	PD_{te}
		pmol mm^{-1} sec^{-1}		mV
Normal	−2 to 0.2	0	− 3	− 1
Normal + ADH	20		− 8	− 6 to − 8
DOC	14 to 35	−2	−14	− 4 to −13
DOC + ADH	58 to 110	−17	−42	−26 to −39

Data are taken from references 3–6

solution increases reversibly all three variables within a few minutes. In tubules dissected from DOC-treated rats the sodium, potassium and rubidium transport rates and transepithelial voltages in the absence of ADH are similar to those in tubules from normal rats in the presence of ADH. Addition of ADH to these DOC-treated tubules, however, leads to a much greater increase in all three variables compared to the ADH effects in tubules from normal rats. Thus, both hormones, the synthetic mineralocorticoid DOC after chronic application and ADH acutely, increase sodium reabsorption and potassium secretion independently in the rat cortical collecting duct. The enhanced effects induced by the combination of both hormones indicates not only additivity but even a synergistic action on these cation transport processes.

Figure 1 shows the effect of ADH on the unidirectional sodium fluxes in normal and DOC-treated animals. Concomitant with the increase in the lumen to bath flux of sodium produced by ADH, the lumen negative voltage increases markedly. In the rabbit a similar enhancement of sodium and potassium transport and transepithelial voltage is observed in tubules dissected from DOC-treated animals compared to those from normal rabbits [1,2,8–10]. ADH, however, only transiently increases sodium reabsorption and transepithelial voltage followed by a sustained inhibition below control levels, presumably due to stimulated prostaglandin production [7,8,10]. In both species sodium reabsorption and transepithelial voltage are sensitive to ouabain in the bath [6, 10,11]. The lumen negative voltage and the net sodium reabsorption (see Figure 1) can also be abolished with low doses (10μM) of luminal amiloride [3,12–14]. These findings suggest a model for sodium reabsorption in the cortical collecting duct with a basolateral Na/K-ATPase as primary active process and an apical sodium conductance. On the other hand, the net potassium secretion induced by ADH or DOC is sensitive to luminal barium [6]. The lumen negative transepithelial voltage hyperpolarizes with luminal barium (2–3mM) and depolarizes with bath barium (2–4mM) [5,6,14], suggesting the presence of potassium conductances in both cell membranes which would allow for the variable rates of potassium secretion seen in the rat.

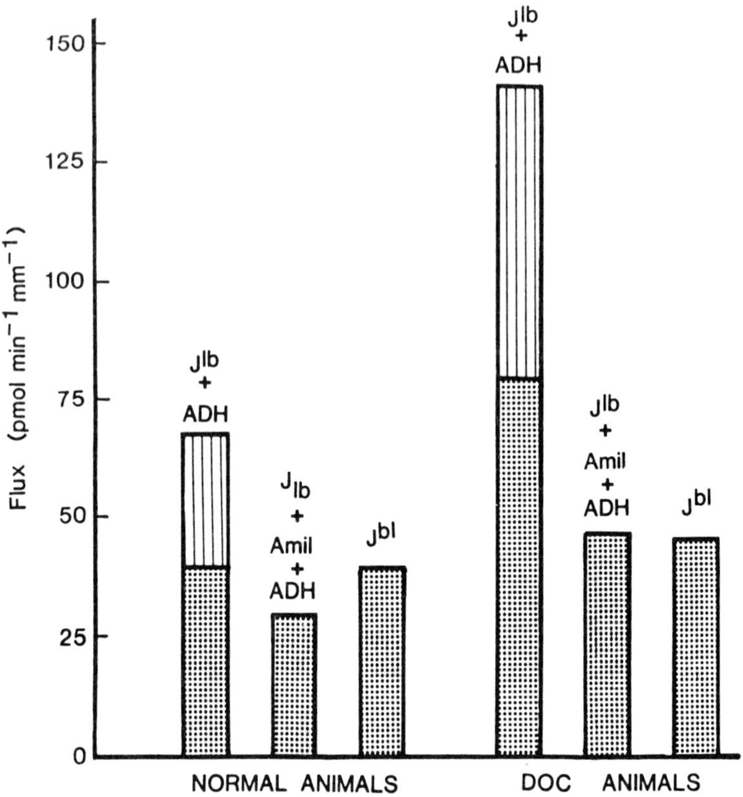

Figure 1. Unidirectional sodium fluxes (J_{lb}=lumen to bath, J_{bl}=bath to lumen) in tubules from normal and DOC-treated animals. Fluxes are shown in the absence (dotted areas) and presence (striped areas) of ADH. The second column of each group shows the inhibition of the lumen to bath flux by luminal amiloride ($10\mu M$) in the presence of ADH

Discrimination of different cell types

The cortical collecting duct of the rat and the rabbit consists of two distinct cell populations, the principal cells and one or more types of intercalated cells. The sodium and potassium transport is thought to occur through the principal cells, whereas the intercalated cells seem to be involved in hydrogen and bicarbonate transport [15,16]. It is possible to distinguish the two cell types optically using light microscopy with a contrast-enhancing procedure such as Hoffman modulation at 400X magnification. In addition, differences in functional parameters, such as opposite responses of the membrane voltages and fractional resistances upon addition of luminal amiloride or bath ADH can be used for cell discrimination, as recently described in detail for the rat cortical collecting duct [14].

Basolateral membrane

Sodium reabsorption and transepithelial voltage are sensitive to ouabain. The principal cells are most likely the only cells involved in this sodium reabsorption and are responsible for developing the lumen negative transepithelial voltage. Thus, inhibition of the Na/K-ATPase by ouabain should also lead to a depolarization of the basolateral membrane in these cells as is typical for many other preparations. Figure 2 shows the effect of 0.5mM ouabain on the basolateral

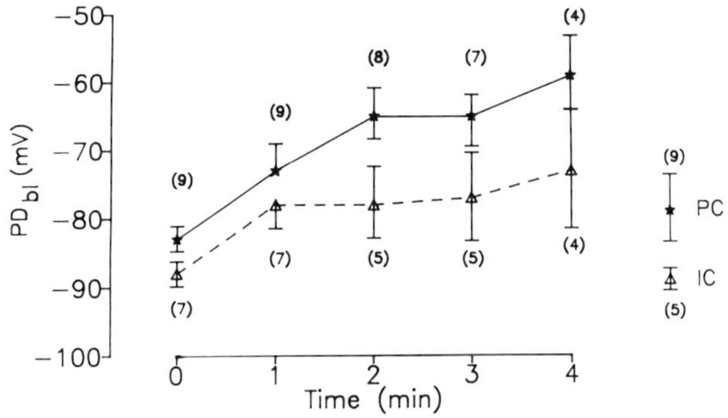

Figure 2. Effect of ouabain (0.5mM, bath, added at time 0) on basolateral membrane potential (PD_{bl}) in principal (PC) and intercalated (IC) cells of rat cortical collecting tubules. The data points on the right of the graph are values after return to control conditions by removal of ouabain from the bath. Mean ± SEM, (n)=number of cells

membrane voltage in both principal and intercalated cells of the isolated perfused rat cortical collecting duct. In both cell types ouabain slowly and reversibly depolarizes the basolateral membrane. The depolarization of the principal cells is greater than in the intercalated cells, possibly indicating a lower Na/K-ATPase activity in the latter cell type. A lower Na/K-ATPase activity in the intercalated cells is consistent with the hypothesis that transepithelial sodium and potassium transport occurs primarily through the principal cells. On the other hand, the presence of the Na/K-ATPase in the basolateral membrane of the intercalated cells is also indicated by their depolarization. Whether this Na/K-ATPase activity is involved in any transcellular ion transport or serves only as a volume regulatory mechanism is an interesting aspect for further examination.

As reported for the rabbit cortical collecting duct [17,18] the basolateral membrane of the principal cells in the rat is also conductive to potassium [14]. However, in contrast to the rabbit, in the rat there is no evidence for a chloride conductance parallel to the potassium conductance in this membrane. The basolateral potassium conductance which has a transference number of 1 in the rat [14] allows potassium to recycle across that membrane. This conductive pathway for potassium is sensitive to barium [6,14] and is also essential to maintain maximal rates of sodium reabsorption [6]. Blocking of this basolateral potassium conductance with barium reduces the unidirectional sodium flux from lumen to bath and thus also the net sodium reabsorption. This is consistent with potassium recycling across the basolateral membrane being necessary to maintain maximal Na/K pump turnover rates and the driving force for the sodium reabsorption.

Basolateral potassium conductance appears to be linked to the Na/K-ATPase in some way because inhibition of the pump reduces this potassium conductance,

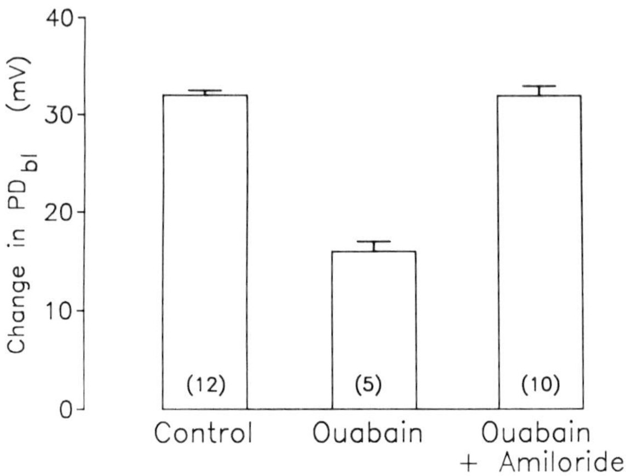

Figure 3. The effect of a potassium concentration step from 5 to 20mM in the bath, on the basolateral membrane voltage (PD_{bl}). Plotted here are the changes of PD_{bl} in control conditions and when ouabain (0.5mM, bath) or ouabain + amiloride (10μM, lumen) were present. Mean ± SEM, (n)=number of cells

as shown in Figure 3 for the rat cortical collecting duct. In this figure the depolarization of the basolateral membrane that is observed when the bath potassium concentration is increased from 5 to 20mM is compared under different conditions. Under control conditions this depolarization amounts to 32mV but is reduced to 16mV in the presence of ouabain. When amiloride (10μM) is added to the lumen before ouabain the depolarization induced by a potassium concentration step change is still identical to that under control conditions. Therefore, the link between the Na/K-ATPase and the basolateral potassium conductance is not the pump rate itself, because stopping the pump by inhibiting the apical sodium entry with amiloride does not change the depolarization induced by the potassium concentration step. Amiloride also prevents the depolarization induced by the potassium concentration step. Amiloride also prevents the depolarization of the basolateral membrane observed in the presence of ouabain alone [14]. Possible candidates for the link between potassium uptake via the pump and recycling across the basolateral membrane are the membrane voltage or the cellular potassium activity. In the presence of ouabain alone the basolateral membrane is depolarized, whereas it stays hyperpolarized in the presence of ouabain and amiloride. Cellular potassium activity may be low after ouabain and unchanged or even higher when ouabain and amiloride are present.

Apical membrane

In both the rabbit and the rat cortical collecting duct the apical membrane has sodium and potassium conductances [14,19]. These conductances are increased by DOC treatment of the animal for several days [20]. The apical potassium channel of the rabbit cortical collecting duct is Ca^{++}, pH, and voltage sensitive [19,21], i.e. its conductance or open probability is reduced with luminal acidification, increased at higher intracellular Ca^{++} levels, and increased by membrane depolarization. In the DOC-treated rat the apical membrane is predominantly potassium conductive [14], with a transference number for potassium of 0.73. This large apical potassium conductance is probably the major route for potassium secretion. The amiloride sensitive transepithelial conductance increases with ADH and the potassium transference number is reduced to 0.5 indicating that the sodium conductance, which probably is the only other sizeable conductance in this membrane, is increased relative to the potassium conductance. The apical sodium conductance seems to be the only pathway for sodium to enter the principal cell since 10μM amiloride is sufficient to prevent the ouabain-induced depolarization of the basolateral membrane [14]. If there were an amiloride insensitive pathway for sodium entry, that entry would depolarize the basolateral membrane during inhibition of the pump by ouabain. In addition, 10μM amiloride abolishes the lumen negative potential difference [3,14] and completely inhibits net sodium reabsorption [3]. The latter effect would not be expected if there were another pathway for sodium reabsorption such as an electroneutral NaCl cotransport system.

Effects of ADH on principal cells

ADH (20nM) enhances sodium reabsorption and potassium secretion in the normal and DOC-treated rat [3,5,6]. The lumen negative transepithelial potential increases concomitantly with a 20 to 25% decrease in the transepithelial resistance. Table II summarizes the effects of ADH in the rat cortical collecting

TABLE II. Effects of ADH and luminal amiloride (10μM) on electrophysiological properties of rat CCT principal cells

Condition	PD_{te}	R_{te}	PD_a	FR_a
	mV	Ωcm^2	mV	
−ADH	− 4.9±0.8	55±5	78±1	0.72±0.04
+ADH	−17.1±1.6	40±3	65±2	0.67±0.05
+ADH + amiloride	+ 1.2±0.4	62±6	85±1	0.86±0.04
(n)	29	20	25	9

Mean ± SEM. All differences in this table between + and − ADH or + and − amiloride are significant ($p<0.05$) on a paired basis.

duct from DOC-treated animals. The increase in the lumen negative voltage is due to the depolarization of the apical membrane which exceeds by far that of the basolateral membrane and is expected if ADH increases the sodium conductance of the apical membrane; thus the fractional resistance of the basolateral membrane would be reduced. Table II also demonstrates that 10μM amiloride in the lumen inhibits all of the baseline and ADH-enhanced lumen-negative transepithelial voltage. The slightly positive transepithelial voltage seen in the presence of amiloride is probably due to hydrogen ion secretion or bicarbonate reabsorption by the intercalated cells. With amiloride, the transepithelial and fractional apical membrane resistances are markedly increased to above baseline values. The apical membrane voltage in the presence of luminal amiloride is dominated by the potassium equilibrium potential across that membrane. These effects of ADH on the apical membrane voltage and resistance of the principal cell are consistent with an increase in the apical membrane sodium conductance.

If ADH primarily increases the sodium conductance of the apical membrane, the above described effects of ADH should be inhibited by luminal amiloride but not by luminal barium. This is indeed the case as demonstrated in Figure 4.

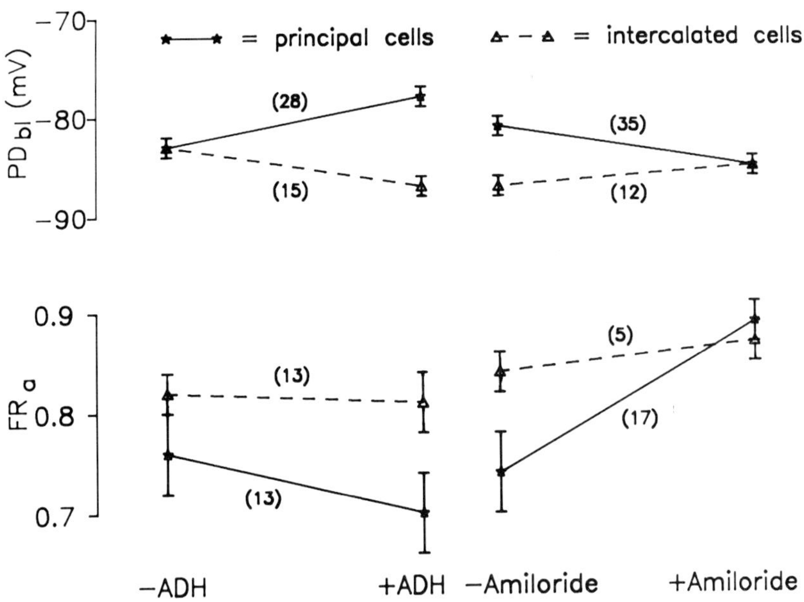

Figure 4. Comparison of the effects of ADH on transepithelial (PD_{te}), apical membrane voltage (PD_a), and fractional resistance of the apical membrane (FR_a) in the presence of either luminal amiloride (10μM) or luminal barium (3mM). Mean ± SEM, (n)=number of tubules or cells

Addition of amiloride to the lumen prior to the addition of ADH to the bath prevents the increase in the lumen negative potential, the depolarization of the apical membrane and the decrease of the fractional resistance of that membrane. After removal of the inhibitor all three variables change in the expected direction. Depolarization of the apical membrane after removal of amiloride, when ADH had been present for several minutes together with the amiloride, is faster compared to ADH addition under control conditions with no amiloride present [14]. This result most likely indicates that ADH activates sodium channels in the apical membrane even in the presence of amiloride, but that the channels are blocked immediately by the inhibitor. After the removal of amiloride there are already more active sodium channels present leading to faster membrane depolarization.

In contrast to the situation with luminal amiloride, luminal barium does not prevent the ADH-induced changes of transepithelial and apical membrane voltages and fractional apical membrane resistance. Since there is also no ADH-induced decrease in the transepithelial resistance when luminal amiloride is present [14], ADH apparently does not change the shunt resistance, the apical potassium conductance of the principal cells or the cellular resistance of the intercalated cells significantly.

Mechanism and regulation of cation transport

The basic mechanisms involved in the cation transport across the principal cells of the cortical collecting duct are similar in the rat and the rabbit. A model for the transport pathways in this cell type is shown in Figure 5. Sodium reabsorption is driven by the activity of the ouabain-sensitive basolateral Na/K-ATPase. The sodium-pump keeps the cellular sodium activity low which provides the driving force for sodium to enter the cell across the amiloride sensitive sodium channel in the apical membrane. Potassium recycles across the barium-sensitive basolateral potassium conductance and also leaves the cell across the barium-sensitive apical potassium conductance, which we assume is the route for net potassium secretion.

The sustained stimulation of both sodium and potassium transport rates by ADH in the rat cortical collecting duct can be explained entirely by a primary increase in the apical sodium conductance, presumably mediated via cAMP. The increase in the apical sodium conductance leads to depolarization predominantly of the apical membrane. The increased sodium entry would then in turn increase the pump rate of the Na/K-ATPase. Because the apical membrane is depolarized to a greater extent than the basolateral membrane, the secretory exit of potassium from the cell across the apical membrane would be increased. This increase in the driving force for the potassium secretory flux could be sufficient to explain the observed increase in net potassium secretion in the presence of ADH without involving an additional change in the apical potassium conductance. The difference in the net transport rates between sodium and potassium is electrically

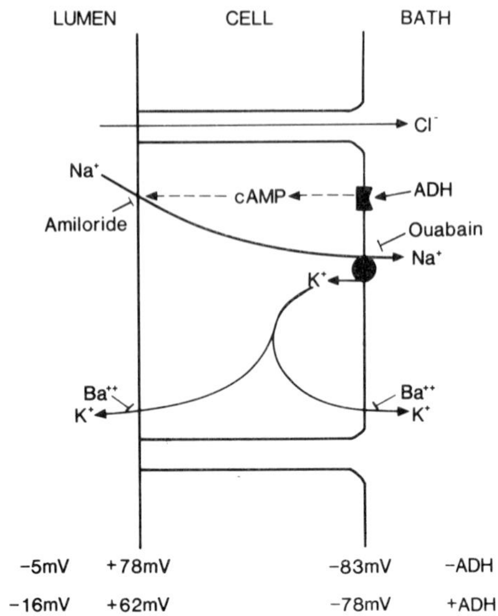

Figure 5. Model for cation transport across the principal cells of the rat cortical collecting tubule. Voltages shown are referenced to the bath. Modified after Figure 14 from [14]
active transport;
diffusion;
interaction of cAMP;
inhibitor;
ADH receptor

compensated by the movement of chloride across the paracellular shunt which, although not very selective for anions over cations, has a comparably high conductance [14,21].

With this model for the principal cell, cation transport in the cortical collecting duct can be explained without involving the intercalated cells. Whether those cells also contribute to the cation transport other than hydrogen ion secretion is not yet known. The reasons for the differences in cortical collecting duct cation transport between the rat and the rabbit especially in their response to ADH is also an important topic for future investigations.

Acknowledgments
The authors acknowledge the expert assistance of SL Troutman and SK Williams in the work cited from the authors' laboratory. Parts of the authors' work were presented at the 19th ASN meeting, Washington DC 1986 and at the 71st FASEB meeting in Washington DC 1987, and is in press in Pflügers Archiv [14]. Dr E Schlatter was recipient of a Fogarty International Fellowship from the NIH No.1-F05-TWO3748-01. This work was also supported in part by NIH Research Grant DK-25519.

References

1 Schwartz GJ, Burg MB. Mineralocorticoid effects on cation transport by cortical collecting tubules in vitro. *Am J Physiol 1978; 235:* F576–F585

2 O'Neil RG, Helman SI. Transport characteristics of renal collecting tubules: influences of DOCA and diet. *Am J Physiol 1977; 233:* F544–F558

3 Reif MC, Troutman SL, Schafer JA. Sodium transport by rat cortical collecting tubule. Effects of vasopressin and desoxycorticosterone. *J Clin Invest 1986; 77:* 1291–1298

4 Tomita K, Pisano J, Knepper MA. Control of sodium and potassium transport in the cortical collecting duct of the rat. Effects of bradykinin, vasopressin, and desoxycorticosterone. *J Clin Invest 1985; 76:* 132–136

5 Schafer JA, Troutman SL. Effect of ADH on rubidium transport in isolated perfused rat cortical collecting tubules. *Am J Physiol 1986; 250:* F1063–1072

6 Schafer JA, Troutman SL. Potassium transport in cortical collecting tubules from mineralocorticoid-treated rats. ADH increases Rb^+ secretory flux. *Am J Physiol 1987; 253:* in press

7 Frindt G, Burg MD. Effect of vasopressin on sodium transport in renal cortical collecting tubules. *Kidney Int 1972; 1:* 224–231

8 Holt WF, Lechene C. ADH-PGE_2 interactions in cortical collecting tubule. Depression of sodium transport. *Am J Physiol 1981; 241:* F452–F460

9 Stokes JB, Ingram MJ, Williams AD, Ingram D. Heterogeneity of the rabbit collecting tubule: localization of mineralocorticoid hormone action to the cortical position. *Kidney Int 1981; 20:* 340–347

10 Schuster VL. Bradykinin and vasopressin actions on rabbit cortical collecting tubule: mechanism of their interaction and effects on Na transport. *Am J Physiol 1987:* in press

11 Stokes JB. Na and K transport across the cortical and outer medullary collecting tubule of the rabbit: evidence for diffusion across the outer medullary portion. *Am J Physiol 1982; 242:* F514–F520

12 Stokes JB. Pathways of K^+ permeation across the rabbit cortical collecting tubule: effect of amiloride. *Am J Physiol 1984; 246:* F457–F466

13 Helman SI, O'Neil R. Model of active transepithelial Na and K transport of renal collecting tubules. *Am J Physiol 1977; 233:* F559–F571

14 Schlatter E, Schafer JA. Electrophysiological studies in principal cells of rat cortical collecting tubules. ADH increases the apical membrane Na^+-conductance. *Pfluegers Arch:* in press

15 Stokes JB. Ion transport by the cortical and outer medullary collecting tubule. *Kidney Int 1982; 22:* 473–484

16 O'Neil RG, Hayhurst RA. Functional differentiation of cell types of cortical collecting duct. *Am J Physiol 1985; 248:* F449–F453

17 Sansom SC, O'Neil RG. Effects of mineralocorticoids on transport properties of cortical collecting duct basolateral membrane. *Am J Physiol 1986; 251:* F743–F757

18 Koeppen BM, Biagi BA, Giebisch GH. Intracellular microelectrode characterization of the rabbit cortical collecting duct. *Am J Physiol 1983; 244:* F35–F47

19 O'Neil RG, Sansom SC. Characterization of apical cell membrane Na^+ and K^+ conductances of cortical collecting duct using microelectrode techniques. *Am J Physiol 1984; 247:* F14–F24

20 Sansom SC, O'Neil RG. Mineralocorticoid regulation of apical cell membrane Na^+ and K^+ transport of the cortical collecting duct. *Am J Physiol 1985; 248:* F858–F868

21 Hunter M, Lopes AG, Boulpaep E, Giebisch G. Regulation of Single potassium ion channels from apical membrane of rabbit collecting tubule. *Am J Physiol 1986; 251:* F725–F733

22 Warden DH, Schuster VL, Stokes JB. The paracellular pathway of rabbit cortical collecting tubule (CCT): a high resistance, non-selective barrier. *Fed Proc 1986; 45:* 517

ELECTROPHYSIOLOGY OF THE OUTER MEDULLARY COLLECTING DUCT

B M Koeppen

University of Connecticut Health Center, Farmington, Connecticut, USA

Introduction

Recent studies of the outer medullary collecting duct of the rabbit have shown that the outer stripe (OMCDo) and inner stripe (OMCDi) portions are functionally distinct. Table I summarizes some of these differences as determined by in vitro microperfusion studies of these two segments.

TABLE I. Transepithelial transport properties of the rabbit outer medullary collecting duct

	Outer stripe	Inner stripe	References
J_{Na} (pmol/mm/min)	7.9±3.2	1.5±2.5	1,2
J_K (pmol/mm/min)	−2.9±0.5	0.7±0.6	1,2
J_{Cl} (pmol/mm/min)	−1.4±4.1*	−9.8±1.2*	1–3
J_{HCO_3} (pmol/mm/min)	8.7±0.7*	10.3±0.4*	3–9
V_T (mV)	−3.4±1.2*	25.3±0.9*	1–14
R_T (kΩcm)	28.5±2.9	58.6±5.3	5,11,12

J is the net flux of the ion; V_T is the transepithelial voltage and R_T the transepithelial resistance of a 1cm length of tubule.
Negative values of net flux denote secretion.
* Calculated as weighted average of published values.

In this report, the electrophysiological properties of the OMCDo and OMCDi will be reviewed. Special emphasis is placed on results obtained using intracellular voltage recording microelectrodes, and the models of cellular ion transport derived from these studies.

Inner stripe (OMCDi)

The OMCDi appears to be specialized for urine acidification. When perfused and bathed with symmetrical solutions there is no net transport of sodium ion (Na^+) or potassium ion (K^+) [1,2], while bicarbonate ion (HCO_3^-) reabsorption occurs under all conditions thus far studied [3–6,8,9]. HCO_3^- secretion has not been observed in the OMCDi.

The specialized role of the OMCDi in urine acidification is also evident in its structure. Specifically, histochemical studies have shown that all cells of the OMCDi contain carbonic anhydrase [15].

The transport properties of the OMCDi have made this segment a convenient model system for studying cellular mechanisms of urine acidification; the electrophysiological properties of this segment also reflect this role.

Cellular electrophysiology

The OMCDi maintains a lumen positive transepithelial voltage (V_T) under all conditions. As indicated in Table I, the average value reported in the literature is +25.3±0.9mV. Several observations support the notion that this lumen positive V_T results from an electrogenic hydrogen ion (H^+) secretory (or HCO_3^- reabsorptive) process. First, H^+ secretion is facilitated by carbonic anhydrase, and inhibition of this enzyme, by acetazolamide for example, reduced both H^+ secretion and V_T [6,8,14]. Similarly, H^+ secretion and the V_T are inhibited by the addition of the disulphonic stilbene SITS (4-acetamide-4′ isothiocyano-stilbene-2,2′ disulphonic acid) to the peritubular bathing medium [3,14]. Finally, manoeuvres which stimulate H^+ secretion, such as reducing the $[HCO_3^-]$ of the peritubular bathing medium, also increase the magnitude of V_T [5].

Intracellular microelectrode studies of the OMCDi indicate that, electrophysiologically, there is only a single cell type [10,11]. Since, as noted above, all cells in this segment contain carbonic anhydrase, such a finding is not surprising. This apparent homogeneity in cell function greatly facilitates the use of intracellular microelectrodes.

The basolateral membrane voltage (V_{bl}) of the OMCDi cell is low in comparison to other renal tubule cells, and averages only −30 to −40mV [5,10]. Since the V_T is approximately +25mV, the apical membrane voltage (V_a) must be 55 to 60mV, cell interior negative with respect to the luminal fluid compartment.

The fractional resistance of the apical membrane ($fRa=R_a/(R_a+R_{bl})$) is near unity indicating that the resistance of the apical membrane is at least 100 times greater than that of the basolateral membrane. The low resistance of the basolateral membrane effectively 'voltage clamps' the apical membrane voltage. As a result, luminal ion substitution experiments, even in the presence of a Nernstian change in the electromotive force of the membrane, result in only a few millivolt change in V_a. Consequently, it is difficult to rule out the existence of specific ion channels in this membrane. Nevertheless it is quite clear that the apical membrane does not represent a significant pathway for passive current flow.

In contrast to the apical membrane, the conductive properties of the basolateral membrane can be readily studied by single ion substitutions of the bath solution. Consequently, its conductive properties are well characterized [11]. The major ion conductance in this membrane is for chloride (Cl^-) (apparent transfer number for chloride ≈ 0.9). A small K^+ conductance has also been identified, but it is difficult to demonstrate in all cells. Conductive pathways for Na^+ or HCO_3^- have not been identified.

It has been assumed that the cells impaled with the microelectrode secrete H^+ into the tubule lumen, and that this is the result of the activity of an electrogenic H^+-ATPase in the apical membrane. Therefore, HCO_3^- must also exit the cell across the basolateral membrane. The results of bath ion substitution experiments indicate that this occurs by an electrically silent mechanism. The studies of Stone et al have provided evidence consistent with a Cl^-/HCO_3^- antiporter

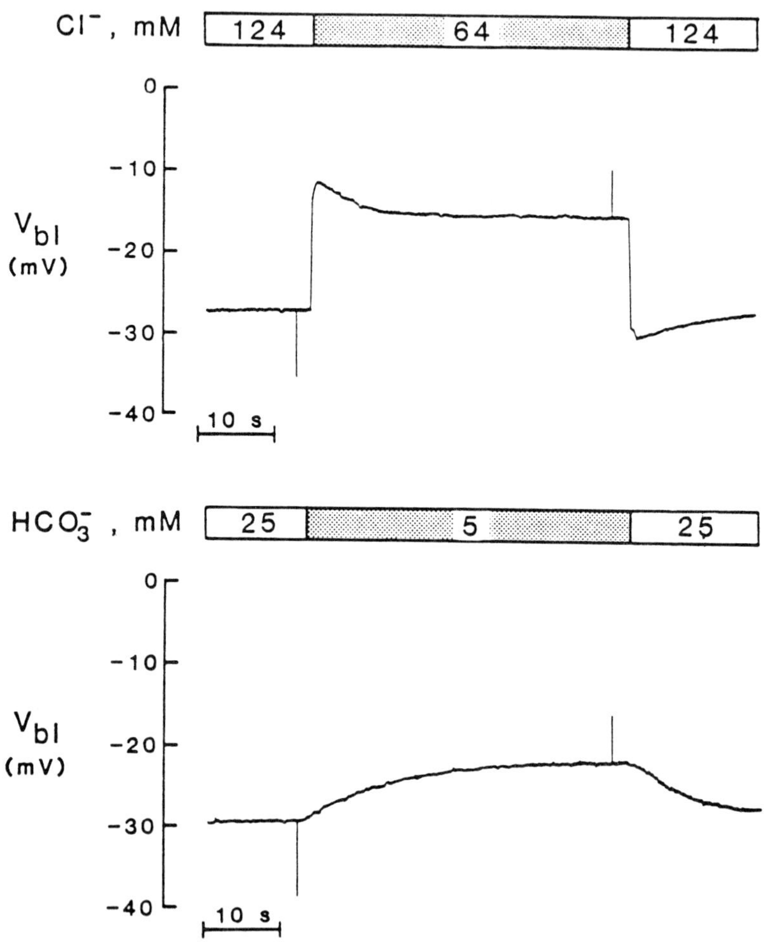

Figure 1. Response of basolateral membrane voltage (V_{bl}) to step changes in the bath Cl^- and HCO_3^- concentrations in the rabbit OMCDi.

[3], and the results of microelectrode studies support such a model [11]. For example, Figure 1 illustrates the response of V_{bl} to rapid (<1 second) step changes in the Cl^- and HCO_3^- concentrations of the bath solution by substituting gluconate for Cl^- or HCO_3^-. When the bath $[Cl^-]$ is reduced, there is a rapid depolarization of V_{bl}, which reflects the Cl^- conductive properties of this membrane. V_{bl} also depolarizes when the bath $[HCO_3^-]$ is reduced. The time course of this depolarization, however, is much slower than can be explained by a conductive pathway for HCO_3^- (compared with the time course for the Cl^- response), and must therefore represent a secondary change in the cell. One likely mechanism for this HCO_3^--induced slow depolarization, is an increase in the intracellular $[Cl^-]$ mediated by the activity of a Cl^-/HCO_3^- antiporter in the basolateral membrane. In the presence of a Cl^-/HCO_3^- antiporter, reducing the $[HCO_3^-]$ of the peritubular bathing medium, would accelerate the efflux of HCO_3^- from the cell. This in turn would lead to increased accumulation of Cl^- within the cell. Since the basolateral membrane is dominated by a Cl^- conductive pathway, and can be considered a 'Cl^- electrode', an increase in the intracellular $[Cl^-]$ would decrease the Nernst potential for Cl^- (E_{Cl}) and thus depolarize V_{bl}.

If the basolateral membrane is modelled as a Cl^-/HCO_3^- antiporter in parallel with a Cl^- conductance, then any manoeuvre which accelerates the process of transcellular H^+ secretion would be expected to depolarize V_{bl}, and any process that inhibits H^+ secretion would be expected to hyperpolarize V_{bl}. This has been observed, at least in studies where H^+ secretion has been inhibited. In particular, inhibition of H^+ secretion with either acetazolamide or SITS markedly hyperpolarizes V_{bl} [14]. The effects of these inhibitors are considered in more detail in a later section.

Jacobson has shown that H^+ secretion by the OMCDi can be accompanied by either the secretion of Cl^- or the reabsorption of K^+ [5]. Given the electrophysiological properties of the cell, the most likely route for this coupling of Cl^- and K^+ movement to that of H^+ is via the paracellular pathway. Since the process of H^+ secretion is electrogenic, and results in the generation of a lumen positive V_T, either the Cl^- secretion or K^+ reabsorption could occur passively by this route. In this regard, studies of the ionic selectivity of the paracellular pathway have provided evidence consistent with significant K^+ and Cl^- permeabilities [11].

Cell model

Figure 2 summarizes the electrophysiological properties of the OMCDi cell in terms of both a mechanistic and electrical equivalent circuit model. The apical membrane contains an electrogenic H^+-ATPase. Because of the high value of fRA, the H^+-ATPase is assumed to have a relatively high internal resistance, and therefore is modelled as a rheogenic pump. HCO_3^- exits the cell across the basolateral membrane in exchange for Cl^-, which in turn recycles across this

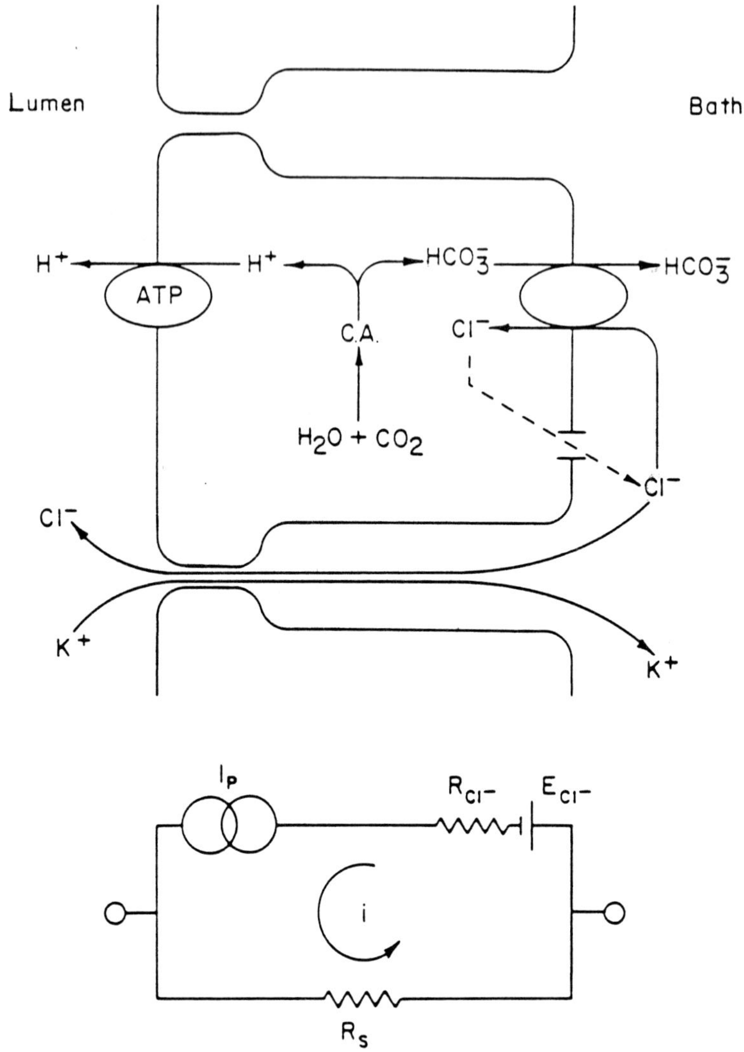

Figure 2. Mechanistic and electrical equivalent circuit model of the H^+ secreting cell of the rabbit OMCDi. Positive intraepithelial current flow (i) is indicated by the arrow. See text for details

membrane via a conductive pathway. Because the basolateral membrane is dominated by a Cl^- conductance, it is modelled electrically as a Thevenin electromotive force (E_{Cl}) and resistance (R_{Cl}) for Cl^-. When the tubule is perfused and bathed with identical solutions, the paracellular pathway is ohmic, and allows the movement of both K^+ and Cl^-.

According to this model, positive current (i) flows from bath-to-lumen through the cell, and from lumen-to-bath through the paracellular pathway. The transcellular current is carried by H^+ across the apical membrane, and by Cl^- across the basolateral membrane (negative current flow out of the cell is equivalent to positive current flow into the cell). Current flow through the paracellular pathway is carried either by the movement of Cl^- from bath-to-lumen, or by the movement of K^+ from lumen-to-bath. Regardless of the current carrying ion, the V_T will be oriented lumen positive due to the internal resistance drop across this pathway. H^+ secretion will be accompanied either by Cl^- secretion or K^+ reabsorption depending on the relative concentrations of these two ions in the lumen and bath. Under in vivo conditions, it is likely that the lumen $[K^+]$ is quite high because of upstream K^+ secretion by the CCD. Thus, the OMCDi would normally be expected to function as an H^+ for K^+ exchange segment.

The magnitude of the V_{bl} is determined by the Cl^- gradient across this membrane and the current flow associated with Cl^- efflux from the cell:

$$V_{bl} = E_{Cl} - iR_{Cl}$$

Normally, Cl^- is maintained above electrochemical equilibrium by the activity of the Cl^-/HCO_3^- antiporter, with the ultimate source of energy being the H^+-ATPase located in the apical membrane. Thus, V_{bl} is hyperpolarized above E_{Cl}, because of the internal resistance drop associated with Cl^- efflux from the cell. Under conditions where net H^+ secretion is stimulated (e.g. reduction of bath $[HCO_3^-]$), more Cl^- would be brought into the cell making E_{Cl} less negative and thus depolarizing V_{bl}. Conversely, under conditions where net H^+ secretion is inhibited (e.g. acetazolamide or SITS), Cl^- will run out of the cell and come to equilibrium. As a result, V_{bl} will hyperpolarize.

This model predicts that the calculated equivalent short circuit current ($I_{sc}=V_T/R_T$) should yield a measure of the H^+ current (I_H), provided that there are no other pathways for conductive ion flow through the H^+ secreting cell, or that other mechanisms for HCO_3^- or H^+ transport do not exist in this segment. Indeed, to a first approximation the calculated I_H is equivalent to the measured rates of net HCO_3^- reabsorption [11]. However, measurements of I_H and net HCO_3^- flux must be made in the same tubule in order to test more rigorously this relationship.

As described above, electrophysiological studies have demonstrated that the apical membrane does not contain appreciable ion conductance pathways. Vesicle studies, however, have reported the existence of a Cl^- channel [16]. The reason(s) for these apparently discrepant results remain to be defined, but two possibilities seem likely. First, the Cl^- channel may be gated. According to recent studies. H^+ secretion by these cells can be regulated by the insertion and retrieval of the H^+-ATPase, together with the Cl^- channel, into and out of the apical membrane [17,18]. It may be that when stored in cytoplasmic vesicles the Cl^- channel has a higher probability of being in the open state than when it is present in the apical membrane. Alternatively, the gating characteristics of the channel may be constant, but because of a relatively low density the overall conductance of the apical membrane is still much less than that of the basolateral membrane. Additional studies, perhaps using patch clamp techniques, will be needed in order to distinguish between these possibilities. Given the measured distribution of apical and basolateral membrane resistance, it seems unlikely, however, that significant transepithelial Cl^- secretion occurs via a conductive

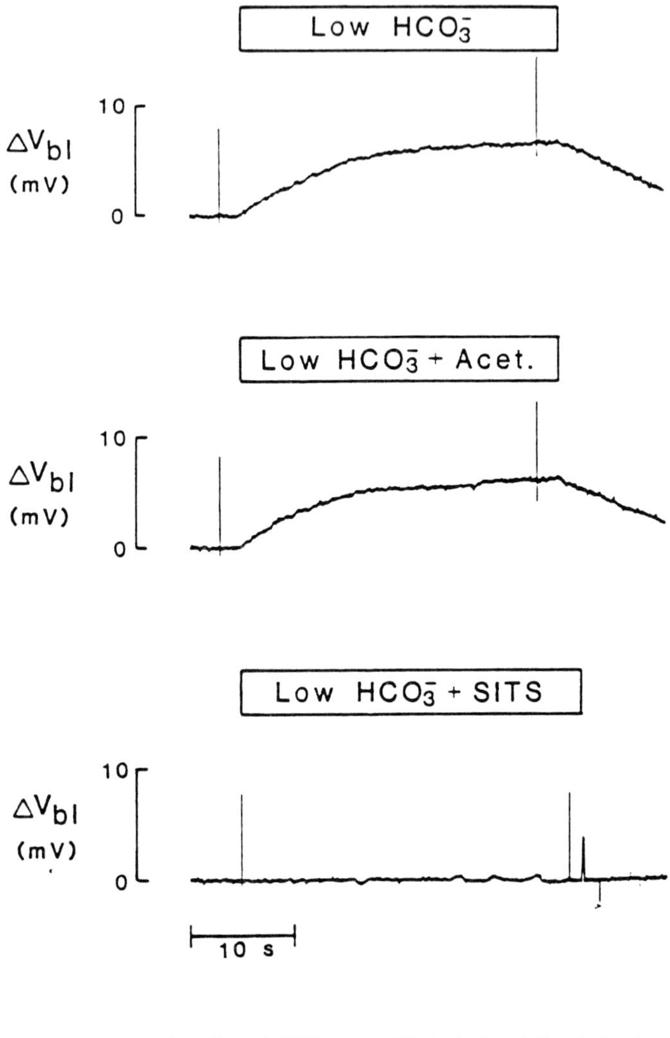

Figure 3. Effect of acetazolamide and SITS on the HCO_3^--induced depolarization of V_{bl} in the rabbit OMCDi. The upper panel illustrates the response in the absence of inhibitor. Acetazolamide did not alter the response (middle panel), although the steady-state value of V_{bl} was hyperpolarized approximately 25mV. SITS completely abolished the response (lower panel), and also hyperpolarized the steady-state V_{bl} by approximately 25mV

pathway in the apical membrane. Indeed, Cl^- secretion by such a route would render a portion of the H^+ secretory process electroneutral, and electroneutral H^+ secretion has not been described in this segment [3,6,8,9].

Effect of inhibitors

The carbonic anhydrase inhibitor acetazolamide and the disulphonic stilbene SITS inhibit H^+ secretion in the OMCDi [3,6]. Both of these inhibitors have a marked effect on the electrical properties of the cell [14]. When either inhibitor is added to the peritubular bathing medium V_{bl} hyperpolarizes. The magnitude of the hyperpolarization is similar for both drugs, averaging 27.3±5.5mV for SITS and 20.7±3.2mV for acetazolamide. This hyperpolarization cannot be attributed to a change in the ionic selectivity of the basolateral membrane, and likely reflects an alteration in the intracellular $[Cl^-]$ (see above).

As illustrated in Figure 3, SITS but not acetazolamide alters the response to reducing the bath $[HCO_3^-]$. Under control conditions, reducing the bath $[HCO_3^-]$ from 25 to 5mM (constant PCO_2) results in a slow depolarization of V_{bl}, which is thought to reflect stimulation of the Cl^-/HCO_3^- antiporter in the basolateral membrane (see above). As can be seen, SITS completely abolishes the response, while acetazolamide is without effect. Thus, it would appear from this that SITS directly inhibits the Cl^-/HCO_3^- antiporter, while acetazolamide does not.

Despite their different mechanisms of action both SITS and acetazolamide hyperpolarize V_{bl}. In terms of the model presented above, this hyper polarization would result from a decrease in the intracellular $[Cl^-]$, which in turn would result from a reduction in the activity of the Cl^-/HCO_3^- antiporter in the basolateral membrane. In the case of SITS, this reduction in antiporter activity results from direct inhibition. With acetazolamide the antiporter is still functional, but its activity is reduced as a result of decreased availability of intracellular HCO_3^-.

Outer stripe (OMCDo)

The OMCDo is similar in some respects to the cortical collecting duct (CCD), but important differences exist. The OMCDo, like the CCD, reabsorbs Na^+ and secretes K^+ [1,2]. The rates of transport of these ions, however, are two to three times lower than those in the CCD. The OMCDo also reabsorbs HCO_3^- secretion [7,8].

The OMCDo is composed of two cell types: the principal cell and the intercalated cell [17]. Based on both physiological and morphological data, it is believed that the principal cell is responsible for Na^+ reabsorption and K^+ secretion, while the intercalated cell is involved in urine acidification [13,17].

Microelectrode studies of the OMCDo are complicated by the existence in this segment of two functionally distinct cell types. However, it has been possible to distinguish between principal cells and intercalated cells based on their electrophysiological properties [13].

Cellular electrophysiology

The transepithelial voltage (V_T) of the OMCDo varies widely, and can be oriented either lumen negative or lumen positive [1,2,7,8,12]. On average, the V_T is slightly lumen negative (see Table I). The polarity of the V_T is determined by two parallel electrogenic transport processes: one for Na^+ reabsorption, and one for H^+ secretion. Figure 4 illustrates the changes in V_T that occur when either of these two electrogenic transport systems are inhibited. Inhibition of electrogenic Na^+ reabsorption, by the addition of amiloride to the luminal fluid,

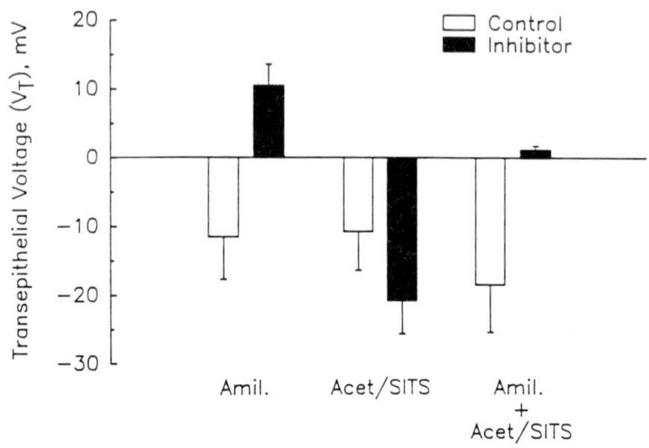

Figure 4. Effect of luminal amiloride and bath acetazolamide or SITS on the transepithelial voltage of the rabbit OMCDo

causes the V_T to become lumen positive. This lumen positive V_T represents electrogenic H^+ secretion, and it can be inhibited by either the carbonic anhydrase inhibitor acetazolamide, or by the disulphonic stilbene SITS, when these agents are added to the peritubular bathing media. Thus, the polarity of the V_T under control conditions will be determined by the relative rates of Na^+ reabsorption and H^+ secretion.

The electrical properties of the principal cell and intercalated cell are summarized in Table II. The intercalated cell has a basolateral membrane voltage (V_{bl}) of -28.5mV. The fractional resistance of the apical membrane (fRa) is near unity, indicating that the resistance of the apical membrane is at least 100 times greater than that of the basolateral membrane. The basolateral membrane contains a large Cl^- conductive pathway (apparent transfer number for chloride ≈ 0.8), and virtually no K^+ conductance. The principal cell has a V_{bl} of -64.0mV. The fRA is high, but measurable (fRa=0.80), indicating the existence of significant ion conductive pathways in the apical membrane. The basolateral membrane of this cell is highly K^+ selective (apparent transport number for potassium ≈ 0.8), but does not contain an appreciable Cl^- conductive pathway. Thus the principal cell of the OMCDo differs from that of the CCD, since in this later segment the basolateral membrane contains conductive pathways for both K^+ and Cl^-.

TABLE II. Electrophysiological properties of cell types in the OMCDo

	V_{bl}, mV	fRa	Bath ion substitution ΔV_{bl}, mV K^+	Cl^-
Intercalated cell	−28.5±2.0	0.99±0.01	0.3±0.2	13.2±0.2
(n)	(13)	(13)	(12)	(13)
Principal cell	−64.0±2.1	0.80±0.02	33.8±1.7	0.4±0.2
(n)	(36)	(36)	(25)	(23)

Values are mean ± SE. Bath [K^+] was stepped from 5 to 50mM, and [Cl^-] from 124 to 64mM. Values of ΔV_{bl} represent depolarization

Additional studies have attempted to identify conductive pathways for other ions in the basolateral membranes of these cells. In this regard, neither Na^+ nor HCO_3^- appear to move across the basolateral membrane of either the intercalated cell or the principal cell by passive electrodiffusive mechanisms.

Identification of cells as either intercalated cells or principal cells can be accomplished using inhibitors of H^+ secretion and Na^+ reabsorption, respectively [13]. In particular, either acetazolamide or SITS can be used as functional probes of the intercalated cell, while amiloride can be used as a functional probe of the principal cell. When amiloride is added to the luminal fluid, the V_{bl} of the principal cell hyperpolarizes by 10.3±2.1mV. Concurrently, fRa increases from 0.82 to 0.98. Both the observed change in V_{bl} and fRa are consistent with the blockade of Na^+ conductive channels in the apical membrane of the cell by amiloride, and serve to identify the cell as a principal cell. In contrast, amiloride does not directly alter the electrical properties of the intercalated cell.

Addition of either acetazolamide or SITS to the peritubular bathing medium does not directly alter the electrical properties of the principal cell. However, both agents hyperpolarize V_{bl} of the intercalated cell. The mean change in V_{bl} induced by acetazolamide and SITS is 26.4±8.2mV. The fRa is unchanged by these inhibitors, as is the ionic selectivity of the basolateral membrane. As already discussed, the hyperpolarization of V_{bl} seen with these inhibitors probably reflects a change in the intracellular [Cl^-] (see above). The fact that these agents alter the electrical properties of this cell type provides evidence that it is involved in urinary acidification, and corresponds to the intercalated cell.

Cell model

Figure 5 summarizes the electrophysiological properties of the principal cell and intercalated cell in terms of mechanistic models.

The apical membrane of the principal cell is dominated by an amiloride inhibitable Na^+ conductive pathway. Since in some tubules luminal barium also

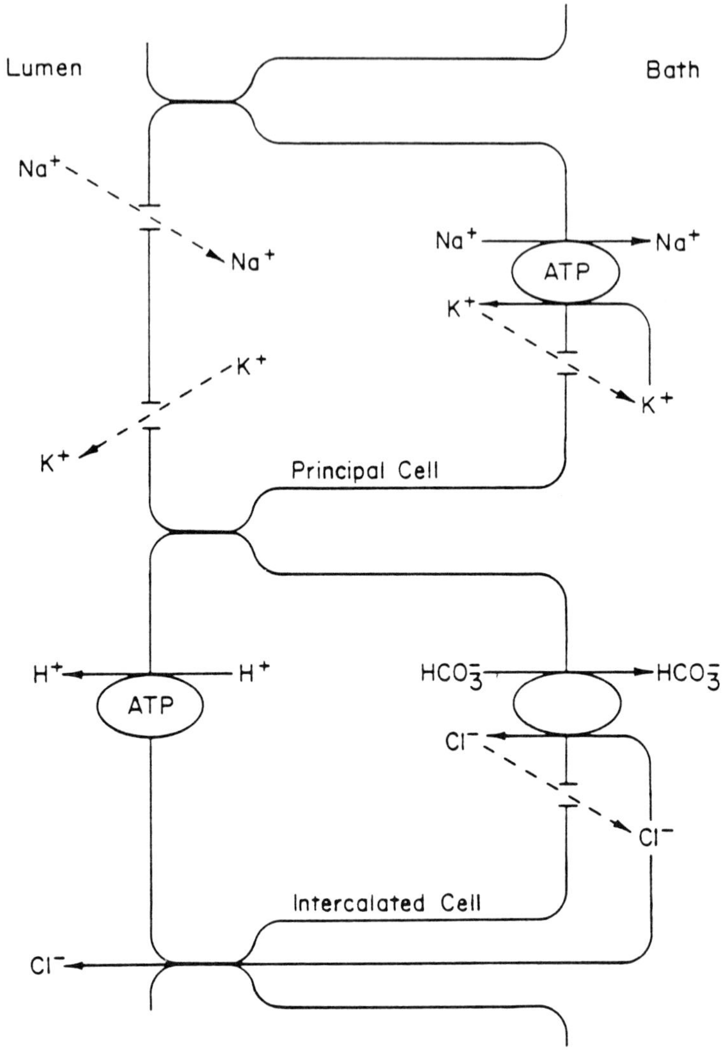

Figure 5. Mechanistic models of the principal cell and intercalated cell of the rabbit OMCDo. See text for details

causes a small increase in fRa, a K^+ conductive pathway is also indicated. It should be emphasized, however, that the existence of this K^+ conductance is highly variable, and it is not observed in all tubules. The basolateral membrane of this cell contains a large K^+ conductance, which serves to recycle the K^+ brought into the cell by the Na^+-K^+-ATPase.

The electrical properties of the intercalated cell are identical to those described above for the H^+ secreting cell of the OMCDi. Because the OMCDo does not secrete HCO_3^- it is assumed that the intercalated cells in this segment only secrete H^+. Thus, the proposed cellular model is identical to that described for the OMCDi.

It is clear from the marked electrophysiological differences between the principal and intercalated cell that they can not be coupled electrically to each other. This does not mean, however, that interaction between the cells cannot occur. For example, changes in Na^+ transport, via changes in the V_T, could effect the secretion H^+ by the intercalated cell. Indeed, recent measurements have shown that amiloride, by altering V_T, can hyperpolarize the voltage across the apical membrane of the intercalated cell by approximately 15mV [13]. Since the H^+-ATPase is electrogenic this could alter H^+ secretion by increasing the electrochemical gradient against which the H^+-ATPase would have to pump.

Summary

The electrophysiological properties of the OMCDo and OMCDi underscore the functional heterogeneity of this region of the collecting duct. The OMCDo reabsorbs Na^+ and secretes H^+ by parallel electrogenic processes; electrophysiological techniques have been used to localize these processes to different cell types. The OMCDi functionally appears to contain only a single cell type, which is involved in electrogenic H^+ secretion. This homogeneity in cell function has made the OMCDi a convenient model system for studying the cellular mechanism of electrogenic H^+ secretion using microelectrode techniques. There is some similarity in transport mechanism between OMCDi and the intercalated cells of OMCDo.

Acknowledgments

Special thanks is to given to P Mitchell for preparation of the figures.

Work from the author's laboratory was supported by NIH grant DK-32489, and an established investigatorship from the American Heart Association.

References

1 Stokes JB. Ion transport by the cortical and outer medullary collecting tubule. *Am J Physiol 1982; 22:* 473–484

2 Stokes JB, Ingram MJ, Williams AD, Ingram I. Heterogeneity of the rabbit collecting tubule: localization of mineralocorticoid hormone action to the cortical portion. *Kidney Int 1981; 20:* 340–347

3 Stone DK, Seldin DW, Kokko JP, Jacobson HR. Anion dependence of rabbit medullary collecting duct acidification. *J Clin Invest 1983; 71:* 1505–1508

4 Hays S, Kokko JP, Jacobson HR. Hormonal regulation of proton secretion in rabbit medullary collecting duct. *J Clin Invest 1986; 78:* 1279–1286

5 Jacobson HR. Medullary collecting duct acidification. Effects of potassium, HCO_3 concentration and Pco_2. *J Clin Invest 1984; 74:* 2107–2114

6 Lombard WE. Kokko JP, Jacobson HR. Bicarbonate transport in cortical and outer medullary collecting tubules. *Am J Physiol 1983; 244:* F289–F296

7 McKinney TD, Davidson KK. Characteristics of bicarbonate transport in collecting tubules from the outer stripe of the outer medulla (OMCTos). *Kidney Int 1987; 31:* 412

8 Star RA, Burg MB, Knepper MA. Distribution of luminal pH disequilibrium along the rabbit outer medullary collecting duct: role in ammonia and bicarbonate transport. *Am J Physiol 1987:* in press

9 Stone DK, Seldin DW, Kokko JP, Jacobson HR. Mineralocorticoid modulation of rabbit medullary collecting duct acidification. A sodium-independent effect. *J Clin Invest 1983; 72:* 77–83

10 Ishibashi K, Sasaki S, Shiigai T, Takeuchi J. Intracellular electrical potentials in the rabbit collecting ducts perfused in vitro. *Jpn J Physiol 1986; 36:* 671–681

11 Koeppen BM. Conductive properties of the rabbit outer medullary collecting duct: inner stripe. *Am J Physiol 1985; 248:* F500–F506

12 Koeppen BM. Conductive properties of the rabbit outer medullary collecting duct: outer stripe. *Am J Physiol 1986; 250:* F70–F76

13 Koeppen BM. Electrophysiological identification of principal and intercalated cells in the rabbit outer medullary collecting duct. *Pfluegers Archiv 1987:* in press

14 Koeppen BM. Proton secretion by the rabbit outer medullary collecting duct: effect of inhibitors. *Kidney Int 1987; 31:* 410

15 Ridderstrale Y, Kashgarian M, Giebisch G et al. Rabbit collecting duct heterogeneity: localization of carbonic anhydrase and Na-K-ATPase. *Kidney Int 1987; 31:* 441

16 Al-Awqati Q. Proton-locating ATPases. *Ann Rev Cell Biol 1986; 2:* 179–199

17 Madsen KM, Tisher CC. Structural-functional relationships along the distal nephron. *Am J Physiol 1986; 250:* F1–F15

18 Steinmetz PR. Cellular organization of urinary acidification. *Am J Physiol 1986; 251:* F173–F187

INNER MEDULLARY COLLECTING DUCT

M A Knepper, J M Sands, H Nonoguchi, *R A Star, †R K Packer

*National Heart, Lung and Blood Institute, National Institutes of Health, Bethesda, Maryland, *Southwestern Medical School, Dallas, Texas, †George Washington University, Washington DC, USA*

Background

The mammalian collecting duct system consists of several morphologically and functionally distinct parts. The functions of the cortical and outer medullary parts of the collecting duct system have been described in other papers in this volume. This article discusses the major functions of the inner medullary part of the collecting duct. The inner medullary collecting duct carries out the final modifications of urinary composition before the urine is discharged into the renal pelvis. As described below, the inner medullary collecting duct itself consists of two morphologically and functionally distinct parts.

Anatomy

The initial part of the inner medullary collecting duct has two cell types: principal cells and intercalated cells [1]. The intercalated cells are of the A subtype, which has been associated with proton secretion in other parts of the collecting duct system [2]. The terminal part of the inner medullary collecting duct contains only one cell type, which is usually referred to as a 'principal cell', although these principal cells differ morphologically from those in the initial inner medullary collecting duct and in other parts of the collecting duct system [3]. The initial inner medullary collecting duct is found in approximately the outer third of the inner medulla, i.e. the part that is adjacent to the outer medulla. The terminal inner medullary collecting duct is found in the inner two-thirds of the inner medulla, i.e. in the papillary cone. The term 'papillary collecting duct' has been applied to the entire inner medullary collecting duct by some investigators and to the terminal inner medullary collecting duct by others. Because of this ambiguity, we recommend that the term 'papillary collecting duct' be avoided.

Throughout the inner medulla collecting ducts join to result in a continually decreasing total number of ducts toward the papillary tip. Such junctions are

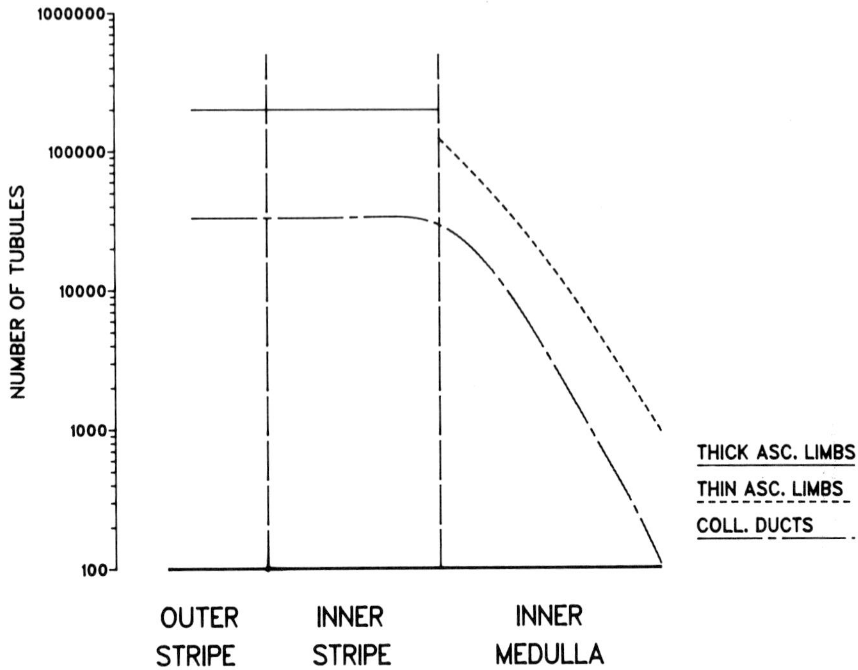

Figure 1. Total numbers of collecting ducts and ascending limbs at various positions along the cortico-medullary axis of the rabbit kidney. Calculated from morphometric data [4]. Modified from Chandhoke et al [5]

present in both initial inner medullary collecting ducts and terminal inner medullary collecting ducts, but are only rarely present in outer medullary collecting ducts (unpublished observations). The total number of collecting ducts at each level of the inner medulla has been enumerated in both rat and rabbit using morphometric techniques [4,5]. Figure 1 shows the total numbers of collecting ducts and ascending limbs plotted as a function of axial position in the rabbit renal medulla [5]. Note that the reduction in the number of collecting ducts in the inner medulla is accompanied by a parallel decrease in the number of loops of Henle. This parallel reduction in the number of collecting ducts and loops of Henle is responsible for the tapered structure of the renal papilla.

Functional studies in vivo

Ullrich and his colleagues were the first to study the in vivo function of the inner medullary collecting duct almost 30 years ago [6]. Their findings using the microcatheterization technique in non-diuretic hamsters subsequently have been confirmed in numerous micropuncture and microcatheterization studies in rats and hamsters [3]. In general, these studies have shown that large amounts of urea, NaCl and water are reabsorbed from the inner medullary collecting duct under non-diuretic conditions. In addition there is substantial ammonium secretion, but little or no net potassium transport.

Functional studies in vitro

In vitro techniques have been very useful in the study of nephron function when the goal has been to study transport mechanisms or control mechanisms. The chief advantage of in vitro methods is that they allow precise control of both the luminal and peritubular environment of the renal tubule. Until recently, the in vitro technique that has yielded most information about the inner medullary collecting duct has been the isolated papilla technique developed in the 1960s by Marsh [7] and by Morgan and his colleagues [8,9]. Despite its intensive use to study other renal tubule segments, there has been relatively little application of the isolated perfused tubule technique of Burg [10] chiefly because it has been perceived as too difficult to apply to the inner medullary collecting duct. Before 1985, only Rocha and his colleagues [11,12] had used it. Recently, we have worked out a technical approach that has allowed us to study isolated perfused inner medullary collecting ducts on a routine basis [13]. Application of this approach has allowed us to make rapid progress toward an understanding of the roles of arginine vasopressin and atrial natriuretic factor in the regulation of water, urea and NaCl transport in the inner medullary collecting duct. In addition, we have been able to demonstrate important functional differences between the two parts of the inner medullary collecting duct: the initial inner medullary collecting duct and the terminal inner medullary collecting duct. In the remainder of this article we review these recent studies.

Functions of the initial and terminal parts of the inner medullary collecting duct

Urea transport

In both rat (Figure 2) and rabbit (not shown), we found that the urea permeability is relatively low in collecting ducts from the outer third of the inner medulla (initial inner medullary collecting duct), but very high in collecting ducts from the inner two-thirds of the inner medulla (terminal inner medullary collecting duct) [13]. The urea permeability in the terminal inner medullary collecting duct is the highest among all renal tubule segments. Furthermore, vasopressin was found to increase the urea permeability of the terminal inner medullary collecting duct and not the initial inner medullary collecting duct (Figure 3) [14]. The vasopressin concentration required for half-maximal stimulation of urea permeability is approximately 10^{-11} M. These data provided the first evidence that the initial and terminal parts of the inner medullary collecting duct have different functional properties.

The difference in urea permeability of the initial and terminal parts of the

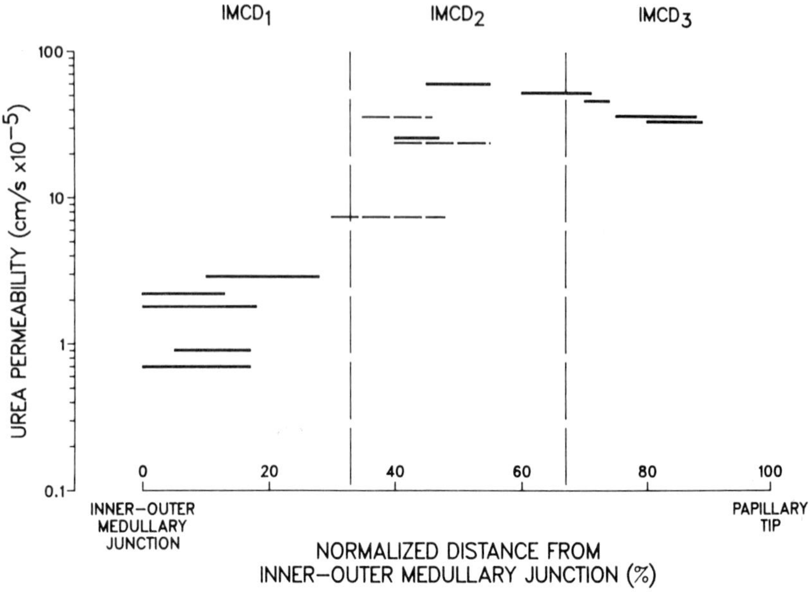

Figure 2. Apparent urea permeabilities in rat inner medullary collecting ducts as a function of distance along the inner medullary axis. The mean permeability for each tubule is represented by a horizontal line that indicates the original position of the tubule in the inner medulla before it was dissected. Tubules were arbitrarily divided into three groups based on position. From Sands and Knepper [13]

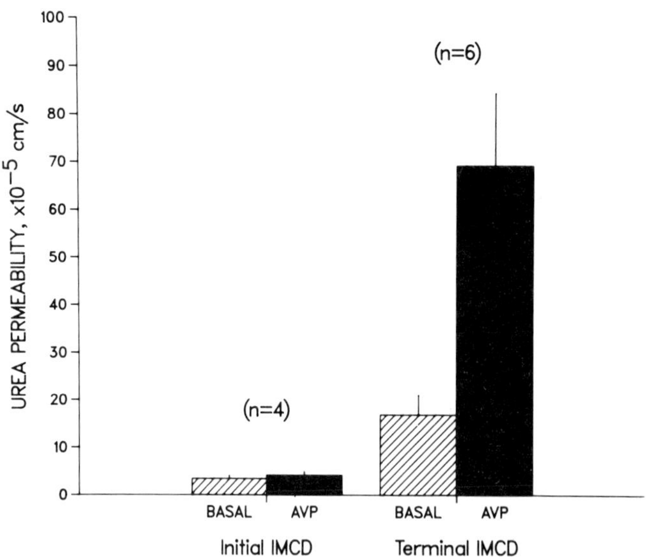

Figure 3. Effect of vasopressin (AVP, 10nM) on urea permeability of initial and terminal parts of the rat inner medullary collecting ducts. Vasopressin increased the urea permeability significantly only in the terminal inner medullary collecting duct. From Sands et al [14]

inner medullary collecting duct is thought to be critical for the urinary concentrating mechanism. During antidiuresis, urea accumulates in the inner medullary interstitium and accounts for a large fraction of the total inner medullary osmolality. Urea enters the inner medullary interstitium chiefly as a result of passive reabsorption from the inner medullary collecting duct [13,15]. Mathematical modelling studies [5] have shown that when a uniformly high urea permeability was assumed along the inner medullary collecting duct (with a step transition from a low to a high value at the inner-outer medullary junction), rapid absorption of urea from the early inner medullary collecting duct was predicted, leaving little urea in the final urine and allowing very little urea accumulation in the inner medulla. In contrast, when a gradual rise in urea permeability to high values in the inner half of the inner medulla is assumed, as we have found experimentally (Figure 2), high concentrations of urea in the final urine and inner medullary interstitium are predicted by the model. That is, urea absorption from the inner medullary collecting ducts must be delayed to the deepest part of the inner medulla (where the effective blood flow is lowest) to achieve maximal urea concentrations in the inner medullary interstitium.

The finding of a non-uniform urea permeability along the inner medullary collecting duct resolves a controversy that arose from a comparison of urea permeabilities measured in rat and rabbit inner medullary collecting ducts. The urea permeability of isolated inner medullary collecting ducts from rabbits [11] was found to be an order of magnitude lower than values measured in inner medullary collecting ducts from rats [8,12]. These results have been widely interpreted to indicate that there is a major species difference between rats and rabbits with regard to urea handling in the inner medulla. However, it is clear from the diameters of the rabbit inner medullary collecting ducts studied by Rocha and Kokko [11] that their tubules were initial inner medullary collecting ducts and thus can be expected to have a low urea permeability, based on our findings. In contrast, the technical descriptions of the studies in rat inner medullary collecting ducts [8,12] indicate that these were undoubtedly terminal inner medullary collecting ducts, which normally have a very high urea permeability. Our measurements in initial and terminal inner medullary collecting ducts of rabbits and rats show that the basic pattern of urea permeabilities along the inner medullary collecting duct is the same in the two species. That is, there is no longer any need to postulate that rats and rabbits concentrate urea in the inner medulla by different mechanisms.

Osmotic water permeability

Figure 4 shows osmotic water permeability coefficients (P_f) measured in initial and terminal inner medullary collecting ducts [14]. The basal osmotic water permeability was significantly higher in the terminal inner medullary collecting duct than in the initial inner medullary collecting duct, a finding that further

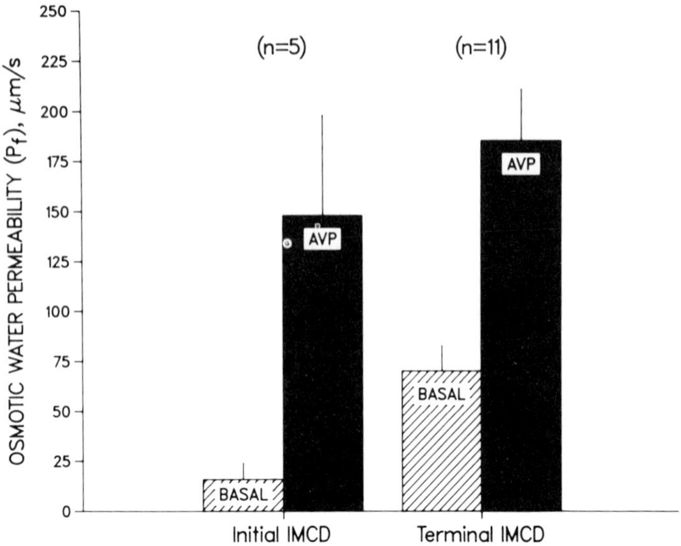

Figure 4. Effect of vasopressin (AVP, 10nM) on osmotic water permeability (P_f) of initial and terminal parts of the rat inner medullary collecting ducts. Increases were statistically significant in both segments. From Sands et al [14]

highlights the functional distinction between the two renal tubule segments. In contrast to the urea permeability, which increased in response to vasopressin only in the terminal inner medullary collecting duct, osmotic water permeability was increased by vasopressin in both the initial and terminal inner medullary collecting duct segments.

The high water permeability of the terminal inner medullary collecting duct in the absence of vasopressin helps to explain the seemingly paradoxical observation in Brattleboro (diabetes insipidus) rats that more water is absorbed from the terminal inner medullary collecting duct during water diuresis than during antidiuresis [16]. Jamison et al [16] observed that the transepithelial osmolality gradient across the terminal inner medullary collecting duct is much greater during water diuresis than during antidiuresis. The high water permeability in the absence of vasopressin allows the large osmotic gradient present during water diuresis to drive a high rate of water absorption. The reduction in inner medullary tissue osmolality that occurs during water diuresis is a consequence not only of a reduction in solute content but also of an increase in water content [17]. The increase in water absorption from the terminal inner medullary collecting duct during water diuresis contributes to the positive inner medullary water balance, and hence to the reduction in tissue osmolality.

Electrolyte permeability

Table I compares the permeability properties of the initial and terminal parts of the inner medullary collecting duct. The Na/Cl permselectivity, determined

TABLE I. Solute permeability of rat inner medullary collecting duct subsegments

	Initial Inner medullary collecting duct	Terminal Inner medullary collecting duct
Solute permeabilities ($x10^{-5}$ cm/s):		
1. Creatinine	0.9 ±0.2	1.3 ±0.5
2. Raffinose	0.3 ±0.1	0.2 ±0.1
3. Chloride	–	2.2 ±0.5
4. Sodium	–	1.1 ±0.3
P_{Na}/P_{Cl} (from dilution potentials):		
Control	0.89±0.05	0.76±0.03*
Arginine vasopressin (10nM)	1.11±0.18	0.80±0.03*

* Terminal inner medullary collecting duct significantly different from initial inner medullary collecting duct. From published sources [13,14] and unpublished observations.

from dilution potential measurements, is greater in the initial inner medullary collecting duct than in the terminal inner medullary collecting duct. The P_{Na}/P_{Cl} in both subsegments is greater than the ratio of free solution mobilities (u_{Na}/u_{Cl}=0.66) suggesting that the tight junctions are relatively sodium selective.

Direct measurements of chloride and sodium permeabilities in the terminal inner medullary collecting duct are also shown in Table I. These measurements were made by imposing an electrochemical gradient across the epithelium and measuring net sodium or chloride fluxes. The P_{Na}/P_{Cl} ratio determined from flux measurement are very roughly in accord with the ratio calculated from dilution potentials. Furthermore the sum of the partial ionic conductances for Na and Cl (calculated from the measured permeabilities) do not exceed the total transepithelial conductance. These results do not provide evidence for a major electrically silent permeation pathway for either ion.

Is the papillary surface epithelium functionally similar to the inner medullary collecting duct?

The papillary surface epithelium covers the outer surface of the renal papilla and separates the inner medullary interstitium from the renal pelvis. Based on morphological similarities between the inner medullary collecting duct and the papillary surface epithelium [18,19], it has often been assumed that the two epithelia are functionally similar. To study the transport properties of the papillary surface epithelium, we have recently developed a technique for isolating the papillary surface epithelium from the kidneys of rabbits and mounting it in a small Ussing chamber [13]. These studies have revealed that the papillary surface epithelium is functionally distinct from the inner medullary collecting duct. Both the urea permeability [13] and osmotic water permeability [20] are relatively low, and in contrast to the terminal inner medullary collecting duct, vasopressin has no effect on either permeability. The rabbit papillary surface epithelium possess an apical Na-K-Cl cotransporter that is stimulated by vasopressin and inhibited by bumetanide at concentrations down to 1nM [21]. We conclude that the papillary surface epithelium is an epithelium with its own unique set of properties, and that it is not a functional extension of the inner medullary collecting duct.

It has been proposed by many investigators that passive transport of urea across the papillary surface epithelium can provide a major fraction of the urea that accumulates in the inner medullary interstitium. However, the low urea permeability and the low surface area of the papillary surface epithelium appear to be incompatible with this hypothesis [13]. Instead the solute that appears to have the greatest ability to penetrate the papillary surface epithelium is NaCl. The measured chloride permeability in isolated rabbit papillary surface epithelium was $6x10^{-5}$ cm/s [20]. A major part of the passive chloride transport appeared to be through the cells, rather than via a paracellular pathway. We propose that transport of NaCl across the papillary surface epithelium may play an important role in removing solute from the medullary interstitium during the transition from antidiuresis to water diuresis [20]. The most likely pathway of urea efflux (i.e. secretion) from the inner medullary interstitium to the urine during medullary washout is via the terminal inner medullary collecting duct which has an extremely high urea permeability (Figure 2).

Mechanism of urea transport across the terminal inner medullary collecting duct

Even in the absence of vasopressin, the urea permeability of the terminal inner medullary collecting duct is extremely high (Figure 2). It is 13-fold higher than the creatinine permeability and 85-fold higher than the raffinose permeability (Table I). Most likely, creatinine and raffinose penetrate the epithelium via the paracellular pathway. The permeability ratios greatly exceed the values that would be expected if urea also penetrated the epithelium via the paracellular pathway. Instead, most of the passive urea transport is likely to be by a transcellular route.

One transcellular transport mechanism that may contribute to urea penetration across the terminal inner medullary collecting duct is simple diffusion through the lipid phase of cell membranes. However, studies in artificial lipid membranes have shown that the urea permeability of lipid bilayers is relatively low, $4x10^{-6}$ cm/s [22]. Assuming this value, the expected epithelial urea permeabilities in the various nephron segments can be calculated, taking into account the extent to which the cell membrane surface areas of each segment are amplified by the presence of microvilli (in apical membranes) and basal infoldings (in basolateral membranes). In Figure 5, the predicted epithelial permeabilities calculated in this manner (solid line) are compared with the actual permeabilities measured in isolated perfused tubules (points). As can be seen, the measured urea permeabilities in proximal convoluted tubules, proximal straight tubules, medullary thick ascending limbs, cortical collecting ducts, and the papillary

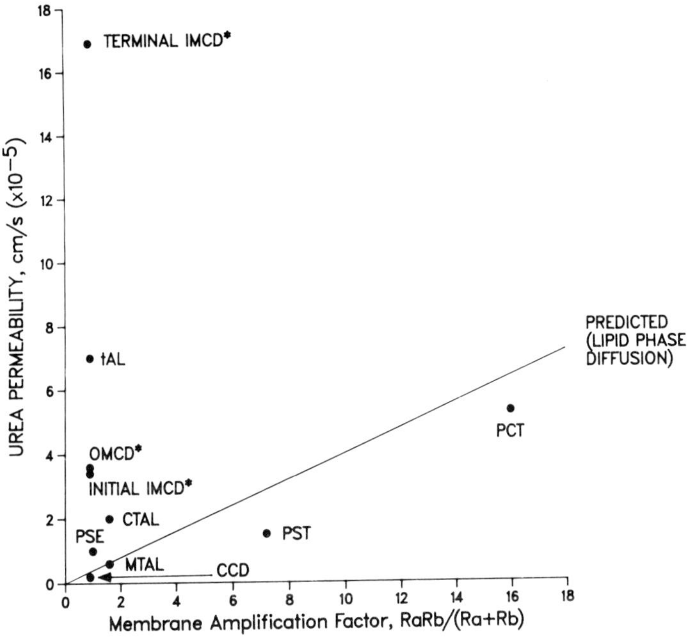

Figure 5. Comparison of measured urea permeabilities (points) with predicted urea permeabilities assuming transport by lipid phase diffusion across cell membranes as the sole mechanism of transepithelial transport (solid line). The predicted values assume that the urea permeabilities of the apical and basolateral membranes are equal to the value found by Galluci et al [22] in lipid bilayers (4×10^{-6} cm/s). Epithelial permeabilities are calculated using a virtual surface area (S_i) calculated from the inner diameter (D_i) and length (L) of the tubule ($S_i = \pi \cdot D_i \cdot L$) rather than the actual membrane surface areas which are amplified due to the presence of apical microvilli and basolateral infoldings. The calculation of the predicted epithelial permeability must take into account the membrane amplification. Membrane amplification is expressed in terms of the ratio of the actual apical membrane area to the virtual inner surface area (R_a) and the ratio of the actual basolateral membrane area to the virtual inner surface area (R_b). The overall membrane amplification factor ($R_a R_b / [R_a + R_b]$) is obtained by considering that the overall resistance to passive urea penetration across the epithelium is determined by two lipid membrane barriers in series. Thus, the predicted epithelial urea permeability is calculated as the lipid membrane permeability (4×10^{-6} cm/s [22]) multiplied by the overall membrane amplification factor.

R_a and R_b were calculated from the data of Welling et al [23–26] for the rabbit proximal convoluted tubule (PCT), the rabbit proximal straight tubule (PST), the rabbit cortical thick ascending limb (CTAL), and the rabbit cortical collecting duct (CCD). R_a and R_b for rat inner medullary collecting ducts were estimated from the data of Rastegar et al [27]. R_a and R_b for the rabbit medullary thick ascending limb (MTAL) were assumed to be the same as values for the CTAL.

The measured permeabilities were obtained from published sources [14,28–33]. All values were from rabbit renal epithelia with the exception of those for the inner medullary collecting ducts which were from rats [14]. Figure adapted from Sands et al [14] surface epithelium approximate the permeabilities predicted on the basis of lipid-phase diffusion. In contrast, the urea permeabilities of several segments exceed the values predicted from lipid-phase diffusion alone. Prominent among these is the terminal inner medullary collecting duct, in which the urea permeability is approximately 85-fold greater than the predicted value even in the absence of vasopressin stimulation. (The vasopressin-dependent urea permeability is approximately 335-fold greater than the predicted value.) Thus, it is unlikely that a major fraction of passive urea transport across the terminal inner medullary collecting duct occurs by lipid-phase diffusion.

The very high apparent urea permeability in the terminal inner medullary collecting duct raises the possibility that the transport is mediated by a facilitated transport process (e.g. a carrier). A saturable carrier for urea has been previously demonstrated in several tissues including red cells [34] and toad urinary bladder [35]. Two observations support the possibility of a urea carrier in inner medullary collecting ducts: a) the apparent urea permeability of the terminal inner medullary collecting duct decreases with increased absolute urea concentration [36] and b) phloretin, which blocks carrier-mediated urea transport in other tissues, decreases passive urea transport across the inner medullary collecting duct [37].

In addition to non-selective paracellular transport, lipid-phase diffusion across cell membranes, and carrier-mediated transport, an additional mechanism of urea transport has been proposed in the inner medullary collecting duct, viz. solvent drag. Reflection coefficients significantly less than unity, which would indicate passage of urea through water channels, have been reported in the rat inner medullary collecting duct [9,12]. The presence of a urea carrier in the terminal inner medullary collecting duct complicates the interpretation of the reflection coefficient measurements, however. The reflection coefficient has been calculated by comparing the water flux resulting from a transepithelial urea gradient to the water flux from an equal gradient of an impermeant reference substance such as mannitol. The apparent reflection coefficient calculated in this way could be artifactually low if the urea gradient were dissipated by the urea carrier. A valid measurement of reflection coefficient requires either that the carrier be blocked, e.g. by phloretin, or that a correction be made for passive urea transport that does not occur via water channels. Thus, it remains unclear whether significant solvent drag occurs in the inner medullary collecting duct.

Second messengers for vasopressin in the inner medullary collecting duct

Recently, we have completed studies of the second messengers involved in vasopressin action in isolated perfused terminal inner medullary collecting ducts [38]. We found that vasopressin increases cyclic AMP production (measured by radioimmunoassay) and the intracellular calcium (measured with the intracellular calcium-sensitive fluorescent dye INDO-1) in isolated terminal inner medullary collecting ducts. The concentration of vasopressin required to produce a half-maximal increase in urea permeability and osmotic water permeability was 10^{-11}M. The dose-response relationship for stimulation of cyclic AMP production was compatible with a role for cyclic AMP as a second messenger for both the urea and water permeability responses. A direct effect of 8-bromo cyclic AMP to increase urea permeability established that cyclic AMP is the second messenger that mediates the permeability response. Relatively high concentrations of vasopressin ($>10^{-10}$M) were required to produce a rise in intracellular calcium. Large increases in urea permeability occurred in response to addition of 10^{-10}M vasopressin or 1mM 8-bromo cyclic AMP without a demonstrable change in intracellular calcium activity. Thus, a change in intracellular calcium was not necessary to elicit a nearly maximal increase in urea permeability.

The increase in intracellular calcium is a transient response to vasopressin. The time course of the response is similar to the time course of the vasopressin-mediated increases in intracellular calcium in hepatocytes and smooth muscle cells. The responses in these tissues occurs as part of the phosphoinositide cascade [39,40]. Occupation of V_1 type vasopressin receptors results in activation of phospholipase C which releases inositol tris-phosphate and diacylglycerol from phosphatidylinositol bis-phosphate in the plasma membrane. Inositol tris-phosphate causes the release of calcium from intracellular stores. Diacylglycerol activates protein kinase C, a response that is abetted by the rise in intracellular calcium. Calcium may activate a variety of enzymes and transport proteins in cells, and thus may regulate several important cell functions.

Shayman and Morrison [41] have demonstrated the presence of a bradykinin-stimulated increase in phosphoinositide turnover in cultured rabbit inner medullary collecting duct cells. They have also shown an associated rise in intracellular calcium in response to bradykinin [42]. Based on their demonstration of a functional phosphoinositide pathway in inner medullary collecting duct cells, we presume that the rise in intracellular calcium demonstrated in our study may be secondary to activation of the phosphoinositide system by vasopressin. If so, it is thus far unclear what physiological processes are regulated as a result of activation of the phosphoinositide pathway by vasopressin in the inner medullary collecting duct. One possibility is that activation of the phosphoinositide pathway in the inner medullary collecting duct mediates vasopressin-induced increases in prostaglandin production as in the toad bladder [43].

Effects of atrial natriuretic factor on inner medullary collecting duct function

The inner medullary collecting duct is an important renal tubular site of atrial natriuretic factor action. Cyclic GMP is a second messenger for atrial natriuretic factor in several tissues. We measured cyclic GMP accumulation in microdissected renal tubule segments from rats to determine which segments are likely sites of atrial natriuretic factor action [44]. Among all renal tubule segments, atrial natriuretic factor (rat ANF_{1-28}) caused the greatest response in the terminal

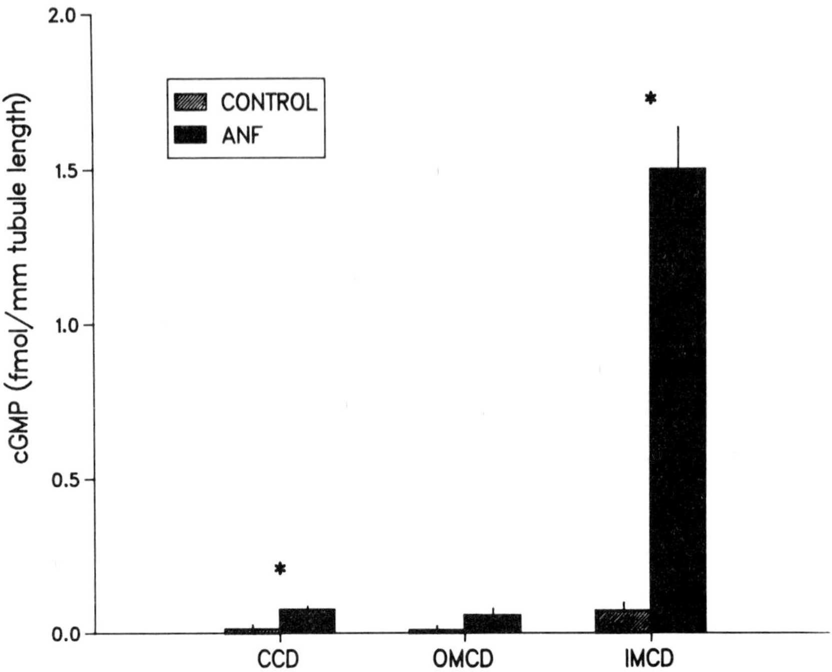

Figure 6. Effect of ANF_{1-28} on cyclic GMP accumulation in microdissected rat collecting duct segments. Asterisk indicates a statistically significant increase. From Nonoguchi et al [44]

inner medullary collecting duct. Figure 6 compares the cyclic GMP response of collecting duct segments. 10^{-6}M atrial natriuretic factor caused a 20-fold increase in cyclic GMP accumulation in the terminal part of the inner medullary collecting duct. Significant responses were seen with much lower concentrations of atrial natriuretic factor, within range of circulating levels of the peptide.

Based on our measurements of cyclic GMP accumulation and previous in vivo studies [45] pointing to the inner medullary collecting duct as a likely site of atrial natriuretic factor action to increase water and NaCl excretion, we have studied the ability of atrial natriuretic factor to alter water, urea, and NaCl transport in isolated perfused terminal inner medullary collecting duct segments [46,47]. Atrial natriuretic factor (ANF_{1-28}, 1–100nM in the peritubular bath) caused a 45–60% decrease in osmotic water permeability in the presence of physiologic concentrations of arginine vasopressin (10^{-11}M) [46]. There was no effect on osmotic water permeability in the absence of vasopressin or in the presence of high concentrations of vasopressin (10^{-8}M).

Several pieces of evidence indicate that the decrease in osmotic water permeability does not result from an effect on cyclic AMP metabolism. First atrial natriuretic factor had no effect on the urea permeability of the terminal inner medullary collecting duct in the presence of 10^{-11} M vasopressin [46]. Since the effect of vasopressin on water and urea permeability are both mediated by cyclic AMP (see above), an effect of atrial natriuretic factor on cyclic AMP production would be expected to decrease both water and urea permeability. Second, when we measured cyclic AMP accumulation in microdissected terminal inner medullary collecting ducts, there was no demonstrable effect of atrial natriuretic factor on cyclic AMP accumulation in the presence of vasopressin at any concentration [44,46]. These observations were repeated both in the presence and the absence of the phosphodiesterase inhibitor IBMX to assess the possibility that atrial natriuretic factor could affect cyclic AMP in the cell by stimulating its phosphodiesterase-mediated degradation. Although cyclic AMP accumulation was low in the absence of IBMX, there is still no demonstrable effect of atrial natriuretic factor on cyclic AMP accumulation. We propose that the effect of atrial natriuretic factor to decrease vasopressin-stimulated osmotic water permeability in the terminal inner medullary collecting duct does not occur via an effect on cyclic AMP metabolism. Rather, in the chain of events that link the receptor binding to an increase in epithelial water permeability, it appears that atrial natriuretic factor exerts its effect by altering some process subsequent to cyclic AMP generation.

Based on results from microcatheterization studies, Sonnenberg and co-workers [45] proposed that atrial natriuretic factor may increase NaCl excretion by increasing the NaCl permeability of the inner medullary collecting duct. An increase in NaCl permeability would allow NaCl to leak passively from the hypertonic medullary interstitium into the urine. To investigate this possibility, we tested whether atrial natriuretic factor increases NaCl permeability in isolated perfused terminal inner medullary collecting ducts. Atrial natriuretic factor at high concentrations (100nM) decreased chloride permeability by 15–25% [47]. The same dose of atrial natriuretic factor had no effect on sodium permeability. Therefore, these results do not support the hypothesis of Sonnenberg and co-workers. The decrease in chloride permeability may be due to an effect of atrial natriuretic factor on a transcellular pathway that may normally be involved in active NaCl absorption from the inner medullary collecting duct.

References

1 Clapp WL, Madsen KM, Verlander JW, Tisher CC. Intercalated cells of the rat inner medullary collecting duct. *Kidney Int 1987; 31:* 1080–1087

2 Madsen KM, Tisher CC. Structural-functional relationship along the distal nephron. *Am J Physiol 1986; 250:* F1–F15

3 Jamison RL, Kriz W. *Urinary Concentrating Mechanism: Structure and Function.* Oxford: Oxford University Press. 1982

4 Knepper MA, Danielson RA, Saidel GM, Post RS. Quantitative analysis of renal medullary anatomy in rats and rabbits. *Kidney Int 1977; 12:* 313–323

5 Chandhoke PS, Saidel GM, Knepper MA. Role of inner medullary collecting duct NaCl transport in urinary concentration. *Am J Physiol 1985; 249:* F668–F697

6 Ullrich KJ. Function of the collecting ducts. *Circulation 1960; 21:* 869–874
7 Marsh DJ. Hypoosmotic reabsorption due to active salt transport in perfused collecting ducts of the rat renal medulla. *Nature 1966; 210:* 1179–1180
8 Morgan T, Berliner RW. Permeability of the loop of Henle, vasa recta, and collecting duct to water, urea, and sodium. *Am J Physiol 1968; 215:* 108–115
9 Morgan T, Sakai F, Berliner RW. *In vitro* permeability of medullary collecting ducts to water and urea. *Am J Physiol 1968; 214:* 574–581
10 Burg MB. Perfusion of isolated renal tubules. *Yale J Biol Med 1972; 45:* 321–326
11 Rocha AS, Kokko JP. Permeability of medullary nephron segments of urea and water: effect of vasopressin. *Kidney Int 1974; 6:* 379–387
12 Rocha AS, Kudo LH. Water, urea, sodium, chloride, and potassium transport in the *in vitro* isolated perfused papillary collecting duct. *Kidney Int 1982; 22:* 485–491
13 Sands JM, Knepper MA. Urea permeability of mammalian inner medullary collecting duct system and papillary surface epithelium. *J Clin Invest 1987; 79:* 138–147
14 Sands JM, Nonoguchi H, Knepper MA. Vasopressin effects on urea and H_2O transport in inner medullary collecting duct subsegments. *Am J Physiol 1987; 253:* in press
15 Knepper MA, Roch-Ramel F. Pathways of urea transport in the mammalian kidney. *Kidney Int 1987; 31:* 629–633
16 Jamison RL, Buerkert J, Lacy F. A micropuncture study of collecting tubule function in rats with hereditary diabetes insipidus. *J Clin Invest 1971; 50:* 2444–2452
17 Schmidt-Nielsen B, Graves B, Roth J. Water removal and solute additions determining increases in renal medullary osmolality. *Am J Physiol 1983; 244:* F472–F482
18 Pfeiffer EW. Comparative anatomical observations of the mammalian renal pelvis and medulla. *J Anat 1968; 102:* 321–331
19 Silverblatt FJ. Ultrastructure of the renal pelvic epithelium of the rat. *Kidney Int 1974; 5:* 214–220
20 Packer R, Sands J, Knepper M. Osmotic water and chloride permeabilities of isolated rabbit renal papillary surface epithelium (abstract). *Physiologist 1987; 30:* in press
21 Sands JM, Knepper MA, Spring KS. Na-K-Cl cotransport in apical membrane of rabbit renal papillary surface epithelium. *Am J Physiol 1986; 251:* F475–F484
22 Galluci E, Micelli S, Lippe C. Non-electrolyte permeability across thin lipid membranes. *Arch Int Physiol Biochim 1971; 79:* 881–887
23 Welling LW, Evan AP, Welling DJ. Shape of cells and extracellular channels in rabbit cortical collecting ducts. *Kidney Int 1981; 20:* 211–222
24 Welling LW, Welling DJ. Surface areas of the brush border and lateral cell walls in the rabbit proximal nephron. *Kidney Int 1975; 8:* 343–348
25 Welling LW, Welling DJ. Shape of epithelial cells and intercellular channels in the rabbit proximal nephron. *Kidney Int 1976; 9:* 385–394
26 Welling LW, Welling DJ, Hill JJ. Shape of cells and intercellular channels in the rabbit thick ascending limb of Henle. *Kidney Int 1978; 13:* 114–151
27 Rastegar A, Biemesderfer D, Kashgarian M, Hayslett JP. Changes in membrane surfaces of collecting duct cells in potassium adaptation. *Kidney Int 1980; 18:* 293–301
28 Burg M, Helman S, Grantham J, Orloff J. Effect of vasopressin on the permeability of isolated rabbit cortical collecting tubules to urea, acetamide, and thiourea. In Schmidt-Nielsen B, ed. *Urea and the Kidney.* Amsterdam: Elsevier. 1968: 193–199
29 Kokko JP. Urea transport in the proximal tubule and the descending limb of Henle. *J Clin Invest 1972; 51:* 1999–2008
30 Schafer JA, Andreoli TE. Cellular constraints to diffusion: the effect of antidiuretic hormone on water flows in isolated mammalian collecting tubules. *J Clin Invest 1972; 51:* 1264–1278
31 Schafer JA, Andreoli TE. The effect of antidiuretic hormone on solute flows in mammalian collecting tubules. *J Clin Invest 1972; 51:* 1279–1286
32 Imai M, Kokko JP. Sodium chloride, urea, and water transport in the thin ascending limb of Henle. Generation of osmotic gradients by passive diffusion of solutes. *J Clin Invest 1974; 53:* 393–402

33 Knepper MA. Urea transport in nephron segments from medullary rays of rabbits. *Am J Physiol 1983; 244:* F622–F627

34 Macey RI. Transport of water and urea in red blood cells. *Am J Physiol 1984; 246:* C195–C203

35 Levine S, Franki N, Hays RM. A saturable, vasopressin-sensitive carrier for urea and acetamide in the toad bladder epithelial cell. *J Clin Invest 1973; 52:* 2083–2086

36 Morgan T, Rayson B, Haberle D. The effects of sodium chloride, urea and mannitol on the permeability *in vitro* of rat papillary collecting ducts to THO, ^{14}C-urea, and ^{22}Na. *Clin Exp Pharm Physiol 1977; 4:* 565–574

37 Kondo Y, Imai M. Effects of gluteraldehyde fixation on renal tubular function. I. Preservation of vasopressin-stimulated water and urea pathways in rat papillary collecting duct. *Pfluegers Arch 1987; 408:* 479–483

38 Star RA, Nonoguchi H, Balaban RB, Knepper MA. Calcium and cyclic AMP as second messengers for vasopressin in rat inner medullary collecting duct (abstract). *Kidney Int 1988; 33:* in press

39 Berridge MJ. Inositol trisphosphate and diacylglycerol as second messengers. *Biochem J 1984; 220:* 345–360

40 Exton JH. Role of calcium and phophoinositides in the actions of certain hormones and neurotransmitters. *J Clin Invest 1985; 75:* 1753–1757

41 Shayman JA, Morrison AR. Bradykinin-induced changes in phosphatidyl inositol turnover in cultured rabbit papillary collecting tubule cells. *J Clin Invest 1985; 76:* 978–984

42 Shayman JA, Hruska KA, Morrison AR. Bradykinin stimulates increased intracellular calcium in papillary collecting tubules of the rabbit. *Biochem Biophys Res Comm 1986; 134:* 299–304

43 Schlondorff D, Satriano JA. Interactions of vasopressin, cAMP, and prostaglandins in toad urinary bladder. *Am J Physiol 1985; 248:* F454–F458

44 Nonoguchi H, Knepper MA, Manganiello VC. Effects of atrial natriuretic factor on cyclic guanosine monophosphate and cyclic adenosine monophosphate accumulation in microdissected nephron segments from rats. *J Clin Invest 1987; 79:* 500–507

45 Sonnenberg H, Honrath U, Chong CK, Wilson DR. Atrial natriuretic factor inhibits sodium transport in medullary collecting duct. *Am J Physiol 1986; 250:* F963–F966

46 Nonoguchi H, Sands JM, Knepper MA. Interaction between atrial peptide and vasopressin in the inner medullary collecting duct (abstract). *Kidney Int 1988; 33:* in press

47 Sands JM, Nonoguchi H, Knepper MA. NaCl permeability of the rat inner medullary collecting duct (abstract). *Kidney Int 1988; 33:* in press

ANATOMY OF THE H^+-SECRETING MECHANISM IN COLLECTING DUCT EPITHELIAL CELLS

D Brown

Massachusetts General Hospital, Harvard Medical School, Boston, Massachusetts, USA

Introduction

Net acid excretion by the kidney is mainly performed by two segments of the urinary tubule – the proximal tubule and the collecting duct. Whereas the entire population of epithelial cells in the proximal tubule appears to be involved in this process, the task of proton-secretion in the collecting duct is largely carried out by a highly specialized subpopulation of epithelial cells known as intercalated cells. The existence of two cell types in the collecting duct was first noted by Seraphima Schachowa in 1876 [1], but interest in these cells was only sporadic until quite recently. It is now clear that intercalated cells are but one member of a family of cells, found in various transporting epithelia, that are collectively known as 'mitochondria-rich' cells [2]; much of our current understanding of the rôle of these cells has resulted from studies using the toad and, particularly, the turtle urinary bladder as model acidifying systems [3]. These cells are, in addition, found in amphibian epidermis and the initial segment of rat epididymis [2].

All mitochondria-rich cells have a set of common, characteristic features that appear to be related to their proton-secretory activity. The first major clue pointing to a rôle in acidification was the discovery that intercalated cells, as well as all other mitochondria-rich cells, contain abundant carbonic anhydrase in their cytoplasm. This has been shown by both enzyme histochemistry [4,5] and immunocytochemistry at the light and electronmicroscope level [6,7] (Figure 1). A second line of evidence came from several morpho-functional studies that showed changes in the morphological appearance of these cells under different physiological conditions that are known to modify proton secretion [8–16]. These modifications of structure are particularly evident at the level of the apical plasma membrane, where the number and size of apical microvilli and microplicae can vary considerably, and the number of characteristic rod-shaped intramembranous particles (IMPs), seen in freeze-fracture, is also highly variable

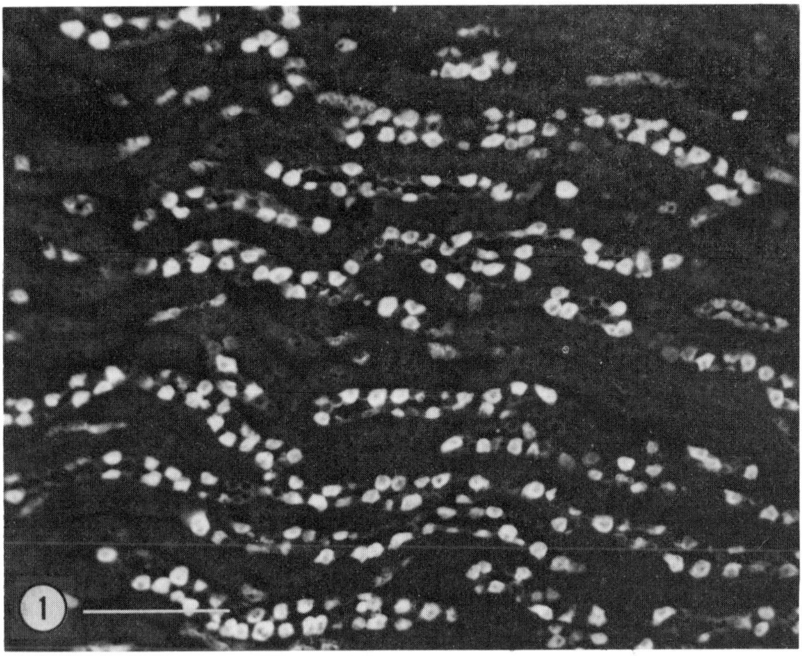

Figure 1. Inner stripe of rat kidney medulla stained with antibodies against rat carbonic anhydrase C, followed by an FITC-labelled secondary antibody. The mosaic pattern of staining in collecting ducts reflects the intense reactivity of intercalated cells, whereas the principal cells are only weakly labelled [taken from 7]. Bar=100μm

[2,16]. In parallel with these alterations in apical membrane structure during stimulation of H^+ secretion, there is a reduction in the number of cytoplasmic vesicles in the apical cytoplasmic region of these cells [11,12].

Thus, when H^+ secretion is stimulated, specialized cytoplasmic vesicles appear to fuse with the apical plasma membrane and deliver proton pumps to this membrane domain. Evidence indicating the presence of proton pumps on the limiting membrane of these vesicles was obtained using the fluorescent pH indicator, acridine orange, which revealed that the vesicles have an internal acidic pH that is sensitive to inhibitors of vacuolar proton pumps [17]. The rôle of membrane fusion events in the stimulation of H^+ secretion by this family of cells has been most clearly shown in the turtle urinary bladder [17,18], but a similar mechanism has more recently been demonstrated in collecting duct intercalated cells [19] (Figure 2).

The vesicles involved in this process have a prominent coat of regularly-arranged dense studs on their cytoplasmic surface [11,12,16]; using anti-clathrin antibodies in conjunction with the protein A-gold immunocytochemical technique we have shown that the coat does not contain clathrin [20] (Figure 3).

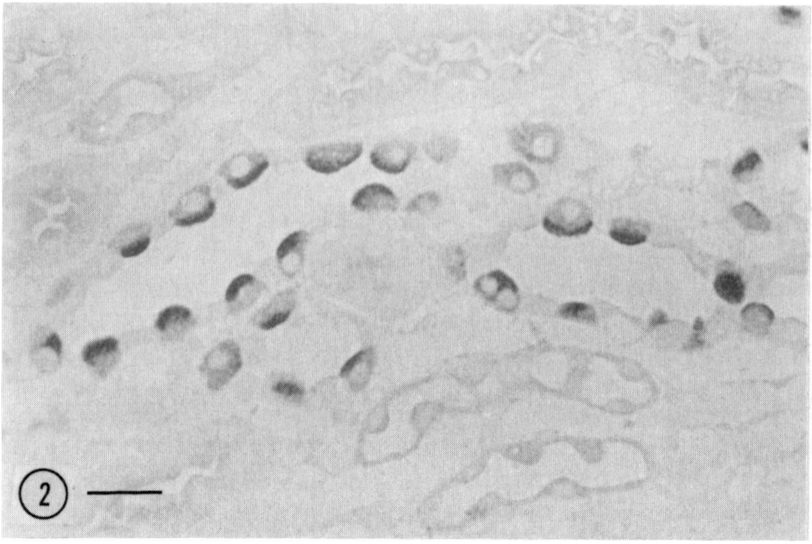

Figure 2. Inner stripe of rat kidney medulla labelled with specific antibody against the 70kD subunit of bovine medullary H^+ATPase, followed by the ABC-peroxidase procedure. Intercalated cells in this region of the collecting duct are intensely stained at their apical pole, indicating antigenic sites associated with the apical plasma membrane, and with a population of apical cytoplasmic vesicles. Bar=20μm

Nevertheless, more recent studies using horseradish peroxidase as a tracer have shown that these vesicles *are* involved in endocytosis in intercalated cells [21] (Figure 4). In view of the known association of clathrin with the endocytosis of surface molecules and ligands in other cell types [22], it became important to determine whether the membrane coat in proton-secreting cells was a material involved in vesicle recycling (by analogy with clathrin) or whether it could be the cytoplasmic domain of a molecule that is transported to and from the plasma membrane by these vesicles; for example, the H^+ATPase. The remainder of this short review will summarize data obtained in collaboration with John Hartwig (Hematology and Oncology Laboratory, Massachusetts General Hospital), and Stephen Gluck (Jewish Hospital, Washington University, St Louis) which shows that the material coating these vesicles and parts of the plasma membrane of proton-secreting cells contains subunits of a proton-pumping ATPase.

Structure of the coat revealed by rapid-freezing and freeze-drying

The structure of the coating material was examined using the rapid-freezing, freeze-drying technique which has been used to reveal the structure of clathrin and components of the cytoskeleton in other cell types [23]. For our study [24], mitochondria-rich cells from toad urinary bladder epithelium were used. Portions of apical plasma membrane were sheared away from the remainder of

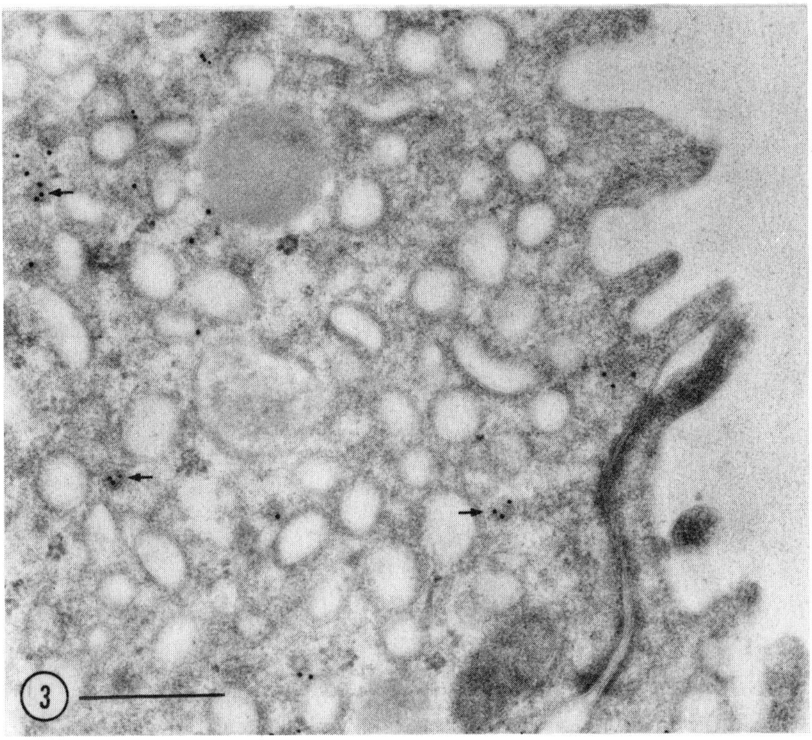

Figure 3. Thin section of Lowicryl K4M-embedded kidney showing the apical region of an intercalated cell. The section was incubated with an affinity-purified anti-clathrin antibody (provided by Dr Daniel Louvard, Paris) followed by protein A-gold. Antigenic sites, revealed by gold particles, are mainly associated with small vesicles (arrows) that are clathrin-coated. The larger, more abundant vesicles that characterize intercalated cells are virtually unlabelled [taken from 20]. Bar=0.5μm

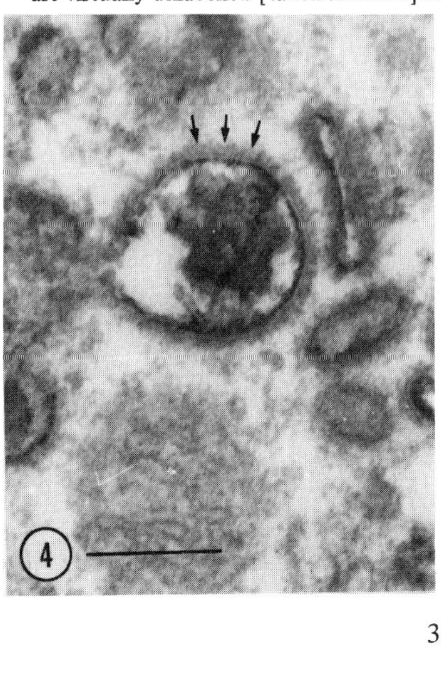

Figure 4. Thin section of intercalated cell from a rat that was injected with horseradish peroxidase for 15 minutes prior to fixation. Peroxidase reaction product, taken into the cell by endocytosis, is present inside vesicles that have an extensive cytoplasmic coat (arrows). This coat does not contain clathrin (Figure 3), but does contain subunits of a proton pump (Figure 5) [taken from 21]. Bar=0.25μm

Figure 5. Thin section of Lowicryl K4M-embedded kidney showing a vesicle in the cytoplasm of an intercalated cell, similar to the vesicle shown in Figure 4. After incubation with the specific antibody against the 70kD subunit of H^+ATPase (see also Figure 2), gold particles indicating H^+ATPase antigenic sites are localized on the cytoplasmic surface of the limiting membrane of the vesicle. These particles are directly overlying the membrane coating material, seen more readily in conventionally embedded and sectioned tissue (Figure 4). Bar=0.25μm

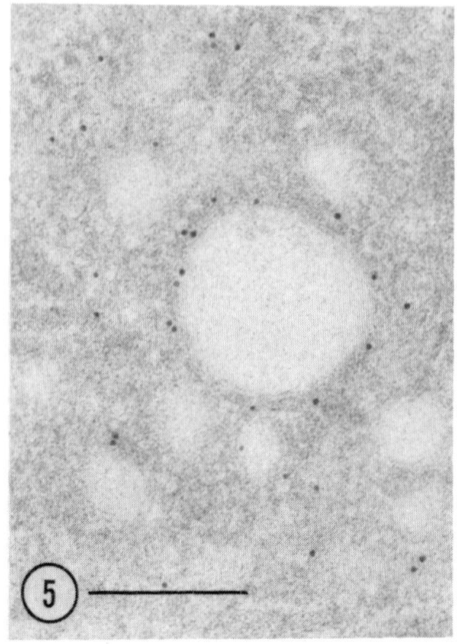

the cell using a polylysine-coated coverslip, and the membrane fragments were rapidly-frozen by slamming against a helium-cooled copper block. After freeze-drying in a Balzers freeze-etch device, platinum-carbon replicas of the underside of the membrane were prepared by rotary-shadowing. As shown in Figures 6 and 7, a striking membrane feature was present on the underside of mitochondria-rich cell plasma membranes, and on the cytoplasmic side of a population of cytoplasmic vesicles. These membranes were decorated with many stud-like projections that were often arranged into regular, hexagonal arrays. Each stud was between 9–10nm in diameter, and there were 16,800 studs per square micron of membrane. This material corresponds to the coating material seen in thin sections of these cells, and has a structure that is quite different from that of clathrin.

Structure of H^+ATPase incorporated into liposomes

We went on to examine directly the structure of proton pumps that had been affinity-purified on a column prepared using a monoclonal antibody directed against partially-purified bovine kidney medullary H^+ATPase [24–26]. This multisubunit protein was capable of ATP-dependent acidification and potential generation when reconstituted into liposomes while still bound to the affinity matrix [24,26]. The immunoaffinity purified protein complex was incorporated into phospholipid liposomes, and the liposomes were examined by rapid-freezing and freeze-drying. Remarkably, the replicas revealed stud-like projections on the liposomes that were identical in size and packing to the coating material found on toad bladder mitochondria-rich cell membranes [24].

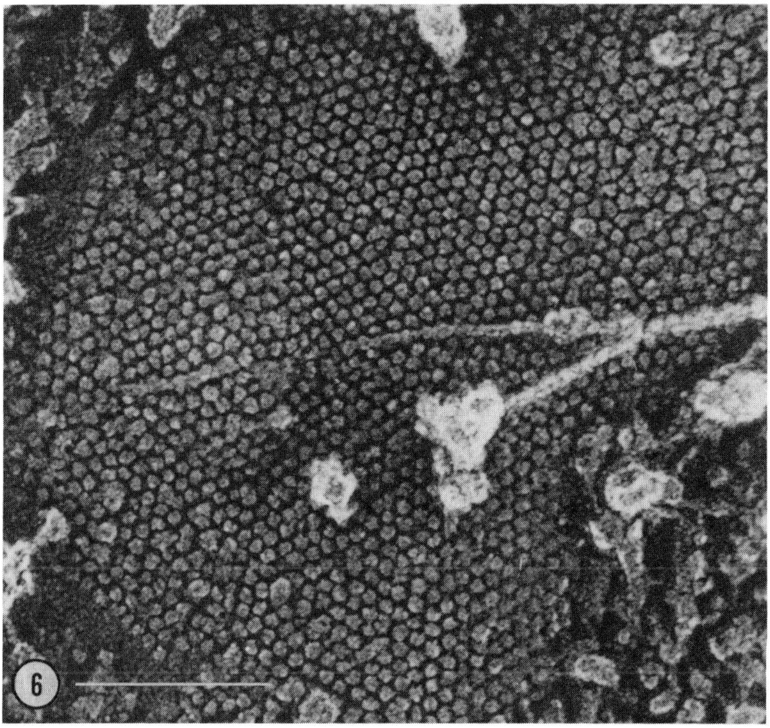

Figure 6. Platinum-carbon replica of the underside of a toad bladder mitochondria-rich cell apical plasma membrane prepared by rapid-freezing and freeze-drying. The membrane coating material is formed by numerous, stud-like projections that are arranged into hexagonally-packed arrays. Each stud is about 10nm in diameter [taken from 24]. Bar=0.1μm

Immunocytochemical localization of H^+ATPase

Using the affinity-purified H^+ATPase protein complex as an immunogen, a polyclonal antiserum was raised in rabbits. This antiserum contained cross-reactivity against multiple subunits of the protein; subunit-specific polyclonal antisera were prepared by absorption of the original antiserum with nitrocellulose filters containing only individual subunits of the protein [24,27]. By light microscopy, immunoperoxidase labelling revealed a population of cells in the inner stripe of the rat kidney collecting duct that were strongly positive. Antibodies against the 3kD, 55kD and 70kD subunits of the protein gave identical results. The label was concentrated at the apical pole of the positive cells. By immunoelectronmicroscopy using the protein A-gold technique [28] on sections cut from Lowicryl K4M-embedded material, gold particles were found on the cytoplasmic side of all stud-coated membrane domains of intercalated cells, including the cytoplasmic vesicles [24,27] (Figure 5). Again, all three antibodies gave similar results.

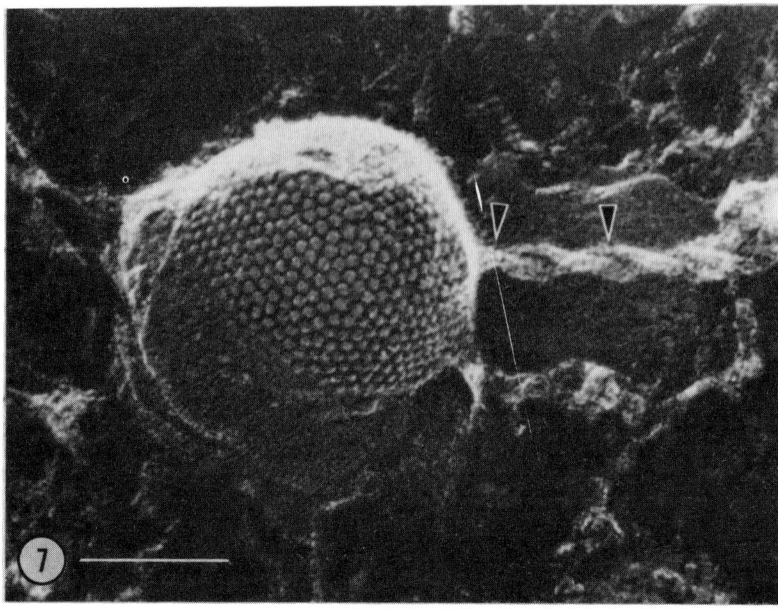

Figure 7. Platinum-carbon replica showing a small, stud-coated vesicle in the cytoplasm of a mitochondria-rich cell from toad urinary bladder. The studs are identical to those found on the plasma membranes of these cells (Figure 6). In many cases, actin filaments, identified by the binding of myosin S1 (arrowheads), are associated with these vesicles [taken from 24]. Bar=0,1μm

Together with the rapid-freeze, freeze-drying data, these observations provide direct evidence that the novel membrane-coating material found on specialized membrane domains in proton-secreting cells contains subunits of a proton-translocating ATPase [24].

It is now considered that while all intercalated cells in the inner stripe are acid-secreting cells, the cortical collecting duct contains intercalated cells that are either H^+-secreting or HCO_3^--secreting [19]. These cells would have proton pumps inserted into their apical or basolateral plasma membranes, respectively. Recent data suggest that some intercalated cells in the cortex can reverse their functional polarity with respect to proton secretion under different acid-base conditions [29]. Although such a reversal of polarity remains to be demonstrated with a specific marker for membrane proteins, our antibodies against subunits of the proton pump clearly show the presence of subpopulations of cortical intercalated cells with either apical or basolateral pumps [27]. Furthermore, mitochondria-rich cells with opposing polarities with respect to rod-shaped IMPs (seen in freeze-fracture) and membrane associated studs have been described in the turtle urinary bladder [30]. These observations raise the intriguing question as to how proton pumps can be targetted to distinct membrane domains in epithelial cells. One factor that appears to be involved in the selective insertion of membrane components is the aminoacid composition of the protein itself [31,32]. It is possible, therefore, that the precise subunit composition of proton pumps may be different at the apical and basolateral poles of subpopulations of intercalated cells. This difference may be responsible for the selective targetting of the enzyme. It is also possible that other factors such as specific properties of transporting vesicles, and their interaction with the microtubular system of the cell, may be important in the trafficking of membrane proteins. In this respect, it has been shown that microtubule-disrupting drugs can alter the domain specificity of viral protein insertion into plasma membranes of cultured cells [33], and it has been suggested that the interior pH of secretory granules in endocrine and exocrine cells may determine from which pole of the cell the protein contents are secreted [34].

The intercalated cell of the kidney collecting duct, and related mitochondria-rich cells in other epithelia, provide a virtually unique system in which a major membrane protein can be localized at opposite poles of adjacent cells. Using our battery of subunit-specific antibodies, together with morphological markers for this protein in thin sections and platinum-carbon replicas, we are now in the process of examining conditions that regulate this targetting process. The results should provide information that is of specific importance to acid-base regulation by the collecting duct, and that is of more general significance to the cell biology of polarized epithelia.

References

1 Schachowa S. *Untersuchungen über die Nieren.* Inaugural dissertation, University of Bern, Switzerland, 13 July 1876

2 Orci L, Humbert F, Brown D, Perrelet A. Membrane ultrastructure in urinary tubules. *Int Rev Cytol 1981; 73:* 183–242

3 Steinmetz PR. Cellular organization of urinary acidification. *Am J Physiol 1986; 251:* F173–F187

4 Rosen S. Localization of carbonic anhydrase activity in the vertebrate nephron. *Histochem J 1972; 4:* 35–38

5 Lonnerholm G, Ridderstrale Y. Intracellular distribution of carbonic anhydrase in rat kidney. *Kidney Int 1980; 17:* 162–174

6 Brown D, Roth J, Kumpulainen T, Orci L. Ultrastructural localization of carbonic anhydrase. Presence in intercalated cells of the rat collecting tubule. *Histochemistry 1982; 75:* 209–213

7 Brown D, Roth J, Kumpulainen T, Orci L. Immunohistochemical localization of carbonic anhydrase in postnatal and adult rat kidney. *Am J Physiol 1983; 245:* F110–F118

8 Evan A, Huser J, Bengele HH, Alexander EA. The effect of alterations in dietary potassium on collecting system morphology in the rat. *Lab Invest 1980; 42:* 668–675

9 Hagege J. Morphologie et histophysiologie des cellules intercalaires du tube urinaire des vertebrés tétrapodes. *Ann Biol 1972; 11:* 105–143

10 Kaissling B. Structural aspects of adaptive changes in renal electrolyte secretion. *Am J Physiol 1982; 243:* F211–F226

11 Madsen KM, Tisher CC. Cellular response to acute respiratory acidosis in rat medullary collecting duct. *Am J Physiol 1983; 245:* F670–F678

12 Madsen KM, Tisher CC. Response of intercalated cells of rat outer medullary collecting duct to chronic metabolic acidosis. *Lab Invest 1984; 51:* 268–276
13 Rastegar A, Biemesderfer D, Kashgarian M, Hayslett JP. Changes in membrane surfaces of collecting duct cells in potassium depletion. *Kidney Int 1980; 18:* 293–301
14 Richet G, Hagege J. Dark cells of the distal convoluted tubules and collecting ducts. II. Physiological significance. *Fortschr Zool 1975; 23:* 299–306
15 Stanton B. Biemesderfer D, Wade JB, Giebisch G. Structural and functional study of rat distal tubule: effects of potassium adaptation and depletion. *Kidney Int 1981; 19:* 36–48
16 Stetson DL, Wade JB, Giebisch G. Morphological alterations in the rat medullary collecting duct following potassium depletion. *Kidney Int 1980; 17:* 45–56
17 Gluck S, Cannon C, Al-Awqati Q. Exocytosis regulates urinary acidification in turtle bladder by rapid insertion of H^+ pumps into the luminal membrane. *Proc Natl Acad Sci USA 1982; 79:* 4327–4331
18 Stetson DL, Steinmetz PR. Role of membrane fusion in CO_2 stimulation of proton secretion by turtle bladder. *Am J Physiol 1983; 245:* C113–C120
19 Schwartz GJ, Al-Awqati Q. Carbon dioxide causes exocytosis of vesicles containing H^+ pumps in isolated perfused proximal and collecting tubules. *J Clin Invest 1985; 75:* 1638–1644
20 Brown D, Orci L. The "coat" of kidney intercalated cell tubulovesicles does not contain clathrin. *Am J Physiol 1986; 250:* C605–C608
21 Brown D, Weyer P, Orci L. Non-clathrin coated vesicles are involved in endocytosis in kidney collecting duct intercalated cells. *Anat Rec:* in press
22 Goldstein JL, Anderson RGW, Brown MS. Coated pits, coated vesicles and receptor-mediated endocytosis. *Nature 1979; 279:* 679–685
23 Heuser J, Kirschner MW. Filament organization revealed in platinum replicas of freeze-dried cytoskeletons. *J Cell Biol 1980; 86:* 212–234
24 Brown D, Gluck S, Hartwig J. Structure of the novel membrane-coating material in proton-secreting epithelial cells and identification as an H^+ATPase. *J Cell Biol:* in press
25 Yurko M, Fitch F, Gluck S. Production and characterization of a monoclonal antibody to H^+ATPase. *Fed Proc 1986; 45:* 652a
26 Gluck S, Caldwell J. Proton translocating ATPase from bovine kidney medulla. Partial purification and reconstitution. *Am J Physiol 1987:* in press
27 Gluck S, Hirsch S, Brown D. Immunocytochemical localization of H^+ATPase in rat kidney. *Kidney Int 1987; 31:* 167a
28 Roth J, Bendayan M, Orci L. Ultrastructural localization of intracellular antigens by the use of protein A-gold complex. *J Histochem Cytochem 1978; 26:* 1074–1081
29 Schwartz GJ, Barasch J, Al-Awqati Q. Plasticity of functional epithelial polarity. *Nature 1985; 318:* 368–371
30 Stetson DL, Steinmetz PR. α and β types of carbonic anhydrase-rich cells in turtle bladder. *Am J Physiol 1985; 249:* F553–F565
31 Kelly RB. From organelle to organelle. *Nature 1987; 326:* 14–15
32 Garoff H. Using recombinant DNA techniques to study protein targetting in the eucaryotic cell. *Ann Rev Cell Biol 1985; 1:* 403–445
33 Rindler MJ, Ivanov IE, Sabatini DD. Microtubule-acting drugs lead to the non-polarized delivery of the influenza hemagglutinin to the cell surface of polarized Madin-Darby canine kidney cells. *J Cell Biol 1987; 104:* 231–241
34 Orci L, Ravazzola M, Anderson RGW. The condensing vacuole of exocrine cells is more acidic than the mature secretory granule. *Nature 1987; 326:* 77–79

VASOPRESSIN RECEPTOR-ADENYLATE CYCLASE INTERACTIONS: A MODEL FOR cAMP METABOLISM IN THE KIDNEY

D A Ausiello

Massachussetts General Hospital and Harvard Medical School, Boston, Massachusetts, USA

Introduction

The antidiuretic action of vasopressin is mediated by the sequential steps of vasopressin binding to its cell surface receptor, followed by the receptor-mediated stimulation of adenylate cyclase. During the last decade it has become clear that adenylate cyclase is a compex enzyme system requiring at least three subunits for hormonal activation [1–3]. These subunits, receptor (R), guanyl nucleotide-regulatory protein (G), and catalytic unit (C), have been characterized in terms of their individual biological properties using a variety of techniques [2,4–8]. The G subunit in turn consists of two major subunits termed α and β, with molecular weights of $(45–52) \times 10^{-3}$ and 35×10^{-3} kDa, respectively [9]. A third subunit of G, the γ protein, interacts with β to form a $\beta\gamma$ complex functionally similar to β alone. For simplicity we will only refer to the α and β subunits. A fundamental question is how the individual subunits are structured in the membrane before and after exposure to activating ligands [4]. In this regard, several possible models for the sequence of subunit interactions involved in the activation of adenylate cyclase have been proposed [8,10].

To address the question of subunit interactions involved in adenylate cyclase activation, we required approaches which could be applied to intact cells, thus avoiding possible disruption of subunit assembly which accompanies solubilization and purification techniques. The model system utilized was the cultured pig kidney epithelial cell line, LLC-PK_1. This cell line demonstrates a 50-fold increase in cAMP production in response to vasopressin [11]. The availability of the LLC-PK_1 cell has allowed study of hormone binding and cAMP production in a homogeneous population of intact cells, as well as correlation of these results with adenylate cyclase activation in membranes [12–14]. More recently target analysis by radiation inactivation has been used, applied to cultured cell monolayers to further characterize the sequence of subunit interactions involved in the hormonal and non-hormonal activation and inhibition of adenylate cyclase in the intact membrane [15–18]. By combining information on the known biochemical characteristics of the individual solubilized subunit components with the results of binding and radiation inactivation studies carried out in intact cells, we arrived at a model for vasopressin stimulation of cyclase. In the following discussion we will describe the details of this comprehensive model.

Model for adenylate cyclase activation

Target analysis data were combined with known biochemical characteristics of the vasopressin-adenylate cyclase system (Table I) to formulate a unique pattern

TABLE I. Characteristics required of a model for adenylate cyclase activation

A. *TARGET ANALYSIS CRITERIA*
1. 'Dissociative' reaction mechanism in which hormone facilitates the disaggregation of subunits into active enzyme.
2. Molecular weight of 'activated' enzyme is 170–180 kDa.
B. *BIOCHEMICAL CRITERIA*
3. High and low affinity hormone binding species exist.
4. Guanine nucleotides lower receptor affinity.
5. Non-linear coupling occurs between receptor occupancy and enzyme activation.
6. Must account for the activation of enzyme by hormone, guanine nucleotides, and forskolin.
7. Any activation mechanism should allow for the addition of an inhibitory pathway.

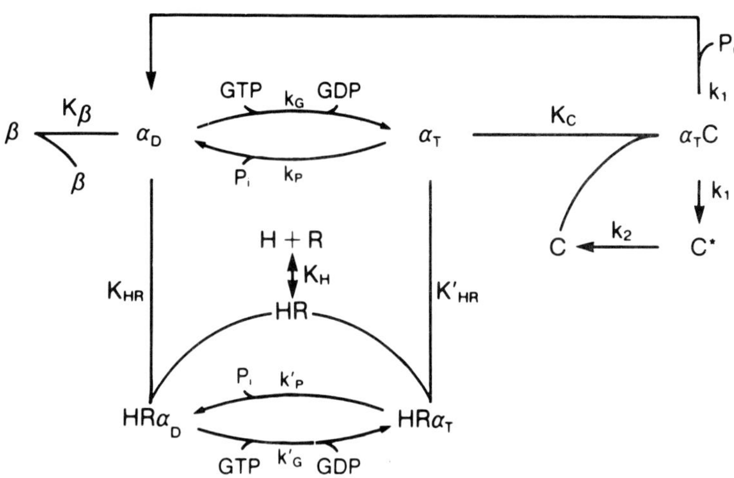

Figure 1. $\alpha\beta$ Cyclic dissociation model for adenylatecyclase activation. H=hormone; R=receptor; α,β=subunits of guanine nucleotide-regulatory protein; C=catalytic unit; GTP and GDP=guanosine triphosphate and diphosphate respectively; P_i=inorganic phosphate; D and T subscript denote GTP- and GDP-associated states of α respectively. K_{HR}, K_{HR}', K_C, and K_β are equilibrium dissociation constants and k_G, k_p', k'_G, k_p, k_1, k_2 are kinetic constants

for the interaction of the vasopressin receptor-adenylate cyclase subunits (Figure 1). It should be noted that the biochemical criteria listed in Table I are general characteristics of a number of hormone receptor-adenylate cyclase systems, and not limited to the enzyme activation by vasopressin.

The model in Figure 1 predicts that hormone (H) interacts with its free receptor to form an HR complex which in turn can interact with either α_{GDP} or α_{GTP}. The α_{GDP} subunit is the high affinity subunit for HR binding, and GTP lowers the affinity of hormonal binding during the formation of $HR\alpha_{GTP}$. The multiple interdependent binding sites for hormone account for the presence of a nonlinear Scatchard plot which, interestingly, could become a linear Scatchard plot as the relative stoichiometry of R and α, and the individual binding affinities are varied. Such a transition in shape of the Scatchard plot for vasopressin binding has been observed [12,14]. The coupling ratio of receptor occupancy to enzyme activation will be a function of the lifetime of activated C* compared to the rate of unbinding of hormone. If C* is long lived, non-linear coupling will occur. The mechanism shown in Figure 1 satisfies the details of the radiation inactivation data [15–17]. The species whose concentration is proportional to enzyme activity is $\alpha_{GTP}C$. This corresponds to the target size of 180 kDa (α=45 kDa; C=120–150 kDa) obtained for the active species for radiation inactivation. It is equally important to note that a number of other plausible models previously suggested in the literature as mechanisms of activation of adenylate cyclase could be excluded on the basis of their inability to satisfy all the criteria in Table I. The models eliminated included those in which $\alpha\beta$ dissociation was assigned as the hormone sensitive step, as well as models in which there was precoupling of either R or C with the $\alpha\beta$ subunits [16,17].

The 'cyclic dissociation model' in Figure 1 also adequately accounts for the activation of adenylate cyclase by guanine nucleotides and forskolin. GTP addition results in increased $\alpha\beta$ dissociation. Therefore, the principles of a dissociative model apply. There are two possible interpretations for forskolin action. Forskolin may act like GTP and cause increased $\alpha\beta$ dissociation. Alternatively, forskolin may decrease k_2, and prolong the lifetime of the activated enzyme. This mechanism of action for forskolin would be consistent with its direct effects on C in the absence of $\alpha\beta$ [6,7]. At the same time, without involving another locus of action, such an effect of forskolin on k_2 would be consistent with the observation that forskolin can also enhance α_{GTP}-mediated activation of the enzyme [6,7].

Incorporation of an inhibitory pathway into the model for adenylate cyclase activity

In recent years it has become known that an independent inhibitory pathway exists for the regulation of adenylate cyclase activity [for review see 19]. In general, this pathway is activated through inhibitory receptors (e.g. opiates, α_2-adrenergic, A_1-adenosine) coupled to an 'inhibitory' guanine nucleotide regulatory unit ($\alpha_i\beta$) which is distinct from its stimulatory counterpart ($\alpha_s\beta$) by the presence of a unique α subunit. Both α_s and α_i share a common β (and γ) subunit. The mechanism by which $\alpha_i\beta$ causes inhibition of adenylate cyclase remains controversial, but likely involves at least two separate processes: 1) $\alpha_i\beta$ dissociation results in increased availability of β which in turn can interact with active α_s to form inactive $\alpha_s\beta$; and 2) free α_i can interact directly with the catalytic unit C, to form an inactive complex, α_iC.

Both α_s and α_i share the characteristics of binding GTP, which results in activation of these proteins, and possess GTPase activity. Both are ADP-ribosylated by toxins, but with opposite results: cholera toxin stimulates the activity of α_s, whereas pertussis toxin inhibits the activity of α_i.

While it is clear that $\alpha_i\beta$ inhibition of adenylate cyclase can occur through the stimulation of inhibitory receptors, it is uncertain whether $\alpha_i\beta$ can tonically modulate $\alpha_s\beta$ function, either in the basal state or in the exclusive presence of stimulatory receptor activity. The possibility of a tonic modulatory rôle of $\alpha_i\beta$ for stimulatory receptors is supported by studies in solubilized and reconstituted systems containing purified β-adrenergic receptors, $\alpha_s\beta$, and $\alpha_i\beta$ [20,21]. These studies demonstrated that the addition of $\alpha_i\beta$ was necessary to express the full stimulatory capacity of the β-adrenergic receptor. However, a similar rôle for $\alpha_i\beta$ has not been demonstrated in intact membranes.

The effect of $\alpha_i\beta$ on vasopressin-sensitive adenylate cyclase was investigated following a series of studies involving the addition to GTP to intact

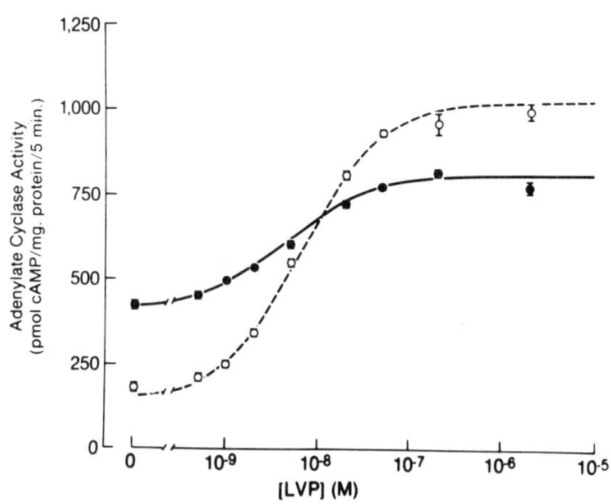

Figure 2. Experimentally-observed hormone concentration dependence of GTP mediated inhibition. Adenylate cyclase activity was determined at each concentration of vasopressin shown without (open circles, broken line) or with (closes circles, solid line) the addition of 100μM GTP. When fitted to a single site binding model the $K_{1/2}$ for activation in the absence of GTP (broken line) was 0.65±0.07nM and in the presence of GTP 0.47±0.04nM

membranes from LLC-PK_1 cells [18]. GTP addition resulted in the stimulation of basal activity, but inhibition of maximal vasopressin-stimulated activity. Of particular interest was the hormone concentration dependence for the inhibitory effect of GTP shown in Figure 2. At concentrations of hormone below the $K_{1/2}$ for enzyme activation, GTP addition enhanced enzyme activity whilst at higher hormone concentrations, GTP was inhibitory. The inhibitory effect of GTP was also observed for a V_2-receptor agonist, dDAVP, and was not abolished by a V_1-receptor antagonist indicating that a distinct V_1-receptor does not mediate the inhibition of vasopressin-sensitive adenylate cyclase.

A rôle for $\alpha_i\beta$ as the effector of the inhibitory response was determined in studies utilizing pertussis toxin (Table II). The addition of 100μM GTP resulted

TABLE II. Effects of GTP and pertussis toxin on basal and vasopressin-stimulated adenylate cyclase activity

	Without pertussis toxin		With pertussis toxin	
	No GTP	100μM GTP	No GTP	100μM GTP
Basal	84±10	350±46	74±7	500±55
Vasopressin, 2μM	1362±122	837±73*	1437±137	1782±113*

Adenylate cyclase activity is expressed as pmol cAMP/mg protein/5 min ± SEM.
*Significantly less than corresponding 'No GTP' ($p<0.01$).

in a several-fold increase in basal adenylate cyclase activity, but a 40% inhibition of maximal vasopressin stimulation. Pertussis toxin treatment of intact cells had little effect on basal or GTP-stimulated activity in the absence of hormone, or on hormone-stimulated activity in the absence of GTP. However, in contrast to the inhibitory effect of GTP on hormone-stimulated activity, there was further stimulation by vasopressin plus GTP in pertussis toxin-treated cells.

We used the above data to incorporate $\alpha_i\beta$ interaction into the overall adenylate cyclase activation mechanism shown in Figure 1, assuming that activation of $\alpha_i\beta$ also occurs by dissociation of its α_i and β subunits, and that GTP binds to the α_i subunit [19]. Illustrated in Figure 3 is a general model which includes the possibility of a direct interaction of the receptor with α_i (dashed lines) as is postulated for a classical inhibitory receptor. Both major mechanisms which have been proposed for the inhibitory action of $\alpha_i\beta$ based on studies in solubilized systems are included (mass action effect of β released upon $\alpha_i\beta$ dissociation; direct inhibitory interaction of α_i with the catalytic unit). By applying the data from the above studies to this general model we examined whether a direct interaction of the receptor with α_i was necessary and secondly, whether a mass action of β released upon dissociation of $\alpha_i\beta$ was sufficient to account for GTP-mediated inhibition in the intact membrane system. We first determined the simplest form of the model which could account for the data on the left side of Table II (absence of pertussis toxin). Parameters used for the stimulatory pathway

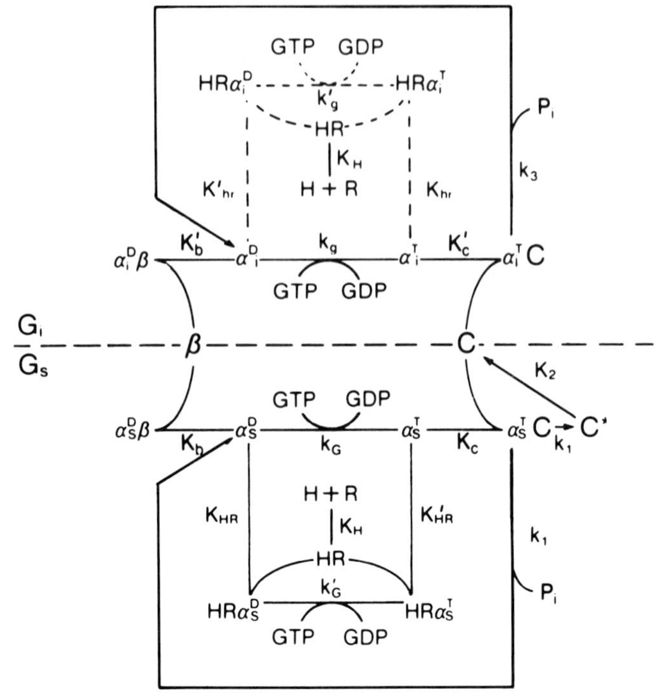

Figure 3. Model for cross-talk between $\alpha_s\beta$ and $\alpha_1\beta$ in the overall activation of adenylate cyclase. Abbreviations are as for Figure 1 with the addition of dissociation and rate constants for the inhibitory pathway. The stimulatory and inhibitory forms of α are expressed as α_s and α_i respectively. Reactions shown as broken lines are not required in applying the models to the experimental results

were taken from previous target analysis experiments [17]. Parameters for the inhibitory pathway were varied systematically to obtain agreement between the pattern of calculated and experimental results. Predicted activities were most

TABLE III. Model predictions for effect of GTP on adenylate cyclase activity

	With $\alpha_i\beta$ input		$\alpha_i\beta$ input eliminated	
	(-) GTP	(+) GTP	(-) GTP	(+) GTP
Basal	100	245	100	304
Vasopressin	1,065	483	1,081	1,727

Basal activity was set at 100 and model parameters chosen to give a 10-fold stimulation with maximal vasopressin, approximately 2–3-fold stimulation of basal activity with GTP, and -50% inhibition of hormone stimulated activity with GTP. Actual values of the total concentrations of subunits and rate and dissociation constants used were as follows: $[\alpha_s]=1$, $[\alpha_1]=10$, $[\beta]=10$, $[C]=1$, $[R]=1$, $K_b=1$, $K_b'=0.1$, $K_C=0.001$, $K_C'=0.0001$, $K_H=K_{HR}=K_{HR}=1$, $K_{hr}=K_{hr}=\infty$, $k_1=100$, $k_2=1$, $k_3=20$, $k_G'=2$, $k_g=10$, $k_g'=0$. GTP addition was incorporated in the model as a five-fold enhancement of the rate of GTP-dependent reaction steps. $\alpha_i\beta$ input was eliminated (right side of table) by setting $K_C'=0.01$ in Figure 3 sensitive to changes in any of the rate constants, as well as to changes in K_b, K'_b, K_C and K'_C (Figure 3). As indicated by the data in Table III, no direct interaction of the receptor with α_i was required (K_{hr}, $K'_{hr} = \infty$) to generate results consistent with those in the left-hand side of Table II. The same parameters were used to generate the predicted hormone concentration dependence for GTP-mediated inhibition and to compare this with the corresponding experimental results (Figure 2). Despite the lack of a direct interaction of α_i with the receptor this model still predicted the inhibitory effect of GTP to be dependent on activator concentration with stimulation by adding GTP at concentrations of hormone below the $K_{1/2}$ for activation, and inhibition at higher concentrations. The predicted leftward shift in the $K_{1/2}$ for enzyme activation with GTP was also observed. The model provides, therefore, a mechanism to explain the activator concentration dependent effects of $\alpha_i\beta$ without requiring its direct interaction with a receptor.

The addition of excess free β in solubilized systems has been shown to inhibit overall adenylate cyclase activity [22]. This is consistent with a mass action effect of excess free β which would oppose $\alpha_s\beta$ dissociation and is consistent with the models shown in Figures 1 and 3. Whether such a mass action effect of β released upon $\alpha_i\beta$ dissociation would be sufficient to explain inhibition of adenylate cyclase by added GTP in our system has been evaluated. Despite setting a 10-fold stoichiometric excess of α_i and β over α_s [20,21], reducing the direct inhibitory interaction of α_i with C (increased K'_C) resulted in loss of GTP-mediated inhibition (Table III). Whilst a β-mass action effect might account for inhibition by classical inhibitory receptors, or in artificial systems, this is apparently not sufficient to account for the modulatory effect of $\alpha_i\beta$ on activation by stimulatory receptors in the native membrane. Elimination of the interaction of α_i with C also suggests this as a possible locus of action for pertussis toxin, since this resulted in reversal of GTP-mediated inhibition. Eliminating $\alpha_i\beta$ dissociation (decreased K'_b), or decreasing guanine nucleotide exchange on α_i (decreased k_g), also reversed GTP-mediated inhibition but were not as sensitive as changes in K'_C. Therefore, this model cannot be used to pinpoint a single locus for pertussis toxin action. Of note, in a recent study Huff and Neer [23] have demonstrated persistent $\alpha_i\beta$ subunit dissociation upon stimulation of ADP-ribosylated $\alpha_i\beta$ in a solubilized system. This observation would be consistent with an effect of pertussis toxin either on k_g or K'_C.

Rôle of G_s and G_i in hormone-induced desensitization

Prior exposure of intact cells to vasopressin results in the attenuation of subsequent adenylate cyclase responsiveness to vasopressin [13, and Figure 4, top panel: 3 versus 1]. Since the magnitude of attenuation of adenylate cyclase responsiveness in the desensitized state is similar to that achieved by GTP addition to non-desensitized membranes (Table II), it was of interest to evaluate pretreatment and GTP addition. As evident in the top panel of Figure 4, pertussis

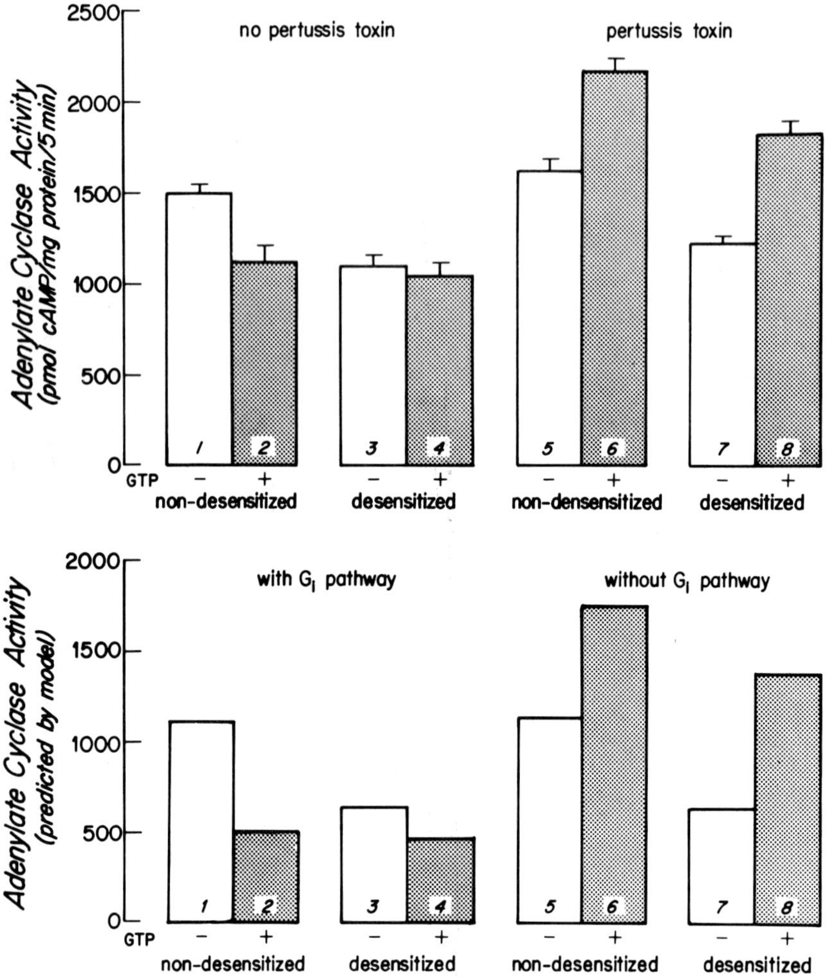

Figure 4. Rôle of G_s and G_i in desensitization. Culture medium was changed without (left) or with (right) pertussis toxin the day prior to assay in experiments in top panel. Where indicated (desensitized), cells were incubated with lysine vasopressin (100nM) at 37°C for 20 minutes prior to assay. Maximum vasopressin-stimulated enzyme activities were measured with or without added 100μM GTP as indicated by the (+) and (−) signs on the horizontal axis. $p<0.01$ for comparisons: 1 versus 3, 2 versus 6, and 4 versus 8. The bottom panel shows the corresponding model predictions for each incubation condition. Model parameters were the same as those used to generate Table III. K'_G was reduced by 50% to simulate the desensitized state (reduced capacity for hormone to accelerate guanyl nucleotide exchange) as discussed in the text

toxin pretreatment failed to abolish desensitization (7 versus 5) but was clearly effective in overcoming the inhibitory effect of GTP addition in both non-desensitized (6 versus 2) and desensitized cells (8 versus 4). This result does not support a rôle for G_i in mediating homologous desensitization in this system and is further consistent with the absence of a direct interaction of the receptor with G_i.

In contrast, homologous desensitization can be attributed to a diminished ability of hormone-occupied receptor to accelerate guanyl nucleotide exchange (GTP-GDP interconversion) on G_s. By use of the same model parameters used to generate Table III, the predicted effects of a 50% decrease in the rate of guanyl nucleotide exchange at G_s were evaluated both in the absence and in the presence of G_i input. As shown in the bottom panel of Figure 4, this resulted in attenuation of hormone-stimulated activity (3 versus 1), corresponding to experimentally observed desensitization. Furthermore, this attenuation persisted when G_i input was eliminated in the model (7 versus 5), corresponding to the lack of a pertussis toxin effect on desensitization observed experimentally. The pattern of observed and predicted results was also in agreement with respect to the observed effects of added GTP. With G_i input intact, the observed (top panel) and predicted (bottom panel) results both indicated no increase in enzyme activity with GTP addition (4 versus 3). With G_i input eliminated, GTP addition was observed (top panel) and predicted (bottom panel) to enhance hormone-stimulated adenylate cyclase activity (8 versus 7), as it does in non-desensitized cells (6 versus 5).

Conclusions

Our understanding of the hormone-receptor adenylate cyclase system has expanded rapidly in the last several years as a direct consequence of the purification and, in some instances, the cloning of the proteins involved in the generation of the cyclic AMP signal. However, our knowledge of the molecular events that occur among these proteins in intact membranes is still limited. The studies described in this paper were designed to develop a minimal model for the sequence of interaction among the stimulatory and inhibitory subunits of the adenylate cyclase complex. We were able to achieve this result by combining traditional biochemical techniques with target analysis and computer modelling. Like any model of a biological process, its worth is measured by its prediction of experimental data. In this regard, the data utilized to define the model in Figure 3 have provided evidence that vasopressin-stimulation of adenylate cyclase in cell membranes involves: 1) sequential interaction of hormone with receptor and high and low affinity states of the α_s subunit; 2) $\alpha\beta$ dissociation; 3) GTP-dependent cross-talk between $\alpha_s\beta$ and $\alpha_i\beta$ without the involvement of an inhibitory receptor; 4) a rôle for both α_i and β in the modulation of enzyme activity; 5) an activated enzyme species consisting of α_sC; and 6) a rôle for α_s but not α_i in homologous desensitization. As discussed in detail elsewhere [18], these model predictions have provided new interpretations to unexplained, and often conflicting data, obtained from vasopressin and other hormone-sensitive adenylate cyclase systems. Whereas the present model is likely to be an oversimplification of all the events involved in adenylate cyclase activity, it does provide a framework from which logical experiments can be devised to probe the molecular mechanisms involved in enzyme activation.

References

1 Rodbell M. The role of hormone receptors and GTP-regulatory proteins in membrane-transduction. *Nature 1980; 284:* 17–22

2 Ross EM, Gilman AG. Biochemical properties of hormone-sensitive adenylate cyclase. *Ann Rev Biochem 1980; 49:* 533–564

3 Stiles GL, Caron MG, Lefkowitz RJ. β-Adrenergic receptors: biochemical mechanisms of physiological regulation. *Physiol Rev 1984; 64:* 661–743

4 Birnbaumer L, Iyengar R. Coupling of receptors to adenylate cyclases. In Nathanson JA, Kebabian JW, eds. *Handbook of Experimental Pharmacoloy, Vol 58.* Berlin: Springer-Verlag. 1982: part I, 153–183

5 Korner M, Gilon C, Schramm M. Locking of hormone in the β-adrenergic receptor by attack on a sulfhydryl in an associated component. *J Biol Chem 1982; 257:* 3389–3396

6 Seamon KB, Padgett W, Daly JW. Forskolin: unique diterpene activator of adenylate cyclase in membranes and in intact cells. *Proc Natl Acad Sci USA 1981; 78:* 3363–3367

7 Smigel MD, Ross EM, Gilman AG. Role of the β-adrenergic receptor in the regulation of adenylate cyclase. In Elson E, Frazier W, Glaser L, eds. *Cell Membranes Methods and Reviews, Vol 2.* New York: Plenum. 1984: 247–294

8 Tolkovsky AM, Levitzki A. Mode of coupling between the β-adrenergic receptor and adenylate cyclase in turkey erythrocytes. *Biochemistry 1978; 17:* 3795–3810

9 Sternweis PC, Northrup JK, Hanski E et al. Purification and properties of the regulatory component (G/F) of adenylate cyclase. *Adv Cyclic Nucleotide Res 1981; 14:* 23–36

10 Tolkovsky AM, Levitzki A. Theories and predictions of models descring sequential interactions between the receptor, the GTP regulatory unit, and the catalytic unit of hormone dependent adenylate cyclases. *J Cyclic Nucleotide Res 1981; 7:* 139–150

11 Goldring SR, Dayer JM, Ausiello DA, Krane SM. A cell strain cultured from porcine kidney increases cyclic AMP content upon exposure to calcitonin or vasopressin. *Biochem Biophys Res Commun 1978; 83:* 434–440

12 Roy C, Ausiello DA. Characterization of (8-lysine) vasopressin binding sites on a pig kidney cell line (LLC-PK_1). Evidence for hormone-induced receptor transition. *J Biol Chem 1981; 256:* 3415–3422

13 Roy C, Hall D, Karish M, Ausiello DA. Relationship of (8-lysine) vasopressin receptor transition to receptor functional properties in a pig kidney cell line (LLC-PK_1). *J Biol Chem 1981; 256:* 3423–3427

14 Roy C, Ausiello DA. Regulation of vasopressin binding to intact cells. *Ann NY Acad Sci 1981; 372:* 91–105

15 Verkman AS, Skorecki KL, Ausiello DA. Radiation inactivation of oligomeric enzyme systems: theoretical considerations. *Proc Natl Acad Sci USA 1984; 81:* 150–154

16 Verkman AS, Skorecki KL, Ausiello DA. Radiation inactivation of multimeric enzymes: application to subunit interactions of adenylate cyclase. *Am J Physiol 1986; 250 (Cell Physiol 19):* C103–C114

17 Skorecki KL, Verkman AS, Jung CY, Ausiello DA. Evidence for vasopressin activation of adenylate cyclase by subunit dissociation. *Am J Physiol 1986; 260 (Cell Physiol 19):* C115–C123

18 Skorecki KL, Verkman AS, Ausiello DA. Cross-talk between stimulatory and inhibitory GTP-binding proteins. Role in activation and desensitization of the adenylate-cyclase response to vasopressin. *Biochemistry 1987; 26:* 639–645

19 Gilman AG. G proteins: transducers of receptor-generated signals. *Ann Rev Biochem 1987; 56:* 615–649

20 Cerione RA, Codina J, Kilpatrick BF et al. Transducin and the inhibitory nucleotide regulatory protein inhibit the stimulatory nucleotide regulary protein mediated stimulation of adenylate cyclase in phospholipid vesicle systems. *Biochemistry 1985; 24:* 4499–4503

21 Cerione RA, Staniszewski C, Caron MG et al. A role for N_i in the hormonal stimulation of adenylate cyclase. *Nature 1986; 318:* 293–295

22 Northrup JK, Sternweis PC, Gilman AG. The subunits of the stimulatory component of adenylate cyclase. Resolution, activity, and properties of the 35,000–dalton (β) subunit. *J Biol Chem 1983; 258:* 11361–11368

23 Huff RM, Neer EJ. Subunit interactions of native and ADP-ribosylated α_{39} and α_{41}, two guanine nucleotide-binding proteins from bovine cerebral cortex. *J Biol Chem 1986; 261:* 1105–1110

PATHOPHYSIOLOGY

HUMAN T-CELL RECEPTORS: A 1987 PERSPECTIVE

E L Reinherz

Dana-Farber Cancer Institute, Harvard Medical School, Boston, Massachusetts, USA

Thymus derived (T) lymphocytes comprise 60–80% of peripheral blood lymphoid cells and serve as both effectors and regulators of the vertebrate immune system. Unlike B-lymphocytes which produce immunoglobulin molecules acting to neutralize antigen in solution, T-lymphocytes express membrane bound receptors which sense perturbations in the context of normal cell surfaces. As viruses, certain bacteria (including the mycobacteria responsible for tuberculosis and leprosy) and many parasitic infections invade host cells and disrupt their function, it is critical for the immune system to be endowed with components capable of identifying pathogens and selectively destroying invading cells. Such mechanisms are presumably important for eliminating tumour cells as well. Therefore the elucidation of the structural basis for T-cell recognition is of basic theoretical and practical significance.

In order to place the T-cell receptor field into an appropriate perspective, let me review some of the salient features of T-cell recognition and its known structural basis. In both human and murine systems, the helper T-cells, which turn on the immune response, and the cytotoxic T-cells, which are responsible for specific destruction of target cells, express a T-cell receptor. This receptor is a molecular complex composed of at least five polypeptide chains [1,2]. These include the disulphide linked Ti α and β subunits, each encoded by a gene assembled by means of somatic rearrangements from pools of separate gene segments [3] and the three monomorphic T3 subunits which are non-covalently associated with the $\alpha\beta$ heterodimer. All of these chains have been cloned and sequenced [reviewed in 4]. There are variable region domains in the α and β subunits created by V, D and J elements in the case of the Ti β gene and V and J segments in the case of the Ti α gene. Combinatorial diversity and joining diversity mechanisms are operative here as they are in Ig genes. In contrast, the T3 subunits are invariant and probably involve signal transduction providing little, if any, contribution to antigen binding. Cell surface expression of the Ti

Up to this point, I have emphasized the Ti γ related developments in the human system where functional and biochemical analyses have proceeded more rapidly. Nevertheless, in the area of ontogeny, murine studies are providing novel insights. One of the most intriguing initial components of the Ti γ story related to the early pronounced expression of γ RNA in immature T lineage cells such as fetal thymocytes. For this reason, Tonegawa and colleagues originally proposed that the γ protein might associate with the β chain to give a binding to self-MHC specificity, thus allowing for selection of self-MHC restricted cells within the thymus [29]. This $\gamma\beta$ heterodimer would then give way to $\alpha\beta$ which would bind self-MHC with weaker affinity, somehow requiring the presence of nominal antigen. This γ swap α notion was not dissimilar to known haemoglobin switching mechanisms.

Recent analyses suggest that this proposal, although imaginative, is probably incorrect but do not rule out the possibility that the γ gene product may be important in thymic education or tolerance induction. The work of Coligan, Pardoll, Bluestone and colleagues [30–32] shows that only the T3 associated γ X proteins are present on surface labelled thymocytes at day 15 of gestation. By day 17½, there is an equivalent amount of surface T3 associated Ti $\alpha\beta$ and Ti γ X protein. Furthermore, on day 20 (the day of birth), no γ X is detected in immunoprecipitates with anti-T3 from the total thymocyte population. At that time, the γ protein is restricted to the surface of $T3^{+}L3T4^{-}Lyt2^{-}$ cells. Anti-γ heteroantisera identify the murine γ chain as a 35kD structure which is disulphide linked to a T3 associated 45kD partner. Thus, during fetal murine thymus development, the appearance of $T3^{+}L3T4^{-}$Lyt2-Ti γ X^{+} cells is first detected on day 15 of gestation, preceding surface T3-Ti $\alpha\beta$ expressing cells by two days. Identification of 35kD γ polypeptides disulphide linked to a 45kD chain has also been observed by Tonegawa's group using antisera generated to λ gt11 produced γ-β galactosidase fusion proteins [33]. Note that in the mouse, non-disulphide linked γ forms have not been detected, consistent with the presence of a membrane proximal cysteine residue in all known constant regions which could be utilized in formation of a putative interchain disulphide. Anti-T3 monoclonal antibody + IL-2 stimulates the $T3^{+}$L3T4-$Lyt2^{-}$ thymocytes to proliferate and mediate cytotoxic activity in a fashion analogous to that observed in the human [31,32].

The γ protein on fetal and adult thymocytes bears N-linked carbohydrates presumably derived from the Cγ1 constant gene product which unlike Cγ2, has a site for these glycans. This is of particular note since in most of the murine T-cell hybridomas and clones studied to the present, there are generally only defective (out of frame joining) Cγ2 gene transcripts in T3-Ti $\alpha\beta$ protein expressing mature T-lymphocytes. Therefore, the T3-Ti γ X receptor may define a separate T-cell lineage whose intrathymic development precedes that of cells expressing T3-Ti $\alpha\beta$. Further support for this view is coming from studies of thymic ontogeny in the chicken within the laboratory of Max Cooper and

Chen-lo Chen [personal communication]. These investigators have produced monoclonal antibodies against the chicken T3, T4 and T8 structures as well as a T-cell receptor framework (TCR1) which identified a putative Ti γ epitope expressed on $T3^+T4^-T8^-$ T lineage cells in the chick and precipitates a disulphide linked T3 associated heterodimer with subunits of molecular weight 50kD and 38kD. In the adult chicken, TCR1 reacts with 10% of thymocytes and 25% of peripheral T-cells. However, oncogenetic studies reveal that the first wave of precursor cells which move into the epithelial thymus and are $T3^-$ rapidly express T3 and TCR1 reactivity but lack T4 and T8 reactivity. The $T3^+TCR1^+$ cells account for 30% of thymocytes by embryonic day 15. Subsequently, the frequency drops to <5% by the day of hatching (day 21), while the frequency of $T3^+T4^+T8^+TCR1^-$ increases. These investigators have also found that subsequent waves of thymic progenitors, although acquiring T3 expression (and probably Ti $\alpha\beta$) infrequently express TCR1 reactivity. The data suggest that the $T3^+$ Ti γ cells are a separate lineage rather than a precursor of the T3-Ti $\alpha\beta$ receptor expressing cells. Conclusive proof of this hypothesis will come when the Cooper group determines whether TCR1 antibody treatment of embryos abrogates expression of T3-Ti γ X cells without inhibiting development of T3-Ti $\alpha\beta$ thymocytes.

Curiously, studies of genomic DNA derived from a panel of fetal liver, fetal thymus and adult thymus hybridoma by the Kappler and Marrack group suggests that immature thymocytes begin to rearrange Ti γ and β genes synchronously [34]. For example, among 81 hybridoma studies, only two had rearranged γ complex in the presence of unrearranged β complexes in both alleles whereas 39 had rearranged γ complexes in the presence of various β gene rearrangements. The nature of this linkage remains unclear but, as speculated by the authors, might be based on common usage of recombinases and synchronized activation of DNA substrates. However, the γ locus completes V-J-C rearrangement in most thymocytes by day 15 when many β locus rearrangements are still incomplete.

It is far from clear what regulates differentiation along T3-Ti γ X versus T3-Ti $\alpha\beta$ pathways. However, generally T3-Ti γ X clones have one functional γ gene rearrangement and usually no β gene rearrangements while, in contrast, T3-Ti $\alpha\beta$ clones have several non-functional γ gene rearrangements and functional β gene rearrangements so that a stochastic model may be applicable. Thus, if γ gene rearrangement is productive, productive β and α gene rearrangement fails to occur. Alternatively, if γ gene rearrangement is unsuccessful in both alleles, β and α rearrangement attempts continue. If such a view were correct, then production of a transgenic mouse expressing a functional γ gene product might inhibit development of Ti $\alpha\beta$ expressing cells. Of course, this speculation does not take into account the contribution of the γ partner, X. Nevertheless, such a model does not readily explain why T3-Ti γ X as opposed to T3-Ti $\alpha\beta$ expression is mostly limited to thymocytes of the $T4^-T8^-$ phenotype. Given the small number of $T3^+$Ti γ X^+ peripheral T-lymphocytes, is functional γ rearrangement selected against, perhaps by a mechanism involving AT dinucleotide additions at the Vγ Jγ junctions?

Why are there several forms of T-cell receptor? Certainly, T3-Ti γ X receptors lack the extensive germline diversity relative to their T3-Ti αβ counterparts, implying that the specificities they encode are more limited. Could this receptor complex have been the phylogenetic precursor of the αβ heterodimer? If so, it is far from vestigial given the precise maintenance of recombination-recognition signals in its various Ti γ elements and the nature of the γ gene protein which has now surfaced over the last six months. Is it possible that the early appearance of T3-Ti γ X receptor in ontogeny may provide important protective immunity to the fetus against common viral or other pathogens prior to development of MHC restricted T3-Ti αβ expressing receptor structures? Moreover, even in the mature peripheral compartment, the T3-Ti γ receptor may encode certain specificities not provided by the T3-Ti αβ repertoire. In this regard, κ and λ light chains have maintained their own utility in contributing to antibody diversity in humans. Whether there are substantially unique characteristics in triggering physiology among these various T3-Ti γ X and T3-Ti αβ receptors remains to be determined. Differences in refractoriness or sensitivity to triggering events may be of importance in functionally diverse and perhaps oncogenetically distinct populations, such as suppressor T-lymphocytes.

Finally, a burning question remains as to the origin of the Ti γ associated X chain. Is this also a structure with a V domain encoded by a rearranging set of genes? Certainly, comparison of X chains from different clones can address the question of peptide variability as was done in the past for Ti α and β subunits. Identification of X will elucidate whether Ti γ associates with only X as opposed to Y or Z to yield a fourth, fifth, etc type of receptor. Materials from PEER or $T3^+Ti\gamma^+L3T4^-$ $Lyt2^-$ thymocytes fused to BW5147 may be sufficient for primary structural analysis. The very recent identification of a rearranging gene locus composed of V, D and J-like elements and a C region located 70 or more Kb 5′ to Cα may represent the X chain locus itself [35]. This C locus is only 9–18% homologous to other T-cell receptor sequences at the aminoacid level. Its features are more similar to Cα than Cγ or Cβ. Furthermore, the early rearrangements which occur during thymic ontogeny within this locus precede Ti α gene rearrangements as does RNA expression. Shortly, it should be possible to know whether this gene encodes X or another class of T-cell receptor.

References

1. Meuer SC, Cooper DA, Hodgdon JC et al. Identification of the receptor for antigen and major histocompatibility complex on human inducer T lymphocytes. *Science 1983; 222:* 1239–1242
2. Borst J, Prendiville MA, Terhorst C. Complexity of the human T lymphocyte – specific cell surface antigen T3. *J Immunol 1982; 128:* 1560–1565
3. Hedrick SM, Nielsen EA, Kavaler J et al. Sequence relationships between putative T-cell receptor polypeptides and immunoglobulins. *Nature 1984; 308:* 153–158

4 Robertson M. The present state of recognition. *Nature 1985; 317:* 768–771
5 Benacerraf B, McDevitt HO. Histocompatibility-linked immune response genes. *Science 1972; 175:* 273–279
6 Zinkernagel RM, Doherty PC. H-2 compatibility requirement for T-cell-mediated lysis of target cells infected with lymphocytic choriomeningitis virus. Different cytotoxic T-cell specificities are associated with structures coded for in H-2K or H-2D. *J Exp Med 1975; 141:* 1427–1436
7 Hunig T, Bevan MJ. Specificity of T-cell clones illustrates altered self hypothesis. *Nature 1981; 294:* 460–462
8 Ritz J, Campen TJ, Schmidt RE et al. Analysis of T-cell receptor gene rearrangement and expression in human natural killer clones. *Science 1985; 228:* 1540–1543
9 Marrack P, Shimonkevitz R, Hannum C et al. The major histocompatibility complex-restricted antigen receptor on T cells. IV. An antiidiotypic antibody predicts both antigen and I-specificity. *J Exp Med 1983; 158:* 1635–1646
10 Dembic Z, Hass W, Weiss S et al. Transfer of specificity by murine α and β T-cell receptor genes. *Nature 1986; 320:* 232–238
11 Saito T, Weiss A, Miller J et al. Specific antigen-Ia activation of transfected human T cells expressing murine Ti alpha beta-human T3 receptor complexes. *Nature 1987; 325:* 125–130
12 Siliciano RF, Hemesath TJ, Pratt JC et al. Direct evidence for the existence of nominal antigen binding sites on T cell surface Ti alpha beta-heterodimers of MHC-restricted T cell clones. *Cell 1986; 47:* 161–171
13 Borst J, van de Griend RJ, van Oostveen JW et al. A T-cell receptor gamma/CD3 complex found on cloned functional lymphocytes. *Nature 1987; 325:* 683–688
14 Brenner MB, McLean J, Scheft H et al. Two forms of the T-cell receptor gamma protein found on peripheral blood cytotoxic T lymphocytes. *Nature 1987; 325:* 689–694
15 Allison JP, McIntyre BW, Bloch D. Tumour-specific antigen of murine T-lymphoma defined with monoclonal antibody. *J Immunol 1982; 129:* 2293–2300
16 Meuer SC, Fitzgerald A, Hussey RE et al. Clonotypic structures involved in antigen-specific human T cell function. *J Exp Med 1983; 157:* 705–719
17 Acuto O, Hussey RE, Fitzgerald KA. The human T cell receptor: appearance in ontogeny and biochemical relationship of alpha and beta subunits on IL-2 dependent clones and T cell tumors. *Cell 1983; 34:* 717–726
18 Haskins K, Kubo R, White J. The major histocompatibility complex-restricted antigen receptor on T cells. 1. Isolation with a monoclonal antibody. *J Exp Med 1983; 157:* 1149–1169
19 Brenner MB, McLean J, Dialynas DP et al. Identification of a putative second T-cell receptor. *Nature 1986; 322:* 145–149
20 Moingeon P, Ythier A, Goubin G et al. A unique T-cell receptor complex expressed on human fetal lymphocytes displaying natural-killer-like activity. *Nature 1986; 323:* 638–640
21 Bank I, De Pinho RA, Brenner MB et al. A functional T3 molecule associated with a novel heterodimer on the surface of immature human thymocytes. *Nature 1986; 322:* 179–181
22 Weiss A, Newton M, Crommie D. Expression of T3 in association with a molecule distinct from the T-cell antigen receptor heterodimer. *Proc Natl Acad Sci USA 1986; 83:* 6998–7002
23 Saito H, Kranz DM, Takagaki Y et al. Complete primary structure of a heterodimeric T-cell receptor deduced from cDNA sequences. *Nature 1984; 309:* 757–762
24 Lanier LL, Weiss A. Presence of Ti (WT31) negative T lymphocytes in normal blood and thymus. *Nature 1986; 324:* 268–270
25 Lefranc MP, Forster A, Rabbitts TH. Genetic polymorphism and exon changes of the constant regions of the human T-cell rearranging gene gamma. *Proc Natl Acad Sci USA 1986; 83:* 9596–9600
26 Littman DR et al. *Nature:* in press

27 Dialynas DP, Murre C, Quertermous T et al. Cloning and sequence analysis of complementary DNA encoding an aberrantly rearranged human T-cell gamma chain. *Proc Natl Acad Sci USA 1986; 83:* 2619–2623

28 Moingeon P, Jitsukawa S, Faure F et al. A gamma-chain complex forms a functional receptor on cloned human lymphocytes with natural killer-like activity. *Nature 1987; 325:* 723–726

29 Raulet DH, Garman RD, Saito H, Tonegawa S. Developmental regulation of T-cell receptor gene expression. *Nature 1985; 314:* 103–107

30 Lew AM, Pardoll DM, Maloy WL et al. Characterisation of T cell receptor gamma chain expression in a subset of murine thymocytes. *Science 1986; 234:* 1401–1405

31 Bluestone JA, Pardoll D, Sharrow SO, Fowlkes BJ. Characterisation of murine thymocytes with CD3-associated T-cell receptor structures. *Nature 1987; 326:* 82–84

32 Pardoll DM, Fowlkes BJ, Bluestone JA et al. Differential expression of two distinct T-cell receptors during thymocyte development. *Nature 1987; 326:* 79–81

33 Nakanishi N, Maeda K, Ito K et al. T gamma protein is expressed on murine fetal thymocytes as a disulphide-linked heterodimer. *Nature 1987; 325:* 720–723

34 Born W, Rathburn G, Tucker P et al. Synchronised rearrangement of T-cell gamma and beta chain genes in fetal thymocyte development. *Science 1986; 234:* 479–482

35 Chien T, Iwashima M, Kaplan KB et al. A new T-cell receptor gene located within the alpha locus and expressed early in T-cell differentiation. *Nature 1987; 327:* 677–682

36 Samelson LE, Harford JB, Klausner RD. Identification of the components of the murine T cell antigen receptor complex. *Cell 1985; 43:* 223–231

37 Kuno M, Goronzy J, Weyand M, Gardner P. Single-channel and whole-cell recordings of mitogen-regulated inward currents in human cloned helper T lymphocytes. *Nature 1986; 323:* 269–273

INTERACTION OF CYTOLYTIC T-LYMPHOCYTES WITH ENDOTHELIUM

A M Krensky, D V Landers, Carol Clayberger

Stanford University, Stanford, California, USA

Introduction

Although circulating lymphocytes are in constant contact with vascular endothelial cells, the interaction between these two cell types is not intimate except under special circumstances. In cases where immune cells perceive the endothelium as foreign (as in organ transplants) or as altered self (as in tumours or viral infection), the endothelium can be a major target for the immune response. During antigenic challenge outside the vascular system lymphocytes must move across the endothelial cell lining into tissue. Understanding the molecules involved in the interaction of lymphocytes with endothelium may allow the development of new therapeutic modalities for the treatment of a variety of human diseases.

The involvement of endothelium in renal disease was initially suggested by pathological examination of renal biopsies and postmortem specimens. These studies indicated that endothelium is involved in: 1) transplant rejection; 2) vasculitis; 3) glomerulonephritis; 4) diabetic glomerulosclerosis; 5) some infections, and 6) some renal tumours [1,2]. In addition, it is generally believed that many renal diseases are immunologically mediated. Immunofluorescence studies and experimental models have indicated that both humoral and cellular mechanisms are involved in the pathogenesis of transplant rejection, vasculitis and glomerulonephritis, among others [3,4]. Renal vascular damage can clearly result from antibodies directed against molecules on the surface of endothelial cells. In addition, during renal transplant rejection, lymphocytes have been found in close proximity to endothelial cells and are recoverable from rejected allografts. Although the cells involved in this endothelial cell damage have not been precisely identified, there is evidence that both cytolytic T-lymphocytes (CTL) and cells mediating antibody dependent cellular cytotoxicity (ADCC) are involved [5,6].

Our studies have centred on the interaction of cytolytic T-lymphocytes with endothelium. Information gained from these studies may allow direct manipulation of CTL in patients with organ transplants. In addition, we hope to define the molecules expressed on endothelial cells which are recognized by T-lymphocytes and other cells of the immune system. We have used the techniques of cellular immunology, protein chemistry, and molecular biology to study the cell surface molecules on both cytolytic T-lymphocytes and endothelial cells. Cytolytic T-lymphocyte lines and clones have been generated by separating the peripheral blood lymphocytes from the blood of normal donors on ficoll-hypaque gradients and stimulating these cells in vitro with Epstein-Barr virus (EBV) transformed B-lymphoblastoid cells or with endothelial cell lines [7]. These cytolytic effector cells are propagated in long-term culture by weekly stimulation with the appropriate stimulator cell line in the presence of medium containing T-cell growth factors. These cell lines are tested for 1) differential cytolysis of a specificity panel of target cells, and 2) inhibition of cytolysis by various monoclonal antibodies (Figure 1).

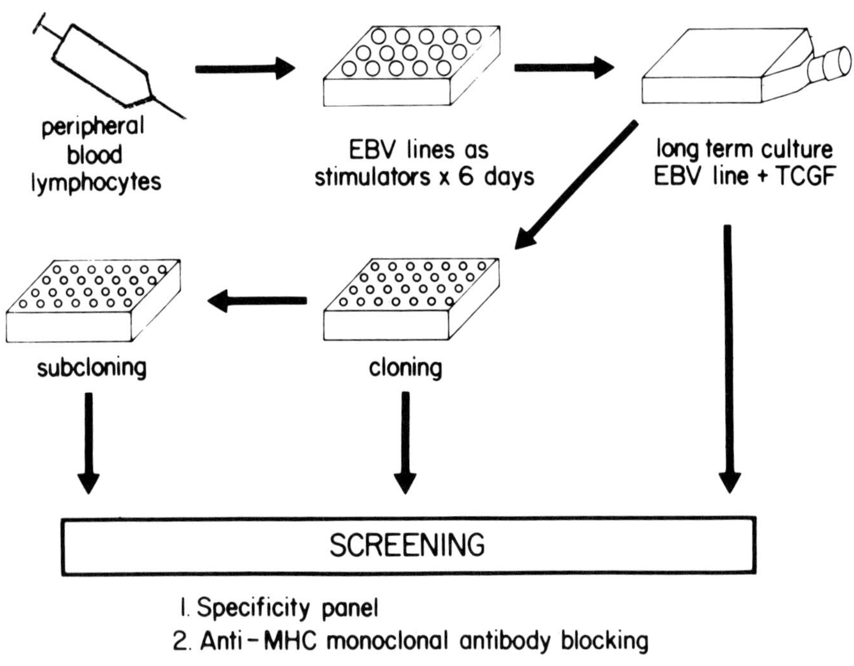

Figure 1. Generation and screening of cytolytic T-lymphocyte lines. Epstein-Barr virus transformed B-lymphoblastoid cell lines or endothelial cells are used as stimulators. The method is detailed elsewhere [7,8]

Target antigens

The major molecules recognized in a human allogeneic response are the class I (HLA-A, B, C) and class II (HLA-DR, DP and DQ) antigens. We use panels of B cell lines of known HLA types to determine the particular HLA molecule which

TABLE I. Lysis of B lymphoblasts and endothelial cells by CTL

Target cell	HLA type				Percent lysis by	
	A	B	C	DR	AH2	AE1
JY	2	7	–	4,6	46	50
Herluff	2	12,35	–	4,7	63	72
WT49	2	17	3	3	54	39
DK1	2,33	44,40			63	71
LB	28	40	3	6	30	88
IDF	26,28*	38,18		5	40	48
PGF	3	7	–	2	2	70
FMB	1,32	44,57	5,6	5	1	40
MANN	29	12	4	7	3	81
A2M1	1	44,17	2,6	2,6	2	50
SB	1,2	12,17			48	56
Daudi	–	–	–	6	0	0
K562	–	–	–	–	9	12
E1211					3	32
E1214					7	36
E1300					48	40
E1298					5	35
E1430					52	53
E1126					9	39

The target cells shown are EBV lines (JY-Daudi), an erythroleukaemia cell line used to detect natural killing (K562), and endothelial cell lines isolated from newborn preputial microvessels (E1211-E1430) or umbilical vein (E1126). HLA types are shown for those targets which have been typed. Values shown are percentage specific release in a four hour ^{51}Cr release assay at effector to target ratios of 5:1 for B-cells and 0.5:1 for endothelial cells. AH2 is an HLA-A2 specific CTL line [8]; AE1 is an MHC unrestricted CTL line generated by stimulating peripheral blood lymphocytes with endothelial cells [7]

is recognized [7]. For example, Table I shows that a cytolytic T-lymphocyte clone that was stimulated by the cell JY (HLA-A2,2; B7,7; DR4,6) caused significant cytolysis only of cells which express HLA-A2. Lysis of an extended panel showed that this CTL line recognized the HLA-A2 molecule. Using similar analyses, we and others have demonstrated CTL specific for a variety of HLA class I and class II antigens [8–12].

CTL specificity can be further proven using monoclonal antibodies which recognize either monomorphic or polymorphic determinants on HLA molecules. As evident in Table II, inhibition of cytolysis by appropriate anti-MHC monoclonal antibodies confirms the specificity determined by panels of target cell lines.

In our initial studies we asked whether allospecific CTL could also recognize and lyse endothelial cells. Table I shows that HLA-A2 specific cytolytic T-lymphocytes generated against HLA-A2$^+$ B lymphoblasts can recognize and lyse endothelial cells which express HLA-A2. Monoclonal antibodies specific for class I molecules inhibited lysis, further demonstrating lysis was in fact directed at the MHC class I molecule (Table II).

TABLE II. Inhibition of cytolysis by anti-HLA monoclonal antibodies

Effector	Target	mAb added (antigen recognized)				
		None	MA2.1 (HLA-A2)	PA2.6 (Class I)	TS1.16 (Class II)	BBM.1 (microglobulin)
AE1	1430	53	54	47	61	52
AE1	JY	56	52	47	58	51
AH2	JY	60	*30*	*21*	62	63
AE1	JY	50	51	49	*16*	54

Monoclonal antibodies were used at 1–10μg/ml. Values are percent lysis. Italic values show significant inhibition of cytolysis. Effector AE1 is an MHC unrestricted anti-endothelial cell CTL line [7]; AH2 is an HLA-A2 specific CTL line [8]. 1430 is a microvascular endothelial cell line [7]; JY is an EBV transformed B lymphoblastoid cell line (HLA-A2,2; B7,7; DR4,6) [8]. The antibodies used have been previously described [7]

We were also interested in the role of class II antigens in the CTL-endothelial cell interaction. Although there is some controversy as to whether endothelial cells express class II antigens in vivo, it is clear that under in vitro conditions endothelial cells normally express little, if any, class II antigens. Several investigators, however, have recently shown that gamma interferon will induce the expression of class II molecules [13]. The experiment in Table III shows that a

TABLE III. Specific lysis of endothelial cells by an HLA-DR6 specific CTL clone

Target	Treatment	Anti-HLA-DR+C	DR6 specific CTL	CTL+Anti-HLA-DR
HUVE No1	Control	7	8	5
	IFN Gamma	64	34	6
HUVE No2	Control	1	2	2
	IFN Gamma	50	25	3
HUVE No3	Control	3	7	6
	IFN Gamma	62	7	5

Values shown are percentage specific release in a 6 hour ^{111}In release assay [13,21]. The Anti-HLA-DR antibody is LB3.1 [13]; the CTL is CF1 [13], and C=baby rabbit complement [13]. IFN gamma was provided by W Fiers (State University of Ghent, Ghent, Belgium)

class II (HLA-DR6) specific CTL did not recognize cultured endothelial cells isolated from an HLA-DR6$^+$ individual. After stimulation with gamma interferon, however, the endothelial cells express HLA-DR molecules and are now recognized by the cytolytic T-lymphocytes. Furthermore, the same T-cell clone which lysed HLA-DR6$^+$ endothelial cells produced a factor (or factors), presumably gamma interferon, which induced class II expression [13].

Thus, both class I and class II molecules can be targets for the human allogeneic response to endothelial cells. The question remained, however, as to whether or not MHC class I and class II antigens would predominate if cytolytic

T-lymphocytes were generated against endothelial cells directly. To address this, we stimulated peripheral blood lymphocytes with allogeneic endothelial cells [7]. Several long-term cytolytic T-lymphocyte lines derived from peripheral blood lymphocytes of at least two donors were analysed for target specificity. CTL generated in this way were broadly specific and apparently unrestricted by HLA molecules. The lytic activity of these cells could be distinguished from natural killing activity since neither Daudi nor K562 cells were lysed (Table I).

Accessory molecules

Reinherz, Schlossman and their colleagues showed that essentially all peripheral blood T-lymphocytes express the CD3 (OKT3, Leu4) antigen [14]. Furthermore, approximately one-third of these cells express CD8 (OKT8, Leu2) and two-thirds express CD4 (OKT4, Leu3) [15]. The CD8 positive subset includes the majority of cytotoxic and suppressor cells whereas the CD4 positive subset includes most helper and inducer cells [16]. Analysis of class II specific CTL showed that they expressed CD4 antigens and were inhibited by monoclonal antibodies against the CD4 cell surface structure. In contrast, CD8 positive CTL recognized class I MHC antigen and lysis could be blocked by anti-CD8 monoclonal antibodies [8]. This led to the hypothesis that CD4 is a recognition structure for MHC class II molecules whereas CD8 is a recognition structure for MHC class I molecules [8–10]. There remains, however, no direct evidence that these T-cell surface molecules actually bind MHC determinants.

A number of other molecules are also involved in the CTL-target cell interaction. The lymphocyte function associated antigens, LFA-1, LFA-2 (CD2) and LFA-3 were originally identified by screening for antibodies which could inhibit cytolysis [17,18]. LFA-1 is a 177,000–95,000 molecular weight heterodimer. LFA-2 is a 49,000 molecular weight molecule and LFA-3 is a molecule of approximately 60–70,000 molecular weight depending on the cell type studied. LFA-1 is present on all human leucocytes but no other cell types. LFA-2 is the sheep erythrocyte receptor present on T-cells and large granular lymphocytes and LFA-3 is found on all cell types studied to date. Recent studies suggest that LFA-2 and LFA-3 interact as a receptor ligand pair important in T-lymphocyte adhesion to a variety of cell types [19]. Springer and co-workers have recently shown that the T-cell LFA-1 molecule binds to the ICAM-1 molecule on endothelial cells but it is clear that LFA-1 binds to other ligands in different systems [20].

We undertook studies to assess the role of these accessory molecules in recognition of endothelial cells by CTL. We found that class I or II specific CTL utilize the same accessory molecules in lysis of endothelial cells and B-lymphoblasts. In contrast, only LFA-1 and LFA-3 are involved in lysis by the MHC unrestricted CTL; no inhibition was observed using antibodies to CD2 (LFA-2), CD3, CD4/CD8, or the T-cell receptor [7]. These results underscore the importance of comparing different types of stimulator cells in such analyses and suggest that in some cases T-cells utilize as yet uncharacterized structures for CTL-target conjugation and effector-function.

Monoclonal antibodies recognizing endothelial cells

One way to identify the molecules involved in MHC unrestricted CTL lysis of endothelial cells is to generate monoclonal antibodies which inhibit lysis of endothelial cells. We immunized mice with human microvascular endothelium, generated hybridomas, and screened the supernatants for binding to a variety of cell types including EBV transformed B-lymphoblasts, human microvascular endothelial cells, SV40 transformed endothelial cells, B-cells, monocytes, smooth muscle, embryonic fibroblasts, CTL lines, and peripheral blood lymphocytes. Thirty-three hybridomas were selected for further analysis. We tested the ability of these antibodies: 1) to bind to endothelial cells in frozen section; 2) to bind to a variety of cells in tissue section; 3) to block CTL-mediated endothelial cell lysis, and 4) to immunoprecipitate radio-iodinated proteins from endothelial cells. Clones were selected based on these parameters and subclones were grown in ascites and purified. The molecules so defined should be useful in defining three groups of endothelial cell antigens: 1) subset antigens; 2) function-associated antigens, and 3) activation/differentiation/injury antigens.

Subset specific antigens will be expressed on some types of endothelial cells and not on others. These could be used to differentiate: 1) microvasculature versus macrovasculature; 2) arteries versus veins versus capillaries, and 3) functional subsets (as defined for lymphocytes). These monoclonal antibodies may be helpful in: 1) pathological diagnosis, for example, identifying certain cell types; 2) purifying endothelial cells from tissue for further study, or 3) studying functional subsets. It appears that existing monoclonal antibodies specific for Factor VIII, and PAL-E as well as the lectin *Ulex europaeus I* may subdivide endothelial cells into useful subsets [20]. Initial screening of our panel of endothelial cell monoclonal antibodies showed that some of the antigens recognized are expressed in varying degrees by different cell types (Table IV). Eight of the monoclonal antibodies stained endothelial cells only. Immunoperoxidase staining studies are in progress to define the subset distribution, if any, of these antigens.

Function associated antigens are so called because monoclonal antibodies which bind them either augment or inhibit a particular function. The lymphocyte function associated antigens LFA-1, -2, and -3 are examples of such molecules [17]. Although LFA-1 and LFA-2 are expressed only on lymphocytes, LFA-3 is also expressed on endothelial cells, and monoclonal antibodies against this antigen inhibit endothelial cell directed cytolysis by binding to the endothelial cell [21]. LFA-3 and the recently identified ICAM-1 [22] are prototypes for these endothelial cell function-associated antigens. Both of these molecules appear to be involved in cell adhesion. Therefore, antibodies which block or augment function may be clinically useful in vivo and/or help define molecules of potential functional relevance.

TABLE IV. Human foreskin endothelial cell antibodies

Mab	Cell binding	Immunoprecipitation	Comments
Group 1 ($E_{10,12,17,20}$)	HFEn only	No	Narrow distribution
Group 2 ($E_{3,14,22,32}$)	HFEn and TransEn	$E_{3.5}$ = 33kd on HUVEC	$E_{3.5}$ may differentiate HUVEC from HFEn
Group 3 ($E_{7,11,15,16,18}$)	HFEn, TransEn plus one other (U937, B-cell, SM or Emb fib)	No	
Group 4 ($E_{1,2,4,5,6,8,9,}$ $_{13,19,21,23-31}$)	Wide distribution, beyond HFEn	$E_{1.5}$ = 72kd (HFEn) E_{28} = 72kd (HFEn) E_{8} = 25kd (HUVEn) = 70kd (HFEn)	

A panel of 33 monoclonal antibodies has been screened as described in the text.
Abbreviations: HFEn: human foreskin endothelial cells; TransEn: SV40 transformed endothelial cells; SM: smooth muscle; Emb fib: embryonic fibroblasts; HUVEC: human umbilical vein endothelial cells. Molecular weights shown were obtained by standard iodination and immunoprecipitation techniques as previously described [18]

Activation antigens are expressed on activated but not on resting cells. Many activation antigens are receptors for growth hormones, such as insulin, transferrin, and interleukin-2 [reviewed in 23]. It is possible that diseased or damaged endothelial cells may express antigens not normally expressed on resting endothelial cells and that these antigens may serve as diagnostic markers or may be used to target therapy. Several of the antigens recognized by our panel of monoclonal antibodies increased in expression upon endothelial activation or injury. The prototype in this category is designated E12 [24]. This molecule is normally expressed by the capillary and small vessel endothelial cells of heart, lung, brain, and kidney. It is expressed, but in lower amounts, by skin and the great vessels, but it is not expressed at all by the liver parenchymal vascular bed. E12 expression is dramatically increased in diseased tissues, including cirrhotic liver and skin involved by mycosis fungoides, vasculitis, or psoriasis. This increase in expression by diseased vessels suggested that antigen expression was induced by injury. We exposed cultured endothelial cells to interleukin-1 for 24 hours and found a dramatic increase in E12 expression. These data suggest that, although we have yet to define the function of this endothelial cell-specific molecule, E12 is a specific marker for endothelial cell activation and/or injury. Pober, Cotran, and their colleagues have also recently identified antigens which increase in expression upon endothelial cell stimulation with IL-1, tumour necrosis factor, and/or interferon [25]. Activation of endothelial cells also results in expression of Fc and C3b receptors, and HLA-DR antigens. Exposure of endothelial cells to IL-1 increased pro-coagulant activity and leucocyte adhesion. Although the precise relationship between these inducible functions and new antigen expression remains unknown, these molecules may prove to be useful markers for clinical states and/or mechanisms of inflammation.

Basic science, diagnostic and therapeutic implications of endothelial cell antigens

Monoclonal antibodies have recently proven useful not only to define the function and cell distribution of antigens as discussed above, but also for the molecular cloning of the genes which encode these molecules. Sequence information can provide clues as to the function of a particular molecule and can also be used to develop new diagnostic and therapeutic modalities. Currently, the three most widely used techniques for cloning genes which encode a molecule recognized by a monoclonal antibody are: 1) using the monoclonal antibody to sort (on the fluorescence activated cell sorter) or to rosette cells which have been transfected with human DNA [26,27]; 2) using the monoclonal antibody to affinity purify enough protein to obtain limited aminoacid sequence and to generate oligonucleotides with which to screen libraries [28], and 3) using the monoclonal antibody to screen an expression library such as lambda gt11 [29]. We are currently applying all of these approaches to the cloning of selected endothelial cell antigens.

Monoclonal antibodies against endothelial cell antigens may prove useful in the diagnosis and/or therapy of renal and/or other diseases. They may be useful diagnostically: 1) to assess the immune status of a tissue: for example, pathological studies may be undertaken to define the state of activation or disease of a biopsy specimen; 2) to provide correlations between pathological specimens and clinical course, or 3) to provide the molecular definition of disease states. Monoclonal antibodies may be used therapeutically to suppress or augment the immune response. For example, they may 1) bind directly to the antigen, thereby removing a potential antigenic stimulus; 2) destroy or activate a functional endothelial cell subset; 3) inhibit an immune response by binding to specific endothelial cell receptors, or 4) inhibit a self-recognition process involved in the immune response, such as MHC restriction. Monoclonal antibodies recognizing human lymphocytes are now widely used for many similar diagnostic and therapeutic purposes.

In conclusion, we have applied the techniques of cellular immunology, protein chemistry, and most recently, molecular biology, to define the cell surface molecules involved in the lymphocyte-endothelial cell interaction. These molecules are thought to be intimately involved in blood clotting, inflammation and tumour growth. Further understanding of the structure of these molecules will allow new insights into these processes and should allow novel diagnostic and therapeutic approaches to human disease.

Acknowledgments

This work is supported by NIH Grant AM35008 and a grant from the American Heart Association of California. AMK is a Clinician-Scientist of the American Heart Association. DVL is supported by a Physician-Scientist Award from NIH (HD00750).

References

1 Hepinstall RH, ed. *Pathology of the Kidney.* Boston: Little Brown. 1983

2 Brenner BM, Rector FC, eds. *The Kidney.* Philadelphia: W B Saunders. 1981

3 Cummings NB, Michael AF, Wilson CB, eds. *Immune Mechanisms in Renal Disease.* New York: Plenum Press. 1983

4 Wilson CB, ed. *Immunologic Mechanisms of Renal Disease.* New York: Churchill Livingstone. 1978

5 Strom TB, Tilney NL, Paradysz JM et al. Cellular components of allograft rejection: identity, specificity, and cytotoxic function of cells infiltrating acutely rejecting allografts. *J Immunol 1977; 118:* 2020–2025

6 Lord EM, Nardella G. The multicellular tumor spheroid model: II. Characterization of the primary allograft response in unsensitized mice. *Transplantation 1980; 29:* 112–132

7 Clayberger C, Uyehara T, Hardy B et al. Target specificity and cell surface structures involved in the human cytolytic T lymphocyte response to endothelial cells. *J Immunol 1985; 135:* 12–18

8 Krensky AM, Reiss CS, Mier JW et al. Longterm human cytolytic T cell lines allospecific for HLA-DR6 antigen are OKT4+. *Proc Natl Acad Sci USA 1981; 79:* 2365–2369

9 Spits HH, Yssel H, Thompson A, DeVries JE. Human $T4^+$ and $T8^+$ cytotoxic T lymphocyte clones directed at products of different class II MHC loci. *J Immunol 1983; 131:* 678–683

10 Biddison WE, Rao PE, Talle MA et al. Possible involvement of the T4 molecule in T cell recognition of class II HLA antigens. *J Exp Med 1984; 159:* 783–797

11 Terhorst C, Van Agthoven A, Reinherz E, Scholossman S. Biochemical analysis of human T lymphocyte differentiation antigens T_4 and T_5. *Science 1980; 209:* 520–523

12 Engleman EG, Benike F, Grumet C, Evans RL. Activation of human T lymphocyte subsets: helper and suppressor/cytotoxic T cells recognize and respond to distinct histocompatibility antigens. *J Immunol 1981; 127:* 2124–2129

13 Pober JS, Collins T, Gimbrone MA et al. Lymphocytes recognize human vascular endothelial and dermal fibroblast Ia antigens induced by recombinant immune interferon. *Nature 1983; 305:* 726–729

14 Reinherz EL, Hussey RE, Schlossman SF. A monoclonal antibody blocking human T cell function. *Eur J Immunol 1980; 10:* 758–762

15 Reinherz EL, Schlossman SF. The differentiation and function of human T lymphocytes. *Cell 1980; 19(4):* 821–827

16 Kung P, Goldstein G, Reinherz EL, Schlossman SF. Monoclonal antibodies defining distinctive human T cell surface antigens. *Science 1979; 206(4416):* 347–349

17 Krensky AM, Sanchez-Madrid F, Robbins E et al. The functional significance, distribution and structure of LFA-1, LFA-2, and LFA-3: cell surface antigens associated with the CTL-target interaction. *J Immunol 1983; 131:* 611–616

18 Sanchez-Madrid F, Krensky AM, Ware CF et al. Three distinct antigens associated with human T lymphocyte-mediated cytolysis: LFA-1, LFA-2, and LFA-3. *Proc Natl Acad Sci USA 1982; 79:* 7489–7493

19 Shaw S, Luce GEG, Quinones R et al. Two antigen-independent adhesion pathways used by human cytotoxic T cell clones. *Nature 1986; 323:* 262–264

20 Paul LC, Baldwin WM, van Es LA. Vascular endothelial alloantigens in renal transplantation. *Transplantation 1985; 40:* 117–123

21 Collins T, Krensky AM, Clayberger C et al. Human cytolytic T lymphocyte interactions with vascular endothelium and fibroblasts. Role of effector and target cell molecules. *J Immunol 1984; 137:* 1878–1884
22 Rothlein R, Dustin ML, Marlin SD, Springer TA. A human intercellular adhesion molecule (ICAM-1) distinct from LFA-1. *J Immunol 1986; 137:* 1270–1274
23 Krensky AM, Clayberger C. Diagnostic and therapeutic implications of T cell surface antigens. *Transplantation 1985; 39:* 339–348
24 Tuder R, Landers DV, Clayberger C et al. Identification and characterization of a novel inducible endothelial cell antigen. Submitted
25 Pober JS, Bevilacqua , Mendrick DL et al. Two distinct monokines, interleukin-1 and tumor necrosis factor, each independently induce biosynthesis and transient expression of the same antigen on the surface of cultured human vascular endothelial cells. *J Immunol 1986; 136:* 1680–1684
26 Littman DR, Thomas Y, Maddon PJ et al. The isolation and sequence of the gene encoding T8: a molecule defining functional classes of T lymphocytes. *Cell 1985; 40:* 237–246
27 Kavathas P, Herzenberg LA. Stable transformation of mouse L cells for human membrane T cell differentiation antigens, HLA and B_2-microglobulin: selection by fluorescence activated cell sorting. *Proc Natl Acad Sci USA 1983; 80:* 524–528
28 Kavathas P, Sukhatme VP, Herzenberg LA, Parnes JR. Isolation of the gene coding for the human T lymphocyte differentiation antigen Leu-2 (T8) by gene transfer and cDNA subtraction. *Proc Natl Acad Sci USA 1984; 81:* 7688–7692
29 Suggs SV, Hirose T, Miyake T et al. Use of synthetic oligodeoxiribononucleotides for the isolation of specific cloned DNA sequences. In Brown DD, ed. *Developmental Biology Using Purified Genes. UCLA Symposia Vol. 23.* New York: Academic Press. 1981: 683–693
30 Young RA, Davis RW. Efficient isolation of genes using antibody probes. *Proc Natl Acad Sci USA 1983; 80:* 1194–1198

RENAL ENDOTHELIAL CELLS AND PERIVASCULAR GROWTH CONTROL

T O Daniel

Vanderbilt University, Nashville, Tennessee, USA

Recent experiments with cultured endothelial cells have provided considerable information about the rôle they may play at vascular interfaces in vivo. A wide range of endothelial cell properties have been described, including surface-expressed anticoagulant and procoagulant activity [1–6], production of prostanoids and other agents affecting vascular smooth muscle contraction and coagulation [7–15], adherence of circulating blood leucocytes [16–20], and production of agents that stimulate proliferation, chemotaxis and matrix deposition [21–27]. Recognition that many pathological proliferative and sclerotic processes occur in vivo at vascular interfaces bounded by epithelial cells has added to the significance of these findings.

Pathological proliferation at vascular and perivascular sites may impair organ function either through obliteration of the vascular lumen of vessels supplying an organ or through destruction of functioning tissue units. These processes may affect tissues in many ways; examples in the kidney ranging from the renovascular lesions of hypertension and scleroderma to the destructive glomerular lesions of focal glomerulosclerosis and proliferative glomerulonephritis. Current understanding of endothelial cell function suggests several ways in which endothelial cells may participate.

Under basal conditions, endothelial cells express surface anticoagulant properties. They synthesize structural determinants and mediators that inhibit thrombogenesis [2–4,6] but in response to specific biochemical mediators the surface may be converted to one with procoagulant activity [2,3,5]. The frequent presence of intracapillary thrombi at sites adjacent to the extracapillary proliferation and sclerosis in proliferative glomerulonephritis suggests that a procoagulant endothelial surface may contribute to proliferative responses at sites adjacent to fibrin deposition.

Specific interactions between endothelial cells and circulating leucocytes are also tightly regulated. Surface expression of adhesion molecules that may be endothelial sites for specific leucocyte margination and mediator release is also regulated by endothelial cell exposure to specific biochemical mediators [18,19]. Thus endothelial cells may participate by targeting circulating leucocytes to marginate at 'initiated' vascular sites, where lymphokines and monokines may be released locally. Endothelial cells may mediate significant events in the progression of vascular and perivascular pathological lesions through influences on vessel wall coagulation and through regulated surface expression of leucocyte adhesion molecules.

For initiating events to provoke pathological proliferation, cell types subjacent to the endothelial barrier must presumably be exposed to biochemical mitogenic signals. These mitogens may either originate from the intravascular compartment, from cells that marginate at the site, or from endothelial cells that form the border between intra- and perivascular compartments. In pathological processes that evolve at perivascular sites where the endothelial cell barrier has not been interrupted, either mitogenic agents must traverse the endothelial cell barrier to reach target cells, or endothelial cells must produce these biochemical mediators. If the endothelial cells themselves are capable of producing the relevant mitogens, increased production may participate in mediating the proliferative perivascular response through a so-called 'paracrine' mechanism.

Just as endothelial cell functions such as surface anticoagulant and leucocyte binding properties are regulated in response to specific biochemical mediators, we have investigated whether growth factor production may similarly be regulated. In collaboration with Drs Lewis Williams and Verna Gibbs at UCSF, our work has tested the hypothesis that agonists available at the intralumenal surface of endothelial cells, whether from marginated cell types, circulating agonists, or products of local events such as coagulation, may stimulate endothelial cell growth factor production.

For several reasons we have focused attention on endothelial cell expression of the potent mesenchymal cell mitogen, platelet-derived growth factor. First, cell types that participate in destructive proliferative perivascular processes are mesenchymally derived, and platelet-derived growth factor is a potent mitogen for these cells which include fibroblasts, smooth muscle cells, and mesangial cells [28]. Secondly, the work of Bowen-Pope, DiCorletto and others has shown that platelet-derived growth factor activity is released by cultured human umbilical vein endothelial cells [29]. Barrett, Collins and others have shown these cells express the mRNA for the B chain of platelet-derived growth factor, encoded by the c-*sis* proto-oncogene [30,31]. Endothelial cell expression of c-*sis* mRNA is reversibly regulated with differentiation of cultured human umbilical vein endothelial cells [32]. Finally, in addition to its action to stimulate proliferation of mesenchymal cells, platelet-derived growth factor is chemotactic for fibroblasts, leucocytes, and stimulates production of extracellular matrix constituents that may constitute part of sclerotic pathological lesions [26–28,33]. The endothelial cells themselves do not express surface platelet-derived growth factor receptors, cytoplasmic platelet-derived growth factor receptor mRNA, nor do they divide in response to platelet-derived growth factor [Daniel, unpublished results], making platelet-derived growth factor an effective 'paracrine' mediator for stimulating adjacent cell and not endothelial cell proliferation.

We have used a preparation of endothelial cells derived from the microvasculature of renal cortex [34]. Donor kidneys otherwise unusable for transplantation are dissected, treated with collagenase, and endothelial cells are recoverable from the outgrowth of glomeruli and other vascular fragments isolated by Percoll gradient centrifugation. This preparation includes greater than 90% endothelial cells as identified by immunohistochemical staining for Factor VIII antigen and expression of angiotensin converting enzyme activity, though the outgrowth endothelial cells are not exclusively of glomerular origin unlike those reported by Striker et al [35].

Reasoning that sustained increases in growth factor production would be most significant in mediating relevant in vivo proliferation, and that sustained increases in production would require increased gene expression, we screened several agonists of possible relevance for effects upon renal microvascular endothelial cell expression of the c-*sis* mRNA, encoding the B chain for platelet-derived growth factor [36,37]. We utilized a hybridization/protection assay of high sensitivity and specificity for specific mRNA species to quantify c-*cis* mRNA in samples of total RNA extracted from confluent endothelial cell monolayers that had been exposed to specific mediators in serum-free media [38].

Our studies have shown that exposure of this preparation of renal microvascular endothelial cells to a variety of agonists including interleukins 1 and 2, platelet activating factor, and bradykinin, does not affect cellular levels of c-*cis* mRNA. In contrast, however, exposure to thrombin induced expression of c-*cis* mRNA by 3–5-fold with a maximal response evident at four hours after exposure [38]. The mechanism by which thrombin induced the c-*sis* expression is apparently independent of its proteolytic activity, as proteolytically inactivated DFP-thrombin caused the same level of c-*sis* induction as native thrombin. The effect of thrombin upon the B chain platelet-derived growth factor message expression in these cells is mimicked by biologically active tumour-promoting phorbol esters, suggesting that thrombin may exert its effect through the phorbol activated kinase C system. The endothelial cell mitogen, fibroblast growth factor, does not induce c-*sis* expression in these cells, showing that the induction seen in response to thrombin and PMA is not a non-specific mitogenic effect.

More recently, using similar experimental approaches, we have demonstrated that transforming growth factor β (TGF-β), an agent present in high concentrations in platelet α-granules and released upon platelet activation, also induces the expression of c-*sis* mRNA in this preparation of renal microvascular endothelial cells [39]. However, the time course of this induction response differs from that seen with thrombin and phorbol ester induction, peaking at 30 hours after stimulation. Similarly c-*sis* induction by TGF has been reported in a murine embryonic fibroblast cell, AKR2B, by Leof et al [40]. In this cell line, it has been suggested that c-*sis* mRNA induction and increased platelet-derived growth factor activity accounts for the mitogenic response to TGF-β, through an 'autocrine' mechanism; induced platelet-derived growth factor production may also activate platelet-derived growth factor receptors to stimulate proliferation of the same cells expressing the platelet-derived growth factor activity. The absence of platelet-derived growth factor receptors on the microvascular endothelial cells distinguishes their response from that of the murine fibroblast cell line. In fact, TGF-β is growth inhibitory for endothelial cells from several sources [41–43], further suggesting that the c-*sis* induction response is unrelated to endothelial cell proliferation.

The distinctions in the time courses of c-*sis* induction by thrombin and TGF-β points toward different transduction mechanisms responsible for transmitting information from surface receptor binding events to the elevation of cellular c-*sis* mRNA levels. Further, the c-*sis* mRNA response to TGF-β stimulation provides a molecularly defined assay for TGF-β action and may help elucidate the biochemical mechanisms effecting responses to TGF-β receptor activation.

The induction of endothelial cell platelet-derived growth factor gene expression may link the mechanisms responsible for intracapillary fibrin deposition and subjacent cellular proliferation in diseases such as proliferative glomerulonephritis. Either locally activated thrombin or local release of the platelet product, TGF-β, or both may potentially induce sustained endothelial cell production of platelet-derived growth factor activity. However, this extrapolation is worthy of further consideration only if the increased gene expression is accompanied by increased production of platelet-derived growth factor activity.

The second assay we have employed allows a specific recognition of biologically active platelet-derived growth factor species released into medium conditioned in vitro by renal microvascular endothelial cells under the conditions mentioned earlier [38]. This assay reconstitutes the essential components of the paracrine growth factor action paradigm. Platelet-derived growth factor activity released from treated endothelial cells is collected and assayed by its activation of platelet-derived growth factor receptors on responder murine fibroblasts. Responder Balb c/3T3 cell proteins, including platelet-derived growth factor receptors, are labelled with [^{35}S]-methionine; upon stimulation with conditioned medium samples containing platelet-derived growth factor activity from either control, thrombin, or TGF-β treated endothelial cells, active platelet-derived growth factor molecules bind to the 185kDa platelet-derived growth factor receptor and stimulate autophosphorylation of tyrosine through activation of intrinsic tyrosine kinase activity. Activated, but not inactivated, platelet-derived growth factor receptors are purified from cell extracts using an antiphosphotyrosine antibody [44]. Platelet-derived growth factor receptor autoradiographic signal serves to quantify the platelet-derived growth factor activity in the endothelial cell conditioned media sample tested when compared to a standard curve generated using purified platelet-derived growth factor.

In this way, we have demonstrated that thrombin induced a 3.5-fold increase in the release of platelet-derived growth factor activity into media conditioned by renal microvascular endothelial cells for 36 hours after stimulation with thrombin compared to the basal amount of activity released by unstimulated cells [38]. Similarly, platelet-derived, TGF-β, also stimulated platelet-derived growth factor activity release by 5-fold over two sequential collections of 24 hours after exposure [39]. The correlation of these findings of stimulated platelet-derived growth factor activity production with the c-*sis* mRNA data supports the possible biological significance of platelet-derived growth factor B chain message induction.

In addition to the induction responses outlined above, we have recognized that the β-adrenergic agents norepinephrine and isoproterenol decrease the basal level of c-*sis* expression in unstimulated cells and block the induction responses to thrombin and TGF-β when administered simultaneously [39]. The β-adrenergic action appears to be mediated through activation of adenylate cyclase, since forskolin, a direct activator of adenylate cyclase, similarly blocks thrombin and TGF-β induction on c-*sis* mRNA expression [39]. Further, forskolin blocks the thrombin- and TGF-β-induced increases in endothelial cell conditioned medium platelet-derived growth factor activity, again correlating with the c-*sis* mRNA response.

Recent data from our laboratory have shown that these renal microvascular endothelial cells also express the mRNA encoding the A chain of platelet-derived growth factor in a manner that is also subject to regulation by thrombin and TGF-β [Daniel, unpublished results]. The relative contributions of A and B chains to the platelet-derived growth factor activity released remains to be determined, as available data suggest that platelet-derived growth factor activity may be found in AA or BB homodimers, as well as in what appears to be the platelet form, AB heterodimer.

In addition to the thrombin mediated increased levels of platelet-derived growth factor B chain mRNA and release of platelet-derived growth factor activity we have reported in the renal microvascular endothelial cells, Harlan et al [45] reported that α-thrombin induces release of platelet-derived growth factor-like molecules from human umbilical vein endothelial cells in a manner independent of new protein synthesis. Exposure to α-thrombin in that system results in greater than 4-fold increase in the release of platelet-derived growth factor binding competition activity beginning within 1.5 hours and proceeding in the absence of new protein synthesis.

Invoking a mechanism independent of thrombin action but still potentially operative in pathological conditions involving endothelial cell surface coagulation, Cadjusek and co-workers [46] have shown that activated Factor X is bound by bovine aortic endothelial cells and increases the release of platelet-derived growth factor binding competition activity. Fox and DiCorleto have shown that endothelial cells injured by exposure to either phorbol myristate acetate or endotoxin release increased amounts of platelet-derived growth factor activity as assayed by a radioreceptor competition assay [47]. They have also recognized that lipid peroxides in modified low density lipoprotein species inhibits release of platelet-derived growth factor activity through a mechanism that is unassociated with changes in c-*sis* mRNA [48,49].

In addition to possible proliferative actions that endothelial cell-released platelet-derived growth factor may have on subjacent cell types, platelet-derived growth factor may also act as a mediator of vasoconstriction [50] or possibly mesangial cell contraction in the renal glomerulus. Its action as a chemotactic agent active upon fibroblasts and leucocytes may participate at local sites as well [28,33].

Additional examples of induction of endothelial cell growth factor production by specific biochemical mediators have been reported recently, further supporting the potential rôle of endothelial cell-derived mediators in vascular and perivascular proliferative pathology. Libby et al [51] have demonstrated that expression of interleukin 1 mRNA and release of interleukin 1 activity are induced following human umbilical vein endothelial cell exposure to both tumour necrosis factor and endotoxin. Interleukin 1 has great potential as a mediator of perivascular proliferative responses, as it is both mitogenic for fibroblasts and mesangial cells (in the presence of platelet-derived growth factor) and induces plasminogen activator expression [52–54]. In addition to platelet-derived growth factor and interleukin 1, endothelial cells synthesize and respond to fibroblast growth factor [22,23] and express mRNA for TGF-β [Daniel, unpublished observations], though regulation of either fibroblast growth factor or TGF-β expression has yet to be identified.

As additional in vitro systems are explored, other endothelial cell functions will be identified that may play intermediary rôles in proliferative vascular responses. Ultimately, links between in vitro results such as those presented here, and in vivo findings at pathological sites must be made to confirm participation of these mediators and responses in disease processes. Other assays such as in situ hybridization could be used to identify whether regulated endothelial cell expression of genes for specific mediator molecules may actually participate in pathological proliferation adjacent to the endothelial cell barrier. As other functions of endothelial cells are discerned through study of cultured cells from specific vascular beds, functional distinctions between endothelial cells from different vascular sites may give clues as to the site specificity of perivascular lesions in pathological states. Co-culture systems may allow more definitive characterizations of intercellular mediator effects and specificity of responses that relate to contiguous cell-cell interactions.

Acknowledgments

This work was supported by the Howard Hughes Medical Institute, PHS Grants HL32898 and DK38517, and the Robert Wood Johnston Foundation.

References

1 Simionescu M, Simionescu N. Functions of the endothelial cell surface. *Ann Rev Physiol 1986; 48:* 279–293

2 Stern D, Nawroth P, Handley D, Kisiel W. An endothelial cell-dependent pathway of coagulation. *Proc Natl Acad Sci 1985; 82:* 2523–2527

3 Nawroth PP, Handley DA, Esmon CT, Stern DM. Interleukin 1 induces endothelial cell procoagulant activity. *Proc Natl Acad Sci 1986; 83:* 3460–3464

4 Marcum JA, Atha DH, Fritze LMS et al. Cloned bovine aortic endothelia cells synthesize anticoagulantly active heparan sulfate proteoglycan. *J Biol Chem 1986; 261:* 7507–7517

5 Bevilaqua MP, Pobert JS, Majeau GR et al. Recombinant tumor necrosis factor induces procoagulant activity in cultured human vascula endothelium: characterization and comparison with the actions of interleukin 1. *Proc Natl Acad Sci 1986; 83:* 4533–4537

6 Stern D, Brett J, Harris K, Nawroth P. Participation of endothelial cells in the Protein C-Protein S anticoagulant pathway: the synthesis and release of Protein S. *J Cell Biol 1986; 102:* 1971–1978

7 Miller DK, Sadowski S, Sodermen DD, Kuehl FA Jr. Endothelial cell prostaglandin production induced by activated neutrophils. *J Biol Chem 1985; 2660:* 1006–1014

8 McIntyre TM, Zimmerman GA, Satoh K, Prescott SM. Cultured endothelial cells synthesize both platelet-activating factor and prostacyclin in response to histamine, bradykinin, and adenosine triphosphate. *J Clin Invest 1985; 76:* 271–280

9 Moncada S, Herman AG, Higgs EA, Vane JR. Differential formation of prostacyclin (PGC or PGI_2) by layers of the arterial wall. An explanation for the anti-thrombotic properties of vascular endothelium. *Thromb Res 1977; 11:* 323–344

10 Moncada S, Vane JR. Arachidonic acid metabolites and the interactions between platelets and blood-vessel walls. *N Engl J Med 1979; 300:* 1142–1147

11 Prescott SM, Zimmerman GA, McIntyre TM. Human endothelial cells in culture produce platelet-activating factor when stimulated with thrombin. *Proc Natl Acad Sci 1984; 81:* 3534–3538

12 Furchgott RF. Role of endothelium in responses of vascular smooth muscle. *Circ Res 1983; 53:* 557–573

13 Gerritsen ME. Eicosanoid production by the coronary microvascular endothelium. *Fed Proc 1987; 46:* 47–53

14 Smith WL. Prostaglandin biosynthesis and its compartmentation in vascular smooth muscle and endothelial cells. *Ann Rev Physiol 1986; 48:* 251–262

15 Ganz P, Davies PF, Leopold JA et al. Short- and long-term interactions of endothelium and vascular smooth muscle in coculture: effects on cyclic GMP production. *Proc Natl Acad Sci 1986; 83:* 3552–3556

16 Pawlowski NA, Abraham EL, Pontier S et al. Human monocyte-endothelial cell interaction in vitro. *Proc Natl Acad Sci 1985; 82:* 8208–8212

17 Wallis WJ, Beatty PG, Ochs HD, Harlan JM. Human monocyte adherence to cultured vascular endothelium: monoclonal antibody-defined mechanisms. *J Immunol 1985; 135:* 2323–2330

18 Gamble JR. Harlan JM, Klebanoff SJ, Vadas MA. Stimulation of the adherence of neutrophils to umbilical vein endothelium by human recombinant tumor necrosis factor. *Proc Natl Acad Sci 1985; 82:* 8667–8671

19 Yu C-L, Haskard D, Cavender D, Ziff M. Effects of bacterial lipopolysaccharide on the binding of lymphocytes to endothelial cell monolayers. *J Immunol 1986; 136:* 569–573

20 Gallatin WM, Weissman IL, Butcher EC. A cell surface molecule involved in organ-specific homing of lymphocytes. *Nature 1983; 304:* 30–34

21 Castellot JJ Jr, Hoover RL, Karnovsky MJ. Glomerular endothelial cells secrete a heparin-like inhibitor and a peptide stimulator of mesangial cell proliferation. *Am J Pathol 1986; 125:* 493–500

22 Vlodavsky I, Folkman J, Sullivan R et al. Endothelial cell-derived basic fibroblast growth factor: synthesis and deposition into subendothelial extracellular matrix. *Proc Natl Acad Sci 1987; 84:* 2292–2296

23 Schweigerer L, Neufeld G, Friedman J et al. Capillary endothelial cells express basic fibroblast growth factor, a mitogen that promotes their own growth. *Nature 1987; 325:* 257–259

24 Bowen-Pope DF, Ross R, Seifert RA. Locally acting growth factors for vascular smooth muscle cells: endogenous synthesis and release from platelets. *Circulation 1985; 72:* 735–740

25 Postlethwaite AE, Smith GN, Mainardi CL et al. Lymphocyte modulation of fibroblast function in vitro: stimulation and inhibition of collagen production by different effector molecules. *J Immunol 1984; 132:* 2470–2477

26 Majack RA, Cook SC, Bornstein P. Platelet-derived growth factor and heparin-like glycosaminoglycans regulate thrombospondin synthesis and deposition in the matrix by smooth muscle cells. *J Cell Biol 1985; 101:* 1059–1070

27 Narayanan AS, Page RC. Biosynthesis and regulation of Type V collagen in diploid human fibroblasts. *J Biol Chem 1983; 258:* 11694–11699

28 Ross R, Raines EW, Bowen-Pope DF. The biology of platelet-derived growth factor. *Cell 1986; 46:* 155–169

29 DiCorleto PE, Bowen-Pope DF. Cultured endothelial cells produce a platelet-derived growth factor-like protein. *Proc Natl Acad Sci 1983; 80:* 1919–1923

30 Barrett TB, Gajdusek CM, Schwartz SM et al. Expression of the *sis* gene by endothelial cells in culture and in vivo. *Proc Natl Acad Sci 1984; 81:* 6772–6774

31 Collins T, Ginsburg D, Boss JM et al. Cultured human endothelial cells express platelet-derived growth factor B chain: cDNA cloning and structural analysis. *Nature 1985; 316:* 748–750

32 Jaye M, McConathy E, Drohan W et al. Modulation of the *sis* gene transcript during endothelial cell differentiation in vitro. *Science 1985; 228:* 882–885

33 Seppa H, Grotendorst G, Seppa S et al. Platelet-derived growth factor is chemotactic for fibroblasts. *J Cell Biol 1982; 92:* 584–588

34 Gibbs VC, Wood DM, Garavoy MR. The response of cultured human kidney capillary endothelium to immunologic stimuli. *Hum Immunol 1985; 14:* 259–269

35 Striker GE, Soderland C, Bowen-Pope DF et al. Isolation, characterization, and propagation in vitro of human glomerular endothelial cells. *J Exp Med 1984; 160:* 323–328

36 Chiu I-M, Reddy EP, Givol D et al. Nucleotide sequence analysis identifies the human c-*sis* protoncogene as a structural gene for platelet-derived growth factor. *Cell 1984; 37:* 123–129

37 Josephs SF, Guo C, Ratner L, Wong-Staal F. Human proto-oncogene nucleotide sequences corresponding to the transforming region of simian sarcoma virus. *Science 1984; 223:* 487–491

38 Daniel TO, Gibbs VC, Milfay DF et al. Thrombin stimulates c-*sis* gene expression in microvascular endothelial cells. *J Biol Chem 1986; 261:* 9579–9582

39 Daniel TO, Gibbs VC, Milfay DF, Williams LT. Agents that increase cAMP accumulation block endothelial c-*sis* induction by thrombin and TGF-beta. *J Biol Chem 1987:* in press

40 Leof EB, Proper JA, Goustin AS et al. Induction of c-*sis* mRNA and activity similar to platelet-derived growth factor by transforming growth factor: a proposed model for indirect mitogenesis involving autocrine activity (1986). *Proc Natl Acad Sci 1986; 83:* 2453–2457

41 Baird A, Durkin T. Inhibition of endothelial cell proliferation by type β-transforming growth factor: interactions with acidic and basic fibroblast growth factors. *Biochem Biophys Res Commun 1986; 138:* 476–482

42 Frater-Schroder M, Muller G, Birchmeier W, Bohlen P. Transforming growth factor-β inhibits endothelial cell proliferation. *Biochem Biophys Res Commun 1986; 137:* 295–302

43 Heimark RL, Twardzik DR, Schwartz SM. Inhibition of endothelial regeneration by type-beta transforming growth factor from platelets. *Science 1986; 233:* 1078–1080

44 Daniel TO, Tremble PM, Frackelton AR Jr, Williams LT. Purification of the platelet-derived growth factor receptor using an antiphosphotyrosine antibody. *Proc Natl Acad Sci 1985. 82:* 2684–2687

45 Harlan JM, Thompson PJ, Ross R, Bowen-Pope DF. Thrombin induces release of platelet-derived growth factor-like molecule(s) by cultured human endothelial cells. *J Cell Biol 1986; 103:* 1129–1133

46 Gajdusek C, Carbon S, Ross R et al. Activation of coagulation releases endothelial cell mitogens. *J Cell Biol 1986; 103:* 419–428

47 Fox PL, DiCorleto PE. Regulation of production of a platelet-derived growth factor-like protein by cultured bovine aortic endothelial cells. *J Cell Physiol 1984; 121:* 298–308

48 Fox PL, DiCorleto PE. Modified low density dipoproteins suppress production of a platelet-derived growth factor-like protein by cultured endothelial cells. *Proc Natl Acad Sci 1986; 83:* 4774–4778

49 Fox PL, Chisolm GM, DiCorleto PE. Lipoprotein-mediated inhibition of endothelial cell production of platelet-derived growth factor-like protein depends on free radical lipid peroxidation. *J Biol Chem 1987; 262:* 6046–6054

50 Berk BC, Alexander RW, Brock TA et al. Vasoconstriction: a new activity for platelet-derived growth factor. *Science 1986; 232:* 87–90

51 Libby P, Ordovas JM, Auger KR et al. Endotoxin and tumor necrosis factor induce interleukin-1 gene expression in adult human vascular endothelial cells. *Am J Pathol 1986; 124:* 179–186

52 Schmidt JA, Mizel SB, Cohen D, Green I. Interleukin 1, a potential regulator of fibroblast proliferation. *J Immunol 1982; 128:* 2177–2182

53 Lovett DH, Ryan JL, Sterzel RB. Stimulation of rat mesangial cell proliferation by macrophage interleukin 1. *J Immunol 1983; 131:* 2830–2836

54 Emeis JJ, Kooistra T. Interleukin 1 and lipopolysaccharide induce an inhibitor of tissue-type plasminogen activator in vivo and in cultured endothelial cells. *J Exp Med 1986; 163.* 1260–1266

PHENOTYPIC CHARACTERISTICS OF CULTURED PROXIMAL TUBULAR EPITHELIUM

R L Tannen, Ming-Jer Tang, Atul Sahai

Internal Medicine (Nephrology), University of Michigan, Ann Arbor, Michigan, USA

The development of established cell lines and of primary cultures with all the phenotypic properties of proximal tubular epithelium in vivo, would provide an invaluable tool for the study of tubular cell biology and pathophysiology.

Significant strides have been made already towards achieving this goal. A variety of established cell lines which express the properties of proximal tubular epithelium have been characterized, for example LLC-PK_1, JTC-12 and OK cells [1–3]. Microdissected proximal tubules from rabbit and humans have been cultured successfully, and macroseparation techniques have also been employed to culture proximal tubular cells from rabbits, rats and dogs [4–9].

A variety of the phenotypic characteristics of proximal tubular epithelium have been demonstrated in these established cell lines and primary cultures. Apical microvilli and brush border enzymes typical of proximal tubular epithelium are expressed [7–10]. Sodium-dependent glucose, phosphate and aminoacid transporters have been identified and transepithelial transport of solutes as well as of glucose and aminoacids are demonstrable [7,8,11–16]. Some of these cells exhibit a parathyroid hormone responsive adenylate cyclase and in OK cells, this is coupled to an inhibition of phosphate transport [6,7,12, 13,17]. Glutamine-dependent and pH responsive ammonia formation has been found in LLC-PK_1 cells by our laboratory [18], and gluconeogenesis has been demonstrated in subclones of LLC-PK_1 cells [19] as well as in primary cultures of canine proximal tubules [20].

Nevertheless, despite these advances, phenotypic expression by cultured epithelium of the precise differentiated features of proximal tubular cells in vivo has yet to be achieved. Apical microvilli are sparser and brush border enzyme activities lower than in vivo [7]. LLC-PK_1 cells do not respond to parathyroid hormone whereas JTC-12 cells increased cAMP levels but is not associated with inhibition of phosphate transport [12,21]. Most cell lines that have been studied extensively express a glycolytic enzyme profile rather than the gluconeogenic pattern typical of proximal epithelium in vivo [10].

Many factors influence the differentiation of cells in culture. These include hormones and possibly other factors in the incubation medium, the substratum upon which the cells are grown, the access of nutrients and potential mediators to the basal surface, the availability of oxygen, and cell-to-cell interactions as well as cell structural features [16,18,22–25].

In the process of attempting to identify a cell culture model for the investigation of renal ammoniagenesis, our laboratory has evaluated some of the factors that modulate differentiation by proximal tubular epithelium.

Our initial studies of ammonia formation were carried out in LLC-PK_1 cells. These cells derived from the Hampshire Pig [1] have several characteristics of proximal tubular epithelium including apical microvilli, high activities of the brush border enzymes gamma glutamyl transpeptidase, leucine amino peptidase and alkaline phosphatase [10]; and they exhibit both sodium-dependent glucose and phosphate transport [11,14]. However, in contrast to proximal epithelium, LLC-PK_1 are unresponsive to parathyroid hormone, and express vasopressin and calcitonin stimulative adenylate cyclase activity [21].

Initially we investigated ammonia production by subconfluent cells cultures in Eagles minimal essential media supplemented with dialysed 10% fetal bovine serum using glutamine as an ammoniagenic substrate [18]. Although the cultured cells produced ammonia, the rate of ammonia formation did not change when the cells were incubated in 4mM rather than 2mM glutamine. Furthermore, as

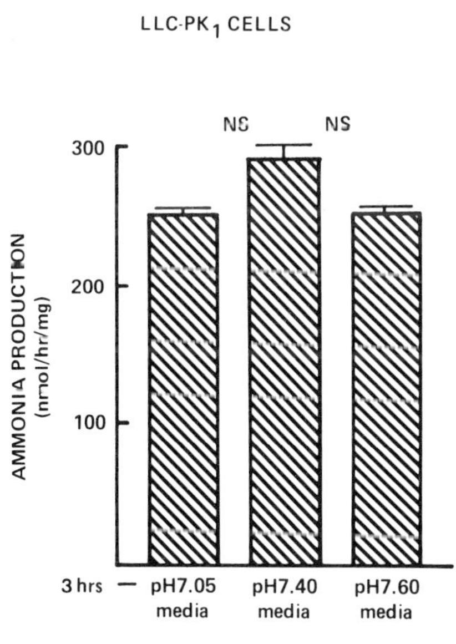

Figure 1. Effect of media pH on NH_3 production by LLC-PK_1 cells grown under still conditions. Incubation for three hours at acidotic and alkalotic pH values had no effect on NH_3 production. Reproduced with permission from *Am J Physiol 1986; 251:* C293–C298

shown in Figure 1, when the cells were incubated for three hours at pH 7.0, 7.4 or 7.6, a pH dependent alteration in NH_3 formation was not detected. This contrasts with a large body of evidence from intact animals, perfused kidneys and incubated tubule experiments, which demonstrate direct stimulation of NH_3 formation by a decrease in pH [26].

Based on both direct measurements of oxygen tension at the surface of cultured cells, as well as theoretical calculations of oxygen diffusion through a layer of still fluid, we speculated that cells cultured under standard still conditions might be deprived of oxygen [27,28]. In order to circumvent this potential problem, cells were grown on a Bellco Rocker at 2.5 rocks/minute, thereby providing intermittent exposure to atmospheric oxygen and constant gentle mixing of the overlying media. Cells cultured in this fashion exhibited growth kinetics similar to those cultured under standard still conditions [29].

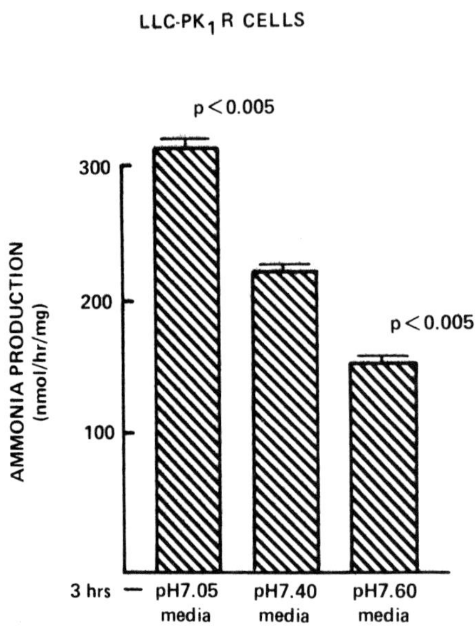

Figure 2. Effect of media pH on NH_3 production by LLC-PK_1 cells grown on a Bellco Rocker. In contrast to cells grown under still conditions, when cells were grown on a Rocker NH_3 production was stimulated by a low pH

When ammonia formation by rocked cells was examined, strikingly different behaviour was found. An increase in glutamine concentration from 2 to 4mM was accompanied by an increase in NH_3 production, thereby providing evidence of glutamine-dependent ammoniagenesis. Furthermore, as shown in Figure 2, pH dependent ammoniagenesis was demonstrable also. Rocked cells incubated for three hours at pH 7.0 produced significantly more ammonia than cells incubated at pH 7.6, while the values for pH 7.4 fell between the acidotic and alkalotic conditions. Thus rocking resulted in expression of the differentiated proximal tubular function of pH regulatable ammoniagenesis in $LLC\text{-}PK_1$ cells.

Subsequently we carried out experiments using $LLC\text{-}PK_1$ cells to determine whether rocking influenced other aspects of cellular differentiation and to delineate the mechanism underlying this effect.

Two aspects of epithelial cell differentiation were assessed: 1) dome formation, which is a reflection of vectorial transepithelial transport by cultured cells, and 2) sodium-dependent glucose transport, a phenotypic property of proximal tubular epithelium which has been shown to parallel differentiation in $LLC\text{-}PK_1$ cells [11].

Cells grown on a rocker exhibited earlier and more copious dome formation than those grown under still conditions in the standard ambient oxygen atmosphere (18% oxygen). In addition, sodium-dependent glucose uptake, measured by measuring cellular accumulation of 14C α-methylgucoside, occurred earlier and in increased magnitude in rocked as opposed to still cultures [30].

Thus three markers of functional differentiation in proximal tubular epithelium were induced by rocking: 1) pH responsive ammonia production; 2) transepithelial transport, as reflected by dome formation, and 3) sodium-dependent glucose transport.

We suspected that the improvement in oxygenation promoted by rocking, might explain the altered behaviour induced by this manoeuvre. This suspicion was supported by a decrease in lactate dehydrogenase activity in rocked cells, which suggested a decrease in glycolytic metabolism.

To test the potential role of oxygen in mediating the effects of rocking, $LLC\text{-}PK_1$ cells were cultured under still conditions in a high oxygen atmosphere (36% oxygen). Cells cultured in this fashion exhibited decreased activity of lactate dehydrogenase, pH responsive ammoniagenesis, enhanced dome formation, and increased capacity for sodium-dependent glucose transport [30]. Thus culture in a high oxygen atmosphere replicated qualitatively all the changes induced by rocking.

These findings indicate increased oxygenation induces differentiated function in $LLC\text{-}PK_1$ cells, and suggest that this mechanism explains the effect of rocking on the behaviour of these cells. It is important to stress, however, that these findings do not exclude the possibility that rocking also may alter cellular behaviour by other mechanisms independent of oxygen provision, as for example by enhanced mixing and dissipation of unstirred layer effects.

These studies also indicate that culture under standard still conditions may provide an hypoxic environment, which can impair the expression of normal cellular differentiation and function.

In view of the findings indicating that culture under standard conditions results in hypoxic environment, we decided to examine whether the development of glycolytic metabolic profile in cultured cells can be explained on this basis. First we investigated carbohydrate metabolism by primary cultures of rabbit proximal tubules, since differentiated proximal tubular epithelium have a gluconeogenic rather than glycolytic metabolic profile in vivo.

Primary cultures of rabbit proximal tubules were obtained using a modification of the method described by Chung et al [7]. The tubules were grown in serum free Dulbecco's modified Eagle's medium supplemented with insulin, transferrin and hydrocortisone and containing 5mM glucose. Cellular outgrowth from the plated tubules began on the second day in culture and a confluent monolayer was achieved on the sixth day in culture.

The cultured cells exhibited cyclic AMP stimulation in response to parathyroid hormone, but were unresponsive to vasopressin and calcitonin [31]. Activities of the brush border enzymes, gamma glutamyl transpeptidase and leucine aminopeptidase were present. Furthermore cultured rabbit proximal tubules demonstrated sodium-dependent glucose transport, as reflected by the phlorizin-inhibitable uptake of 14C α-methylglucoside and vectorial transport of solutes and water reflected by dome formation. Thus, similar to the findings by Chung et al, relatively purified proximal tubules plates in a hormonally defined serum-free media resulted in cultured cells with the phenotypic properties of proximal tubular epithelium [7].

Daily glucose consumption and lactate production, assessed per milligram of cell protein, increased dramatically from the fourth to the sixth day in culture, when confluency was achieved. This metabolic evidence of increased glycolysis was accompanied by changes in the enzymatic profile, which also indicated a shift to a glycolytic pattern. For the first four days in culture, pyruvate kinase activity was equivalent to the levels measured in freshly isolated tubules, but then increased dramatically from day four to day six in parallel with the change in glucose uptake and lactate formation. Similarly the activity of lactate dehydrogenase was substantially greater on the sixth day of culture than in fresh tubules.

To determine whether these changes were caused by hypoxia, we also examined primary cultures grown on a rocker. We detected no effect from improved oxygenation either on glucose uptake and lactate production or on the activity of the glycolytic enzymes, pyruvate kinase and lactate dehydrogenase. Thus it appears that hypoxia does not account for the conversion from gluconeogenic to glycolytic behaviour when these cells are grown in culture.

The capacity of these cells for oxidative metabolism was assessed on day six, by placing scraped cells suspended in culture media in a chamber with a Clark type oxygen electrode. Both basal rates of oxygen consumption and uncoupled rates following the addition of the uncoupler carbonyl cyanide m-chlorophenylhydrazone (CCCLP), were significantly lower than freshly isolated proximal tubules. Thus the cultured cells had an impaired capacity for oxidative metabolism. However, no differences in the oxidative profile were detected between cells grown under still and rocked conditions. Thus the reduced oxidative capacity is not a response to provision of inadequate oxygen.

In view of the diminished capacity for oxygen utilization by cultured proximal tubular cells, it is possible that the increase in glycolytic metabolism is caused by declining adenosine triphosphate (ATP) levels. Therefore, cellular ATP content was measured in both still and rocked cells on day six and compared to the values obtained in freshly isolated tubules incubated in a substrate replete media with 95% oxygen [32]. ATP content of both still and rocked culture cells was significantly higher than in the fresh tubules and so the high rate of glycolytic metabolism cannot be explained by reduction in ATP levels. In fact ATP feedback regulation of glycolysis, which is a characteristic of differentiated cells, appears to be either lacking or strikingly modified in cultured proximal tubular epithelium.

We also examined whether the glycolytic profile was related in some fashion to the availability of glucose in the culture medium. Cells were grown in 0.5, 5.0 or 25mM glucose and the activity of pyruvate kinase was measured. Cells grown in the lowest glucose concentration exhibited the highest pyruvate kinase activity. Thus an abundance of glucose does not account for the induction of the glycolytic profile.

Finally we examined the behaviour of two gluconeogenic enzymes, phosphoenolpyruvate carboxykinase (PEPCK) and fructose 1,6-bisphosphatase. To our surprise PEPCK behaved in a fashion very similar to pyruvate kinase. Until the fourth day in culture the levels in cultured cells were similar to fresh tubules. Then they increased strikingly from the fourth to the sixth day. Fructose 1,6-bisphosphatase levels on the other hand, declined in culture and by day six were lower than the levels in fresh tubules. Thus as might be anticipated the gluconeogenic enzyme fructose 1,6-bisphosphatase is down regulated at a time when glycolytic metabolism is stimulated. Unexpectedly PEPCK activity appears to parallel the change in glycolytic metabolism. Presumably its role in the metabolism of proliferating cultured cells differs from its predominant function as a gluconeogenic enzyme in differentiated proximal tubules.

These studies indicate that the development of glycolysis in proliferating proximal tubular cells in culture is not a response to hypoxia or energy deprivation. Rather it appears to be an integral metabolic feature of proliferating cells, although the specific functional role played by heightened glycolytic metabolism is unexplained.

The factors that transform these cultured cells into differentiated epithelium with a gluconeogenic metabolic profile are currently undefined. A preliminary report suggests that canine proximal tubular cells in culture can become gluconeogenic during the confluent phase [20]. To date, we have not been able to achieve this switch in metabolic profile in cultured rabbit proximal tubular epithelium.

Although the provision of adequate oxygen did not modify the profile of carbohydrate metabolism in rabbit primary cultures during the proliferative phase, it was not without effect. Indeed rocking promoted dome formation in these cells similar to its effects in LLC-PK_1 cells. Thus provisions of adequate oxygen, can impact on the differentiated function of more than one cell line.

The molecular mechanism whereby oxygen promotes differentiation, and those factors that dictate the conversion from an immature glycolytic to a differentiated gluconeogenic profile in cultured proximal tubular epithelium are areas worthy of future investigation.

References

1 Hull RN, Cherry WR, Weaver W. The origin and characteristics of a pig kidney cell strain, LLC-PK. *In Vitro 1976; 12:* 670–677

2 Ishizuka I, Tadcno K, Nagata N et al. Hormone-specific responses and biosynthesis of sulfolipids in cell lines derived from mammalian kidney. *Biochim Biophys Acta 1978; 541:* 467–482

3 Koyama H, Goodpasture C, Miller MM et al. Establishment and characterization of a cell line from the American Opossum (Didelphys Virginiana). *In Vitro 1978; 14:* 239–246

4 Horster M. Hormonal stimulation and differential growth response of renal epithelial cells cultivated in vitro from individual nephron segments. *Int J Biochem 1980; 12:* 29–35

5 Horster M. Primary culture of mammalian nephron epithelia requirements for cell outgrowth and proliferation from defined explanted nephron segments. *Pfluegers Arch 1979; 382:* 209–215

6 Wilson PD, Dillingham MA, Breckon R, Anderson RJ. Defined human renal tubular epithelia in culture: growth, characterization, and hormonal response. *Am J Physiol 1985; 248:* F436–F443

7 Chung SD, Alavi N, Livingston D et al. Characterization of primary rabbit kidney cultures that express proximal tubule functions in a hormonally defined medium. *J Cell Biol 1982; 95:* 118–126

8 Hruska KA, Goligorsky M, Scoble J et al. Effects of parathyroid hormone on cytosolic calcium in renal proximal tubular primary cultures. *Am J Physiol 1986; 251:* F188–F198

9 Harris RC, Seifter J, Lechene C. Coupling of Na/H exchange and Na/K pump activity in cultured rat proximal tubule cells. *Am J Physiol 1986; 251:* C815–C824

10 Gstraunthaler G, Pfaller W, Kotanko P. Biochemical characterization of renal epithelial cell cultures (LLC-PK_1 and MDCK). *Am J Physiol 1985; 248:* F536–F544

11 Amsler K, Cook JS. Development of Na^+-dependent hexose transport in a cultured line of porcine kidney cells. *Am J Physiol 1982; 242:* C94–C101

12 Malmstrom K, Murer H. Parathyroid hormone inhibits phosphate transport in OK cells but not in LLC-PK_1 and JTC-12.P3 cells. *Am J Physiol 1986; 251:* C23–C31

13 Takuwa Y, Ogata E. Characterization of Na^+-dependent phosphate uptake in cultured kidney cells (JTC-12) from monkey. *Biochem J 1985; 230:* 715–721

14 Rabito CA. Phosphate uptake by a kidney cell line (LLC-PK_1). *Am J Physiol 1983; 245:* F22–F31

15 Saier MH Jr, Boerner P, Grenier FC et al. Sodium entry pathways in renal epithelial cell lines. *Mineral Electrolyte Metab 1986; 12:* 42–50

16 Lever JE. Expression of differentiated functions in kidney epithelial cell lines. *Mineral Electrolyte Metab 1986; 12:* 14–19

17 Caverzasio J, Rizzoli R, Bonjour JP. Sodium-dependent phosphate transport inhibited by parathyroid hormone and cyclic AMP stimulation in an opossum kidney cell line. *J Biol Chem 1986; 261:* 3233–3237

18 Cole LA, Scheid JM, Tannen RL. Induction of mitochondrial metabolism and pH-modulated ammoniagenesis by rocking LLC-PK_1 cells. *Am J Physiol 1986; 251:* C293–C298

19 Gstraunthaler G, Handler JS. Isolation, growth and characterization of a gluconeogenic strain of renal cells. *Am J Physiol 1987; 252:* C232–C238

20 Goligorsky MS, Hruska KA, Karl I. Hormonal control of gluconeogenesis in primary cultures of renal proximal tubular cells: role of calcium. *Clin Res 1986; 34:* 596A

21 Meier KE, Insel PA. Hormone receptors and response in cultured renal epithelial cell lines. In Taub M, ed. *Tissue Culture of Epithelial Cells.* New York: Plenum Press. 1985: 145–178

22 Green N, Algren A, Hoyer J et al. Differentiated lines of cells from rabbit renal medullary thick ascending limbs grown on amnion. *Am J Physiol 1985; 249:* C97–C104

23 Valentich JD, Stokols MF. An established cell line from mouse kidney medullary thick ascending limb. I. Cell culture techniques, morphology, and antigenic expression. *Am J Physiol 1986; 251:* C299–C311

24 Lang MA, Muller J, Preston AS, Handler JS. Complete response to vasopressin requires epithelial organization in A6 cells in culture. *Am J Physiol 1986; 250:* C138–C145

25 Taub M. Importance of hormonally defined, serum-free medium for in vitro studies concerning epithelial transport. In Taub M, ed. *Tissue Culture of Epithelial Cells.* New York: Plenum Press. 1985: 255–280

26 Tannen RL, Sastrasinh S. Response of ammonia metabolism to acute acidosis. *Kidney Int 1984; 25:* 1–10

27 Werrlein RJ, Glinos AD. Oxygen microenvironment and respiratory oscillations in cultured mammalian cells. *Nature 1974; 251:* 317–319

28 McLimans WF et al. Kinetics of gas diffusion in mammalian cell culture systems. I. Experimental. *Biotechnol Bioeng 1968; 10:* 725–740

29 Cole LA, Jaskoski B, Tannen RL. Rocking, a promoter of improved metabolism and continuous differentiation in renal tubule cultures. *Clin Res 1986; 34:* 695A

30 Sahai A, Clarke D, Tannen RL. Rocking promotes differentiation in LLC-PK_1 cells by improved oxygenation. *Clin Res 1987; 35:* 637A

31 Tang MJ, Tannen RL. The primacy of glycolytic induction in the adaptation of proximal tubule cells to the culture environment. *Kidney Int 1987; 31:* 402

32 Weinberg JM, Humes HD. Increases of cell ATP produced by exogenous adenine nucleotides in isolated rabbit kidney tubules. *Am J Physiol 1986; 250:* F720–F733

INFLAMMATORY MEDIATORS: IN VITRO ASSESSMENT ON CULTURED GLOMERULAR CELLS

G Camussi, J R Brentjens

School of Medicine, State University of New York at Buffalo, Buffalo, New York; Renal Research Laboratory of the Buffalo General Hospital, Buffalo, New York, USA; Laboratory of Renal Immunopathology, University of Torino, Italy

Inflammation is the reaction of vascularized tissue to exogenous or endogenous noxious stimuli. It constitutes a protective response which localizes tissue injury and promotes repair and healing, but which in doing so, may interfere transiently or permanently with the function of the affected tissue. Inappropriate or sustained activation of the mechanisms involved in the inflammatory response may result not in protection, but in destruction of tissue integrity.

The glomerulus is directly exposed to a variety of circulating stimuli, whether immunologic, toxic or metabolic in nature, that may cause injury of glomerular structures and lead to an inflammatory reaction. The interaction of intrinsic glomerular components with humoral and/or cellular mediators of inflammation may initiate and propagate structural and functional glomerular alterations. Qualitative and quantitative aspects of this interaction may determine the characteristics of the various nephropathies. Increasing awareness of the information that can be obtained from tissue culture has stimulated nephrologists to use cultures of glomerular cells to analyse the biological events involved in glomerular injury. The use of well-defined populations of glomerular cells under controlled culture conditions promises to provide more direct and specific information on the mechanisms and mediators that play a rôle in glomerular inflammatory reactions [1–4]. In the present paper we will discuss the usefulness of glomerular cell cultures in attempts to investigate:

1. the mechanisms of immunologically mediated glomerular injury;
2. the ability of glomerular cells to produce mediators of inflammation; and
3. the response of the various glomerular cell types to mediators of inflammation.

Mechanisms of immunologically mediated glomerular injury

Interaction of antibodies with cell surface antigens

Cultured glomerular visceral epithelial cells of Lewis rat have been used to study the pathogenesis of Heymann glomerulonephritis [5]. Heymann glomerulonephritis is a model of membranous nephropathy that develops in Lewis rats after immunization with antigens obtained from the brush-border of proximal convoluted tubules of rat kidneys [6]. Glomerular lesions result from the accumulation within the capillary wall of immune deposits formed by interaction of antibody with an antigen gp330 [7], which is found in coated pits and the plasma membrane of glomerular visceral epithelial cells as well as in the brush-border [7]. Studies performed in vitro support the hypothesis that the sequence of events leading to the formation of these immune deposits involves antibody-binding to a cell surface antigen. This causes redistribution of the nephritogenic antigen on the plasma membrane of podocytes and subsequent shedding of immune complexes between the epithelium and the glomerular basement membrane [5].

Rabbits were immunized with brush-border vesicles or with gp330 to produce polyclonal antibodies. Mice were also immunized to produce monoclonal mouse antibodies to gp330. Rat glomerular visceral epithelial cells were incubated with the various antibody preparations at 4°C. The Heymann antigen was found mainly on the plasma membrane of microvilli and in coated pits. After incubation at 37°C, the polyclonal antibodies induced a rapid clustering of antigen-antibody complexes on the free surface of living cells to form patches and caps. After prolonged incubation, there was temporary disappearance of Heymann antigen from the cell surface. This 'antigenic modulation' was explained by the shedding of immune complexes from the microvilli and to a lesser extent, internalization of the complex by coated pits. Redistribution and modulation of Heymann antigen appeared to be active processes requiring metabolic energy, activation of the cytoskeleton, and crosslinking of the antigen by divalent antibodies [5]. Specific monovalent Fab fragments did not alter the distribution of Heymann antigen unless they were subsequently crosslinked. Drugs that affect the intracellular concentration of calcium, like Ca^{++} ionophore, or affect the cytoskeleton, like cytocalasin B, colchicine or chlorpromazine, blocked the redistribution of Heymann antigen [5,8]. Additional evidence that the redistribution of Heymann antigen was related to the contractile activity of the cytoskeleton was provided by experiments showing co-capping of Heymann antigen with actin and myosin [5]. Experiments performed in vivo have demonstrated that Heymann antigen is present in the immune deposits [9], and that Fab antibodies do not produce subepithelial immune deposits [5] but that chlorpromazine inhibits the development of membranous nephropathy [8]. These all support the notion that the phenomenon of antigenic modulation is a basic component of the pathogenesis of Heymann glomerulonephritis.

Interaction of immune complexes with cell surface receptors

Little is known about the interaction between various glomerular cell types and immune complexes in vitro. Bone marrow derived mesangial cells have been shown to interact with immune complexes through Fc and C3b surface receptors [3]. The resulting phagocytosis of the immune complexes is associated with an oxidative burst [10]. In contrast, conflicting results have been reported on the ability of smooth muscle-like mesangial cells to phagocytose immune complexes or complement opsonized zymosan [3,10,11]. Glomerular visceral epithelial cells in culture may bind preformed immune complexes through surface C3b receptors [12–14]. Preliminary results indicate that binding is followed by a rapid cytoskeleton-dependent redistribution and patching of the receptor-ligand complexes on the surface of the cells, a series of events that is similar to that described for Heymann antigen. Aggregation of immune complexes on the surface of the cells is normally followed by internalization but when antibodies against the IgG component of the immune complexes were added, they were shed into the medium [unpublished observations]. These results suggest an active rôle of glomerular visceral epithelial cells in the local accumulation of immune complexes in discrete subepithelial electron dense deposits in vivo.

Ability of glomerular cells to produce mediators of inflammation

Glomerular cells in culture are able to produce a wide variety of inflammatory mediators (Table I). In vivo, these mediators participate in the development

TABLE I. Products made by glomerular cells in culture

Endothelial cells	– Coagulation factors – Anti-thrombogenesis factors – Angiotensin converting enzyme
Mesangial cells	– Extracellular matrix constituents – Neutral proteinases – Cytokines – Eicosanoids – Platelet activating factor – Reactive oxygen metabolites
Epithelial cells	– Extracellular matrix constituents – Heparin-like substances – Eicosanoids

of inflammatory reactions. It is likely that they also play a key rôle in the regulation of glomerular ultrafiltration and the microvascular circulation, and that inappropriate production in response to injury may be responsible for significant structural and functional glomerular lesions.

Mediators produced by cultured glomerular cells include the eicosanoids, platelet activating factor, reactive oxygen metabolites and cytokines.

Eicosanoids

Under this term are grouped the biologically active metabolites of arachidonic acid. Glomerular cells can generate several eicosanoids either via the cyclo-oxygenase pathway (PGE_2, prostacyclin, thromboxane A_2) or via the lipoxygenase pathway (hydroxyeicosa-tetraenoic acids and leukotrienes) [15–20]. However, there are quantitative and qualitative differences in the production of arachidonic acid metabolites between cultured glomerular mesangial and visceral epithelial cells [2,3,10,17,21]. In addition, these cells may react to the same stimulus in different ways. Eicosanoids may have an important rôle in modulating glomerular inflammation. Cyclo-oxygenase and lipoxygenase products of arachidonic acid may be pro-inflammatory or anti-inflammatory [22]. For example, when combined with leukotrienes, histamine, bradykinin or C5a, PGE_2 markedly increases vascular permeability [23,24]. On the other hand, stable analogues of PGE have an anti-inflammatory effect in several models of immunologically mediated glomerular injury [25,26]. While PGI_2 induces vasodilation, increases glomerular filtration and inhibits the recruitment of inflammatory cells, TxA_2 produces vasoconstriction and promotes adhesion and intravascular aggregation of leucocytes and platelets [22]. LTC_4 and LTD_4 act as vasoconstrictors and increase vascular permeability [27,28], while LTB_4 not only increases permeability but also enhances leucocyte adherence, chemotaxis, phagocytosis, and the release of mediators from leucocytes [22,29,30].

Increased eicosanoid production was found in glomeruli isolated from animals with immune-mediated, diabetic or adriamycin glomerulopathies [31–34]. These observations, together with the results of experiments in vivo using pharmacological manipulation of synthesis or action of eicosanoids, demonstrate their involvement in haemodynamic alterations and in interactions between different glomerular cell types and between glomerular and inflammatory cells.

Platelet activating factor

Platelet activating factor (PAF) represents a 1-alkyl-2-acetyl-sn-glycero-3-phosphorylcholine with a wide range of biological actions [35,36]. The biological activity requires an alkyl chain linked by an ether bond at the sn-1 position (usually at C15 to C18 saturated carbon chain), a short-chain acyl group (acetyl or propionyl) at the sn-2 position and a polar head group of phosphocholine at the sn-3 position of glycerol. PAF is a mediator of cell-to-cell communication. Its actions are related to the function of the target cells. Its physiological rôle is kept in control by potent humoral and cellular inactivators. When released in vascularized tissue during an inflammatory response, PAF may mediate many of the local vasoactive phenomena and may recruit and activate inflammatory cells and platelets. PAF is released, after appropriate stimulation, from cells of the monocyte-macrophage series, neutrophils, platelets and endothelial cells. As a consequence, PAF appears to be involved in many different types of immunopathological reaction [37].

Renal tissue and isolated glomeruli have been shown to generate PAF when incubated at pH 10.6 or when stimulated by Ca^{++} ionophore A23187. More recently, in cell culture experiments Schlondorff and co-workers have identified rat glomerular mesangial cells as the main source of PAF and 1-0-hexadecyl-2-acetyl-sn-glycerol-3-phosphorylcholine as the major species of PAF synthetized in glomeruli [38,39]. Additional studies with more physiological stimuli, should be performed to define the rôle of this mediator in immunological injury of glomeruli.

Reactive oxygen metabolites

Several studies suggest that reactive oxygen metabolites produced by activation of neutrophils are important mediators in models of neutrophil-dependent glomerular injury [40–42]. Furthermore, it has been shown that mesangial cells in culture produce reactive oxygen metabolites in response to a number of stimuli including the membrane attack complex of the complement system (MAC), opsonized zymosan and preformed immune complexes [10,11,43,44]. These findings raise the possibility that production of oxygen radicals by resident glomerular cells may participate in the induction of glomerular pathology.

Cytokines

Cytokines are biologically active polypeptides secreted by a variety of cells, which are capable of modulating locally the growth and biosynthetic activities of target cells.

Interleukin I (IL-I) is produced by several cell types including monocytes/macrophages, endothelial cells and epidermal keratinocytes [45–47]. IL-I has an immunodulatory action on T-cell activation [45,46] and is a major mediator of inflammatory reactions [45,46]. IL-I induces leucocyte adherence and chemotaxis, target cell proliferation, release of eicosanoids, enhancement of collagen synthesis, and production of PAF and of procoagulant activity from endothelium [45,46]. Recently it has been reported that mesangial cells produce an autocrine that closely resembles IL-I [42,48].

It has been proposed that increased production of IL-I is an important determinant of the hypercellularity commonly observed in glomerular diseases [4]. Proliferation of glomerular cells, in vivo, may also be stimulated by a platelet derived growth factor (PDGF)-like substance, which has been shown to be produced by mesangial cells in vitro [49]. Additional studies employing the various glomerular cell types in culture should help to clarify the rôle of IL-I, PDGF and related cytokines in the development of glomerular proliferative diseases.

Response of the various glomerular cell types to mediators of inflammation

The cellular response to stimuli studied in vitro include cytolysis, contraction, phagocytosis, proliferation, production of matrix and intracellular signal transduction.

It has been reported that the development of proteinuria in Heymann nephritis is complement-dependent and leucocyte-independent [50,51]. Using cultured cells, we tested the possibility that this might be due to an antibody- and complement-mediated injury of glomerular visceral epithelial cells accompanied by fixation of complement. The third component of complement, C3, was co-redistributed with IgG-Heymann antigen complexes, while membrane attack complex remained diffusely bound to the cell surface, indicating that MAC was not associated with the immune complexes. The lytic rôle of MAC was shown by the binding of MAC to the surface of epithelial cells, the presence of focal clusters of 110Å ring-like structures seen by electronmicroscopy on negatively stained membranes of visceral epithelial cells exposed to antibody and complement, by the absence of lysis and of ring-like structures when epithelial cells were exposed to Heymann antibodies in the presence of C6 deficient rabbit serum, and by the restoration of lytic activity to deficient sera when purified C6 was added. The majority of cultured epithelial cells, however, were able to protect themselves from lysis by shedding MAC from their surface by a process of vesiculation with release of fragments of plasma membrane with MAC into the supernatant. This mechanism was most effective when epithelial cell cultures were exposed only for a short period to antibody and complement or at low concentrations of complement.

Another cellular response that has been studied in vitro is cell contraction. This is characteristic of mesangial cells, which contract when stimulated with angiotensin II, vasopressin, eicosanoids, PAF or immune complexes [52–56]. Contraction of mesangial cells in vivo may result in reduction of glomerular filtration surface area and thus of the glomerular ultrafiltration coefficient [57]. Stimuli that induce mesangial cell contraction may at the same time elicit production of mediators. These mediators, in turn, will modulate the response of mesangial cells. PAF, for instance, causes a rapid and dose-dependent stimulation of prostaglandin synthesis that can be inhibited by specific PAF receptor antagonists [54]. In isolated rat glomeruli PAF causes a decrease in the planar surface area of the glomeruli, probably because of mesangial cell contraction [39]. PGE_2 produced upon stimulation with PAF may provide a feedback inhibition of the PAF-induced contraction of mesangial cells, because, when added exogenously PGE_2 partially reverses the effect of PAF. A similar mechanism has been proposed to explain the actions of vasoactive peptides such as angiotensin II and vasopressin, which stimulate both mesangial cell contraction and production of prostaglandins [58]. PAF also generates reactive oxygen radicals from cultured mesangial cells [59] and in preliminary results was found to markedly increase their phagocytic activity [unpublished observations]

Cell proliferation and accumulation of newly formed matrix are typical findings in several progressive glomerular diseases [60]. Studies on cultured glomerular cells indicate that mesangial and epithelial cell proliferation are enhanced by monocyte conditioned media [61] and by IL-I [62]. The proliferation of visceral epithelial cells was found to be augmented by leukotrienes LTC_4 and LTD_4 [63]. PDGF is required for proliferation of glomerular endothelial cells in culture [64]. In contrast, a heparin-like factor secreted by epithelial cells inhibits the growth of cultured mesangial cells [65]. Inflammatory stimuli may, in addition, modulate the amount and nature of extracellular matrix synthetized. Glomerular cells in culture are suitable for testing this possibility. Recent studies, for example, reveal that IL-I increases the synthesis of collagen [61] and that long-term cultures of mesangial cells in medium containing a high concentration of serum results in the formation of matrix nodules composed of fibronectin and collagen types I, II, IV and V [66]. Finally, cultures of defined populations of glomerular cells may form ideal substrata for the study of intracellular signal transduction following surface receptor-mediator interaction. Investigations on the rôle of intracellular cyclic AMP or cyclic GMP systems [67] on the metabolism of phosphatidyl inositol [68] and on cytosolic free calcium concentrations [69] have already been reported.

Conclusions

The steady progress made in the area of tissue culture coupled with the fact that mediators of inflammation and their inhibitors are increasingly available, promises to provide in the future information essential for the understanding of glomerular inflammatory injury.

Acknowledgment

This work was supported by Grant AM-36807 of the National Institute of Arthritis, Diabetes, Digestive and Kidney Diseases; and by the Ralph Hochstetter Medical Research Fund on honour of Dr Henry C and Bertha H Buswell.

References

1 Foidart JB, Dechenne C, Dubois C et al. Tissue culture of isolated renal glomeruli: present and future. *Adv Nephrol 1981; 10:* 267–292

2 Kreisberg JI, Karnovsky MJ. Glomerular cells in culture. *Kidney Int 1983; 23:* 439–447

3 Striker GE, Striker LJ. Biology of disease: glomerular cell culture. *Lab Invest 1985; 53:* 122–131

4 Lovett DH, Sterzel RB. Cell culture approaches to the analysis of glomerular inflammation. *Kidney Int 1986; 30:* 246–254

5 Camussi G, Brentjens JR, Noble B et al. Antibody-induced redistribution of Heymann antigen on the surface of cultured glomerular visceral epithelial cells: possible role in the pathogenesis of Heymann glomerulonephritis. *J Immunol 1985; 135:* 2409–2416

6 Edginton TS, Glassock RJ, Dixon FJ. Autologous immune complex nephritis induced with renal tubular antigen. I. Identification and isolation of the pathogenic antigen. *J Exp Med 1968; 127:* 555–572

7 Kerjaschki D, Farquhar MG. Immunocytochemical localization of the Heymann nephritis antigen (gp330) in glomerular epithelial cells of normal Lewis rats. *J Exp Med 1983; 157:* 667–686

8 Camussi G, Noble B, Van Liew J et al. Pathogenesis of passive Heymann glomerulonephritis: chlorpromazine inhibits antibody mediated redistribution of cell surface antigens and prevents development of the disease. *J Immunol 1986; 136:* 2127–2135

9 Bhan AK, Schneeberger EE, Baird LG et al. Studies with monoclonal antibodies against brush border antigens in Heymann nephritis. *Lab Invest 1985; 53:* 421–432

10 Baud L, Hagege J, Sraer J et al. Reactive oxygen production by cultured rat glomerular mesangial cells during phagocytosis is associated with stimulation of lipoxygenase activity. *J Exp Med 1983; 158:* 1836–1852

11 Adler S, Baker PJ, Johnson RJ et al. Membrane attack complex (C5b-9) stimulates production of reactive oxygen species by rat mesangial cells. *J Clin Invest 1986; 77:* 762–767

12 Killen PD, Striker GE. Human glomerular visceral epithelial cells synthesize a basal lamina collagen in vitro. *Proc Natl Acad Sci USA 1979; 76:* 3518–3522

13 Striker GE, Killen PD, Farin FM. Human glomerular cells in vitro: isolation and characterization. *Transplant Proc 1980; 12:* 88–99

14 Kasinath BS, Maaba M, Lewis EJ. Demonstration and characterization of C3 receptors in rat glomerular cells in culture. *Kidney Int 1985; 27:* 214–223

15 Sraer J, Sraer JD, Chansel D et al. Prostaglandin synthesis by isolated rat renal glomeruli. *Mol Cell Endocrinol 1979; 16:* 29–37

16 Hassid A, Konieczkowski M, Dunn MJ. Prostaglandin synthesis in isolated rat kidney glomeruli. *Proc Natl Acad Sci USA 1979; 76:* 1155–1159

17 Kreisberg JI, Karnovsky MJ, Levine L. Prostaglandin production by homogeneous cultures of rat glomerular epithelial and mesangial cells. *Kidney Int 1982; 22:* 355–359

18 Lianos EA, Glomerular leukotriene biosynthesis and degradation in the rat: effects of immune injury. *Kidney Int 1986; 29 (Abstract):* 339

19 Sraer J, Bens M, Ardaillou R, Sraer JD. Sulfidopeptide leukotriene biosynthesis and metabolism by rat glomeruli and papilla. *Kidney Int 1986; 29 (Abstract):* 346

20 Schlondorff D, Perez J, Satriano JA. Differential simulation of PGE_2 synthesis in mesangial cells by antiotensin and A23187. *Am J Physiol 1985; 248:* C119

21 Jim K, Hassid A, Sun F, Dunn MJ. Lopoxygenase activity in rat kidney glomeruli, glomerular epithelial cells, and cortical tubules. *J Biol Chem 1982; 257:* 10294–10299

22 Davies P, Bailey J, Goldenberg MM. The role of arachidonic acid oxygenation products in pain and inflammation. *Am Rev Immunol 1984; 2:* 335–357

23 Williams TJ, Peck MJ. Role of prostaglandin-mediated vasodilation in inflammation. *Nature 1977; 270:* 530–532

24 Williams TJ, Jose PJ. Mediation of increased vascular permeability after complement activation: histamine-independent action of rabbit C5a. *J Exp Med 1981; 153:* 136–153

25 Fantone JC, Kunkel SL, Ward P, Zurier RB. Suppression by prostaglandin E_1 of vascular permeability induced by vasoactive inflammatory mediators. *J Immunol 1980, 125:* 2591 2596

26 Kunkel S, Thrall R, Kunkel R et al. Suppression of immune complex vasculitis in rats by prostaglandin. *J Clin Invest 1979; 64:* 1525–1529

27 Peck MJ, Piper PJ, Williams TJ. The effect of leukotrienes C4 and D4 on the microvasculature of guinea pig skin. *Prostaglandins 1981; 21:* 315–321

28 Dahlen SE, Bjork J, Hedquist P et al. Leukotrienes promote plasma leakage and leukocyte adhesion in postcapillary venules: in vivo effects with relevance to the acute inflammatory response. *Proc Natl Acad Sci USA 1981; 78:* 3887–3891

29 Bray MA, Cunningham FM, Ford-Hutchinson AW, Smith MJ. Leukotriene B4: a mediator of vascular permeability. *Br J Pharmacol 1981; 72:* 483–486

30 Samuelson B. Leukotrienes: mediators of immediate hypersensitivity reactions and inflammation. *Science 1983; 220:* 568–575

31 Lianos EA, Andres GA, Dunn MJ. Glomerular prostaglandin and thromboxane synthesis in rat nephrotoxic serum nephritis. *J Clin Invest 1983; 72:* 1439–1448

32 Lianos EA. Biosynthesis and role of arachidonic acid metabolites in glomerulonephritis. *Nephron 1984; 37:* 73–77

33 Kreisberg JI, Patel PY. The effects of insulin, glucose, and diabetes on prostaglandin production by rat kidney glomeruli and cultures glomerular mesangial cells. *Prostaglandins Leukotrienes Med 1983; 11:* 431–442

34 Stahl R, Kudelka S, Paravicini M, Schollmeyer P. Prostaglandin and thromboxane formation in glomeruli from rats with reduced renal mass. *Nephron 1986; 42:* 252–257

35 Camussi G. Potential role of platelet-activating factor in renal pathophysiology. *Kidney Int 1986; 29:* 469–477

36 Schlondorff D, Neuwirth R. Platelet activating factor and the kidney. *Am J Physiol 1986; 20:* F1–F11

37 Camussi G, Brentjens J, Bussolino F. Tetta C. Role of platelet activating factor in immunopathological reactions. In Otternes I et al, eds. *Advances in Inflammation Research, Volume 11.* New York: Raven Press. 1986: 97–109

38 Schlondorff D, Goldwasser P, Neuwirth R et al. Production of platelet-activating factor in glomeruli and cultured glomerular mesangial cells. *Am J Physiol 250 [Renal Fluid Electrolyte Physiol 19] 1986:* F1123–F1127

39 Schlondorff D, Goldwasser P, Satriano JA. Synthesis of platelet-activating factor by isolated glomeruli and cultured mesangial cells of rat kidney. *Clin Res 1985; 33 (Abstract):* 588A

40 Rehan A, Johnson KJ, Wiggins RC et al. Evidence for the role of oxygen radicals in acute nephrotoxic nephritis. *Lab Invest 1984; 51:* 396–403

41 Rehan A, Johnson KJ, Kunkel RG, Wiggins RC. Role of oxygen radicals in phorbol myristate acetate induced glomerular injury. *Kidney Int 1985; 27:* 503–511

42 Rehan A, Johnson KJ, Wiggins RC, Ward PA. Oxygen free radical induced glomerular injury following intravascular activation of complements. *Fed Proc 1985; 44 (Abstract):* 1546

43 Shah SV. Light emission by isolated rat glomeruli in response to phorbol myristrate acetate. *J Lab Clin Med 1981; 98:* 46–57

44 Shah SV. Effect of enzymatically generated reactive oxygen metabolites on the cyclic nucleotide content in isolated rat glomeruli. *J Clin Invest 1984; 74:* 393–401

45 Durum SK, Schmidt JA, Oppenheum JJ. Interleukin 1: an immunological perspective. *Ann Rev Immunol 1985; 3:* 265–289

46 Dinarello CA. Interleukin 1. *Rev Infect Dis 1984; 6:* 51–95

47 Lovett DH, Ryan JL, Sterzel RB. A thymocyte activating factor derived from glomerular mesangial cells. *J Immunol 1983; 130:* 1796–1801

48 Lovett DH, Szamel M, Ryan JL et al. Interleukin 1 and the glomerular mesangium. I. Purification and characterization of a mesangial cell-derived autogrowth factor. *J Immunol:* in press

49 Abboud HE, Poptic E, Dicorleto P. Rat mesangial cells secrete a platelet-derived growth factor-like molecule. *Kidney Int 1986; 29 (Abstract):* 263

50 Salant DJ, Belok S, Madaio MP, Couser WG. A new role for complement in experimental membranous nephropathy in rats. *J Clin Invest 1980, 66:* 1339–1350

51 Adler S, Salant DJ, Dittmer JE et al. Mediation of proteinuria in membranous nephropathy due to a planted glomerular antigen. *Kidney Int 1983; 23:* 807–817

52 Kreisberg JI. Insulin requirement for contraction of cultured rat glomerular mesangial cells in response to angiotensin II: possible role for insulin in modulating glomerular hemodynamics. *Proc Natl Acad Sci USA 1982; 79:* 4190–4192

53 Scharschmidt LA, Dunn MJ. Prostaglandin synthesis by rat glomerular mesangial cells in culture: effects of angiotensin II and arginine vasopressin. *J Clin Invest 1983; 71:* 1756–1764

54 Schlondorff D, Satriano JA, Hagege J. Effect of platelet-activating factor and serum-treated zymosan on prostaglandin E_2 synthesis, arachidonic acid release and contraction of cultured rat mesangial cells. *J Clin Invest 1984; 73:* 1227–1231

55 Kreisberg JI, Ventatachalam M, Troyer D. Contractile properties of cultured glomerular mesangial cells. *Am J Physiol 1985; 243:* F457–463

56 Simonson MS, Dunn MJ. Leukotriene C4 and D4 contract rat glomerular mesangial cells. *Kidney Int 1986; 30:* 524–431

57 Dworkin LD, Ichikawa I, Brenner BM. Hormonal modulation of glomerular function. *Am J Physiol 1983; 244:* F95–F104

58 Schlondorff D, Ardaillou R. Prostaglandins and other arachidonic acid metabolites in the kidney. *Kidney Int 1986; 29:* 108–119

59 Sedor JR, Abboud HE. Platelet activating factor stimulates oxygen radical release by cultured rat mesangial cells. *Kidney Int 1985; 27 (Abstract):* 222A

60 Striker GE, Killen PD, Farin FM et al. Mesangial matrix and inflammatory cells. *Proc 8th Int Congr Nephrol.* Athens. 1981: 879–887

61 Melcion C, Lachman L, Killen PD et al. Mesangial cells, effect of monocyte products on proliferation and matrix synthesis. *Transplant Proc 1982; 141:* 559–564

62 Lovett DH, Ryan JL, Sterzel RB. Stimulation of rat mesangial cell proliferation by macrophage interleukin 1. *J Immunol 1983; 131:* 2830–2836

63 Bond L, Sraer J, Perez J et al. Leukotriene C4 binds to human glomerular epithelial cells and promotes their proliferation in vitro. *J Clin Invest 1985; 76:* 374–377

64 Striker GE, Soderland C, Lowen-Pope DF et al. Isolation, characterization and propagation in vitro of human glomerular endothelial cells. *J Exp Med 1984; 160:* 323–328

65 Castellot JJ, Hoover RL, Harper PA, Karnovsky MJ. Heparin and glomerular epithelial cell-secreted heparin-like species inhibit mesangial cell proliferation. *Am J Pathol 1985; 120:* 427–435

66 Sterzel RB, Lovett DH, Foellmer HG et al. Mesangial cells hillocks: nodular foci of exaggerated growth of cells and matrix. *Am J Pathol:* in press

67 Scharschmidt L, Simonson M, Dunn MJ. Glomerular prostaglandins, angiotensin II and non steroidal anti-inflammatory drugs. *Am J Med 1986; 81 (2B):* 30–42

68 Troyer DA, Kreisberg JI, Schwertz DW, Venkatachalam MA. Effects of vasopressin on phosphoinositides and prostaglandin production in cultured mesangial cells. *Am J Physiol 1985; 249:* F139–147

69 Bonventre JV, Cheung JY. Cytosolic free calcium concentration in cultured renal epithelial cells. *Am J Physiol 1986; 250:* F329–338

INFECTION OF HUMAN GLOMERULAR CELLS IN VITRO WITH Ad5-SV40; IMPROVED LIFE SPAN

MaryAnn Lange, Liliane J Striker, K Bernstein, S J Elliot, K Van Doren, G E Striker

Metabolic Diseases Branch, National Institute of Diabetes and Digestive and Kidney Diseases, National Institutes of Health, Bethesda, Maryland, USA

Introduction

Cell culture has proved to be a valuable tool for delineating the properties of the individual cell types that make up the glomerulus. The three major cell types have been propagated and partially characterized from normal man, rats, and mice [1–6]. However the individual glomerular cells have been difficult to culture as purified populations in large numbers and have not been propagated in vitro for prolonged periods. Thus it has often been difficult to compare results from one laboratory to the next. In experimental animals, particularly rats, the difficulty in obtaining large numbers of cells has been partially overcome by preparing glomeruli from many animals and using early passage cells. In man, however, few normal kidneys suitable for culture are available and so other means of obtaining large numbers of cells have to be found.

Although considerable data have been obtained using animal cells in culture, further studies are needed to relate these findings to humans. There are substantial interspecies differences which have been emphasized by studies of the prostaglandin profiles of mesangial cells [7]. There are also many differences in the expression of cell surface proteins. Finally, one of the most interesting applications of glomerular cell culture is as a way to study human genetic and metabolic disorders, most of which do not have satisfactory experimental animal counterparts. For these reasons we sought to develop methods to prolong the life, and expand the number, of human glomerular cells in culture. We report the infection of human glomerular cells by the hybrid recombinant virus adeno5-SV40. The resulting transfected cells had a prolonged lifespan in vitro, could be greatly expanded in number, and maintained some in vivo phenotypic characteristics. Of the three resident glomerular types, visceral epithelial cells were most readily obtained.

Methods

Isolation of human glomerular cells

Fragments from human kidneys were minced through a metal screen. The resulting brei was washed until glomeruli were the main component (more than 90%). The isolates were plated into 100mm plastic dishes coated with fibronectin and grown in Waymouth's medium supplemented with fetal bovine serum and platelet-derived growth factor (2ng/ml) or Nu serum (Collaborative Research). The outgrowth was left undisturbed for 10 to 14 days. The number of attached glomeruli varied widely between isolates.

Infection of cells

Cells were infected using an adeno5-SV40 recombinant virus which contained the early region of SV40 and the late region of adeno virus 5 [8]. The virus was propagated in an embryonic kidney 293 cell line, which is permissive for the adenovirus. The infection was carried out in medium supplemented with gamma-free serum. Glomerular cells were washed in serum-free medium and incubated for one hour at 37°C with the hybrid virus. The multiplicity of infection was calculated by estimating the number of cells in a dish and attempting to add a ratio of 10 viral particles for each cell.

Viral titre

Viral titre was measured by both a detachment and plaque assay using 293 cells. The original viral titre was then diluted to obtain a multiplicity of infection which was approximately 10:1.

Isolation and characterization of transfected cells

The cells were dilute plated and then patch cloned in serial fashion. The cells were characterized by phase microscopic morphology and immunofluorescence microscopy. The antibodies used were mouse monoclonal antiserum to SV40 T-antigen, mouse monoclonal antibody to human cytokeratin, polyclonal antiserum to human factor VIII-related antigens, and the appropriate secondary antibodies labelled with FITC. Actin was visualized using rhodamine phalloidin [6].

Results

Transfected cells were isolated from five of seven kidneys attempted. From these five kidneys a total of six individual culture dishes from 24 initial plates were successfuly transfected. We were able to isolate all three cell types from most of the culture dishes. The development of transfected epithelial, endothelial, or mesangial cells did not appear to be dependent on the culture conditions, i.e. the presence of serum additives such as platelet-derived growth factor, EGF, Nu serum or fetal bovine serum concentration. The development of transfected cells appeared to be related to the length of time in culture, in that primary or early passage cells yielded the best results. In most cultures infection was signalled by the loss of cell integrity and detachment of the cell layer. The isolated transfected cell populations were obtained from the remaining small patches of adherent cells. The cells were encircled with a cloning ring, dilute plated and propagated.

SV40 T-antigen expression as demonstrated by nuclear staining was found in all three cell types: mesangial, epithelial, and endothelial. Epithelial cells formed monolayers of polygonal or pavementous cells which developed shallow dome-like structures after confluence was reached. They also contained characteristic cytoplasmic cytokeratin filaments. Transfected mesangial cells grew in an elongated configuration and became multilayered. They had the distribution of actin filaments characteristic for non-transfected mesangial cells in vitro. Endothelial cells contained large cytoplasmic granules which stained positively with an antibody to factor VIII-related antigen.

The different types of transfected glomerular cells were separated from one another using the patch cloning technique. Epithelial cells could be isolated as homogeneous, purified populations. One isolate has undergone a minimum of 40 population doublings yielding a large number of cells. Several other isolates obtained from a single, small fragment of renal cortex have been passaged 15 times. Thus, large populations of epithelial cells have been obtained. Transfected mesangial cells have also been isolated as homogeneous populations. They have undergone more than 23 serial passages. Smaller numbers of mesangial cell isolates have been studied, but they differ from epithelial cells with respect to the ability to isolate them or perform multiple population doublings. Endothelial cells have been multiply passaged; however we have not been able to derive populations with greater than 80 to 90% purity despite multiple, repetitive patch cloning. One issue which remains unresolved, for all transfected cell types, is that we have not been able to isolate them as single cell clonal populations.

Discussion

Transfected populations of human epithelial cells have been obtained in relatively purified form. Mesangial and endothelial cells have also been obtained but they remain at 80 to 90% purity. The vector chosen for infection was an adenovirus SV40 hybrid because it is missing DNA necessary for viral replication [8,9].

The transfected cells could be obtained in large numbers, and had a significantly prolonged in vitro lifespan. Thus this method has potential for providing large numbers of well characterized cells for replicate studies within and between laboratories.

References

1 Quadracci LJ, Striker GE. Growth and maintenance of glomerular cells in vitro. *Proc Soc Exp Biol Med 1970; 135:* 947–950

2 Fish AJ, Michael AF, Vernier RL, Brown DM. Human glomerular cells in tissue culture. *Lab Invest 1975; 33:* 330–341

3 Striker GE, Killen PD, Farin FM. Human glomerular cells in vitro: isolation and characterization. *Transplant Proc 1980; 12:* 88–99

4 Striker GE, Soderland DF, Bowen-Pope AM et al. Isolation, characterization, and propagation in vitro of human glomerular endothelial cells. *J Exp Med 1984; 160:* 323–328

5 Kreisberg JI, Karnovsky M. Glomerular cells in culture (editorial review). *Kidney Int 1983; 23:* 439–447

6 Striker GE, Striker LJ. Biology of disease: glomerular cell culture. *Lab Invest 1985; 53:* 122–131

7 Ardaillou N, Sraer J, Melcion C et al. Prostaglandin synthesis by isolated human glomeruli and human glomerular cells in vitro. In Samuelsson B, Paolette R, Ramwell P, eds. *Advances in Prostaglandin, Thromboxane, and Leukotriene Research, Volume II.* New York: Raven Press. 505–512

8 Van Doren K, Gluzman Y. Efficient transformation of human fibroblasts by adenovirus-simian virus 40 recombinants. *Mol Cell Biol 1984; 4:* 1653–1656

9 Rhim JS, Trimmer R, Arnstein P et al. Neoplastic transformation of chimpanzee cells induced by adenovirus type 12-simian virus 40 hybrid virus. *Proc Natl Acad Sci 1981; 78:* 313–317

IMMUNOPATHOLOGY OF NEPHRITIS

EXPERIMENTAL GLOMERULONEPHRITIS

Ph J Hoedemaeker

University of Leiden, Leiden, The Netherlands

> Die experimentelle Pathologie gibt uns noch keine klare Antwort, unter welchen Bedingungen die verschiedenen Erreger so gleichartige, die gleichen Erreger so verschiedene wirkungen entfalten.
>
> F Volhard, 1914 [1]

HISTORICAL OVERVIEW

Since the turn of the century many investigators have been engaged in the study of experimental models of glomerulonephritis. In imitation of Bright [2] whose major concern was to correlate clinical symptoms with morphological changes in the kidneys, many tried to induce renal disease in animals to study pathogenetic mechanisms. Since it was believed that glomerular disease was invariably associated with bacterial infections, most investigators tried to induce glomerulonephritis by injecting bacteria or bacterial products [3,4]. Following the suggestion of Lohlein [5] who claimed that renal changes in the majority of the cases were due to the action of toxins, injections of chemical compounds were used to induce renal lesions [3,4]. None of these disease-inducing protocols, however, were successful and they were abandoned, although recently some successes were reported on the induction of glomerulonephritis in rabbits with streptococci [6,7].

When Schick and von Pirquet [8] introduced their theory that glomerulonephritis was caused by a local allergic reaction to bacterial products, considerable effort was made to induce allergic reactions in glomeruli through local or systemic injections of heterologous serum [9], or purified serum proteins [10]. Lindemann [12] was the first to induce a proliferative glomerulonephritis in rats with injections of a rabbit antiserum directed to components of the rat kidney, which was further characterized by Masugi [12]. For many years this was the only effective model of glomerulonephritis.

In the fifties further progress was made. In 1953 Germuth and Dixon developed an experimental serum sickness associated with glomerulonephritis [13,14]. Aided by the development of new techniques such as immunofluorescence [15] and electronmicroscopy [16], they demonstrated convincingly that antibodies could become localized in the glomeruli as part of immune complexes deposited from the circulation. Binding and activation of complement components subsequently caused glomerular damage and inflammation. This pathogenetic mechanism was generally accepted, in spite of the fact that injection of preformed immune complexes in animals (passive serum sickness) hardly ever resulted in glomerular disease [17].

In 1951 Heymann [18] induced an autoimmune glomerulonephritis by immunizing Long Evans rats with homologous or heterologous kidney homogenates. The disease was associated with glomerular immune aggregates and with the nephrotic syndrome. In later studies Edgington et al [19] demonstrated that the immune aggregates contained a tubular auto-antigen which was called Fx1A. In the early seventies a passive variant of this experimental glomerulonephritis was reported which was induced by injections with heterologous anti-Fx1A antibody [20]. It was this passive Heymann nephritis that subsequently challenged the theory that immune complexes causing glomerulonephritis were deposited from the circulation, since in this model glomerular immune complexes were shown to be formed in situ by antibody binding to glomerular antigens [21,22]. Later in situ formation of immune complexes was also demonstrated in other models of immune complex glomerulonephritis [23, 24].

Having established the major pathogenetic mechanisms for experimental glomerulonephritis and probably also for glomerulonephritis in man, the investigation of models shifted towards aetiological factors. From these studies it became clear that immune dysregulation resulting in autoimmune reactions associated with anti-idiotypic responses [25] and with polyclonal B-lymphocyte activation could cause glomerulonephritis [26].

Recent studies of experimental glomerulonephritis have centred around the rôle of inflammatory mediators such as complement components, prostanoids and the effects of treatment. In addition the rôle of genetic factors in the induction and morphology of experimental glomerulonephritis has become apparent and will be important in future research.

Animal models of glomerular disease important for our understanding of the pathogenesis or aetiology of their human counterpart are listed in Table I. The rôle of mediators in glomerulonephritis will not be discussed in this chapter, while the rôle of genetics are discussed by Grunfeld in the section on Inherited Renal Diseases.

TABLE I

GLOMERULONEPHRITIS INDUCED BY ANTIBODIES
- A. Glomerular antigens
  - 1. Basement membrane antigens
    - a. Nephrotoxic serum nephritis
    - b. Experimental allergic glomerulonephritis
  - 2. Other glomerular antigens
    - a. Heymann nephritis
    - b. Mesangial nephritis
    - c. Spontaneous nephritis in NZW rabbits
- B. Non-glomerular antigens
  - 1. Deposition of circulating immunecomplexes
    - a. Serum-sickness glomerulopathy
    - b. Passive serum sickness
  - 2. Antigens planted or trapped in the glomerulus
    - a. Charged antigens
    - b. Concanavalin-A nephritis
    - c. Other models

GLOMERULONEPHRITIS INDUCED BY CELLULAR IMMUNE REACTIONS

GLOMERULONEPHRITIS MEDIATED BY AUTOIMMUNE REACTIONS
- A. SLE-like glomerulonephritis
- B. Glomerulonephritis associated with polyclonal activation of B-lymphocytes
  - 1. Drugs and toxic substances
  - 2. Graft-versus-host disease

GLOMERULONEPHRITIS INDUCED BY NON-IMMUNE MECHANISMS
- A. Toxic mechanisms
  - 1. Aminonucleoside of puromycin
  - 2. Adriamycin
- B. Progressive glomerulosclerosis
- C. Protein overload glomerulopathy

GLOMERULONEPHRITIS MODELS MEDIATED BY ANTIBODIES

The majority of glomerular diseases is caused by immunological mechanisms involving antibodies either directed against glomerular or non-glomerular antigens [27].

Antibodies directed against glomerular antigens

Basement membrane antigens

Nephrotoxic serum nephritis. The classical example of glomerulonephritis resulting from a reaction between antibody and glomerular basement membrane antigen(s), is nephrotoxic serum nephritis [28]. This model was introduced almost 90 years ago by Lindemann [12], characterized by Masugi [29] and studied by many others [30–32]. This glomerulonephritis results from a binding of heterologous antibody to antigens in the glomerular basement membrane, resulting in a linear pattern of deposit by immunofluorescence [28] and immunoelectronmicroscopy [33]. The amount is proportional to the severity of the disease [34]. Since heterologous antibody is used, the injected animal develops an autologous phase in which antibodies are formed directed against the injected IgG which are also bound to the glomerular basement membrane [35]. In addition non-immune IgG might be bound to the glomerular basement membrane [36].

Nephrotoxic serum nephritis can be induced in rats [29,30], mice [37], monkeys [38], chickens [39], guinea pigs [40], rabbits [41], and sheep [42], and is characterized by a proliferative glomerulonephritis and an influx of polymorphonuclear leucocytes, platelets and macrophages [43,44]. There is a variable degree of extracapillary proliferation associated with fibrin deposition [45]. The lesions develop either directly after the injection of the antibodies [27] or indirectly through neutrophils and macrophages attracted by activated complement [43]. Evidence exists that eicosanoids produced by inflammatory cells play an important rôle in causing glomerular lesions [46].

Rats preimmunized with IgG from the species used to prepare the anti-glomerular basement membrane antibody, develop severe crescentic glomerulonephritis with an increased influx of mononuclear phagocytes on induction, the so-called accelerated form [47]. Jennings et al [48] and Downie et al [49] demonstrated that anti-glomerular basement membrane antibody injected in rats, reacted with alveolar basement membrane when the lungs of the animals had been exposed to pure oxygen. Recently Yamamoto and Wilson [50] demonstrated a similar binding in rabbits after the animals had been exposed to gasoline. These findings are interesting with respect to the lung involvement of anti-glomerular basement membrane nephritis in man.

Although the antigen(s) responsible for the anti-glomerular basement membrane glomerulonephritis have been identified in man [51], attempts to isolate the glomerular basement membrane antigen(s) responsible for the induction of nephrotoxic nephritis in rats have not been successful. Most investigators agree that the antigen(s) reside in the non-collagenous protein fraction of the glomerular basement membrane [52,53]. Shibata et al [54] isolated a non-collagenous glycopeptide from the glomerular basement membrane, termed nephritogenoside, which is present in a linear distribution on the endothelial aspect of the glomerular basement membrane. Immunization of normal rats with this antigen [55] results in a sclerosing glomerulonephritis associated with proteinuria. Induction of glomerulonephritis with polyclonal or monoclonal antisera directed against isolated components of the glomerular basement membrane, led to varying results. Antibodies directed to collagen type IV bind to the glomerular basement membrane and remain detectable for at least one year, but do not induce glomerulonephritis [Hoedemaeker, unpublished observations]. Antibodies to laminin also bind linearly to the glomerular basement membrane, although in addition subendothelial deposits are formed, presumably through rearrangement of the antigen [56]. Anti-collagen IV antibodies injected simultaneously with anti-laminin antibodies [56], result in a segmental proliferative glomerulonephritis, associated with immune aggregates in both laminae rarae and a slight proteinuria in the autologous phase [57]. Antibodies directed to heparan sulphate are able to induce lesions characterized by an influx of leucocytes, activation of complement and an associated dose-dependent proteinuria, typical of anti-glomerular basement membrane nephritis [58].

Experimental allergic glomerulonephritis. In 1962 Steblay [59] induced a severe crescentic glomerulonephritis by immunizing animals with homologous or heterologous glomerular basement membrane, which he called experimental allergic glomerulonephritis. The disease is mediated by anti-glomerular basement membrane antibodies [42] and is sometimes associated with pulmonary haemorrhage resembling Goodpasture's syndrome in man [60]. It can be transferred to naive animals with antibodies present in the circulation. The disease results almost invariably in renal failure and death of the animals. It can be induced in sheep [59], rats [61], monkeys [62], rabbits [63], goats [64] and mice [37].

In the rat experimental allergic glomerulonephritis usually runs a mild course [65].

Other glomerular antigens

Heymann nephritis. In 1951 Heymann and Lund [18] induced an autoimmune glomerulonephritis in rats by immunization with homologous kidney cortex homogenate. The disease, associated with the nephrotic syndrome, is non-inflammatory and characterized by glomerular immune aggregates localized exclusively at the epithelial side of the glomerular basement membrane, similar to membranous nephropathy in man. Edgington et al [66] and Glassock et al [67] demonstrated that the antigen involved in this glomerulopathy (Fx1A) is present in the brush border of the proximal tubules of normal rat kidneys [19]. Heymann nephritis can be induced in several rat strains but not in mice [68], or dogs [69]. The increased permeability of the glomeruli is thought to be caused by damage to the glomerular basement membrane through complement activation [70], and is neutrophil independent [71] and associated with increased glomerular prostanoid biosynthesis. Stahl et al [72] demonstrated that the increased production of prostaglandins as well as the proteinuria can be inhibited by decomplementation by cobra venom factor.

In the early seventies a passive variant of Heymann nephritis was introduced [20,73,74] in rats by one injection of heterologous antibodies directed against Fx1A, resulting in an immediate appearance of glomerular aggregates [21,22]. This glomerulopathy is also associated with the nephrotic syndrome in the autologous phase and is also complement dependent [75]. Since injection of eluates from rat kidneys with Heymann nephritis results in a pattern identical to that of passive Heymann nephritis it was concluded that in both models probably identical antigens were involved [76]. In the passive Heymann nephritis Van Damme et al [21] and Couser et al [22] showed that perfusion of isolated rat kidneys with anti Fx1A antibodies, in the absence of circulating immune complexes, resulted in immune complex glomerulopathy, indicating that the glomerular immune aggregates were formed in situ. Later in situ formation was shown to operate in Heymann nephritis as well as in other forms of immune complex glomerulopathies [23,24].

Kerjaschki and Farquhar [77] purified the antigen involved and characterized it as a glycoprotein with a molecular weight of 330,000 (gp330). They showed that this antigen was present on the cell membranes of glomerular visceral epithelial cells, especially in coated pits [78]. The function of gp330 is still unknown, but may be related to a defined system of receptor-mediated endocytosis [79].

Camussi et al [80] demonstrated that in vitro binding of antibody to gp330 caused clustering and subsequent shedding of the immune complexes, which could be prevented by pretreatment with chlorpromazine [81]. Extrapolating to the in vivo situation they suggested that in Heymann nephritis a similar mechanism might operate after binding of the antibody to the epithelial antigens, resulting in a shedding of immune complexes in the space between glomerular epithelial cells and the glomerular basement membrane, thus forming the immune aggregates as observed in Heymann nephritis. So far, although the gp330 antigen has been shown to be present in rats and dogs it has been impossible to induce Heymann nephritis in the latter species [69]. Rabbits do not possess the antigen [82].

Many investigators have confirmed the results of Kerjaschki and Farquhar but the question remains whether gp330 is the only antigen involved in Heymann nephritis, because while injections with polyclonal anti-gp330 antibodies result in electron dense aggregates along the epithelial side of the glomerular basement membrane, monoclonal anti-gp330 antibodies do not [83]. Recently, however, it was demonstrated that monoclonal anti-gp330 antibodies from mice [84] or rats [85] could induce passive Heymann nephritis. De Heer et al [85] suggested that this was caused through crosslinking of gp330, because the monoclonal antibody also bound to epitopes on gp300 which is also present on the epithelial cell membrane [85]. Bagchus et al [86] showed that eluates from rat kidneys with passive Heymann nephritis, in addition to antibodies directed against gp330, contained antibodies reacting with a glycoprotein with a molecular weight of 90kd. Ronco et al [68] and Bagchus et al [87] demonstrated that anti-gp90 antibodies bound transiently to the glomerular basement membrane following intravenous injection. Moreover Bagchus et al [37] showed that anti-Fx1A antisera from which the anti-gp90 activity had been removed, did not localize in rat glomeruli after perfusion. This led to the conclusion that anti-gp90 played a rôle in the crosslinking of gp330. Interesting results in this respect were obtained by Hogendoorn et al [88], who demonstrated that polyclonal antibody directed against Fx1A, contains activity against the glomerular basement membrane components type IV collagen and laminin, while monoclonal antibodies do not. This provides additional proof for the necessity of crosslinking gp330 to form immune aggregates and an explanation for the earlier mentioned difference between the passive Heymann nephritis-inducing capacity of polyclonal and monoclonal anti-gp330 antibodies.

In 1979 Thoenes et al [89] reported on a glomerulonephritis following kidney transplantation in rats. Kidney transplantation from congenic Lewis 1N rats, which possess the major histocompatibility complex haplotype of Brown Norway rats combined with a Lewis background, into normal Brown Norway recipients resulted after one to four months in an immune complex glomerulopathy in the transplanted kidney but not in the kidneys of the recipient. Although the glomerulopathy resembled Heymann nephritis, the antigen involved had a different localization than gp330. It was present in the cytoplasm of epithelial cells of the mid-portion of the proximal tubules and presumably cross-reacted with a glomerular antigen. The characteristics of this epithelial antigen have not been established.

Mesangial nephritis. A new model of experimental glomerulopathy resulting from a binding of antibody to mesangial antigens was reported by Bagchus et al [90] and later confirmed by Yamamoto and Wilson [91]. They showed that a monoclonal antibody directed against the Thy-1 antigen present on normal rat mesangial cells [93], resulted in a glomerulopathy characterized by mesangiolysis and heavy proteinuria. In later stages mesangial proliferation is present which is sometimes associated with crescent formation. The observed mesangiolysis is complement dependent. Some features of this experimental glomerulopathy resemble the mesangiolysis obtained after an injection of Agistrodon venom [93].

Mendrick and Rennke [94] recently described an intrinsic mesangial antigen which they characterized with a monoclonal antibody. Intravenous administration of this antibody led to immune aggregate formation in the mesangial area, similar to that in human IgA glomerulopathy, but no proteinuria or haematuria was observed.

Nephritis in New Zealand White rabbits. In 1978, Neale and Wilson [95] found a spontaneously occurring glomerulonephritis in New Zealand White rabbits. This membranoproliferative glomerular lesion was not associated with the deposition of electron dense material in the glomerular basement membrane. They showed that the disease was caused by antibodies to an intrinsic antigen present on the epithelial foot processes and giving rise to glomerular basement membrane damage, glomerulonephritis, and, in a small percentage of the cases, to proteinuria. Although its localization bears resemblance to that of laminin in the glomerular capillary wall, the characteristics of the antigen are unknown at present.

Antibodies directed against non-glomerular antigens

Antibodies directed against non-glomerular antigens either form immune complexes in the circulation, which subsequently can be deposited in glomeruli, or react with antigens that are planted or trapped in glomeruli.

Glomerular deposition of circulating immune complexes

Serum sickness glomerulopathy. The serum sickness glomerulopathy introduced by Germuth and Dixon [13,14] has two forms.

Acute serum sickness or the 'one shot' serum sickness is induced in rabbits by one intravenous injection of a large dose of bovine serum albumin [14]. Approximately nine days after the injection during immune elimination of bovine serum albumin from the serum, glonerulonephritis can be observed which is thought to be caused by the deposition of immune complexes from the circulation [96]. Studies of Germuth and Rodriguez [97] showed that especially immune complexes formed in antigen excess, which remain relatively small, become deposited in the glomerular filter. Large immune complexes formed in equivalence or in antibody excess are deposited in the mesangial area or removed from the circulation by the mononuclear phagocytic system. The glomerular lesions consist of swelling and proliferation of endothelial cells and mesangial cells [98] and show an influx of polymorphonuclear leucocytes and macrophages [99]. At the ultrastructural level, large electron-dense immune aggregates are found subepithelially [98].

Chronic serum sickness glomerulonephritis is induced in rabbits according to two protocols. The first of these involves daily injections of a fixed dose of bovine serum albumin. The results depend on the immune response of the injected rabbits [97]. Animals with a high immune response develop a transient acute glomerulonephritis similar to that observed in acute serum sickness. Rabbits with no detectable antibody production develop no signs of glomerulonephritis. Rabbits with a moderate immune response develop chronic immune complex glomerulonephritis, probably since under these conditions immune complexes are formed in slight antigen excess [97].

The second protocol involves daily injections of variable amounts of bovine serum albumin, adjusted to the serum antibody titre of the animal [97]. In this way a continuous state of antigen excess can be created. This second protocol leads to a glomerulonephritis [96] with detectable antigen, antibody and complement in the glomerular immune aggregates which by electron microscopy are subepithelial.

When immune aggregates are present in the subendothelial or mesangial space of the glomerulus, polymorphonuclear leucocytes and macrophages are attracted by activated complement components. Subsequent phagocytosis will lead to the generation of toxic oxygen products and halides [100] with subsequent damage to the glomerular filter resulting in proteinuria and haematuria. The activation of complement per se may also lead to filter damage and increased permeability as demonstrated in other models [70]. Izumino et al [101] demonstrated an abrogating effect on the nephritis with antiplatelet drugs.

Chronic serum sickness glomerulopathy can also be induced in rats [102,103]. Recent studies by Hogendoorn et al [104] demonstrated that the site of localization of glomerular immune aggregates is directly related to the immune response of the animals. Animals with a high immune response do not develop a glomerulonephritis and show a mesangial deposition. Animals with a low immune response or animals in which the immune response was inhibited with triple drug administration [105] showed a membranous localization, resulting in a membranous glomerulopathy.

Passive serum sickness. Studies on injections of preformed immune complexes (passive serum sickness) have shown that the site of localization of glomerular immune aggregates, i.e. mesangial, subendothelial, or subepithelial, depends on the physicochemical properties of the immune complexes, influenced by the nature of the antigen-antibody reactions. Koyama et al [106] showed that the size of immune complexes formed between cationized bovine serum albumin and antibodies to native bovine serum albumin was approximately 7S, whereas that of immune complexes formed between anti-bovine serum albumin antibodies and native or anionized bovine serum albumin was approximately 19S. Moreover, the 7S immune complexes appeared to be of low avidity compared with the 19S immune complexes. Iskander and Jenette [107], and Lew and Steward [108] showed that high-affinity immune complexes were deposited exclusively in the mesangial area, whereas the low affinity immune complexes were localized in the glomerular capillary wall. Under conditions of low affinity, the immune complexes might easily dissociate according to the equilibrium $(AgAb)n \rightleftarrows AgAb \rightleftarrows Ag+Ab$ and reform in situ in the glomerular capillary wall [24,109]. If immune complexes are formed with antibodies of low avidity the equilibrium shifts to the right, thus fulfilling a prerequisite for the in situ formation of immune complexes in tissues. This hypothesis is consistent with results obtained by various investigators [108,110], who showed that in chronic serum sickness, membranous glomerulonephritis – in which glomerular immune aggregates are believed to be formed in situ [21,22] – develops only in animals producing low affinity antibodies [111]. Other reactants have been shown to bind to immune complexes or immunoglobulin aggregates present in the glomerulus. These reactants include albumin [112], non-specific proteins [113], free antibodies [114], anti-IgG antibodies [115], rheumatoid factor [115], anti-Fab [116], and anti-idiotypic antibodies [25,117]. Circulating immune complexes can also be bound by glomerular deposits especially, but not exclusively [118], if they are of the same species and the glomerular deposits are formed in antibody excess [119]. Antigen can also bind to glomerular aggregates where small amounts of antigen bound to immune complexes formed in antibody excess can result in lattice formation, whereas large amounts can lead to dissolution of the deposits [114]. The finding that it becomes progressively more difficult to remove glomerular immune aggregates by the use of an excess of antigen in the later stages of chronic serum sickness [120], gives additional support to the idea that different antigen/antibody systems participate in glomerular aggregate formation in the late stages of immune complex glomerulopathies.

In several models of glomerulonephritis the mesangial area is specifically involved in the entrapment of immune complexes. Protein aggregates, immune complexes [121] or other substances such as polyvinyl alcohol [122], are taken up by the glomerular mesangium depending on their biological activity or their size [123]. This uptake may be associated with variable degrees of hypercellularity caused by a mesangial influx of monocytes [124], or with a specific reaction with antibodies as shown by Mauer et al [125]. The uptake varies with the functional activity of the mesangium [126,127].

Recently experimental models of IgA nephropathy have been reported. IgA glomerulopathy is associated with virus-like respiratory tract infections or gastrointestinal syndromes [128] and a significant elevation of IgA in serum and exocrine fluids may occur in response to oral immunization [129]. Emancipator et al [130] tried to induce an experimental IgA glomerulopathy by oral immunization of mice with ovalbumin. This resulted in electron dense IgA-containing mesangial deposits in 73% of the cases, associated with complement induced haematuria but not with an influx of leucocytes. Recently, Sato et al [131] succeeded in inducing an IgA-like glomerulonephritis in mice by the administration of oral lactalbumin combined with a RES blockade with colloidal carbon. After 30 weeks, more than 90% of the animals had developed mesangial IgA-containing electron dense deposits.

Since polymeric IgA and immune complexes containing IgA are known to be transported through the hepatocyte by secretory component and excreted in the bile, Melvin et al [132] tried to induce an IgA glomerulopathy in rats by ligating bile ducts. This ligation resulted in a selective increase of IgA, C3, and secretory component in the mesangial area, but these changes were not accompanied by signs of glomerulonephritis.

Antibodies reacting with antigens planted or trapped in the glomerulus

Based on the finding that glomerular immune complexes can be formed in situ, Fleuren et al [133] studied the possibility of in situ formation involving non-renal antigens. They showed that alternating perfusion of rat kidneys with lysozyme and anti-lysozyme or with bovine serum albumin and anti-bovine serum albumin resulted in local formation of immune complexes in the glomeruli.

In 1982, Hoyer et al [134] demonstrated that alternating renal perfusion with heparin and protamine sulphate resulted in complexes with localizations in the glomerular capillary wall roughly indicating the negatively charged sites. The in situ formation of these spherical protamine-heparin complexes was shown to be unrelated to the observed proteinuria [135].

Charged antigens. The establishment of fixed negative charged sites in the glomerular capillary wall [136], had important implications for the pathogenesis of immunologically induced glomerular injury [137]. Whether immune deposits originate from in situ formation or from deposition from the circulation, the anionic charge of the glomerular capillary wall plays a significant rôle either by providing a charge barrier or a site for planted antigen, especially when the antigen possesses a positive charge [109]. These results suggested that cationic proteins can be considered as candidates for nephritogenic antigens [138]. This led to a series of investigations in which a variety of cationic proteins were planted in the glomerular basement membrane and allowed to react with their respective antibodies to obtain immune aggregates [137,139,140]. Border et al [139] showed that immune aggregates were formed between cationized albumin molecules planted in the glomerular capillary wall and anti-albumin antibodies, but not with neutral or anionized albumin. Thaiss et al [141] were able to induce formation of immune aggregates in the glomerular capillary wall by injecting first cationized human IgG and then anti-IgG antibody. Oite et al [140] infused cationized human IgG to rats pre-immunized for human IgG, which resulted in a severe crescentic glomerulonephritis. Similar results were obtained with injections of cationized ferritin into pre-immunized animals [142]. Sawtell et al [143] induced an immune complex glomerulopathy associated with the nephrotic syndrome by giving cationic bovine gammaglobulin to pre-immunized mice. Negatively charged antigens such as DNA have also been shown to act as planted antigens, albeit through different mechanisms.

Gallo et al [144] and Koyama et al [106] showed convincingly that immune complexes bearing a cationic charge could react with anionic sites of the glomerular capillary wall. The more cationic these complexes are, the more they become localized in the subepithelial space and the more nephritogenic they are. Recently Kanwar et al [145] demonstrated that cationic immune complexes are bound by heparan sulphate in the glomerular basement membrane, while neutral immune complexes are non-specifically trapped in the mesangium. Gauthier and Mannik [146] showed that injection of protamine sulphate or cationized rabbit serum albumin prevented the deposition of cationized immune complexes in this region. These authors also showed that once bound to the glomerular capillary wall, cationized immune complexes are readily replaced by these substances, if the latter were injected not later than one minute after the administration of immune complexes. After one hour, however, this replacement appeared to be impossible, which implies that once the immune complexes in glomeruli condense to form larger deposits, other forces besides charge-charge interactions are responsible for their retention [146].

Concanavalin-A nephritis. In 1979, Golbus and Wilson [147] showed that animals injected with the lectin concanavalin-A developed an immune complex glomerulopathy. It is known that concanavalin-A has an affinity for a glycopeptide localized at the endothelial side of the glomerular basement membrane [55]. Once bound to the glomerular basement membrane, the concanavalin-A can react with anti-concanavalin-A antibodies either administered systemically or actively formed by the recipient, resulting in immune aggregate formation and glomerulonephritis.

Other models. Other models involving antibody reaction with planted antigens probably are the forms of glomerulonephritis associated with viral infections. These infections, which include lymphocytic choriomeningitis virus [148,149], parvovirus infections of Aleutian mink [150], cytomegalovirus infections of mice [151] or adenovirus infection of dogs, will not be discussed further.

MODELS MEDIATED BY CELLULAR IMMUNE REACTIONS

Evidence for the rôle of cellular immunity in the induction of glomerular injury is not as clear as that of antibody-mediated mechanisms [27], and is often circumstantial. In experimental glomerulonephritis a rôle of cellular immunity has been suggested in nephrotoxic nephritis and experimental allergic glomerulonephritis. Moorthy and Abreo [153] found that proteinuria in rats receiving subnephritic doses of nephrotoxic serum was due to lymphocytes sensitized to the nephrotoxic IgG. Macrophages play an important rôle in the accelerated form of nephrotoxic nephritis [47]. This accumulation is thought to occur through adherence to the Fc portion of glomerular bound IgG. Tipping et al [154] showed that in this model an accumulation of T-helper cells preceded the influx of macrophages, and that treatment with cyclosporin prevented the influx of both T-helper lymphocytes and monocytes. Recently Boyce et al [155] demonstrated macrophage inhibition activity of these lymphocytes, indicating an·active rôle of these cells in accelerated nephrotoxic nephritis. Bhan et al [156] showed that transfer of sensitized lymphocytes from rats with accelerated nephrotoxic nephritis to naive animals, caused an influx of macrophages into the glomerulus. This possible rôle of cellular immunity expressed through macrophages is intriguing in view of the idea that Ia-positive resident macrophages in the glomerular mesangium may play a rôle in the afferent limb of the immune response [157].

In experimental allergic glomerulonephritis induced in chickens the rôle of cellular immunity has been shown beyond doubt. Bolton et al [39] immunized chickens with bovine glomerular basement membrane in Freund's complete adjuvant, which resulted in a proliferative glomerulonephritis, occasionally with crescent formation and an increase of mesangial cells. Lymphoid cells are thought to attract macrophages through the action of lymphokines, although proteinuria is not observed. In these animals bursectomy abrogated the antibody response completely, but did not influence the incidence of experimental allergic glomerulonephropathy [158]. Moreover these authors demonstrated that the disease could be transferred to naive animals with sensitized lymphocytes.

MODELS MEDIATED BY AUTOIMMUNE REACTIONS

In recent years increasing attention has been given to glomerulonephritis associated with generalized autoimmune phenomena. In addition to the autoimmune responses involving the kidney following immunization (experimental allergic glomerulonephritis, Heymann nephritis) autoimmune responses discussed in this section originate from a polyclonal stimulation of B-lymphocytes, either occurring spontaneously as in SLE-like diseases or resulting from an immunoregulatory disturbance induced by external factors such as toxic agents, or in association with graft-versus-host reaction.

In this section these three examples will be discussed.

Systemic lupus erythematosus-like glomerulonephritis

It has long been known that the mouse strains NZB, NZW, BXB, MRL (NZB x SWR)F1, and especially (NZB x NZW)F1 (B/W) rats, spontaneously develop an SLE-like disease associated with an autoimmune response to DNA and an immune complex glomerulonephritis [159]. The disease is characterized by glomerular hypercellularity, and thickening of the glomerular basement membrane and is occasionally associated with fibrinoid necrosis. Mouse IgG is invariably present in the mesangial area but seldom along the glomerular capillary wall. The disease always progresses towards glomerulosclerosis and renal insufficiency. Gunn et al [160] reported that treatment with cyclosporin reduces the incidence of glomerulonephritis and proteinuria in B/W mice. After Koffler et al [161] reported that in human SLE the glomerular immune complexes were composed of DNA and anti-DNA, similar findings were reported in the above mentioned mouse strains [159] in addition to generalized autoimmunity involving haemolytic anaemia and lupus erythematosus cells. After Izui et al [162] demonstrated an affinity of DNA molecules for the collagen moiety of the glomerular basement membrane in vitro, and Faaber et al [163] found cross-reactivity between DNA and heparan sulphate, it was believed that the glomerular DNA-anti-DNA immune complexes were formed locally. However some doubts were raised against this pathogenesis. O'Regan and Turgeon [164] showed that infusion of DNA into normal mice resulted in mesangial binding and not in a binding to the glomerular capillary wall. Infusion of preformed DNA and anti-DNA immune complexes in rabbits, resulted only in a mesangial localization [165]. Cavallo et al [166] showed that the DNA-anti-DNA content was low in eluates from glomeruli of B/W mice. Izui et al [167] found that the presence of serum antibodies to single- or double-stranded DNA was not significantly associated with glomerulonephritis. All of these studies led to the conclusion that other immune complex systems besides DNA-anti-DNA played a rôle in the pathogenesis of lupus nephritis. Izui et al [167] found a correlation between the development of fatal glomerulonephritis in B/W mice, and the presence of gp70-containing immune complexes. The same investigators found that in BXSB mice glomerulonephritis was significantly correlated with abnormally elevated gp70 serum levels and with the occurrence of gp70 anti-gp70 immune complexes [168]. This was confirmed in B/W mice by Maruyama et al [169].

Gp70 is a serum glycoprotein structurally related to the envelope glycoprotein of murine leukaemia virus [170]. Although this virus has a virtually ubiquitous occurrence in rodents, only lupus-prone animals develop autoantibodies against gp70 spontaneously [171]. Izui et al [167] concluded from these findings that gp70-anti gp70 systems fulfil a pathogenic rôle in experimental lupus nephritis.

Andrews et al [172] recently questioned the essentiality of the anti-gp70 immune response in murine SLE. Using a low gp70 MRL/1 congenic line they could demonstrate that elimination of most of the serum gp70 and virtually all of the immune complex gp70 had no observable effect on the course or nature of the disease.

Treatment of mice susceptible to develop lupus nephritis with cyclosporin or with drugs which prevent polyclonal activation of B-cells [173] reduced the incidence of glomerular lesions and proteinuria, suggesting a pathogenetic mechanism.

Glomerulonephritis associated with polyclonal activation of B-cells

Altered recognition in immune regulation constitutes the basis for a polyclonal stimulation of B-lymphocytes which can be induced by a graft-versus-host reaction [26], injection of bacterial products [174,175], resulting in hypergammaglobulinaemia and circulating autoantibodies and immune complexes as well as a renal localization of immunoreactants. Chronic administration of lipopolysaccharides to mice induced a diffuse proliferative glomerulonephritis associated with the appearance of various autoantibodies such as anti-DNA. Recently Sumazaki et al [176] demonstrated a cross reaction between anti-lps antibodies and DNA histones, explaining in part the pathogenesis. Bruijn et al [177] showed that experimental infection of BX IX rats with Trypanosoma brucei induced the formation of autoantibodies directed against laminin and collagen IV. These authors assumed that these autoimmune phenomena were caused by a restricted polyclonal stimulation of B cells, which is a well-known feature of trypanosomiasis. Such polyclonal stimulation of B-lymphocytes is also found after viral infections [178]. A similar mechanism has been postulated to operate in the induction of glomerulonephritis in newborn mice following treatment with interferon [179].

Polyclonal activation of B-lymphocytes induced by drugs or toxic substances [180] or by an experimental graft-versus-host disease (GvHR) [181] have been studied on a larger scale.

Drugs

In 1971, Bariety et al [182] reported that repeated injections of low doses of mercuric chloride to Wistar rats induced a membranous glomerulonephritis. A similar lesion was induced in PVG/c rats by Weening et al [183] associated with the occurrence of circulating antinuclear antibodies, and a dysregulation of the immune response [184]. A mercury induced disease was also found in Brown Norway rats [185], and shown to be associated with polyclonal B-lymphocyte activation, hypergammaglobulinaemia, high serum IgE, anti-glomerular basement membrane antibodies and proteinuria [185]. The ability to induce polyclonal activation of B-cells as well as the type of the resulting glomerulopathy appeared to be genetically restricted [186]. The induction of these autoimmune phenomena is thought to be T-lymphocyte dependent since treatment with cyclosporin during administration of mercuric chloride prevents the disease [187]. Moreover Pelletier and co-workers [188] showed that congeneic athymic Brown Norway rats and T-lymphocyte deprived Brown Norway rats do not develop autoimmune glomerulonephritis upon $HgCl_2$ administration while reconstitution with normal T-lymphocytes restored the ability to develop the disease. Recently Pelletier et al [189] showed that the proliferation of autoreactive T-lymphocytes in vitro was caused by $HgCl_2$-pretreated T-lymphocytes of the helper/inducer phenotype, in the presence of normal MHC class II antigen bearing cells. The nature of these cells has not been elucidated yet. The pathogenesis of the proteinuria in this model is unknown at present. Both humoral and cellular mechanisms may play a rôle in its induction. Complement activation is not necessary for the development of proteinuria in this model [186]. Ultrastructural study of glomeruli revealed influx of polymorphonuclear leucocytes and monocytes during the proteinuric phase after $HgCl_2$ administration but not lymphocytes [190]. Besides the kidney other organs may be involved as a target in the mercuric chloride induced autoimmune syndrome as shown by extra-renal deposition of immune complexes [191]. In addition Aten et al [192] found an increased expression of MHC class II antigens on renal and non-renal epithelial cells and on dendritic cells. Recently, Lymberi et al [193] established polyclonal stimulation in $HgCl_2$-treated rats by fusing their spleen cells with rat myeloma cells and demonstrating autoantibodies against TNP and HRP, both of the D23 idiotype. An $HgCl_2$-associated membranous glomerulopathy can be induced in Balb/c mice and is associated with the development of antibodies directed against an epitope of gp330 [194].

Graft-versus-host disease

In 1968 Lewis et al [195] described an immune complex glomerulonephritis following the injection of Balb/c lymphocytes into (Balb/c-A/jax) F1 hybrid mice. Later, Gleichmann and Gleichmann [196] showed that this type of glomerulonephritis was associated with the development of various autoantibodies due to a polyclonal stimulation of B-lymphocytes. Rolink et al [176] had shown that small differences between MHC class II antigens suffice to trigger the alloreactive donor T-helper cells to stimulate the autoreactive B-cells.

As in mercury-induced polyclonal activation, GvHR in mice was shown to be associated with an increase of expression of host MHC class II antigens, especially on tubular cells [197]. This observation raises the possibility of a rôle for such altered expression in autoimmune or alloimmune responses involving the kidney.

In our laboratory GvHR was studied in rats as well as in mice with injection of parental thoracic duct lymphocyte into F1 hybrids. Lewis/Brown Norway F1 hybrids injected by Lew cells resulted in a chronic GvHR leading to a variety of autoantibodies, including glomerular basement membrane antibodies which bound in glomeruli [198]. The resulting glomerulonephritis is associated with a transient proteinuria as much as 600mg/24 hours. Hoedemaeker et al [199] reported that injection of low dosages of Lewis lymphocytes into (Lew/BN) F1 hybrid rats led after eight months to a membranous nephropathy associated with proteinuria.

In (C57Bl/10xDBA/2) F1 hybrids injection of DBA/2 lymphocytes led to a membranous glomerulopathy and the nephrotic syndrome, sometimes associated with segmental proliferation resembling SLE-nephritis [200].

GLOMERULONEPHRITIS MODELS MEDIATED BY NON-IMMUNE MECHANISMS

Toxic substances

Aminonucleoside of puromycin

In 1955 Frenk et al [201] induced a proteinuria in rats associated with the nephrotic syndrome by injections of the aminonucleoside of puromycin. In these cases glomerular morphology is only slightly changed and shows protein reabsorption droplets, epithelial cell blebs and a discrete expansion of the mesangial area which may show an increased uptake of macromolecular substances [202]. There is a marked reduction in colloidal iron reactive polyanion at the height of proteinuria [203] and a focal detachment of the epithelium from the underlying glomerular basement membrane can be observed [204]. Puromycin nephrosis can also be induced in monkeys whereas mice, rabbits, guinea pigs and dogs are resistant [205].

Nephrotoxicity results from a direct effect of puromycin on the kidney. Hoyer et al [206] showed that increased permeability was confined to the perfused kidney. Moreover, a kidney transplanted from a donor which had been injected with puromycin, developed proteinuria [207]. The nephrotoxic effect of puromycin can be inhibited by administration of N-methyladenosine, a structural analogue of puromycin [208].

Two variants of puromycin nephrosis have been described: the acute and the chronic model.

In the acute model multiple subcutaneous or one intravenous injection of 50 to 150mg/kg body weight is given, which results in massive proteinuria and the nephrotic syndrome after 7 to 14 days [201,203]. After about three weeks proteinuria decreases and disappears after five to six weeks. The chronic model nephrosis is induced by repeated injections of low doses and is associated with chronic proteinuria and changes in plasma proteins and lipids [209]. Morphological tracer studies visualized increased passage of macromolecular tracers at the sites of detachment of the epithelium from the glomerular basement membrane, whereas a normal restriction in transport across the glomerular capillary wall was found along the intact portions [210]. The structural basis for the defect in puromycin nephrosis is still unknown. A reduction in the charge density of the glomerular basement membrane in puromycin nephrosis was reported [211] although this could not be confirmed by others [212]. A similar controversy exists concerning a loss of heparan sulphate proteoglycans from the glomerular basement membrane in puromycin nephrosis [213] whereas glomerular laminin and collagen IV have been shown to be normally present [214]. Fishman and Karnovsky [215] recently described the effects of puromycin on glomerular epithelial cells in vitro. They found both direct effects on cell membrane, possibly through protein-lipid disorganization, and long-term metabolic derangements such as increased heparan sulphate proteoglycan turnover without a net gain (but possibly with changes in distribution) and decreased glucosamine and sulphate in the cell surface [215].

Adriamycin

Adriamycin (doxorubicin) is an anthracyclin which inhibits RNA and DNA synthesis. Toxicity studies have shown that adriamycin and daunorubicin can cause massive proteinuria in rabbits and rats [216]. Bertani et al [217] described the natural history of the disease in rats and reported morphological changes very similar to those found in puromycin nephrosis. The proteinuria starts within two weeks of administration, plateaus at around four weeks, but – in contrast to puromycin nephrosis – remains at high levels, even after several months. The animals develop a severe nephrotic syndrome with oedema and ascites and coagulation disturbances [218]. Electronmicroscopy shows epithelial cell damage similar to puromycin nephrosis, including focal detachment from the glomerular basement membrane [217,219]. By histochemical stains a marked reduction in colloidal iron reactive polyanion is found [217,219]. Anionic sites in both laminae rarae are intact when stained with PEI [219]. Functional studies have shown that adriamycin nephrosis is associated with modest changes in renal plasma flow and glomerular filtration rate [219] in contrast to puromycin nephrosis [202]. The normal charge barrier function in adriamycin nephrosis was supported by the finding of a normal binding pattern of protamine-heparin aggregates to the glomerular capillary wall in adriamycin nephrotic rats [135]. In addition, a normal binding of heterologous anti-tubular brush border antibodies to the glomerular capillary wall of adriamycin-diseased rats was described [135] indicating the preservation of the Heymann antigen(s) on the surface of adriamycin damaged epithelial cells. Rats which had been severely proteinuric for 12 weeks, showed no signs of focal and segmental sclerosis [220]. After six months of severe proteinuria, sclerotic glomerular lesions develop [221], possibly as a result of extensive tubular cast formation leading to loss of nephrons.

Progressive glomerulosclerosis

Progressive glomerulosclerosis delineates a histological description of glomerular injury in rodents associated with progressive loss of renal function and which resembles focal and segmental glomerulosclerosis in man which was described by Rich in 1957 [222].

A number of experimental studies devoted to the natural history of progressive sclerosis and to influence the glomerular lesions in rats have given insight into its pathogenesis. It is now believed that different pathways may lead to the occurrence of the lesions, which can occur in rabbits and in dogs but which have been studied most frequently in rats.

Progressive glomerulosclerosis develops spontaneously with ageing in several rat strains [223], a process which can be accelerated by a reduction of renal mass [224], high protein feeding [225], by stretozotocin-induced diabetes mellitus [226] and by desoxycorticosterone-salt-induced hypertension [227]. In addition the glomerulosclerosis may develop in chronic aminonucleoside nephrosis [209] and adriamycin nephrosis [221]. Most studies involving pathogenesis have been performed in unilaterally nephrectomized rats or in rats with an even further reduction of renal mass, the so-called remnant kidney model in which five-sixths of the kidney mass is (functionally) removed. Recent studies using micropuncture and morphological techniques demonstrated a central rôle for elevated intraglomerular pressures and flows in the pathogenesis [225, 228], resulting in a process of endothelial, epithelial and mesangial cell damage [229]. Besides these haemodynamic factors, genetic [230], metabolic [231] and coagulation [232] factors have been shown to be important. Proteinuria per se does not seem to induce these focal sclerosis lesions as evidenced by models of chronic proteinuria without mesangial sclerosis such as Heymann nephritis [233]. In several models dietary or pharmacological intervention has been applied to retard or prevent glomerular disease. Protein restriction was found to have a beneficial effect in ablation models [225], in experimental diabetes [234] and hypertension [227]. Anticoagulant drugs were also effective in models of ablation [232] and hypertension [235].

Antihypertensive treatment using converting enzyme inhibitors, introduced shortly after the induction of glomerular hyperperfusion was remarkably effective in reducing glomerulosclerosis in the remnant kidney model [236]. Recently Meyer et al [237] showed that reversal of glomerular hypertension either by converting enzyme inhibition or by protein restriction stabilized established glomerular injury in the remnant kidney model.

In contrast Beukers et al [238] found no beneficial effect of converting enzyme inhibition on the progression of glomerulosclerosis in uninephrectomized rats, once proteinuria and glomerular lesions had developed.

Protein overload glomerulopathy

Parenteral administration of large amounts of protein may result in proteinuria in dogs and rats [239]. In most studies hyperalbuminaemia is induced by administration of human or bovine serum albumin in the range of 0.6–1.5gm protein per day, for five consecutive days. The proteinuric response to this hyperalbuminaemia develops within two days and reaches levels of 400–500mg/24 hours. The amount of urinary protein loss is related to the type and amount of protein administered [240] and depends on the sex and strain of the animal [241]. Measurement of exogenous and endogenous proteins in serum and urine of proteinuric animals revealed that hyperalbuminaemia leads to a highly selective proteinuria, consisting of albumin, both exogenous and endogenous, in a ratio of 2:1, for approximately 90% [241]. After cessation of protein administration, the excretion of exogenous protein disappeared at day 22, but urinary loss of endogenous albumin persisted and was found to be associated with glomerular mesangial proliferation and sclerosis [242].

In the acute phase of massive proteinuria, glomerular changes are usually minor and consist of protein reabsorption droplets in epithelial cells [243] and loss of epithelial foot processes to a varying extent [243,244]. Only few areas of epithelial cell detachment are observed [243]. Immunofluorescence studies remain negative, thus ruling out antibody or immune complex mediation of the increased glomerular permeability in this model. In rats receiving homologous albumin no alterations in glomerular permeability to macromolecules larger than albumin were found as studied by measuring haemoglobin clearances and by electronmicroscopy using native ferritin as a tracer [245]. Functional studies [244] performed in the acute phase of bovine serum albumin-induced proteinuria in rats have produced conflicting results regarding changes in sieving properties of the glomerular capillary wall. Both studies describe minor changes in glomerular filtration rate and renal plasma flow, but while dextran clearances do not reveal changes in size selective properties [246], protein clearances indicate the presence of large pore defects [244], which is in concordance with studies revealing focal epithelial detachment and transcapillary passage of high molecular weight macromolecules [244].

Concluding remarks

For almost a century investigators have tried to reproduce human glomerulonephritis in animal models. Although many models show glomerular changes similar to those found in man, they also demonstrate characteristic features which are difficult to attribute to the immunological mechanisms operating in experimental disease [27]. Moreover glomerular lesions unrelated to immunological mechanisms were shown to express a similar variety of histological features. In addition the induction of glomerulonephritis often is non-physiological. Many models are based on immunization of animals with large doses of antigen, which is not likely to occur in man. Furthermore, the use of heterologous nephritogenic antisera always induces an immune reaction in the injected animal, which complicates the induced glomerulonephritis considerably.

In spite of these disadvantages the use of models of glomerulonephritis has shown to be very useful to study and unravel pathogenetic details which may be extrapolated to the human situation, and which have brought an understanding of various forms of glomerulonephritis.

Nephrotoxic serum nephritis was the first model of glomerulonephritis to be developed, but it took a long time before its human counterpart was established. In spite of the fact that much is known about various pathogenetic mechanisms operating in this disease, the complement independent glomerular basement membrane damage is still poorly understood. Further unravelling of the rôle of cellular immunity and rearrangement of basement membrane components by immunological reactions, undoubtedly will solve this problem, and may shed new light on human anti-glomerular basement membrane disease.

Heymann nephritis is generally regarded as a unique model of human membranous glomerulopathy. It is likely that in the human counterpart immune complexes are formed in situ as in the experimental models. Although in some cases of membranous nephropathy the antigens involved have been identified [22,247], a tentative rôle for Fx1A antigens has not been firmly established [248]. However the concept originating from experimental nephrology that epithelial antigens are clustered and shed to form glomerular aggregates [80,81] provides us with an original working hypothesis which will stimulate the search for the epithelial antigen(s) operating in human membranous nephropathy.

Nephrotic syndrome induced by aminonucleoside has been regarded as a model for human minimal change glomerulopathy. The relevance of this model for human nephropathology, however, also has been questioned because no firm evidence has been presented which holds toxic products responsible for the induction of this disease in humans. However Lagrue [249] proposed that lymphokines may play a rôle in induction, while Bakker et al recently [250] demonstrated that concanavalin-A activated peripheral lymphocytes from patients with minimal change glomerulopathy are able to affect the glomerular polyanion coat in culture. This might indicate that somehow cellular products may affect the charge selective barrier in the human situation.

Glomerulopathy based on autoimmune phenomena also deserves some comment. An autoimmune reaction associated with glomerular disease demonstrating many characteristics of serum lupus erythematosus glomerulonephritis [26] can be induced by toxic products or by an experimental graft-versus-host reaction [26,198,199]. Undoubtedly such a mechanism in which altered structures of lymphocyte membranes lead to a dysregulation of the immune response and to a polyclonal activation of B-lymphocytes is operating in man. Viral infections and even drugs [251,252] might prove important as aetiological factors in human glomerulonephritis [199]. Therefore these models should be studied intensively in the near future to give us the ultimate opportunity to prevent some of the forms of human glomerulonephritis.

References

1 Volhard F, Fahr Th. *Die Brightsche Nierenkrankheiten. Klinik, Patholgie und Atlas.* Berlin: Springer Verlag. 1914

2 Bright R. *Reports of Medical Cases Selected with a View of Illustrating the Symptoms and Cure of Diseases by a Reference to Morbid Anatomy, Volume 1.* London: Longman. 1827: 1

3 Horn H. The experimental nephropathies I. *Arch Pathol 1937; 23:* 71–121

4 Horn H. The experimental nephropathies II. *Arch Pathol 1937; 23:* 241–264

5 Lohlein M. Uber die entzundlichen Veranderungen der Glomeruli der menschlichen Nieren und ihre Bedeuting fur die Nephritis. In *Arbeiten aus dem pathologischen Institut zu Leipzig.* Leipzig: Hirzel. 1907: 1

6 Bergholm AM, Holm SE. Experimental poststreptococcal glomerulonephritis in rabbits. *Acta Path Microbiol Immunol Scand (Sect C) 1983; 91:* 263–270

7 Albini B, Nisengard RJ, Glurich BS et al. Streptococcus mutans-induced nephritis in rabbits. *Am J Pathol 1985; 118:* 408–418

8 Pirquet CE, von Schick B. *Die Serumkrankheit.* Vienna: Deuticke. 1905

9 Longcope WT. The production of experimental nephritis by repeated proteid intoxication. *J Exp Med 1913; 18:* 678–703

10 More RH, Waugh D. Diffuse glomerulonephritis produced in rabbits by massive injections of bovine serum gamma globulin. *J Exp Med 1949; 89:* 541–554

11 Lindemann W. Sur le mode d'action de certains poisons renaux. *Annales de l'institut Pasteur 1900; 14:* 49–59

12 Masugi M. Ueber das Wesen der spezifischen Veranderungen der Niere und der Leber durch das Nephrotoxin bzw das Hepatotoxin. *Beitr Path Anat Alg Path 1933; 91:* 82–112

13 Germuth FG. A comparative histologic and immunologic study in rabbits of induced hypersensitivity of the serum sickness type. *J Exp Med 1953; 97:* 257–282

14 Dixon FJ, Feldman JD, Vazguez JJ. Experimental glomerulonephritis. The pathogenesis of a laboratory model resembling the spectrum of human glomerulonephritis. *J Exp Med 1961; 113:* 899–920

15 Coons AH, Kaplan MH. Localization of antigen in tissue cells. II. Improvement in a method for the detection of antigen by means of fluorescent antibody. *J Exp Med 1950; 91:* 1–13

16 Farquhar MG, Vernier RL, Good RA. Electron microscope study of glomerulus in nephrosis, glomerulonephritis and lupus erythematosus. *J Exp Med 1951; 106:* 649

17 Benacerraf B, Potter JL, McCluskey RT, Miller F. The pathologic effects of intravenously administered soluble antigen-antibody complexes. II. Acute glomerulonephritis in rats. *J Exp Med 1960; 111:* 195–200

18 Heymann W, Lund HZ. Nephrotic syndrome in rats. *Pediatrics 1951; 7:* 691–706

19 Edgington TS, Glassock RJ, Dixon FJ. Autologous immune-complex pathogenesis of experimental allergic glomerulonephritis. *Science 1967; 155:* 1432–1434

20 Feenstra K, Lee R v.d., Greben HA et al. Experimental glomerulonephritis in the rat induced by antibodies directed against tubular antigens. I. The natural history: a histologic and immunohistologic study at the light microscopic and the ultrastructural level. *Lab Invest 1975; 32:* 235–242

21 Damme BJC van, Fleuren GJ, Bakker WW et al. Experimental glomerulonephritis in the rat induced by antibodies directed against tubular antigens. V. Fixed glomerular antigens in the pathogenesis of heterologous immune complex glomerulonephritis. *Lab Invest 1978; 38:* 502–510

22 Couser WG, Steinmuller DR, Stilmant MM et al. Experimental glomerulonephritis in the isolated perfused rat kidney. *J Clin Invest 1978; 62:* 1275–1287

23 Couser WG, Salant DJ. In situ immune complex formation and glomerular injury. *Kidney Int 1980; 17:* 1–13

24 Hoedemaeker PhJ, Fleuren GJ, Weening JJ. In situ formation of glomerular immune aggregates. *Transplant Proc 1982; 14:* 469–471

25 Lambert PH, Goldman M, Rose LM, Morel PA. A possible role for idiotypic interactions in the pathogenesis of immune complex glomerulonephritis. *Transplant Proc 1982; 14:* 543–546

26 Gleichmann E, Pals ST, Rolink AG et al. Graft-versus-host reactions: clues to the etiopathology of a spectrum of immunological diseases. *Immunol Today 1984; 5:* 324–332

27 Wilson CB, Dixon FJ. The renal response to immunological injury. In Brenner BM, Rector FC, eds. *The Kidney, II.* Philadelphia: W B Saunders. 1981: 1237–1350

28 Wilson CB. Immune complex glomerulonephritis. *Proc Vth Int Congress Nephrology, Mexico, I.* Basel: Karger. 1974: 68

29 Masugi M. Ueber die experimentelle Glomerulonephritis durch das spezifischen Antinierenserum. *Beitr Path Anat Alg Path 1934; 92:* 429–466

30 Kay CF. The mechanism by which experimental nephritis is produced in rabbits injected with nephrotoxic duck serum. *J Exp Med 1940; 72:* 559–572

31 Krakower CA, Greenspon SA. Localization of the nephrotoxic antigen within the isolated renal glomerulus. *Arch Pathol 1951; 51:* 629–639

32 Unanue R, Dixon FJ. Experimental glomerulonephritis. V. Studies on the interaction of nephrotoxic antibodies with tissues of the rat. *J Exp Med 1965; 121:* 697–714

33 Hoedemaeker PhJ, Feenstra K, Nijkeuter A, Arends A. Ultrastructural localization of heterologous nephrotoxic antibody in the glomerular basement membrane of the rat. *Lab Invest 1972; 26:* 610–613

34 Weening JJ, Prins FA, Fransen JAM et al. Ultrastructural localization and quantitation of nephritogenic antibodies in experimental glomerulonephritis. *Lab Invest 1986; 55:* 372–376

35 Unanue ER, Dixon FJ. Experimental glomerulonephritis. VI. The autologous phase of nephrotoxic serum nephritis. *J Exp Med 1965; 121:* 715–725

36 Kawachi H, Oite T, Shimizu F. Studies on the 'linear pattern' in renal glomeruli demonstrated with immunofluorescence. *Nephron 1985; 39:* 36–39

37 Avasthi PS, Avasthi P, Tokuda S et al. Experimental glomerulonephritis in the mouse. I. The model. *Clin Exp Immunol 1971; 9:* 667–676

38 Battifora HA, Markowitz AS. Nephrotoxic nephritis in monkeys. Sequential light, immunofluorescence and electron microscopic studies. *Am J Path 1969; 55:* 267–282

39 Bolton WK, Tucker FL, Sturgill BC. Experimental autoimmune glomerulonephritis in chickens. *J Clin Lab Immunol 1980; 3:* 179–184

40 Couser WG, Stilmant M, Lewis EJ. Experimental glomerulonephritis in the guinea pig. I. Glomerular lesions associated with antiglomerular basement membrane antibody deposits. *Lab Invest 1973; 29:* 236–243

41 Lerner RA, Dixon EJ. The induction of acute glomerulonephritis in rabbits with soluble antigens isolated from normal homologous and autologous urine. *J Immunol 1968; 100:* 1277–1287

42 Steblay RW, Rudofsky U. In vitro and in vivo properties of autoantibodies eluted from kidneys of sheep with autoimmune glomerulonephritis. *Nature 1968; 218:* 1269–1271

43 Cotran RS. Monocytes, proliferation, and glomerulonephritis. *J Lab Clin Med 1978; 92:* 837–840

44 Holdsworth SR, Neale TJ, Wilson CB. The participation of macrophages and monocytes in experimental immune complex glomerulonephritis. *Clin Immunol Immunopathol 1980; 15:* 510–524

45 Silva FG, Hoyer JR, Pirani CL. Sequential studies of glomerular crescent formation in rats with antiglomerular basement membrane induced glomerulonephritis and the role of coagulation factors. *Lab Invest 1984; 51:* 404–415

46 Bertani T, Benigni A, Cutillo F et al. Effect of aspirin and sulindac in rabbit nephrotoxic nephritis. *J Lab Clin Med 1986; 107:* 261–268

47 Schreiner GF, Cotran RS, Pardo V, Unanue ER. A mononuclear cell component in experimental immunological glomerulonephritis. *J Exp Med 1978; 147:* 369–384

48 Jennings L, Roholt OA, Blau M et al. Experimental anti-alveolar basement membrane antibody-mediated pneumonitis. I. The role of increased permeability of the alveolar capillary wall induced by oxygen. *J Immunol 1981; 127:* 129–134

49 Downie GH‘ Roholt OA, Jennings L et al. Experimental anti-alveolar membrane antibody-mediated pneumonitis. II. Role of endothelial damage and repair, induction of autologous phase, and kinetics of antibody deposition in Lewis rats. *J Immunol 1982; 129:* 2647–2652

50 Yamamoto T, Wilson CB. Binding of anti-basement membrane antibody to alveolar basement membrane after intratracheal gasoline instillation in rabbits. *Am J Pathol 1987; 126:* 497–505

51 Wieslander J, Barr J, Butkowski R et al. Goodpasture antigen of the glomerular basement membrane: localization to non collagenous region of type IV collagen. *Proc Natl Acad Sci USA 1984; 81:* 3838–3842

52 Abrahamson DR. Recent studies on the structure and pathology of basement membranes. *J Pathol 1986; 149:* 257–278

53 Mendrick DL, Rennke HG, Cotran RS et al. Methods in laboratory investigation. Monoclonal antibodies against rat glomerular antigens: production and specificity. *Lab Invest 1983; 49:* 107–117

54 Shibata S, Sakaguchi H, Nagasawa T. Exfoliation of endothelial cytoplasm in nephrotoxic serum nephritis. A study using antiserum against water-soluble glycoprotein isolated from the glomerular basement membrane. *Lab Invest 1978; 38:* 201–207

55 Shibata S, Natori Y. Nephritogenic glycoprotein X. Correlation between the purity of nephritogenic glycopeptide, nephritogenoside, and morphological manifestation of glomerulonephritis. *Nephron 1984; 37:* 85–93

56 Abrahamson DR, Caulfield JP. Proteinuria and structural alterations in rat glomerular basement membranes induced by intravenously injected anti-laminin immunoglobulin G. *J Exp Med 1982; 156:* 128–145

57 Yaar M, Foidart JM, Brown KS et al. The Goodpasture-like syndrome in mice induced by intravenous injections of anti-type IV collagen and anti-laminin antibody. *Am J Pathol 1982; 107:* 79 91

58 Miettinen A, Stow JL, Mentone S, Farquhar MG. Antibodies to basement membrane heparan sulfate proteoglycans bind to the laminae rarae of the glomerular basement membrane (GBM) and induce subepithelial GBM thickening. *J Exp Med 1986; 163:* 1064–1084

59 Steblay RW. Glomerulonephritis induced in sheep by injections of heterologous glomerular basement membrane in Freund's complete adjuvant. *J Exp Med 1962; 116:* 253 272

60 Sado Y, Okigaki T, Takamiya H, Seno S. Experimental autoimmune glomerulonephritis with pulmonary hemorrhage in rats. The dose-effect relationship of the nephritogenic antigen from bovine glomerular basement membrane. *J Clin Lab Immunol 1984; 15:* 199–204

61 Heymann W, Hackel DB, Harwood S et al. Production of nephrotic syndrome in rats by Freund's adjuvant and rat kidney suspension. *Proc Soc Exp Biol Med 1959; 100:* 660–664

62 Steblay RW. Glomerulonephritis induced in monkeys by injections of heterologous glomerular basement membrane and Freund's adjuvant. *Nature 1963; 197:* 1173–1176
63 Unanue ER. Immunopathology of rabbits immunized to kidney fractions. *Fed Proc 1966; 25 (Abstract):* 659
64 Williams R, Steblay R. Glomerulonephritis induced in goats by injections of human glomerular basement membrane (HGBM) and Freund's adjuvant (FA). *Fed Proc 1965; 24 (Abstract):* 243
65 Fleuren GJ, Hoedemaeker PhJ. Experimental anti-basement membrane renal disease: a linear glomerular and tubular immunofluorescence pattern caused by antibodies directed against endothelial antigens. *Proc Xth Int Congr Nephrol.* Athens. 1981 (Abstract)
66 Edgington TS, Glassock RJ, Dixon FJ. Autologous immune complex glomerulonephritis induced with renal tubular antigen. I. Identification and isolation of the pathogenetic antigen. *J Exp Med 1968; 127:* 555–572
67 Glassock RJ, Edginton TS, Watson JI, Dixon FJ. Autologous immune complex nephritis induced with renal tubular antigen. II. The pathogenetic mechanism. *J Exp Med 1968; 127:* 573–588
68 Ronco P, Allegri L, Melcion C et al. A monoclonal antibody to brushborder and passive Heymann nephritis. *Clin Exp Immunol 1984; 55:* 319–332
69 Behar M, Katz A, Silverman M. Biochemical investigation of the pathogenesis of Heymann nephritis. *Kidney Int 1986; 30:* 9–15
70 de Heer E, Daha MR, Bhakdi S et al. Possible involvement of terminal complement complex in active Heymann nephritis. *Kidney Int 1985; 27:* 388–393
71 Couser WG. In situ formation of immune complexes and the role of complement activation in glomerulonephritis. *Clin Immunol Allergy 1986; 6:* 287–306
72 Stahl RAK, Adler S, Baker PJ et al. Enhanced glomerular prostaglandin formation in experimental membranous glomerulopathy. *Lab Invest 1987; 31:* 1126–1131
73 Hoedemaeker PhJ. Een vorm van experimentele immuun-complex-glomerulonefritis. *Ned Tijdschr Geneesk 1972; 116 (Abstract):* 1802
74 Barabas AZ, Lannigan R. Induction of an autologous immune-complex glomerulonephritis in the rat by intravenous injection of heterologous anti-rat kidney tubular antibody. I. Production of chronic progressive immune-complex glomerulonephritis. *Br J Exp Pathol 1974; 55:* 47–55
75 Cybulski AV, Quigg RJ, Salant DJ. The membrane attack complex in complement-mediated glomerular epithelial cell injury: formation and stability of C4b-9 and C5b-7 in rat membranous nephropathy. *J Immunol 1986; 137:* 1511–1516
76 Madaio MP, Salant DJ, Cohen AJ et al. Comparative study of in situ immune deposit formation in active and passive Heymann nephritis. *Kidney Int 1983; 23:* 498–506
77 Kerjaschki D, Farquhar MG. The pathogenic antigen of Heymann nephritis is a membrane glycoprotein of the renal proximal tubule brush border. *Proc Natl Acad Sci USA 1982: 79:* 5557–5561
78 Kerjaschki D, Noronha-Blob L, Sacktor B, Farquhar MG. Microdomains of distinctive kidney proximal tubule brush border. *J Cell Biol 1983; 98:* 1505–1513
79 Chatelet F, Brianti E, Ronco P et al. Ultrastructural localization by monoclonal antibodies of brush border antigens expressed by glomeruli. I. Renal distribution. *Am J Pathol 1986; 122:* 500–511
80 Camussi G, Brentjens JR, Noble B et al. Antibody-induced redistribution of Heymann antigen on the surface of cultured glomerular visceral epithelial cells: possible role in the pathogenesis of Heymann glomerulonephritis. *J Immunol 1985; 135:* 2409–2416
81 Camussi G, Noble B, Liew JB van et al. Pathogenesis of passive Heymann nephritis: chlorpromazine inhibits antibody-mediated redistribution of cell surface antigens and prevents development of the disease. *J Immunol 1986; 136:* 2127–2135
82 Assmann KJM, Ronco P, Tangelder MM et al. Comparison of antigenic targets involved in antibody-mediated membranous glomerulonephritis in the mouse and rat. *Am J Pathol 1985; 121:* 112–122

83 Allegri L, Brianti E, Chatelet F et al. Polyvalent antigen-antibody interactions are required for the formation of electron-dense immune deposits in passive Heymann's nephritis. *Am J Pathol 1986; 126:* 1–6

84 Ronco P, Neale TJ, Wilson CB et al. An immunopathologic study of a 330-kD protein defined by monoclonal antibodies and reactive with anti-RTE alpha 5 antibodies and kidney eluates from active Heymann nephritis. *J Immunol 1986; 136:* 125–130

85 Heer E de, Deelder AM, Fleuren GJ et al. Passive Heymann's nephritis induced by rat monoclonal antibodies. *J Immunol:* submitted for publication

86 Bagchus WM, Vos JTWM, Hoedemaeker PhJ, Bakker WW. The specificity of nephritogenic antibodies. III. Binding of anti-Fx1a antibodies in glomeruli is dependent on dual specificity. *Clin Exp Immunol 1986; 63:* 639–645

87 Bagchus WM, Donga J, Hoedemaeker PhJ, Bakker WW. The specificity of nephritogenic antibodies. II. Immune complex glomerulopathy in rats induced by heterologous antithymocyte serum. *Transplantation 1984; 38:* 165–169

88 Hogendoorn PCW, Bruijn JA, Heer E de et al. Antibodies to purified renal tubular epithelial antigens contain activity against glomerular basement membrane components laminin, fibronectin and type IV collagen. *Xth Int Congr Nephrology.* London. 1987

89 Thoenes GH, Pielsticker K, Schubert G. Transplantation-induced immune complex kidney disease in rats with unilateral manifestation in the allografted kidney. *Lab Invest 1979; 41:* 321–333

90 Bagchus WM, Hoedemaeker PhJ, Rozing JJ, Bakker WW. Glomerulonephritis induced by monoclonal anti-Thy 1.1 antibodies. A sequential histological and ultrastructural study in the rat. *Lab Invest 1986; 55:* 680–687

91 Yamamoto T, Wilson CB. Quantitative and qualitative studies of antibody-induced mesangial cell damage in the rat. *Kidney Int 1987:* in press

92 Paul LC, Rennke HG, Milford EL, Carpenter CB. Thy-1.1 in glomeruli of rat kidneys. *Kidney Int 1984; 25:* 771–778

93 Cattell V, Bradfield JWB. Focal mesangial proliferative glomerulonephritis in the rat caused by Habu snake venom. A morphologic study. *Am J Pathol 1977; 87:* 511–524

94 Mendrick DL, Rennke HG. Immune deposits formed in situ by a monoclonal antibody recognizing a new intrinsic rat mesangial matrix antigen. *J Immunol 1986; 137:* 1517–1526

95 Neale TJ, Woodroffe AJ, Wilson CB. Spontaneous glomerulonephritis in rabbits: role of a glomerular capillary antigen. *Kidney Int 1984; 26:* 701–712

96 Dixon FJ. Tissue injury produced by antigen-antibody complexes. In *Mechanism of Cell and Tissue Damage Produced by Immune Reactions. Second International Symposium on Immunopathology.* Basel: Benno Schwabe and Co. 1962: 71

97 Germuth FG, Rodriguez E. *Immunopathology of the Renal Glomerulus.* Boston: Little Brown. 1973

98 Feldman JD. Electron microscopy of serum sickness. *J Exp Med 1958; 28:* 108–162

99 Shigematsu H, Kobayashi Y. Accelerated serum sickness in the rabbit. II. Glomerular ultrastructural lesions in transient proliferative and progressive disorganizing glomerulonephritis. *Virchows Arch [Pathol Anat Histol] 1976; 369:* 269–282

100 Johnson KJ, Ward PA. Newer concepts in the pathogenesis of immune complex induced tissue injury. *Lab Invest 1982; 47:* 218–226

101 Izumino K, Iida H, Asaka M et al. Effect of the antiplatelet agents ticlopidine and dipyridamole on experimental immune complex glomerulonephritis in rats. *Nephron 1986; 43:* 56–61

102 Fennell RH, Pardo VM. Experimental glomerulonephritis in rats. *Lab Invest 1967; 17:* 481–488

103 Arisz L, Noble B, Milgrom M et al. Experimental chronic serum sickness in rats. A model of immune complex glomerulonephritis and systemic immune complex deposition. *Int Arch Allergy Appl Immunol 1979; 60:* 80–88

104 Hogendoorn PCW, Dorst EBL van, Daha MR, Fleuren GJ. Chronic serum sickness induced by bovine serum albumin (BSA), human IgG, or human IgM: the role of antigen in localization in the rat glomerulus. *24th Congress EDTA–ERA.* Berlin 1987

105 Fleuren GJ, Hoedemaeker PhJ. Triple-drug treatment of autologous immune complex glomerulonephritis. *Clin Exp Immunol 1980; 41:* 218–224

106 Koyama A, Inage H, Kobayashi M et al. Role of antigenic charge and antibody avidity on the glomerular immune complex localization in serum sickness of mice. *Clin Exp Immunol 1986; 64:* 606–614

107 Iskandar SS, Jennette JC. Influence of antibody avidity on glomerular immune complex localization. *Am J Pathol 1983; 112:* 155–159

108 Lew AM, Steward MW. Glomerulonephritis: the use of grafted hybridomas to investigate the role of epitope density, antibody affinity and antibody isotype in active serum sickness. *Immunology 1984; 52:* 367–376

109 Vogt A, Rohrbach R, Shimizu F et al. Interaction of cationized antigen with rat glomerular basement membrane: in situ immune complex formation. *Kidney Int 1982; 22:* 27–35

110 Kuriyama T. Chronic glomerulonephritis induced by prolonged immunisation in the rabbit. *Lab Invest 1973; 28:* 224–235

111 Germuth FG, Rodriguez E, Lorelle GA et al. Passive immune complex glomerulonephritis in mice: Models for various lesions found in human disease. II. Low avidity complexes and diffuse proliferative glomerulonephritis with subepithelial deposits. *Lab Invest 1979; 41:* 366–371

112 Schneeberger EE, O'Brien A, Grupe WE. Altered glomerular permeability in Munich-Wistar rats with autologous immune complex nephritis. *Lab Invest 1979; 40:* 227–235

113 Bellon B, Belair MF, Kubin J et al. Trapping of circulation proteins in immune deposits of Heymann nephritis. *Lab Invest 1982; 46:* 306–309

114 Wilson CB, Dixon FJ. Quantitation of acute and chronic serum sickness in the rabbit. *J Exp Med 1971; 134:* 7s–8s

115 Ford PM, Kosatka I. In situ immune complex formation in the mouse glomerulus: reactivity with human IgM rheumatoid factor and the effect on subsequent immune complex deposition. *Clin Exp Immunol 1983; 51:* 285–291

116 Kano K, Milgrom F. Immune complex disease. *Vox Sang 1980; 38:* 121–137

117 Rose LM, Goldman M, Lambert PH. The production of anti-idiotypic antibodies and of idiotype-anti-idiotype immune complexes after polyclonal activation induced by bacterial LPS. *J Immunol 1982; 128:* 2126–2133

118 Schneeberger EE, Leber PD, Karnosvky MJ, McCluskey RT. Altered functional properties of the renal glomerulus in autologous immune complex nephritis. *J Exp Med 1974; 139:* 1283–1302

119 Ford PM, Kosatka I. The effect of in situ formation of antigen-antibody complexes in the glomerulus on subsequent glomerular localization of passively administered immune complexes. *Immunology 1980; 39:* 337–344

120 Haakenstad AO, Striker GE, Mannik M. Removal of glomerular immune complex deposits by excess antigen in chronic mouse model of immune complex disease. *Lab Invest 1983; 48:* 323–331

121 Sterzel RB, Lovett DH, Stein HD, Kashgarian M. The mesangium and glomerulonephritis. *Klin Wochenschr 1982; 60:* 1077–1094

122 Sterzel RB, Eisenbach GM, Seiler MW, Hoyer JR. Uptake of polyvinyl alcohol by macrophages in the glomerular mesangium of rats. Histological and functional studies. *Am J Pathol 1983; 111:* 247–257

123 Latta H, Fliegel S. Mesangial fenestrations, sieving, filtration, and flow. *Lab Invest 1985; 52:* 591–598

124 Seiler MW, Hoyer JR, Sterzel RB. Role of macrophages in the glomerular mesangial uptake of polyvinyl alcohol in rats. *Lab Invest 1983; 49:* 26–37

125 Mauer SM, Sutherland DER, Howard RJ et al. The glomerular mesangium. III. Acute immune mesangial injury: a new model of glomerulonephritis. *J Exp Med 1973; 137:* 553–570

126 Mauer SM, Fish AJ, Blau EB, Michael AF. The glomerular mesangium. I. Kinetic studies of macromolecular uptake in normal and nephrotic rats. *J Clin Invest 1972; 51:* 1092–1101

127 Keane WF, Raij L. Relationship among altered glomerular barrier permselectivity, angiotensin II, and mesangial uptake of macromolecules. *Lab Invest 1985; 52:* 599–604
128 Berger J. IgA glomerular deposits in renal disease. *Transplant Proc 1969; 1:* 939
129 Crabbe PA, Nash DR, Bazin H et al. Antibodies of the IgA type in intestinal plasma cells of germfree mice after oral or parenteral immunization with ferritin. *J Exp Med 1979; 130:* 723
130 Emancipator SN, Gallo GR, Lamm ME. Experimental IgA nephropathy induced by oral immunization. *J Exp Med 1983; 157:* 572–582
131 Sato M, Ideura T, Koshikawa S. Experimental IgA nephropathy in mice. *Lab Invest 1986; 54:* 377–384
132 Melvin T, Burke B, Michael AF, Kim Y. Experimental IgA nephropathy in bile duct ligated rats. *Clin Immunol Immunopath 1983; 27:* 369–377
133 Fleuren GJ, Grond J, Hoedemaeker PhJ. In situ formation of subepithelial complexes in passive serum sickness. *Kidney Int 1980; 17:* 631–637
134 Hoyer JR, Krueger ThE, Seiler MW. Kinetics of protamine-heparin complex formation in rat glomeruli during renal perfusion. *Kidney Int 1982; 21:* 102–105
135 Weening JJ, Grond J, Hoedemaeker PhJ. Effect of increased glomerular permeability on the localization of immune aggregates and protamine-heparin aggregates in the rat. *Lab Invest 1983; 49:* 619–625
136 Venkatachalam MA, Rennke HG. The structural and molecular basis of glomerular filtration. *Circulation Res 1978; 43:* 337–347
137 Ward HJ, Cohen AH, Border WA. In situ formation of subepithelial immune complexes in the rabbit glomerulus: requirement of a cationic antigen. *Nephron 1984; 36:* 257–264
138 Batsford SR, Oite T, Takamiya H, Vogt A. Anionic binding sites in the glomerular basement membrane: possible role on the pathogenesis of immune complex glomerulonephritis. *Renal Physiol 1980; 3:* 336–340
139 Border WA, Ward H, Kamil E, Cohen AH. Induction of membranous nephropathy in rabbits by administration of an exogenous cationic antigen. Demonstration of a pathogenic role for electrical charge. *J Clin Invest 1982; 69:* 451–461
140 Oite T, Shimizu F, Kihara I et al. An active model of immune complex glomerulonephritis in the rat employing cationized antigen. *Am J Path 1983; 112:* 185–194
141 Thaiss F, Batsford S, Mihatsch J et al. Mediator systems in a passive model of in situ immune complex glomerulonephritis. Role for complement, polymorphonuclear granulocytes. *Lab Invest 1986; 54:* 624–635
142 Oite T, Shimizu F, Suzuki Y, Vogt A. Ultramicroscopic localization of cationized antigen in the glomerular basement membrane in the course of active, in situ immune complex glomerulonephritis. *Virchows Arch [Cell Pathol] 1985; 48:* 107–118
143 Sawtell NM, Weiss MA, Pesce AJ, Michael JG. An immune complex glomerulopathy associated with glomerular capillary thrombosis in the laboratory mouse. A highly reproducible accelerated model utilizing cationized antigen. *Lab Invest 1987; 56:* 256–263
144 Gallo GR, Caulin-Glaser T, Lamm ME. Charge of circulating immune complexes as a factor in glomerular basement membrane localization in mice. *J Clin Invest 1981; 67:* 1305–1313
145 Kanwar YS, Caulin-Glaser T, Gallo GR, Lamm ME. Interaction of immune complexes with glomerular heparan sulfate-proteoglycans. *Kidney Int 1986; 30:* 842–851
146 Gauthier VJ, Mannik M. Only the initial binding of cationic immune complexes to glomerular anionic sites is mediated by charge-charge interactions. *J Immunol 1986; 136:* 3266–3271
147 Golbus SM, Wilson CB. Experimental glomerulonephritis induced by in situ formation of immune complexes in glomerular capillary wall. *Kidney Int 1979; 16:* 148–157
148 Oldstone MBA, Dixon FJ. Pathogenesis of chronic disease associated with persistent lymphocytic choriomeningitis viral infection. *J Exp Med 1969; 3:* 483–505
149 Oldstone MBA, Dixon FJ. Susceptibility of different mouse strains to lymphocytic choriomeningitis virus. *J Immunol 1968; 100:* 355

150 Muller-Peddinghaus R, Trautwein G. Studies on the pathogenesis of Aleutian disease of mink. XII. Immunopathological determination of immune complex glomerulonephritis. *Zbl Vet Med 1983; 30:* 487–501
151 Smith RD, Wehner RW. Acute cytomegalovirus glomerulonephritis. An experimental model. *Lab Invest 1980; 43:* 278–286
152 Wright NG, Cornwell HJC. Experimental canine adenovirus glomerulonephritis: histological, immunofluorescence and ultrastructural features of the early glomerular changes. *Br J Exp Path 1983; 64:* 312–319
153 Moorthy AV, Abreo K. Potentiation of nephrotoxic serum nephritis in Lewis rats by Freund's complete adjuvant – possible role for cellular immune mechanisms. *Clin Immunol 1983; 28:* 383–394
154 Tipping PG, Neale TJ, Holdsworth SR. T lymphocyte participation in antibody-induced experimental glomerulonephritis. *Kidney Int 1985; 27:* 530–538
155 Boyce NW, Tipping PG, Holdsworth SR. Lymphokine (MIF) production by glomerular T-lymphocytes in experimental glomerulonephritis. *Kidney Int 1986; 30:* 673–677
156 Bhan AK, Collins AB, Schneeberger EE, McCluskey RT. A cell mediated reaction against glomerular bound immune complexes. *J Exp Med 1979; 150:* 1410–1420
157 Schreiner GF, Unanue ER. Origin of the rat mesangial phagocyte and its expression of the leukocyte common antigen. *Lab Invest 1984; 51:* 515–523
158 Bolton WK, Tucker FL, Sturgill BC. New avian model of experimental glomerulonephritis consistent with mediation by cellular immunity. Nonhumorally mediated glomerulonephritis in chickens. *J Clin Invest 1984; 73:* 1263–1276
159 Miyasato F, Manaligod JR, Pollak VE. Auto-immune disease in NZB and NZB-NZW F1 mice. *Arch Pathol 1967; 83:* 20–30
160 Gunn HC, Ryffel B. Successful treatment of autoimmunity in (NZBxNZW)F1 mice with cyclosporin and (Nva2)-cyclosporin. II. Reduction of glomerulonephritis. *Clin Exp Immunol 1986; 64:* 234–242
161 Koffler D, Agnello V, Thorburn R, Kunkel HG. Systemic lupus erythematosus; prototype of immune complex nephritis in man. *J Exp Med 1971; 134:* 169s
162 Izui S, Lambert PM, Miescher PA. In vitro demonstration of a particular affinity of glomerular basement membrane and collagen for DNA. A possible basis for a local formation of DNA-anti-DNA complexes in systemic lupus erythematosus. *J Exp Med 1976; 144:* 428–443
163 Faaber P, Rijke TPM, Putte LBA van der et al. Cross-reactivity of human and murine anti-DNA antibodies with heparan sulfate. The major glycosaminoglycans in glomerular basement membrane. *J Clin Invest 1986; 77:* 1824–1830
164 O'Regan S, Turgeon C. Unilateral glomerular DNA-anti-DNA complex formation in situ. *J Clin Lab Immunol 1984; 15:* 101–104
165 Natali PG, Tan EM. Experimental renal disease induced by DNA-anti-DNA immune complexes. *J Clin Invest 1972; 51:* 345
166 Cavallo T, Graves K, Granholm NA. Murine lupus nephritis. Effects of glucocorticoid on circulating and tissue-bound immunoreactants. *Lab Invest 1983; 49:* 476–481
167 Izui S, McConahey PJ, Clark JP et al. Retroviral gp70 immune complexes in NZBx NZW F2 mice with murine lupus nephritis. *J Exp Med 1981; 154:* 517–528
168 Izui S, Hara I, Ming Hang et al. Association of elevated serum glycoprotein gp70 with increased gp70 immune complex formation and accelerated lupus nephritis in autoimmune male BXSB mice. *Clin Exp Immunol 1984; 56:* 272–280
169 Maruyama N, Furukawa F, Nakai Y et al. Genetic studies of autoimmunity in New Zealand mice. IV. Contribution of NZB and NZW genes to the spontaneous occurrence of retroviral gp70 immune complexes in (NZBxNZW)F1 hybrid and the correlation to renal disease. *J Immunol 1983; 130:* 740–746
170 Nagy I, Bajtai G, Brasch H et al. The role of hepatitis B surface antigen in the pathogenesis of glomerulonephritis. *Clin Nephrol 1979; 12:* 109–116
171 Izui S, McConahey PJ, Theofilopoulos AN, Dixon FJ. Association of circulating retroviral gp70-anti-gp70 immune complexes with murine systemic lupus erythematosus. *J Exp Med 1979; 149:* 1099–1116

172 Andrews J, Hang L, Theophilopoulos AN, Dixon FJ. Lack of relationship between serum gp70 levels and the severity of systemic lupus erythematosus in MRL/1 mice. *J Exp Med 1986; 163:* 458–462

173 Dueymes M, Fournie GJ, Mignon-Conte M et al. Prevention of lupus diseases in MRL/1, NZBxNZW, and BXSB mice treated with a cyclophosphazene derived drug. *Clin Immunol Immunopathol 1986; 41:* 193–205

174 Cavallo T, Goldman M, Lambert PH. Animal model of human disease. Proliferative glomerulonephritis associated with polyclonal B-cell activation. *Am J Path 1984; 114:* 346–349

175 Izui S, Lambert PH, Fournie GJ et al. Features of systemic lupus erythematosus in mice injected with bacterial liposacchariden. Identification of circulating DNA and renal localization. *J Exp Med 1977; 145:* 1115–1130

176 Sumazaki R, Fujita T, Kabashima T et al. Monoclonal antibody against bacterial lipopolysaccharide cross-reacts with DNA-histone. *Clin Exp Immunol 1986; 66:* 103–110

177 Bruijn JA, Oemar BS, Ehrich JHH et al. Antibasement membrane glomerulopathy in experimental trypanosomiasis. *J Immunol 1987:* in press

178 Zinkernagel RM. H-2 restriction of cell-mediated virus-specific immunity and immunopathology: self-recognition, altered self, and auto-aggression. In Talal N, ed. *Autoimmunity.* New York: Academic Press. 1977: 363

179 Morel-Maroger L, Sloper JC, Vinter J et al. An ultrastructural study of the development of nephritis in mice treated with interferon in the neonatal period. *Lab Invest 1978; 39:* 513–522

180 Druet P, Bernard A, Hirsch F et al. Immunologically mediated glomerulonephritis induced by heavy metals. *Arch Toxicol 1982; 50:* 187–194

181 Rolink AG, Pals ST, Gleichmann E. Allosuppressor and allohelper T cells in acute and chronic graft-vs-host disease. II. F1 recipients carrying mutations at H-2K and/or I-A. *J Exp Med 1983; 157:* 755–771

182 Bariety J, Druet P, Laliberte F, Sapin C. Glomerulonephritis with y and B1C-globulin deposits induced in rats by mercuric chloride. *Am J Pathol 1971; 65:* 293–302

183 Weening JJ, Fleuren GJ, Hoedemaeker PhJ. Demonstration of antinuclear antibodies in mercuric chloride-induced glomerulopathy in the rat. *Lab Invest 1978; 39:* 405–411

184 Weening JJ, Hoedemaeker PhJ, Bakker WW. Immunoregulation and antinuclear antibodies in mercury-induced glomerulopathy in the rat. *Clin Exp Immunol 1981; 45:* 64–71

185 Sapin C, Druet E, Druet P. Induction of anti-glomerular basement membrane antibodies in the Brown-Norway rat by mercuric chloride. *Clin Exp Immunol 1977; 28:* 173–179

186 Aten J, Bosman CB, Rozing J et al. HgC12-induced autoimmune glomerulonephritis (GN) in the BN rat. *6th Int Congress of Immunology.* Toronto 1986

187 Prummel B, Aten J, Bosman CB et al. Modulation by cyclosporin A (CyA) of toxin-induced autoimmune reactions and glomerulonephritis in the BN rat. *Kidney Int 1985; 28 (Abstract):* 696

188 Pelletier L, Pasquier R, Vial MC et al. Mercury-induced autoimmune glomerulonephritis: requirement for T-cells. *Nephrol Dial Transplant 1987; 1:* 211–218

189 Pelletier L, Pasquier R, Hirsch F et al. Autoreactive T cell in mercury-induced autoimmune disease: in vitro demonstration. *J Immunol 1986; 137:* 2548–2553

190 Hinglais N, Druet P, Grossetete J et al. Ultrastructural study of nephritis induced in BN rats by mercuric chloride in the BN rat. *Lab Invest 1979; 41:* 150–159

191 Bernaudin JF, Druet E, Belair MF et al. Extrarenal immune complex type deposits induced by mercuric chloride. *Clin Exp Immunol 1979; 38:* 265–273

192 Aten J, Bosman CB, Rozing J et al. Cellular kinetics and MHC II antigen expression in HgC12 induced glomerulonephritis in the BN rat. *8th Eur Immunol Meeting.* Zagreb 1987

193 Lymberi P, Hirsch F, Kuhn J et al. Autoimmunity induced by HgC12 in Brown-Norway rats. II. Monoclonal antibodies sharing specificities and idiotypes with mouse natural monoclonal antibodies. *J Immunol 1986; 136:* 3277–3281

194 Fleuren GJ, de Heer E, v Burgers J et al. Mercuric chloride-induced autoimmune glomerulopathy in Balb/c mice. *Kidney Int 1985; 28 (Abstract):* 702
195 Lewis RM, Armstrong MYK, Andre-Schwartz J et al. Chronic allogenic disease. I. Development of glomerulonephritis. *J Exp Med 1968; 128:* 653–679
196 Gleichmann E, Gleichmann H. Diseases caused by reactions of T lymphocytes to incompatible structures of the major histocompatibility complex. I. Autoimmune hemolytic anemia. *Eur J Immunol 1976; 6:* 899–906
197 Takacs L, Szende B, Rot A, Diamanstein T. Expression of MHC class II antigens on bile duct epithelium in experimental graft versus host disease. *Clin Exp Immunol 1985; 60:* 449–456
198 Fleuren GJ, Vries L de, Nieuwenhuis P, Hoedemaeker PhJ. Antibodies directed against renal antigens and graft-versus-host reactions in rats. *Nephrologie 1982; 3 (Abstract):* 93
199 Hoedemaeker PhJ, Fleuren GJ, Weening JJ. Etiologic factors in immunologically mediated glomerulonephritis. In Robinson E, ed. *Nephrology.* New York: Springer. 1984: 540–549
200 Bruijn JA, Elven EH van, Hogendoorn PCW et al. Murine graft-versus-host disease as a model for lupus nephritis. *Xth Int Congr Nephrol.* London 1987
201 Frenk S, Antonowicz I, Craig JM, Metcoff J. Experimental nephrotic syndrome induced in rats by aminonucleoside. Renal lesions and body electrolyte composition. *Proc Soc Exp Biol Med 1955; 89:* 424–427
202 Grond J, Elema JD. Glomerular mesangium: analysis of the increased activity observed in experimental acute aminonucleoside nephrosis in the rat. *Lab Invest 1981; 45:* 400–410
203 Olson JL, Rennke HG, Venkatachalam MA. Alterations in the charge and size selectivity barrier of the glomerular filter in aminonucleoside nephrosis in rats. *Lab Invest 1981; 44:* 271–279
204 Caulfield JP, Reid JJ, Farquhar MG. Alterations of the glomerular epithelium in acute aminonucleoside nephrosis: evidence for formation of occluding junctions and epithelial cell detachment. *Lab Invest 1976; 34:* 43–59
205 Wilson SGF, Hackel DB, Harwood S et al. Aminonucleoside nephrosis in rats. *Pediatrics 1958; 21:* 963–973
206 Hoyer JR, Mauer SM, Michael AF. Unilateral renal disease in the rat. I. Clinical morphologic and glomerular mesangial functional features in the experimental model produced by renal perfusion with aminonucleoside. *J Lab Clin Med 1975; 85:* 756–768
207 Hoyer JR, Ratte J, Potter AH, Michael AF. Transfer of aminonucleoside nephrosis by renal transplantation. *J Clin Invest 1972; 51:* 277–280
208 Derr RF, Loechler DK, Alexander CS, Nagasawa HT. Inhibition of aminonucleoside nephrosis in rats. IV. Prevention by N6-methyladenosine. *J Lab Clin Med 1968; 72:* 363–369
209 Glasser RJ, Velosa JA, Michael AF. Experimental model of focal sclerosis. I. Relationship to protein excretion in aminonucleoside nephrosis. *Lab Invest 1977; 36:* 519–526
210 Messina A, Davies DJ, Dillane PC, Ryan GB. Glomerular epithelial abnormalities associated with the onset of proteinuria in aminonucleoside nephrosis. *Am J Pathol 1987; 126:* 220–229
211 Caulfield JP, Farquhar MG. Loss of anionic sites from the glomerular basement membrane in aminonucleoside nephrosis. *Lab Invest 1978; 39:* 505–512
212 Kanwar YS, Rosenzweig LJ, Kerjaschki DI. Glycosaminoglycans of the glomerular basement membrane in normal and nephrotic states. *Renal Physiol 1981; 4:* 121–130
213 Lelong B, Makino H, Gibbons JT, Kanwar YS. Distribution of heparan-sulfate proteoglycans in aminonucleoside nephrosis. *Kidney Int 1986; 29 (Abstract):* 281
214 Abrahamson DR, Hein A, Caulfield JP. Laminin in glomerular basement membranes of aminonucleoside nephrotic rats. Increased proteinuria induced by antilaminin immunoglobulin G. *Lab Invest 1983; 49:* 38–47

215 Fishman JA, Karnovsky MJ. Effects of aminonucleoside of puromycin on glomerular epithelial cells in vitro. *Am J Pathol 1985; 118:* 398–407

216 Sternberg SS, Philips FS. Biphasic intoxication and nephrotic syndrome in rats given daunomycin. *Proc Am Ass Cancer Res 1967; 8:* 64

217 Bertani T, Poggi A, Pozzoni R et al. Adriamycin-induced nephrotic syndrome in rats. Sequence of pathologic events. *Lab Invest 1982; 46:* 16–23

218 Poggi A, Kornblihtt, Delaini F et al. Delayed hypercoagulability after a single dose of adriamycin to normal rats. *Thromb Res 1979; 16:* 639–650

219 Weening JJ, Rennke HG. Glomerular permeability and polyanion in Adriamycin nephrosis in the rat. *Kidney Int 1983; 24:* 152–160

220 Grond J, Weening JJ, Elema JD. Glomerular sclerosis in nephrotic rats. Comparison of the long term effects of Adriamycin and aminonucleoside. *Lab Invest 1984; 51:* 277–285

221 Bertani T, Rocchi G, Mecca G et al. Adriamycin induced chronic proteinuria: a new model of glomerular focal sclerosis. *Kidney Int 1983; 23 (Abstract):* 211

222 Rich AR. A hitherto undescribed vulnerability of the juxtamedullary glomeruli in lipid nephrosis. *Bull Johns Hopkins Hosp 1957; 100:* 173–186

223 Elema JD, Arends A. Focal and segmental hyalinosis and sclerosis in the rat. *Lab Invest 1975; 33:* 554–561

224 Olson JL, Hostetter Th, Rennke HG et al. Altered glomerular permselectivity and progressive sclerosis following extreme ablation of renal mass. *Kidney Int 1982; 22:* 112–126

225 Brenner BM, Meyer TW, Hostetter TH. Dietary protein intake and the progressive nature of kidney disease: the role of hemodynamically mediated glomerular injury in the pathogenesis of progressive glomerular sclerosis in aging, renal ablation and intrinsic renal disease. *N Engl J Med 1982; 307:* 651–659

226 Hostetter TH, Troy JL, Brenner BM. Glomerular hemodynamics in experimental diabetes mellitus. *Kidney Int 1981; 19:* 410–415

227 Dworkin LD, Hostetter TH, Rennke HG, Brenner BM. Hemodynamic basis for glomerular injury in rats with desoxycortico-sterone-salt hypertension. *J Clin Invest 1984; 73:* 1448–1461

228 Brenner BM. Nephron adaptation to renal injury or ablation. *Am J Physiol 1985; 249:* F324–F337

229 Rennke HG. Structural alterations associated with glomerular hyperfiltration. In Mitch WE, Stein J, Brenner BM, eds. *The Progressive Nature of Renal Disease.* New York: Churchill Livingstone Inc. 1986: 111

230 Weening JJ, Beukers JJB, Grond J, Elema JD. Genetic factors in focal segmental sclerosis. *Kidney Int 1986; 29:* 789–798

231 Alfrey AC. Thyroid and parathyroid hormones in experimental renal failure. In Mitch WE, Stein J, Brenner BM, eds. *The Progressive Nature of Renal Disease.* New York: Churchill Livingstone Inc. 1986: 37

232 Olson JL. Role of heparin as a protective agent following reduction of renal mass. *Kidney Int 1984; 25:* 376–382

233 Schneeberger EE, Collins AB, Latta H, McCluskey RT. Diminished glomerular accumulation of colloidal carbon in autologous immune complex nephritis. *Lab Invest 1977; 37:* 9–19

234 Zatz R, Meyer TW, Rennke HG, Brenner BM. Predominance of hemodynamic rather than metabolic factors in the pathogenesis of diabetic glomerulopathy. *Proc Natl Acad Sci USA 1985; 82:* 5963–5967

235 Purkerson ML, Valdes A, Yates J et al. Inhibition of thromboxane synthesis ameliorates the progressive kidney disease of rats with subtotal renal ablation. *Proc Natl Acad Sci USA 1985; 82:* 193–197

236 Anderson S, Meyer TW, Rennke HG, Brenner BM. Control of glomerular hypertension limits glomerular injury in rats with reduced renal mass. *J Clin Invest 1985; 76:* 612–619

237 Meyer TW, Anderson S, Rennke HG, Brenner BM. Reversing glomerular hypertension stabilizes established glomerular injury. *Kidney Int 1987; 31:* 752–759

238 Beukers JJB, Wal Avd, Hoedemaeker PhJ, Weening JJ. Converting-enzyme inhibition and progressive glomerulosclerosis in the rat. *Kidney Int:* in press

239 Terry R, Hawlins DR, Chuck EH, Whipple GH. Proteinuria related to hyperproteinemia in dogs following plasma given parenterally. *J Exp Med 1948; 87:* 561–573

240 Lawrence GB, Brewer DB. Normal urinary protein composition in the female Wistar rat and its relationship to the proteinuria induced by intraperitoneal bovine albumin. *Clin Sci Mol Med 1981; 60:* 693–702

241 Lawrence GB, Brewer DB. Effect of strain and sex on the induction of hyperalbuminaemic proteinuria in the rat. *Clin Sci Mol Med 1981; 61:* 751–756

242 Davies DJ, Brewer DB. Irreversible glomerular damage following heterologous serum albumin overload. *J Pathol 1977; 123:* 45–52

243 Lawrence GM, Brewer DB. Studies on the relationship between proteinuria and glomerular ultrastructural change in hyperalbuminaemic female Wistar rats. *J Pathol 1982; 138:* 365–383

244 Weening JJ, Guldener C van, Daha MR. The pathophysiology of protein overload nephrosis in the rat. *Am J Pathol 1987:* in press

245 Fisher ER, Hellstrom HR. Mechanism of proteinuria: functional and ultrastructural correlation of effects of infusion of homologous and heterologous protein (bovine serum albumin) in the rat. *Lab Invest 1962; 11:* 617–637

246 Bliss DJ, Brewer DB. Increased albumin and normal dextran. Clearances in protein-overload proteinuria in the rat. *Clin Sci 1985; 69:* 321–326

247 Ito H, Hattori S, Matusda I et al. Hepatitis B antigen-mediated membranous glomerulonephritis. Correlation of ultrastructural changes with Hbe Ag in the serum and glomerulus. *Lab Invest 1981; 44:* 214–221

248 Whitworth JA, Leibowitz S, Kennedy MC et al. Absence of glomerular renal tubular epithelial antigen in membranous glomerulonephritis. *Clin Nephrol 1976; 5:* 159–162

249 Lagrue G, Xheneumont S, Branallec A et al. A vascular permeability factor elaborated from lymphocytes. I. Demonstration in patients with nephrotic syndrome. *Biomedicine 1975; 23:* 37–40

250 Bakker WW, Luijk WHJ v, Hene RJ et al. Loss of glomerular polyanion in vitro induced by mononuclear blood cells from patients with minimal-change nephrotic syndrome. *Am J Nephrol 1986; 6:* 107–111

251 Hoorntje SJ, Kallenberg CGM, Weening JJ et al. Immune complex glomerulopathy in patients treated with Captopril. *Lancet 1980; i:* 1212–1215

252 Gleichmann H. Studies on the mechanism of drug sensitization: T-cell-dependent popliteal lymphnode reaction to diphenyl-hydantoin. *Clin Immunol Immunopathol 1981; 18:* 203–211

NEW CONCEPTS IN THE IMMUNOPATHOLOGY OF NEPHRITIS

A Fukatsu, G Salvidio, X-J Zhou, G Andres

State University of New York at Buffalo,
Renal Research Laboratory of the Buffalo General Hospital,
Buffalo, New York, USA

Introduction

The idea that immunological mechanisms may cause kidney disease was first suggested more than 70 years ago by von Pirquet [1], and confirmed after 1955 by the application of immunofluorescence technique to the study of renal tissues obtained from laboratory animals or from patients affected by glomerulonephritis [2]. At the end of 1960 the use of these techniques allowed identification of two immunofluorescence patterns of immune deposits in glomeruli: the first was 'linear', resulting from binding of antibodies to fixed structural antigens, such as the glomerular basement membrane (GBM); the second was 'granular' resulting from passive trapping of circulating immune complexes devoid of immunological specificity for glomerular structures. The main example of the first type of injury is Goodpasture's syndrome, and an example of the second is the glomerulonephritis of patients with systemic lupus erythematosus. This view of the pathogenesis of glomerulonephritis was prevalent for over two decades [3].

Recent advances in understanding the immunological basis of nephritis have led to a partial revision of these classical concepts. Progress has been achieved in several areas. We have a deeper insight of renal pathophysiology. Relevant kidney antigens are now biochemically and immunologically characterized. It is evident that, besides passive trapping of circulating immune complexes, circulating antibodies reactive with structural antigens, or with 'planted' non-glomerular autologous or exogenous antigens, can induce 'granular' immune deposits in renal structures. Some alterations of regulatory mechanisms leading to autoimmunity, and new mediators and new mediator pathways of tissue injury have been identified. There is evidence that T-cell mediated hypersensitivity can induce, alone or associated with other mechanisms, glomerular and tubulo-interstitial lesions. Most of these acquisitions derive from studies performed in laboratory animals. In this review some recent data pertinent to the pathogenesis of experimental and human kidney diseases mediated by hypersensitivity reactions are discussed, as they are presently understood. A more detailed review of this topic can be found in other recent publications [4–8].

Renal diseases induced by circulating antibodies

Circulating antibodies interacting in different tissue sites result in variable types of injury which may be explained by the special anatomical and physiological conditions in the target tissue. When antibodies react with fixed renal antigens, such as those in the GBM or in the tubular basement membrane (TBM), the resulting immune deposits are restricted to these structures and, thus, have a 'linear' immunofluorescence pattern. By way of contrast, when antibodies react with antigens expressed on the plasma membrane of cells, with 'planted' antigens which can be redistributed on the cell surface or rearranged in the extracellular matrix, the resulting immune deposits appear 'granular' by immunofluorescence and electron microscopy techniques.

Glomerulonephritis and tubulointerstitial nephritis induced by antibodies reactive with 'fixed' basement membrane antigens

The identification of human renal diseases associated with basement membrane antibodies was preceded by decades of studies performed in animals with nephrotoxic glomerulonephritis [9] or with Steblay's autoimmune glomerulonephritis or tubulointerstitial nephritis [10,11]. The human counterpart of Steblay's glomerulonephritis was identified by Lerner et al [12]. The responsible antigen has a molecular weight of ≈26,000 [13,14] and is localized in the globular domain of type IV collagen, which exists in a hexameric form, comprising monomeric and dimeric subunits [13]. The epitope is sequestered inside the hexamer, but becomes exposed, binding the specific antibody, when the hexamer is dissociated into subunits [15]. The sequestered antigen might provide an explanation for the observation that basement membranes, except GBM, react weakly with Goodpasture's antibodies in tissue sections unless the sections are pretreated with reagents which expose the antigen. It is conceivable that infections or toxic agents may contribute to the exposure of otherwise inaccessible antigen in a variety of tissues, thereby initiating, in genetically predisposed individuals [16], the antibody production.

There is convincing evidence that anti-TBM disease occurs in man, although it is rare. Anti-TBM tubulointerstitial nephritis is well documented in association with anti-GBM glomerulonephritis [17]. Moreover, TBM antibodies have been detected in the sera and in TBM of a few patients with severe acute tubulointerstitial nephritis apparently not associated with concomitant factors [18]. Attempts to transfer the disease to Brown Norway rats or to other mammals by intravenous injections of serum antibodies have been unsuccessful and only minimal binding of human IgG to TBM was found, suggesting that the antigen is not readily accessible to circulating IgG. TBM antibodies may occur in recipients of renal allografts. In some of these patients the antibodies react with the TBM of both the graft and the native kidneys and, therefore, behave like autoantibodies. In other patients, however, the antibodies react only with the TBM of the grafted kidney, suggesting that they may have been generated by an alloimmune response to a foreign TBM antigen present in the graft but not in the recipient [17,18]. Using a monoclonal TBM antibody affinity column the antigen responsible for the autoimmune response was isolated from human TBM. It is a 48,000 molecular weight protein [19–21] similar to the 48,000 molecular weight glycoprotein responsible for Steblay's tubulointerstitial nephritis in guinea pigs [22]. These studies show that TBM target epitopes and their immunological recognition are highly conserved among mammals.

Some of the mechanisms involved in the production and in the disappearance of anti-basement membrane antibodies were studied in animals injected with mercuric chloride ($HgCl_2$). This procedure induces a biphasic, systemic disease first characterized by autoantibodies reactive with the basement membranes and, then, by circulating antigen-antibody complexes containing the same kind of antibodies [23]. The autoimmune response depends upon two or three genes, one of which is H-1 linked [24]. The level of antibodies present in the serum reaches a peak two to three weeks after the beginning of injection of $HgCl_2$ and then rapidly declines. The synthesis of autoantibodies is generated by autoreactive T-cells and by a polyclonal stimulation of B-cells. Helper T-cells exposed to $HgCl_2$ induce both in vitro and in vivo a proliferation of normal autologous T lymphocytes in presence of Ia-positive syngeneic cells [25]. The self-limiting production of autoantibodies is probably related to the emergence of a clone of T-suppressor cells [26] and to the development of anti-idiotypic antibodies [27]. The studies show that the synthesis of autoantibodies is due to a drug-induced dysregulation of the immune response, similar to that observed in chronic graft-versus-host reactions [28].

Mesangial immune deposits, and concomitant lesions, are usually associated with circulating antigen-antibody complexes [4,5,17] or by circulating antibodies reactive with exogenous antigens 'planted' in the mesangium [28]. However, persistent immune deposits also develop in the mesangium of rats injected with a monoclonal antibody that exhibits specificity for an 81,000 molecular weight antigen present exclusively in the mesangial matrix [30]. Patients with IgA glomerulonephritis have circulating IgA antibodies against collagen IVα chains. The epitope appears located in the triple helical part of collagen IV. Inhibition studies demonstrate that the IgA antibodies are directed against epitopes present in collagen type I and II. The titres of these autoantibodies are correlated to disease activity [31]. Therefore, autoantibodies reactive with mesangial collagen might cooperate in the induction of glomerular lesions in man. Evidence that this indeed happens is lacking.

Glomerulonephritis and tubulointerstitial nephritis induced by antibodies reactive to cell surface antigens

When cultured cells, expressing surface antigens to receptors, are exposed to specific ligands in appropriate conditions, a redistribution of molecules takes place in the fluid mosaic of the plasma membrane with patching, capping and shedding and/or internalization of the complexes [32]. Similar events may occur in vivo. The prototype of this interaction is Heymann nephritis in which the pathogenic antigen (gp 330) is localized in the subapical brush border domain of proximal convoluted tubules, and along the glomerular visceral epithelial cell membrane, in the coated pits and in the endoplasmic reticulum [33]. When divalent antibodies react with the antigen expressed on the surface of glomerular epithelial cells the resulting immune complexes are redistributed at the cell surface and shed into the adjacent lamina rara externa and filtration slits [7]. The hydrodynamic forces of filtration prevent migration of immune complexes toward the endothelium, following the turnover rate of the GBM. The process of immune complex shedding requires an intact cytoskeleton. It is presently unknown whether shedding of the antigen (antigenic modulation) induces a temporary loss of target molecules at the cell surface that might account for the relatively slow accumulation of immune deposits, as compared to anti-GBM glomerulonephritis [29], another situation where glomerular immune deposits form in situ. This mechanism may also explain the capacity of protein synthesis inhibitors, such as aminonucleoside of puromycin, to prevent deposit formation in Heymann glomerulonephritis [5].

In Heymann glomerulonephritis and in immune complex oophoritis immune complexes are shed into basement membranes or basement membrane-like structures suitable for precipitation and aggregation of immune complexes resulting in large, granular, immune deposits. The outcome of antibody-cell surface antigen interaction, however, is different when shedding of immune complexes occurs at the bloodstream interface [7]. For instance, a rapid redistribution of endothelial immune complexes occurs in the lungs of rabbits injected into a vein of the ear with antibodies to angiotensin converting enzyme. The complexes are dispersed into the circulation and there is no formation of immune deposits in the alveolar capillary walls. In contrast, when endothelial immune complexes are shed from the renal endothelia a mild and transient glomerulonephritis with discrete subepithelial deposits ensues [34]. It is conceivable that the different results in the two experimental conditions are due to hydrodynamic forces operating in a vascular bed specialized in filtration. This hypothesis is consistent with the finding of larger subendothelial immune deposits containing endothelial immune complexes (angiotensin converting enzyme, and specific antibodies) when the glomerular permeability is artificially increased [34].

Heymann glomerulonephritis mimics some morphological and clinical aspects of human idiopathic membranous glomerulonephritis. Therefore, the possibility that an Heymann-like mechanism may operate in man has arisen considerable interest. Several laboratories have searched for evidence of brush border antigens or antibodies in human idiopathic membranous glomerulonephritis. With rare exceptions these have not been found [4,7,17]. Recent studies have shown that the main antigen of Heymann glomerulonephritis (gp 330) [33] is expressed on human tubular brush border, but not on glomerular epithelial cells. Moreover, when monkeys are actively (or passively) immunized with antigens (or antibodies) of human glomerular epithelial cells, membranous lesions are not observed despite evidence that the antibodies recognize antigens expressed on the surface of cultured monkey glomerular epithelial cells (personal observations). An Heymann-like mechanism might also be postulated to account for the membranous form of lupus glomerulonephritis where the polyspecific reactivity of some DNA antibodies results in antibody binding to renal cell membrane antigens [35,36], and also in localization in glomerular structures in mice [37]. It is obvious that antibodies unrelated to Heymann antigens or DNA, but specifically reactive with unknown glomerular epithelial cell antigens, might have a rôle in the pathogenesis of idiopathic or lupus membranous glomerulonephritis.

Rat mesangial cells share epitopes with T-cells [38]. When rats are injected intravenously with monoclonal (mouse) anti-rat Thy-1.1 antibody an acute glomerulonephritis with transient proteinuria occurs. The disease is characterized by immediate activation of complement and by lysis and proliferation of mesangial cells [39].

Antibody-cell surface antigen interactions, leading to in situ formation of immune deposits, can be experimentally induced in the renal tubules when a well characterized antigen-antibody system is available. In rabbits injected with heterologous antibodies to angiotensin converting enzyme granular immune deposits develop between the epithelial cells of proximal convoluted tubules (personal observation). In rats injected with heterologous antibodies to Tamm-Horsfall protein, similar changes occur between the epithelial cells of the ascending limb of Henle's loop [40]. Both angiotensin-converting enzyme and Tamm-Horsfall protein are expressed on the plasma membranes of epithelial cells in two diverse segments of the nephron. Similar lesions have not been described in humans.

Glomerulonephritis induced by antibodies reactive with 'planted' non-glomerular autologous, or exogenous, antigens

Aggregated γ-globulins, or preformed immune complexes, can be readily localized in the mesangium but there is little evidence of histological or functional changes. If, however, immune deposits are formed in situ by subsequent injection of specific antibodies a focal proliferative glomerulonephritis, similar to that seen in certain human glomerular diseases, occurs [41].

Glomerulonephritis can result from interaction of circulating antibodies with antigens mainly 'planted' on the endothelial side of the GBM. The antigens may be large and cationic, such as ferritin, which do not readily penetrate the capillary wall. The immune deposits subsequently dissociate across the GBM to reform in a subepithelial pattern [8]. Similar lesions occur when antibodies react with antigens which display affinity for certain molecules, such as lectins for the carbohydrate moieties of glycoproteins, which can result in localization along the inner surface of the capillary wall [42].

Membranous glomerulonephritis can be produced when antibodies react with cationic antigen bound by electrical charge to the 'fixed' anionic sites of the GBM, primarily heparan sulfate proteoglycans [5,8]. The subepithelial localization of the deposits probably reflects a coalescence of anionic structures that may occur after interaction with cationic molecules, as well as rearrangement of complexes which contain multivalent antigens and antibodies to condense into larger aggregates detectable by electron microscopy [5,8]. Treatment with polycations, to reduce glomerular negative charges, diminishes deposit formation in these models [5]. Glomerular lesions characterized by immune deposits containing exogenous anionic, rather than cationic antigens, such as DNA, probably also occur on a charge basis. In this situation the process which initiates the formation of immune deposits may be the localization of relatively cationic antibodies, rather than antigens, as suggested by perfusion studies, and by elution studies demonstrating a predominance of cationic antibodies in mice with lupus-like syndrome [5]. Alternatively, a variety of non-immune cationic proteins are released from neutrophils and from platelets following immune reaction and may localize on an electrical basis in the glomerulus [5]. Two studies have implicated an interaction of circulating antibodies with 'planted' cationic antigens in human post-streptococcal glomerulonephritis [43,44].

An important and frequently ignored feature of immune complexes is their continuing capability to react with free antigen or antibody [45], as well as with complement [46], rheumatoid factor [47] and anti-idiotypic antibodies [48], long after their initial formation. Such continuing interaction may modify or perpetuate the phlogogenic stimulus.

Glomerulonephritis and tubulointerstitial nephritis induced by antibodies reactive with antigens possibly secreted by, or leaking out of, cells

When circulating antibodies react with antigens secreted by or leaking out of cells the resulting 'granular' deposits tend to be localized at the site of interaction, although not as sharply so as when the antigen is structurally fixed to the site (basement membrane or cell surface). The classic experimental example of this form of injury is the Arthus reaction [49]. An Arthus-type injury develops around spermatogenic tubules following vasectomy [50], about thyroid follicles in thyroiditis [51], and in the basal part of proximal convoluted tubules in animals receiving multiple renal allografts or immunized with tubular cell homogenates [52]. Similar lesions were seen in some human renal allografts [53]. It is unknown in which conditions the antigens are secreted or released from cells.

It is also unknown whether such immune deposits develop in glomeruli. Possible candidates are the subepithelial deposits of animals injected with $HgCl_2$. Antibodies eluted from nephritic glomeruli react with basement membrane component secreted in vitro by glomerular visceral epithelial cells. Thus, it may be postulated that, in time, complexes of circulating antibodies and secreted basement membrane antigens condense into large subepithelial aggregates. Since immune complexes are present in the circulation of these animals it is difficult, or impossible, to separate the relative rôles of circulating immune complex from in situ immune complex formation [5,7].

Renal diseases induced by circulating antigen-antibody complexes

The most convincing evidence that certain types of glomerulonephritis are induced by passive trapping of antigen-antibody complexes formed in the circulation is based on the demonstration that the same reactants localized in glomerular structures (usually the mesangium and the subepithelial part of the capillary wall) are also detectable, in complex form, in the blood [6]. The observation that certain variables of immune complexes influence their deposition in structures specialized in filtration (renal glomeruli, choroid plexus, mesothelial capillaries) strengthen this evidence. The variables are: concentration of immune complexes in the circulation, lattice form, precipitability, electric charge, and role of the macrophage-phagocytic system (MPS) [6]. In spontaneous disease of laboratory animals and in human diseases the rates of immune complex formation and of removal are practically unknown. Experiments of injection of preformed immune complexes into mice indicate that the total load is a parameter, but that only a small amount of immune complexes deposit in glomeruli. Small-latticed immune complexes do not localize in tissues whereas lattices larger than $Ag_2{-}Ab_2$ deposit and persist in the mesangium. Formation of detectable immune deposits requires condensation of immune complexes into large aggregates and only non cross-linked complexes of precipitating antigen-antibody systems are capable of forming dense deposits visible by electron microscopy. Cationic immune complexes preferentially localize in the subepithelial part of the capillary wall. When the function of the MPS is impaired immune complexes persist longer in the circulation and induce severe tissue lesions. Genetic deficiencies of the complement system [54] and alterations of complement receptors on erythrocytes and on polymorphonuclear leucocytes appear to predispose to tissue injury [6]. Several forms of diseases experimentally induced or developing spontaneously in laboratory animals appear to originate from passive trapping of circulating immune complexes in a vascular bed specialized in filtration. Proliferative and exudative glomerulonephritides, with predominant mesangial and subendothelial deposits, occurring in animals with acute and chronic serum sickness [49], graft-versus-host [28,55] and host-versus-graft [56,57] reactions belong to this category. Mice and dogs with lupus-like syndromes also develop proliferative and exudative glomerular lesions probably related to circulating immune complexes [49]. Discrete or diffuse subepithelial immune deposits can be found in all these conditions suggesting that in situ formation of immune deposits may also occur [5]. Since in any systemic immune complex disease a dynamic equilibrium exists between antigen and antibody in free and immune complex form [45], the relationship between the two mechanisms is difficult or impossible to separate [5,7]. It is likely that both may cooperate, with variable preponderance, in the pathogenesis. When large amounts of immune complexes are present in the circulation for prolonged periods of time, a systemic disease may result, like in some high responder rabbits injected for months with foreign proteins, or in mice with lupus-like syndromes [17]. Human glomerulonephritides in which circulating antigen-antibody complexes are likely to have a preponderant pathogenic rôle are those associated with systemic lupus erythematosus or following bacterial infections [49].

Renal diseases induced by, or associated with, cell-mediated hypersensitivity
Several types of experimental or human proliferative glomerulonephritides are characterized by hypercellularity, but the nature and source of the cells infiltrated in the glomeruli have been only in part, identified. The first studies were performed testing in vitro the stimulatory effect of human GBM antigens on lymphocytes obtained from nephritic patients. It was found that the lymphocytes of patients with 'linear' deposits of human IgG in the GBM were particularly sensitive to the antigen and it was suggested that these cells had a rôle in the pathogenesis of the disease [58]. Other investigators found monocytes and macrophages in glomeruli of rats with nephrotoxic glomerulonephritis [59]. A similar mononuclear cell infiltration was seen in glomeruli of animals with renal allograft rejection, especially when the animals were injected with phytohaemagglutinin, a lectin with a stimulatory effect on T-cells. It was then proposed that the lymphocytes and macrophages are the effector cells, and the endothelium is the target structure [60]. The importance of these observations was better understood when the existence of cellular hypersensitivity to GBM antigens in human glomerulonephritis was confirmed [61,62], and when it was shown that the cells emerging from cultures of glomeruli obtained from patients [63] or from experimental animals [64] with crescentic glomerulonephritis are macrophages. It was subsequently discovered that the mesangium of the rat contains a subpopulation of monocytes with Ia-like determinants, and that these cells can specifically react with antigenic stimuli [65,66]. Other studies have shown that a cell-mediated reaction occurs in glomeruli of rats with nephrotoxic glomerulonephritis [67] or when immune complexes are 'planted' in the mesangium and the rats are subsequently injected with sensitized lymphocytes [68]. The evidence that cell-mediated hypersensitivity cooperates in the induction of antibody or immune complex-mediated injury is strengthened by the observations that exudative glomerular lesions of rabbits with acute serum sickness are abrogated by

administration of anti-macrophage serum [69], and that functional T-cells are required for the development of autoimmune GBM glomerulonephritis in humorally incompetent chickens [70]. The importance of these findings for the interpretation of human glomerulonephritis is shown by the presence of mononuclear cells in glomeruli of patients with a variety of proliferative glomerular diseases [71], and by the identification in renal allografts of patients with cytomegalovirus infection of a distinct form of glomerulonephritis in which the endothelium is the primary target and T-helper are the effector cells (RB Colvin et al, personal communication).

The results of the studies described above are consistent with the hypothesis that cell-mediated hypersensitivity has a rôle in the pathogenesis of glomerular injury initiated by antibodies reactive with structural glomerular antigens or by local deposition of circulating immune complexes. More detailed information concerning the nephritogenic immune response in general and, more specifically, the rôle of T-cell-mediated hypersensitivity results from investigations regarding the pathogenesis of experimental tubulointerstitial nephritis mediated by TBM antibodies. In this condition the nephritogenic immune response, initiated by TBM aautoantibodies includes the generation of antigen-reactive T-cells within the kidney. Concomitantly, there is development of a polyclonal T-cell suppression, a non-specific effect which might influence the further generation of associated immune responses, including the development of anti-idiotypic immunity. The polyclonal T-cell suppression could impair the host's ability to down regulate the production of TBM antibodies and the T-cell-mediated reaction [72].

Acknowledgements
The work was supported by US Public Health Service Grant AM-36807 of the National Institute of Diabetes, Digestive and Kidney Diseases, Bethesda, MD. GS was supported by a grant of the North Atlantic Treaty Organization (NATO), and the Consiglio Nazionale delle Ricerche (CNR) of Italy. X-J Z was supported by a grant of the China Medical University, People's Republic of China.

References

1 von Pirquet CE. *Allergy Arch Inter Med 1911; 7:* 259
2 Mellors RC, Ortega LG, Holman HR. Role of gamma globulin in the pathogenesis of renal lesions in systemic lupus erythematosus and chronic membranous glomerulo nephritis, with an observation on lupus erythematosus cell reaction. *J Exp Med 1957; 106:* 191–199
3 Dixon FJ. The pathogenesis of glomerulonephritis. *Am J Med 1968; 44:* 493–494
4 Couser WG, Salant DJ. Immunopathogenesis of glomerular capillary wall injury in nephrotic states. *Contemp Issues Nephrol 1982; 9:* 47 83
5 Couser WG. In situ formation of immune complexes and the role of complement activation in glomerulonephritis. *Clin Immunol Allergy 1986; 6:* 267–285
6 Wener MH, Mannik M. Mechanisms of immune deposit formation in renal glomeruli. *Springer Semin Immunopath 1986; 9:* 219–235
7 Andres G, Brentjens JR, Caldwell PRB et al. Biology of disease. Formation of immune deposits and disease. *Lab Invest 1986; 55:* 510–520
8 Vogt A. New aspects of the pathogenesis of immune complex glomerulonephritis: formation of subepithelial deposits. *Clin Nephrol 1984; 21:* 15–20

9 Unanue ER, Dixon FJ. Experimental glomerulonephritis: immunological events and pathogenetic mechanisms. *Adv Immunol 1967; 6:* 1–90

10 Steblay RW. Glomerulonephritis induced in sheep by injections of heterologous glomerular basement membrane and Freund's complete adjuvant. *J Exp Med 1962; 116:* 253–272

11 Steblay RW, Rudofsky U. Renal tubular disease and autoantibodies against tubular basement membrane induced in guinea pigs. *J Immunol 1971; 107:* 589–594

12 Lerner R, Glassock RJ, Dixon FJ. The role of antiglomerular basement membrane antibody in the pathogenesis of human glomerulonephritis. *J Exp Med 1967; 126:* 989–1004

13 Wieslander J, Barr JF, Butkowski RJ et al. Goodpasture antigen of the glomerular basement membrane: localization in the noncollagenous regions of type IV collagen. *Proc Natl Acad Sci USA 1984; 81:* 3838–3842

14 Fish AJ, Lockwood MC, Wong M, Price RG. Detection of Goodpasture antigen in fractions prepared from collagenase digests of human glomerular basement membrane. *Clin Exp Immunol 1984; 55:* 58–66

15 Wieslander J, Langeveld J, Butkowski R et al. Physical and immunochemical studies of the globular domain of type IV collagen. *J Biol Chem 1985; 260:* 8564–8570

16 Rees A, Peters DK, Compston DAS, Batchelor JR. Strong association between HLA-DRw2 and antibody-mediated Goodpasture's syndrome. *Lancet 1978; i:* 966–968

17 Wilson CB, Dixon FJ. Renal injury from immune reactions involving antigens in or of the kidney. In Brenner, Stein, eds. *Immunologic Mechanisms of Renal Disease, Contemporary Issues in Nephrology 3.* New York: Churchill Livingstone. 1979: 35–48

18 Andres GA, McCluskey RT. Tubular and interstitial renal disease due to immunologic mechanisms. *Kidney Int 1975; 7:* 271–289

19 Clayman MD, Michaud L, Brentjens J et al. Isolation of the target antigen of human anti-tubular basement membrane antibody-associated interstitial nephritis. *J Clin Invest 1986; 77:* 1143–1147

20 Yoshioka K, Marimoto Y, Iseki T, Maki S. Characterization of tubular basement membrane antigens in human kidney. *J Immunol 1986; 136:* 1654–1660

21 Butkowski RJ, Wieslander G, Brentjens JR et al. Identification of a target antigen in human anti-tubular basement membrane nephritis. *Kidney Int 1987; 31:* 800–807

22 Clayman MD, Martinez-Hernandez A, Michaud L et al. Isolation and characterization of the nephritogenic antigen producing anti-tubular basement membrane disease. *J Exp Med 1985; 161:* 290–305

23 Roman-Franco AA, Turiello M, Albini B et al. Anti-basement membrane antibody and immune complexes in rabbits injected with mercuric chloride ($HgCl_2$). *Kidney Int 1976; 10:* 549A

24 Druet E, Sapin C, Gunther E et al. Mercuric chloride-induced antiglomerular basement membrane antibodies in the rat. Genetic control. *Eur J Immunol 1977; 7:* 348–351

25 Pelletier L, Pasquier R, Hirsh F et al. Autoreactive T cells in mercury-induced autoimmune disease: in vitro demonstration. *J Immunol 1986; 137:* 2548–2554

26 Bowman C, Mason DW, Pusey CD, Lockwood CM. Auto-regulation of auto-antibody synthesis in mercuric chloride nephritis in the Brown Norway rat. I. A role for T suppressor cells. *Eur J Immunol 1984; 14:* 464–470

27 Chalopin JM, Lockwood CM. Autoregulation of autoantibody synthesis in mercuric chloride nephritis in the Brown Norway rat. II. Presence of antigen-augmentable plaque-forming cells in the spleen is associated with humoral factors behaving as auto-anti-idiotypic antibodies. *Eur J Immunol 1984; 14:* 470–475

28 Gleichmann E, Rolink AG, Pals ST, Gleichmann H. Graft-versus-host reactions (GVHRs): clues to the pathogenesis of a broad spectrum of immunologic diseases. *Transplant Proc 1983; 15:* 1436–1440

29 Mauer SM, Sutherland DER, Howard RJ et al. The glomerular mesangium. III. Acute immune mesangial injury: a new model of glomerulonephritis. *J Exp Med 1973; 137:* 553–570

30 Mendrick DL, Rennke HG. Immune deposits formed in situ by monoclonal antibody recognizing a new intrinsic rat mesangial matrix antigen. *J Immunol 1986; 137:* 1517–1526
31 Cederholm B, Wieslander J, Bygren P, Heingard D. Patients with IgA nephropathy have circulating anti-basement membrane antibodies reacting with structures common to collagen I, II, and IV. *Proc Natl Acad Sci USA 1986; 83:* 6151–6155
32 Schreiner GI, Unanue ER. Membrane and cytoplasmic changes in B lymphocytes induced by ligand-surface immunoglobulin interaction. *Adv Immunol 1976; 24:* 37–165
33 Kerjaschki D, Farquhar MG. Immunocytochemical localization of the Heymann antigen (gp330) in glomerular epithelial cells of normal Lewis rats. *J Exp Med 1983; 157:* 667–686
34 Matsuo S, Fukatsu A, Taub ML et al. Glomerulonephritis induced in the rabbit by antiendothelial antibodies. *J Clin Invest 1987:* in press
35 Eilat D. Cross-reaction of anti-DNA antibodies and the central dogma of lupus nephritis. *Immunol Today 1985; 6:* 123–127
36 Jacob L, Lety M-A, Louvard D, Bach J-F. Binding of a monoclonal anti-DNA autoantibody to identical protein(s) present at the surface of several human cell types involved in lupus pathogenesis. *J Clin Invest 1985; 75:* 315–317
37 Madaio MP, Carlson JA, Hodder S. Monoclonal anti-DNA antibodies bind directly to intrinsic glomerular antigens and form immune deposits. *Kidney Int 1985; 27:* 216A
38 Paul LC, Rennke HG, Milford EL, Carpenter CB. Thy-1.1 in glomeruli of rat kidney. *Kidney Int 1984; 25:* 771–778
39 Bagchus WM, Hoedemaeker PhJ, Rozing J, Bakker WW. Glomerulonephritis induced by monoclonal anti-Thy 1.1 antibodies. *Lab Invest 1986; 55:* 680–687
40 Hoyer J. Tubulointerstitial immune complex nephritis in rats immunized with Tamm-Horsfall protein. *Kidney Int 1980; 17:* 284–290
41 Mauer SM, Sutherland DER, Howard RJ et al. The glomerular mesangium. III. Acute immune mesangial injury: a new model of glomerulonephritis. *J Exp Med 1973; 137:* 553–570
42 Globus SM, Wilson CB. Experimental glomerulonephritis induced by in situ formation of immune complexes in the glomerular capillary wall. *Kidney Int 1979; 16:* 148–157
43 Lange K, Seligson G, Cronin W. Evidence for the in situ origin of post-streptococcal glomerulonephritis: glomerular localization of endostreptosin and the clinical significance of the subsequent antibody response. *Clin Nephrol 1983; 19:* 3–16
44 Vogt A, Betsford S, Rodriguez-Iturbe B, Garcia R. Cationic antigens in poststreptococcal glomerulonephritis. *Clin Nephrol 1983; 20:* 271–279
45 Lambert P-H, Bricteux N, Salmon J, Miescher PA. Dynamics of immune complex nephritis during antibody excess. *Int Arch Allergy 1973; 45:* 185–189
46 Miller GW, Nussenzweig V. A new complement function: solubilization of antigen-antibody aggregates. *Proc Natl Acad Sci USA 1975; 72:* 418–422
47 McIntosh RM, Griswold WR, Chernack WB et al. III. Further studies on the nature, incidence, clinical diagnostic, prognostic, and immunopathologic significance of cryoproteins in renal disease. *QJ Med 1975; 174:* 285–307
48 Goldman M, Rose LM, Hochmann A, Lambert P-H. Deposition of idiotype-anti-idiotype immune complexes in renal glomeruli after polyclonal B cell activation. *J Exp Med 1982; 155:* 1385–1399
49 Cochrane CG, Koffler D. Immune complex disease in experimental animals and man. *Adv Immunol 1973; 16:* 185–264
50 Bigazzi PE, Kosuda LL, Hsu KC, Andres GA. Immune complex orchitis in vasectomized rabbits. *J Exp Med 1976; 143:* 382–404
51 Clagett JA, Wilson CB, Weigle WO. Interstitial immune complex thyroiditis in mice: the role of autoantibody to thyroglobulin. *J Exp Med 1974; 140:* 1439–1452
52 Klassen J, Milgrom F. Autoimmune concomitants of renal allografts. *Transplant Proc 1969; 1:* 605–607
53 Andres GA, Accinni L, Hsu KC et al. Human renal transplants. III. Immunopathologic studies. *Lab Invest 1970; 22:* 588–604

54 Schifferli JA, Ng YC, Peters KD. The role of complement and its receptor in the elimination of immune complexes. *N Engl J Med 1986; 315:* 488–495
55 Lewis RM, Armstrong MYK, Andre-Schwartz J et al. Chronic allogeneic disease. I. Development of glomerulonephritis. *J Exp Med 1968; 128:* 653–680
56 Hard RC, Moncure CW, Still WJS. Renal lesions with organized deposits and lipid as part of the host versus graft syndrome in parent/F1 mouse chimeras. *Lab Invest 1973; 28:* 468–476
57 Goldman M, Feng H-M, Engers H. Autoimmunity and immune complex disease after neonatal induction of transplantation tolerance in mice. *J Immunol 1983; 131:* 251–258
58 Rocklin RE, Lewis EJ, David JR. In vitro evidence for cellular hypersensitivity to glomerular basement membrane antigens in human glomerulonephritis. *N Engl J Med 1970; 283:* 497–501
59 Kondo Y, Sigematsu H, Kobayashi Y. Cellular aspects of rabbit Masugi nephritis. II. Progressive glomerular injuries with crescent formation. *Lab Invest 1972; 27:* 620–631
60 Andres GA, Cerra F, Elti G et al. Lymphocyte and blast cell glomerulonephritis in renal allografts of rats injected with phtyohaemagglutinin. *Cell Immunol 1974; 13:* 146–163
61 Mahieu P, Dardenne M, Bach JF. Detection of humoral and cell-mediated immunity to kidney basement membranes in human renal diseases. *Am J Med 1972; 53:* 185–192
62 Fillit H, Read SE, Sherman RL et al. Cellular reactivity to altered glomerular basement membrane in glomerulonephritis. *N Engl J Med 1978; 298:* 862–868
63 Atkins RC, Glasgow EF, Holdsworth SR, Matthews FE. The macrophage in human rapidly progressive glomerulonephritis. *Lancet 1976; i:* 830–832
64 Holdsworth SR, Thomson NM, Glasgow et al. Tissue culture of isolated glomeruli in experimental crescentic glomerulonephritis. *J Exp Med 1978; 147:* 98–109
65 Schreiner GF, Cotran RS, Prado V, Unanue ER. A mononuclear cell component in experimental immunological glomerulonephritis. *J Exp Med 1978; 147:* 369–384
66 Schreiner GF, Kiehly JM, Cotran RS, Unanue ER. Characterization of resident glomerular cells in the rat expressing Ia determinants and manifesting genetically restricted interaction with lymphocytes. *J Clin Invest 1981; 68:* 920–931
67 Bhan AK, Schneeberger EE, Collins AB, McCluskey RT. Evidence for a pathogenic role of a cell-mediated immune mechanisms in experimental glomerulonephritis. *J Exp Med 1978; 148:* 246–260
68 Bhan AK, Collins AB, Schneeberger EE, McCluskey RT. A cell mediated reaction against glomerular-bound immune complexes. *J Exp Med 1979; 150:* 1410–1420
69 Holdsworth SR, Neale TJ, Wilson CB. Abrogation of macrophage-dependent injury in experimental glomerulonephritis in the rabbit. *J Clin Invest 1981; 68:* 686–698
70 Bolton WK, Tucker FL, Sturgill BC. New avian model of experimental glomerulonephritis consistent with mediation by cellular immunity. *J Clin Invest 1984; 73:* 1263–1276
71 Monga G, Mazzucco G, di Belgioioso GB, Busnach G. The presence and possible role of monocyte infiltration in human chronic proliferative glomerulonephritis. *Am J Path 1979; 94:* 271–284
72 Neilson EG, Zakheim B. T cell regulation anti-idiotypic immunity, and the nephritogenic immune response. *Kidney Int 1983; 24:* 289–302

PATHOPHYSIOLOGICAL EFFECTS OF IMMUNE RENAL INJURY

R C Blantz, F B Gabbai, S Thomson, *C B Wilson

*University of California, San Diego and Veterans Administration Medical Center, San Diego, California, *Research Institute of Scripps Clinic, La Jolla, California, USA*

Introduction

Large reductions in the rate of glomerular filtration can result from both proliferative glomerulonephritis and from membranous nephropathy, two important causes of renal disease in man. Immunopathologists have described these two types of glomerulonephritis in great detail and much is known regarding their immunopathogenesis. Recently, physiologists have begun to study the mechanisms whereby glomerular filtration is altered in these two distinct immune-mediated diseases [1,2]. The purpose of this paper is to summarize the current state of knowledge, comparing and contrasting the effects of proliferative and membranous glomerulonephritis on the process of glomerular filtration [3–18].

Experimental micropuncture techniques are currently available which allow for the calculation from direct measurement of each of the determinants of glomerular filtration. These techniques involve the measurement of glomerular capillary and Bowman's space hydrostatic pressures (P_G and P_{BS}), systemic and efferent glomerular arteriolar plasma protein concentrations, and single nephron glomerular filtration rate . From these measurements, the rate of single nephron plasma flow and the hydraulic conductivity or glomerular ultrafiltration coefficient (LpA) of the glomerular capillary network can be calculated. Experiments generally employ Munich-Wistar rats which contain glomeruli accessibly located on the surface of their kidneys. Fortuitously, this same strain of rat serves well in experimental models of membranous and proliferative glomerulonephritis which closely mimic human diseases. The application of micropuncture to the study of the pathophysiology of immune renal injury has provided insight into the mechanisms whereby immune insults can alter glomerular haemodynamics thereby lowering glomerular filtration rate.

Proliferative glomerulonephritis

Animal models of proliferative glomerulonephritis were first subjected to renal micropuncture in the mid-1970s. These studies were performed in rats infused with antibody to glomerular basement membrane (anti-GBM Ab) [3–6]. Infusion of this antibody incites an inflammatory reaction within the kidney which leads rapidly to a diminution of single nephron glomerular filtration rate, causing it to fall by more than 50% within 60–90 minutes [4,5]. Glomerular haemodynamic measurements in this model have consistently implicated a decline in glomerular ultrafiltration coefficient as the predominant cause of this decrease in single nephron glomerular filtration rate. More variably, anti-GBM Ab, particularly when administered in high doses, has been associated with a reduction in single nephron plasma flow. In contrast to changes in LpA and single nephron plasma flow, which conspire to suppress filtration, the glomerular capillary hydrostatic pressure gradient (P_G-P_{BS} or ΔP) is consistently elevated above normal in animal models of proliferative glomerulonephritis. This increase in ΔP tends to ameliorate the effect of declining LpA and single nephron plasma flow on single nephron glomerular filtration rate. Even in mild forms of proliferative glomerulonephritis, where single nephron plasma flow is unaffected and single nephron glomerular filtration rate relatively well preserved, LpA is depressed and ΔP elevated [6].

The reduction in LpA observed acutely after an infusion of anti-GBM Ab may in part be explained by the rheological effect of polymorphonuclear leucocytes accumulating within the glomerular capillary bed (Figure 1). Electron micrographs demonstrate an increased number of neutrophils in glomerular capillary lumina within 15 minutes of anti-GBM Ab administration. Cytoplasmic projections from these cells extend into endothelial fenestrae, implying a relatively strong adherence of polymorphonuclear leucocytes to capillary wall and resultant localized increase in vascular resistance [4]. The presence of available shunts thereby facilitates the adherence of white blood corpuscles to capillary walls in response to leucotactic stimuli.

Furthermore, when a capillary segment contains a localized partial obstruction and the flow through it is diminished, each element of plasma traversing that segment does so more slowly, being exposed for a longer time to the forces of filtration while moving any given axial distance. If flow within a segment decreases to a sufficient degree, filtration pressure equilibrium will occur within that segment when ΔP meets equal opposition from a rising intracapillary oncotic pressure. The remaining endothelial surface downstream from the point where filtration pressure equilibrium occurs is 'lost' as effective filtering surface area. The lower the flow, the more area is lost.

Conversely, unobstructed segments conduct a greater proportion of the total nephron plasma flow without exposing that plasma to any greater filtering surface area. Filtration pressure equilibrium is not achieved within these segments which become more disequilibrated the greater the flow.

When plasma from multiple pathways combines at the efferent arteriole, the protein concentration of the resultant mixture is less than that leaving a capillary network where flow is better matched to surface area. The diminished whole

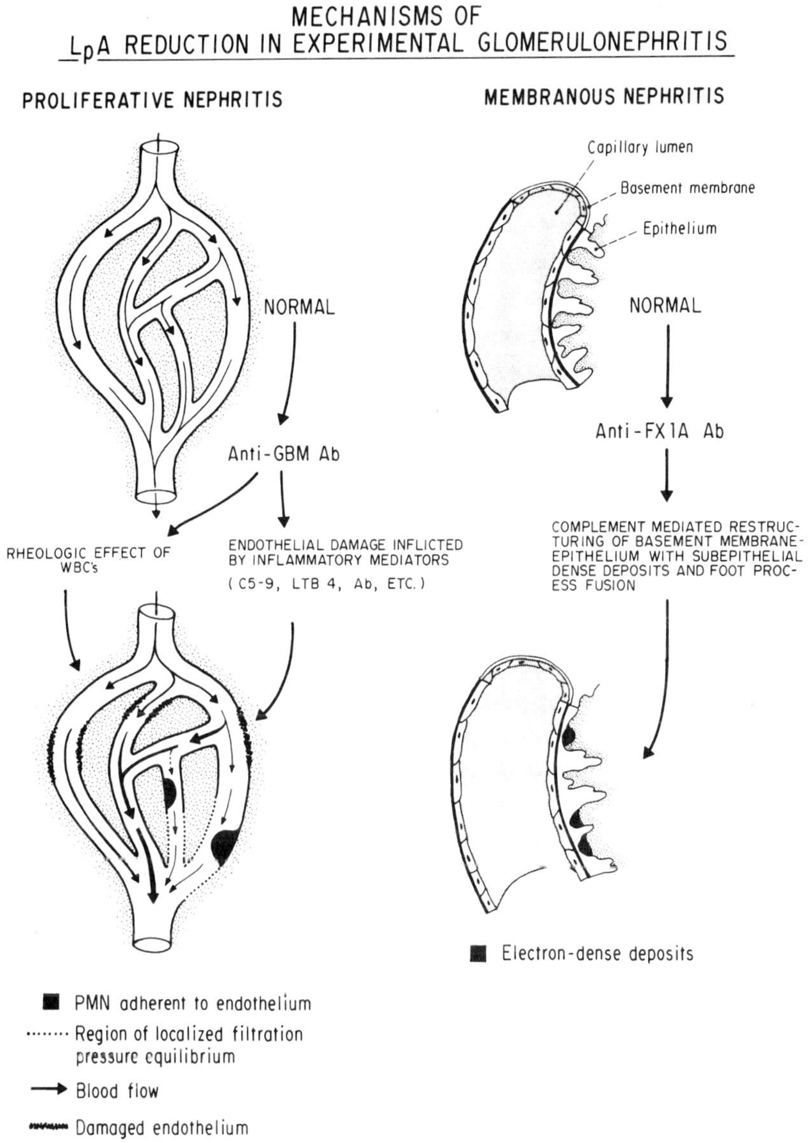

Figure 1. Several factors contribute to the reduction in glomerular ultrafiltration coefficient (LpA) and increase in glomerular capillary hydrostatic pressure gradient (ΔP) in experimental models of proliferative glomerulonephritis (anti-GBM antibody induced) and membranous nephropathy (passive Heymann nephritis, five days after anti-Fx1A antibody). Adherence of inflammatory cells to glomerular capillary wall may divert glomerular blood flow (designated direction of flow by arrows) and/or lead to local filtration pressure equilibrium, leading to loss of effective capillary surface area after administration of anti-GBM Ab. In experimental membranous nephropathy, deposition of anti-Fx1A Ab on the surface of glomerular epithelial cells may lead to formation of electron dense deposits (by 'capping and shedding') and fusion of epithelial cell foot processes, which may provide a partial physical explanation for the reduction in LpA. Although both models of glomerular immune injury exhibit reductions in LpA and increased ΔP, the physical events contributing to the alterations differ significantly

nephron filtration fraction will result in a lower computed LpA independent of any actual change in the structure or intrinsic filtering properties of the capillary membrane.

Additionally, Badr and associates have preliminarily demonstrated that by administering an antagonist to leukotriene D4 (LTD4), one can ameliorate the acute reduction in LpA seen following anti-GBM Ab infusion. This effect may be achieved with no apparent reduction in the numbers of polymorphonuclear leucocytes accumulating within glomerular capillary lumina [10]. These data suggest that white blood corpuscles function humorally via liberation of LTD4, as well as mechanically to impair LpA in anti-GBM Ab nephritis.

White blood corpuscles are not the only notable participants in the derangement of LpA in this model. Studies from our laboratory strongly implicate a rôle for the complement system in the early phases of anti-GBM Ab-induced glomerular injury [5]. Depletion of complement by prior treatment with cobra venom factor improves single nephron plasma flow and partially mitigates the effect of anti-GBM Ab on LpA. This attenuation, however, is associated with a significant decrease in the number of polymorphonuclear leucocytes observed within glomerular capillaries, suggesting an important role for complement components as leucoattractants in this model. Additionally, Pelayo et al have demonstrated that, when infused into the renal artery of normal rats, C5a exerts direct effects on the renal vasculature, primarily causing efferent arteriolar vasoconstriction, thereby causing P_G to rise and single nephron plasma flow to fall [27]. Still others have identified deposits containing membrane attack complex (C5b-9) within glomerular capillaries in experimental proliferative glomerulonephritis [28].

In addition to leucocytes and complement, studies have been performed to evaluate the role of angiotensin II and the adrenergic nervous system in modulating glomerular haemodynamics in anti-GBM Ab nephritis. To date. no rôle has been demonstrated for angiotensin while alpha adrenergic blockade will increase single nephron plasma flow in those instances in which anti-GBM Ab has lowered it [9].

In summary, experimental acute proliferative glomerulonephritis is characterized by a reduction in glomerular ultrafiltration coefficient and an increase in glomerular capillary hydrostatic pressure and these changes are mediated by leucocytes and complement.

Membranous nephropathy

Membranous nephropathy is a disorder characterized by damage to the glomerular capillary wall which occurs in the absence of any inflammatory cellular infiltrate [29]. The human form of this condition is closely approximated by Heymann nephritis, an experimental model generated by immunizing rats with Fx1A, a renal epithelial antigen localized to the brush border of the proximal tubule [12,29]. Proteinuria, fusions of epithelial foot processes and subepithelial electron dense deposits appear simultaneously several weeks after active immunization with Fx1A. These findings bear close resemblance to those in human membranous nephropathy.

The elapsed time required to produce proteinura can be shortened considerably by substituting heterologous anti-Fx1A Ab for active immunization [11,14, 15,25]. This latter model, termed 'passive Heymann nephritis', follows a reproducible time course characterized by the abrupt onset of proteinuria on the fifth day after antibody administration [15,25].

Current understanding of the pathogenesis of experimental membranous nephropathy stems largely from the work of Couser and Salant [13,14,25]. Led on by the finding of intraglomerular complement deposits in Heymann nephritis, these investigators demonstrated that complement depletion will prevent proteinuria from developing on the fifth day after anti-Fx1A Ab, and have provided evidence that the terminal complement components (C5b–C9) play a critical rôle in the development of proteinuria and glomerular injury in this model.

Given this information, questions arose regarding the time course of glomerular injury and the temporal relationship between histological and functional abnormalities in passive Heymann nephritis. We recently reported studies examining the evolution of glomerular haemodynamic changes, glomerular antibody deposition and morphological alterations in passive Heymann nephritis. Experiments were performed both on the third day and concurrent with the onset of overt proteinuria on the fifth day after administration of anti-Fx1A Ab [15]. On day three, LpA, ΔP, single nephron plasma flow and single nephron glomerular filtration rate all remained within the limits of normal. Quantitative determination of anti-Fx1A Ab binding yielded 38.0±0.9μg Ab/7.6x10^4 glomeruli, and kidneys appeared normal under light microscopy. Electron microscopy demonstrated few and small subepithelial electron dense deposits with modest foot process fusion. On day five, commensurate with the onset of proteinura, LpA was diminished by 70% while ΔP was elevated significantly above its measured value on day three. Anti-Fx1A binding had increased by 35% to 51.8±4.2μg Ab/7.6x10^4 glomeruli. Light microscopy still revealed normal glomeruli without inflammatory infiltrate but, on electron microscopy, subepithelial dense deposits were larger and more prominent and zones surrounding these deposits exhibited more extensive epithelial cell foot process fusion (Figure 1).

This association, as observed between dense deposits, foot process fusion and LpA reduction remains purely correlative and as such cannot confirm a cause and effect relationship among these factors, but coincident evidence has accumulated which would support a cause and effect hypothesis. The evolution over time of morphological change implies that alterations in epithelial cell architecture are not an immediate consequence of antibody fixation in passive Heymann nephritis. Matsuo, Andres and co-workers [30] have related the gradual remoulding of epithelial cell structure to a 'capping and shedding' phenomenon whereby antigen-antibody complexes undergo redistribution on the cell surface followed by elimination from the cell membrane. Capping and shedding can be prevented by the administration of chlorpromazine which also has been found to prevent proteinuria in passive Heymann nephritis [18]. Conceivably, capping and shedding requires cytoskeletal rearrangement within the epithelial cell which in turn leads to foot process fusion, increased permeability to protein and decreased permeability to water and small solutes.

In addition to the effects of deranged epithelial structure on glomerular haemodynamics, LpA and ΔP may also undergo functional alterations in passive Heymann nephritis. In a model of chemically induced nephrotic syndrome, infusion of saralasin, an angiotensin II receptor agonist, normalized glomerular filtration rate [31]. Angiotensin II, whether infused into or generated locally within the kidney leads to a lowering of LpA and an elevation of ΔP [32]. Yoshioka has observed that proteinuria can be diminished in experimental membranous nephropathy by using angiotensin II antagonists to lower ΔP [33]. We have further examined the rôle of angiotensin II by measuring the glomerular haemodynamic response before and after acute infusion of angiotensin converting enzyme inhibitor and after chronic treatment with angiotensin converting enzyme inhibitor in rats which had received anti-Fx1A Ab five days previously. We found that angiotensin converting enzyme inhibitor modified the haemodynamic response to the antibody by lowering renal vascular resistance thereby allowing for an increase in single nephron plasma flow. LpA, however, remained unimproved [16].

As previously noted, Couser and Salant have established a role for complement in the evolution of membranous nephropathy [13,25]. Gabbai and co-workers from our laboratory have performed glomerular haemodynamic measurements in animals depleted of complement and given anti-Fx1A Ab. On day five, proteinuria was absent, ΔP was not elevated and LpA, though still lower than normal, was significantly improved over values obtained in non-complement depleted rats with passive Heymann nephritis [17]. Morphological analysis of tissue from antibody treated rats with and without complement depletion revealed only minor differences between the two groups with slightly less epithelial foot process fusion in the complement depleted group. These morphological differences were not considered sufficient to account for the improvement in LpA achieved by administering cobra venom factor to rats with passive Heymann nephritis.

Despite their disparate pathogeneses, proliferative glomerulonephritis and membranous nephropathy bear much in common with respect to altered determinants of glomerular filtration. In both conditions, LpA is diminished while ΔP is increased. These findings hold over a broad range of nephron plasma flows and have been seen in all models of immune-induced glomerular injury studied to date [1]. One tenable hypothesis which may account for the general association between increased ΔP and decreased LpA involves the loss of a path of egress for fluid from the glomerular capillary. Under normal circumstances, the capillary membrane and efferent arteriole serve as parallel impediments to plasma flow of the same order of magnitude. When LpA diminishes, the total resistance to flow out of the glomerulus increases. If blood pressure and afferent resistance remain constant, then P_G varies in direct proportion to this 'effective efferent resistance' which rises as LpA falls. Therefore, some increase in ΔP may be a natural and passive consequence of a reduced LpA, the primary haemodynamic abnormality in immune-reduced glomerular injury.

A more testable hypothesis to explain changes in glomerular hydrostatic pressure invokes the suppression of tubuloglomerular feedback in response to a diminution of tubular flow past the macula densa [34] in glomerulonephritis, leading in turn to renal afferent arteriolar vasodilation. This notion has been investigated by workers from different laboratories with no strong evidence forthcoming to implicate this mechanism in the elevation of P_G in proliferative glomerulonephritis [35,36].

In summary, immune-induced glomerular injury of both proliferative and membranous varieties is characterized by large reductions in the glomerular ultrafiltration coefficient, Lpa, which are partially neutralized by an increase in the hydrostatic pressure gradient, ΔP. Changes in nephron plasma flow are variable and inconsistent. These glomerular haemodynamic abnormalities are common to diverse models of immune injury with disparate pathogenetic mechanisms. In both proliferative and membranous diseases, complement mediates a significant portion of the observed reduction in LpA. In the future, other functional mediators may come to light which will enable the tailoring of specific therapies to alter the course and improve the prognosis of persons afflicted with immune-induced glomerulonephritis.

Acknowledgments

These studies were supported through grants from the National Institutes of Health (DK28602, DK20043 and DK32353) and funds from the Research Service of the Veterans Administration. Dr Gabbai was supported by a grant from the Fogarty International Center of the National Institutes of Health. Dr Thomson is supported by a Physician-Scientist Award (NIH 1 K12 AM01408). This is Publication No IMM-4925 from the Department of Immunology, Research Institute of Scripps Clinic, La Jolla, CA 92037, USA.

References

1 Wilson CB, Blantz RC. Nephroimmunopathology and pathophysiology. *Am J Physiol 1985; 248.* F319–F331

2 Blantz RC, Hostetter TM, Brenner BM. Functional adaptations of the kidney to immunological injury. In Wilson CB, Brenner BM, Stein JH, eds. *Immunologic Mechanisms of Renal Disease.* New York: Churchill Livingstone. 1979: 122–143

3 Allison M, Wilson CB, Gottschalk CW. Pathophysiology of experimental glomerulonephritis in rats. *J Clin Invest 1974; 53:* 1402–1423

4 Blantz RC, Wilson CB. Acute effects of anti-glomerular basement membrane antibody on the process of glomerular filtration in the rat. *J Clin Invest 1976; 58:* 899–911

5 Blantz RC, Tucker BJ, Wilson CB. The acute effects of anti-glomerular basement membrane antibody on the process of glomerular filtration in the rat: the influence of dose and complement depletion. *J Clin Invest 1978; 61:* 910–921

6 Maddox DA, Bennett CM, Deen WM et al. Determinants of glomerular filtration in the rat. *J Clin Invest 1975; 55:* 305–318

7 Tucker BJ, Wilson CB, Gushwa LC, Blantz RC. Effect of leukocyte depletion on glomerular dynamics during acute glomerular immune injury. *Kidney Int 1985; 28:* 28–35

8 Wilson CB, Gushwa LC, Peterson OW et al. Glomerular immune injury in the rat. The effect of antagonists of histamine activity. *Kidney Int 1981; 20:* 628–635

9 Blantz RC, Tucker BJ, Gushwa L et al. Glomerular immune injury in the rat. The influence of AII and α-adrenergic inhibitors. *Kidney Int 1981; 20:* 452–461

10 Badr KF, Gung A, Schreiner GF et al. Reversal of antiglomerular basement membrane-antibody (a-GBM Ab)-induced fall in the glomerular ultrafiltration coefficient (Kf) by leukotriene D4 (LTD4) antagonist Sk&F 104353. *Kidney Int 1987; 31:* 363 (abstr)

11 Ichikawa I, Hoyer JR, Seiler MW, Brenner BM. Mechanism of glomerular injury. Preservation of a close functional linkage between individual nephrons and surrounding microvasculature. *J Clin Invest 1982; 69:* 185–198

12 Heymann W, Hackel DB, Harwood S et al. Production of the nephrotic syndrome in rats by Freund's adjuvants and rat kidney suspension. *Proc Soc Exp Med 1959; 100:* 660–664

13 Groggel GC, Adler S, Rennke HG, Couser WG. Role of the terminal complement pathway in experimental membranous nephropathy in the rabbit. *J Clin Invest 1983; 72:* 1948–1957

14 Adler S, Baker PJ, Pritzl P, Couser WG. Detection of terminal complement components in experimental immune glomerular injury. *Kidney Int 1984; 26:* 830–837

15 Gabbai F, Gushwa L, Wilson CB, Blantz RC. An evaluation of the development of experimental membranous nephropathy. *Kidney Int 1987; 31:* 1267–1278

16 Gabbai FB, Blantz RC. Role of angiotensin II in experimental membranous nephropathy. *Am J Physiol 1987:* submitted for publication

17 Gabbai FB, Mundy CA, Wilson CB, Blantz RC. An evaluation of the role of complement depletion in experimental membranous nephropathy in the rat. *Lab Invest 1987:* submitted for publication

18 Camussi G, Noble B, VanLiew J et al. Pathogenesis of passive Heymann nephritis: chlorpramazine inhibits antibody mediated redistribution of cell surface antigens and prevents development of the disease. *Kidney Int 1986; 29:* 268 (abstr)

19 Brenner BM, Troy JL, Daugharty TM. The dynamics of glomerular ultrafiltration in the rat. *J Clin Invest 1971; 50:* 1776–1780

20 Tucker BJ, Blantz RC. An analysis of the determinants of nephron filtration rate. *Am J Physiol 1977; 232:* F477–F483

21 Blantz RC. Effect of mannitol on glomerular ultrafiltration in the hydropenic rat. *J Clin Invest 1974; 54:* 1135–1143

22 Blantz RC, Gabbai FB. Effect of angiotensin II on glomerular hemodynamics and ultrafiltration coefficient. *Kidney Int 1987; 31(S20):* S108–S111

23 Blantz RC, Tucker BJ. Measurements of glomerular dynamics. In Martinez-Maldonado M, ed. *Methods in Pharmacology, Renal Pharmacology Vol 4B.* New York: Plenum Press. 1978: 141–163

24 Hoyer JR. Tubulointerstitial immune complex nephritis in rats immunized with Tamm-Horsfall protein. *Kidney Int 1980; 17:* 284–292

25 Salant DJ, Belok S, Madiao MP, Couser WG. A new role for complement in experimental membranous nephropathy in rats. *J Clin Invest 1980; 66:* 1339–1350

26 Aeikens B, Ecxboom A, Bohle A. Untersuchungen zur structur des glomerulum. *Virchows Arch A 1979; 381:* 283–293

27 Pelayo JC, Chenoweth DE, Hugli TE et al. Effects of the anaphylatoxin, C5a, on renal and glomerular hemodynamics in the rat. *Kidney Int 1986; 30:* 62–67

28 Perkinson DT, Baker PJ, Couser WG et al. Membrane attack complex deposition in experimental glomerular injury. *Am J Pathol 1985; 120:* 121–128

29 Edgington TS, Glassock RJ, Dixon FJ. Autologous immune complex nephritis induced with renal tubular antigen. I. Identification and isolation of the pathogenetic antigen. *J Exp Med 1968; 127:* 555–572

30 Matsuo S, Caldwell PRB, Brentjens JR, Andres G. In vivo interaction of antibodies with cell surface antigens. A mechanism responsible for in situ formation of immune deposits in the zona pellucida in rabbit oocytes. *J Clin Invest 1985; 75:* 1369–1380

31 Ichikawa I, Rennke HG, Hoyer JR et al. Role of intrarenal mechanisms in the impaired salt excretion of experimental nephrotic syndrome. *J Clin Invest 1983; 71:* 91–103

32 Blantz RC, Konnen KS, Tucker BJ. Angiotensin II effects upon the glomerular microcirculation and ultrafiltration coefficient of the rat. *J Clin Invest 1976; 57:* 419–434

33 Yoshioka T, Rennke HG, Salant DJ et al. Hemodynamic alterations modulate the expression of the glomerular sieving defect in rat membranous glomerulopathy (MGM). *Kidney Int 1986; 29:* 390 (abstr)

34 Blantz RC, Pelayo JC. A functional role for the tubuloglomerular feedback mechanism. *Kidney Int 1985; 25:* 739–746

35 Sakai T, Harris FH Jr, Marsh DJ et al. Extracellular fluid expansion and autoregulation in nephrotoxic serum nephritis in rats. *Kidney Int 1984; 25:* 619–628

36 Gushwa LC, Peterson OW, Wilson CB, Blantz RC. Evaluation of tubuloglomerular feedback (TGF) activity in marked antiglomerular basement membrane antibody nephritis (GN). *Kidney Int 1987; 31:* 386 (abstr)

TOXIC IMMUNE NEPHROPATHY

Ph Druet, L Pelletier, F Hirsch, E Druet, C Sapin

Hôpital Broussais, Paris, France

Introduction

Increasing attention has been given during the past 10 years to chemically-induced immune nephropathy. One obvious reason is that there is an impressive number of drugs able to induce such states; environmental pollutants may also be responsible for autoimmune abnormalities. Experimental models have been developed which may help understanding of the mechanisms involved and the rôle of heredity. Another justification of the recent interest in drug-induced autoimmunity is the light it throws on abnormalities responsible for spontaneous autoimmune disease.

In this chapter we will summarize briefly our knowledge in the human situation as this aspect has been extensively reviewed recently [1,2]. We will discuss more thoroughly experimental data.

TOXIC IMMUNE NEPHROPATHY IN HUMANS

Very little is known about the mechanisms of induction of drug-induced glomerulonephritis or interstitial nephritis of immune origin. The most frequently encountered glomerular lesion is an immune complex type glomerulonephritis and mainly a membranous glomerulonephritis [1,2]. In addition, several cases of drug-induced nephrotic syndrome with minimal glomerular changes have been reported [1,2]. This lesion is similar to the one observed in the idiopathic nephrotic syndrome and could also be T-cell mediated [3]. There is indirect evidence that most cases of drug-induced acute interstitial nephritis are cell-mediated while very few cases seem to be antibody-mediated [1,2].

Several features (Table I) raise the suspicion that a drug-induced nephropathy is immunologically mediated.

TABLE I. Features suggesting the immune origin of a drug-induced nephropathy

- Genetic predisposition (small percentage affected).
- Not dose related.
- Remission after withdrawal.
- Extrarenal manifestations (rash, fever . . .).
- Laboratory findings (hyper-IgE, anti-drug antibodies, eosinophiluria, eosinophilia . . .).
- Renal biopsy (including immunofluorescence study).
- A given drug may induce different nephropathies depending upon genetic background.

Toxic immune glomerulonephritis (Table II)

Glomerulonephritis induced by heavy metals

Gold salts are used to treat patients with rheumatoid arthritis, but cause proteinuria in 6–17.2% of cases and the nephrotic syndrome in 2.6–5.3%. Patients who have inherited the HLA DR3 antigen are at higher risk [4]. Nearly 90% of rheumatoid patients treated with gold salts who develop proteinuria have a membranous glomerulonephritis and 9.6% with the nephrotic syndrome have minimal glomerular changes [1,2,5]. Renal insufficiency is quite rare, and the proteinuria subsides within 4–18 months. Gold therapy has usually been stopped when proteinuria appears; reintroduction has rarely been attempted.

TABLE II. Drugs or toxins that have been found associated with immunlologically mediated glomerulonephritis

Well documented or likely

- Heavy metals (gold, mercury).
- Drugs with a sulphydryl group (D-penicillamine, thiopronine, 5-thiopyridoxine, pyrithioxine, captopril).
- Lithium salts.
- Non-steriodal anti-inflammatory drugs.
- Rifampicin.
- Drugs responsible for lupus-like syndrome (hydralazine, D-penicillamine, anti-convulsants).
- Hydrocarbon exposure.

Not well documented or few cases.

- Toxin-induced connective tissue disease (silica, toxic-oil syndrome, cosmetic surgery).
- Ampicillin, probenecid, phenindione, carbutamide, tolbutamide, chlorpropamide, potassium chlorate, quinidine, dapsone, PUVA, levamisole, nifedipine, interferon.

Mercury-induced membranous glomerulonephritis has been described in patients treated with organomercurial diuretics, ammoniated mercury unguents, mercurous chloride-containing laxatives and in women using mercury-containing skin lightening creams. Such situations should be encountered much less frequently as mercury-containing drugs are rarely used nowadays but cases have also been reported following environmental or occupational exposure to mercurials. It is possible that undiagnosed mercury exposure might account for some cases of apparently idiopathic membranous glomerulonephritis. Besides membranous glomerulonephritis, the nephrotic syndrome with minimal glomerular changes or glomerular linear IgG deposits, suggestive of the presence of anti-glomerular basement membrane antibodies have been observed in few patients [1,2].

Glomerulonephritis induced by drugs with sulphydryl groups
D-penicillamine is used in the treatment of rheumatoid arthritis, Wilson's disease, cystinuria, chronic active hepatitis and systemic sclerosis. Proteinuria has been reported in 7–20% of rheumatoid patients treated with penicillamine and occasionally when it is taken in other situations [1,2]. Emery et al [6] have shown the rôle of HLA DR3 antigens and of sulphoxidation status. Renal biopsies in 82.5% of the patients showed membranous glomerulonephritis; less frequently the patients had mesangioproliferative glomerulonephritis (10.4%). Nephrotic syndrome with minimal glomerular changes, focal necrotizing glomerulonephritis and rapidly progressive glomerulonephritis have also been reported. It is of note that while a linear pattern of deposition of IgG along the glomerular capillary wall has been occasionally observed, circulating anti-GBM antibodies have not been detected [1,2].

Other drugs with a sulphydryl group (Table II) have also been associated with a membranous glomerulonephritis.

Drugs inducing lupus-like syndromes
Several drugs are known to induce lupus-like syndromes. Renal involvement is usually absent, but there are exceptions [1,2]. D-penicillamine can induce a lupus-like syndrome associated with renal involvement. Renal manifestations are very rare after treatment with procainamide, but are less so in patients treated with hydralazine [1,2,7]. Renal biopsy in most instances has shown focal and segmental glomerulonephritis with crescents and necrotizing glomerulonephritis. Patients with the HLA DR4 antigen and slow-acetylators are at higher risk [8,9]. Various anti-convulsant drugs are also able to induce lupus-like syndrome with occasional renal involvement [1,2].

Connective tissue diseases associated with occupational or accidental exposure, or cosmetic surgery
Connective tissue disorders such as scleroderma, systemic lupus erythematosus, and rheumatoid arthritis have been reported following silica exposure, in the toxic-oil syndrome recently described in Spain, and after cosmetic surgery involving injections of silicone or paraffin. Cases of biopsy proven glomerulonephritis have been observed. Circulating anti-glomerular basement membrane antibodies have also been reported but no renal biopsies were taken [2].

Hydrocarbon and agrochemical exposure
A causal relation between hydrocarbon exposure and development of glomerulonephritis has been suggested from case reports and from case control studies.

Immunofluorescent studies were performed in 11 of 12 cases of proliferative necrotizing glomerulonephritis associated with hydrocarbon exposure [2]. All had linear IgG deposits and circulating anti-glomerular basement membrane antibodies were found in eight cases. There is therefore a strong suspicion of a causal association between hydrocarbon exposure and anti-glomerular basement membrane-mediated glomerulonephritis.

Polla et al [10] reported one case of anti-glomerular basement membrane-mediated glomerulonephritis after exposure to herbicides and insecticides.

Other drugs

Rare cases of glomerulonephritis have been reported in association with other drugs listed in Table II, but a causal relation is difficult to establish from so few cases.

Drugs responsible for the nephrotic syndrome with minimal glomerular changes

The nephrotic syndrome has been observed in at least 10 patients treated with lithium salts [1,2]. A causal relation was established in three patients who had recovered from a first episode but relapsed when rechallenged. Serum lithium levels were in the therapeutic range. Proteinuria rapidly disappeared after withdrawal of the drug. Renal biopsies exhibited minimal glomerular changes with negative immunofluorescent findings and/or without electron-dense deposits in most patients. Non-steroidal anti-inflammatory drugs (NSAIDs) and rifampicin have also been responsible for the nephrotic syndrome with minimal glomerular changes but in these situations, the nephrotic syndrome is usually associated with acute interstitial nephritis.

Toxic immune interstitial nephritis

Recent reviews [2,11] have been devoted to drug-induced immune acute interstitial nephritis. Only general considerations will be given. Allergic interstitial nephritis is a well-known side-effect of drug therapy. More than 40 different drugs have been associated with immunological acute interstitial nephritis (Table III). This accounts for 0.8% to 8% of all causes of acute renal failure.

The clinical signs develop usually within 15 days (2–44 days) after initiation of therapy, but the interval may be shorter after rechallenge with the same drug. The onset of acute renal failure is not dose-dependent. Diuresis is preserved in 30–40% of cases. The diagnosis may be missed as 30–40% of cases are not oliguric; this is especially true when the drug has a potential direct nephrotoxic effect, or if it was introduced to treat an illness with possible kidney involvement. Fever, rash, and arthralgia suggest an allergic drug reaction, but these symptoms are only found in 10–40% of patients.

Microscopic or macroscopic haematuria, and mild proteinuria may occur. Nephrotic range proteinuria is common with acute interstitial nephritis induced by NSAIDs [1,2,12] and in some cases after treatment with penicillin, ampicillin,

TABLE III. Drug-induced immunologically-mediated acute interstitial nephritis

1. Antibacterial therapy	2. Diuretics
(a) Penicillin derivatives	Chlorothiazide
Methicillin	Cyclothiazide
Ampicillin	Hydrochlorothiazide
Oxacillin	Tienilic acid
Carbenicillin	Chlorthalidone
Penicillin G	Triamterene
Nafcillin	Frusemide
Amoxycillin	
(b) Cephalosporin	3. Analgesics
Cephalothin	Glafenine
Cephalexin	Floctafenine
Cephradine	Anthrafenine
Cephoxitin	Aminopyrine
	Noramidopyrine
(c) Others	*Clometacine*
Rifampicin	Phenazone
Piromic acid	Sulphinpyrazone
Erythromycin	Paracetamol
Minocycline	
Vancomycin	4. Others
Salicylazosulphapyridine	*Phenindione*
Sulphonamides	*Cimetidine*
	Allopurinol
	Diphenylhydantoin
	Carbamazepine
	Clofibrate

The most frequently incriminated drugs are in italics. Drugs which induce acute interstitial nephritis with the nephrotic syndrome are listed in the text

and thiazides. Eosinophiluria is present in more than half of the patients and seems to be the most reliable diagnostic marker. Eosinophilia is observed in 60–100% of cases and increased serum IgE concentrations in about 50%. Although in many circumstances there is strong evidence for a major rôle of cellular immunity, anti-drug antibodies have been demonstrated with several drugs. Circulating anti-tubular basement membrane antibodies have been detected after methicillin [13], cephalothin, and diphenylhydantoin treatment [1,2].

Histological examination of the kidney shows diffuse or focal interstitial infiltration with lymphocytes, plasmocytes and most often eosinophils. Interstitial oedema and varying degrees of tubular damage are usually found but glomeruli and vessels are almost normal. Granulomas with epithelial cells and giant cells are observed in 32% of the patients and the association of granulomas and acute interstitial nephritis is almost specific to drug-induced acute interstitial nephritis [11,14]. Prognosis is usually good after drug withdrawal but sclerosing transformation of the interstitial infiltrate may lead to permanent renal failure in some patients and thus steroid treatment may be justified in severe cases.

Toxic immune interstitial nephritis and glomerulopathy

The association of acute interstitial nephritis and the nephrotic syndrome has been attributed to several drugs but principally to NSAIDs [12]. Fenoprofen, which belongs to the propionic acid family has been the culprit in more than half of the 50 reported cases. Females (the male:female ratio is 1:4) and the elderly are particularly at risk (mean age of the reported patients is 64 years, range 50–84). Mean duration of exposure to fenoprofen was 7.9 months (range 1–36 months) before presentation and the daily dose in reported cases has always been in the therapeutic range. Except for the rare patient with eosinophilia there have been no extrarenal symptoms of hypersensitivity. Immunological tests are negative. Renal failure has been present in every case and was sometimes severe enough to necessitate dialysis. Renal function returned to normal and proteinuria resolved in the vast majority of patients after the drug was withdrawn. However, renal failure persisted in some patients until steroid therapy was started. A few patients have continued to have some degree of renal failure or proteinuria for several months.

Glomeruli are normal by light microscopy and immunofluorescence. The interstitium is oedematous and infiltrated with numerous mononuclear cells and associated in 40% of cases with eosinophils. Studies of the lymphocyte subpopulations [15] have shown that T-cells constitute about 80% and B-cells about 20% of the lymphocyte population. Cytotoxic/suppressor T-cells predominated over helper/inducer T-cells. The great majority of B-cells are IgE bearing cells.

Less frequently other NSAIDs (zomepirac, piroxicam, fenclofenac, ibuprofen, phenylbutazone, tolmetin, aclofenac, indomethacin and naproxen) can induce an acute interstitial nephritis with minimal glomerular changes. Acute renal failure has been attributed to rifampicin in few patients in whom interstitial and glomerular lesions coexist.

RENAL VASCULITIS

Few cases of renal vasculitis have been reported after penicillin and allopurinol therapy. Cases of Henoch-Schonlein purpura have been associated with piroxicam therapy and of focal cortical necrosis with zomepirac [2].

TOXIC IMMUNE EXPERIMENTAL NEPHROPATHY

Mercury-induced autoimmune disease in the Brown Norway rat

Description of the disease

The glomerulonephritis observed following injections of $HgCl_2$ (thrice weekly at a dose of 100μg/100g body weight) is species and strain-dependent. In Brown

Norway rats, a lymphoproliferation is observed one week after the first injection resulting in a striking polyclonal increase of IgG and IgE concentrations and in the production of autoantibodies including anti-glomerular basement membrane and anti-ss DNA antibodies [16–18]. These autoimmune abnormalities reach a peak (day 15–20) and then decline progressively even if $HgCl_2$ injections are continued [17]. Anti-glomerular basement membrane antibodies deposited in the kidney are identified by immunofluorescence in a typical linear and smooth pattern along the glomerular basement membrane [19]. The circulating and kidney-bound antibodies are directed towards collagenase-digested glomerular basement membrane, laminin, fibronectin [17], proteoglycan, and entactin [20]. Anti-glomerular basement membrane antibody deposition is associated with the occurrence of heavy proteinuria and the nephrotic syndrome [19] but not with significant renal insufficiency. Light and electronmicroscopy showed a mild influx of monocytes without extracapillary proliferation [21]. Rats may die at this time, probably as a consequence of intravascular coagulation due to antibody deposition [20].

When rats survive this phase of the disease, glomerular linear IgG deposits diminish progressively and granular IgG deposits are superimposed along the glomerular capillary wall [19] and in a subepithelial position. Granular IgG deposits are also found in the mesangium and in the vascular walls in the kidneys and in several other organs. Transient circulating immune complexes of unknown composition can be detected but their rôle in glomerular immune complex formation has not been elucidated.

All the mercurials tested (mercurous chloride, methylmercury and various pharmaceutical agents containing mercury), have been found to induce various degrees of autoimmunity [21]. The route of administration of the compound (parenteral injections, oral route, digestive route, topically applied) does not influence the manifestations observed. Mercurials, present in the environment, may therefore be responsible for cases of apparently idiopathic glomerulonephritis in man.

Genetic control of susceptibility

The Brown Norway rat strain is the only one among those tested (Table IV) to develop such autoimmune abnormalities. Interestingly the four strains with the RT1-l haplotype (equivalent to the HLA complex in man) were completely resistant [22]. We have assessed the susceptibility of Lewis rats extensively, including the response of segregants between the resistant Lewis (RT1-l) strain and the susceptible Brown Norway (RT1-n) strain. Their RT1 haplotype was determined as well as the occurrence of linear and granular IgG deposits and total serum IgE level in response to $HgCl_2$. We were thus able to demonstrate that susceptibility was inherited as an autosomal dominant trait and depended upon three or four genes, one of which was RT1 linked [23,24]. This is of interest since, as mentioned above, MHC-linked genes are also involved in drug-induced membranous glomerulonephritis in humans.

TABLE IV. Induction and regulation of mercury-induced autoimmunity in Brown Norway rats

Induction

- Emergence or expansion of frequent autoreactive T-cells including anti-self Ia T-cells.
- Defect at the suppressor T-cell level (?).
- T-dependent polyclonal activation of B-cells.
- Autoimmunity transferred into normal Brown Norway rats with autoreactive T-cells.

Regulation

- Rôle for suppressor T-cells.
- Rôle for auto anti-idiotypic antibodies.
- Decreased frequency of autoreactive T-cells.

The resistance of Lewis rats is not due to the absence of the corresponding glomerular basement membrane antigen, because 1) kidney acid eluate from Brown Norway rats stained Lewis rat glomerular basement membrane by immunofluorescence [23]; 2) when a Lewis rat kidney was transplanted into binephrectomized F1 hybrids (later injected with $HgCl_2$), both linear and granular glomerular IgG deposits were observed [25]; and 3) Lewis rats became susceptible when lethally irradiated and rendered chimaeric by reconstitution with bone marrow cells from susceptible (Lewis x Brown Norway)F1 hybrids [26].

Mechanisms of induction of mercury-induced autoimmune disease in Brown Norway rats (Table IV)

Findings described above in $HgCl_2$-injected Brown Norway rats strongly suggest the polyclonal activation of B-cells. Moreover, using a plaque-forming cell assay to assess antibody synthesis in vitro we observed that the number of anti-TNP and anti-sheep red blood cells plaque-forming cells produced by spleen of $HgCl_2$-injected Brown Norway rats was increased when compared to controls [16]. Similarly, normal Brown Norway rat spleen cells exposed in vitro to non-cytotoxic doses of $HgCl_2$ also produced anti-TNP and anti-sheep red blood cell antibodies; T-cells were required for this polyclonal activation.Finally when spleen cells from diseased Brown Norway rats were fused with the non-secreting IR 983 F rat myeloma cell line, numerous clones were obtained which produced IgG antibodies with various specificities including anti-glomerular basement membrane and antinuclear antibodies, or which secreted IgE of unknown specificity [27]. All these experiments therefore showed that $HgCl_2$ was responsible for T-dependent polyclonal activation of B-cells. T cells are also required for the induction of mercury-induced autoimmunity. Brown Norway rats with the nude mutation or Brown Norway rats thymectomized, irradiated and reconstituted with fetal liver cells (Brown Norway 'B' rats) are profoundly T-cell depleted. Neither develop any autoimmune abnormality when injected with $HgCl_2$ unless reconstituted with T-cells [28].

Recently the mechanisms responsible for polyclonal activation of B-cells in this model have been partly elucidated. First it was observed that T-cells from $HgCl_2$-injected Brown Norway rats as well as normal T-cells incubated with non-toxic amounts of $HgCl_2$ were able to stimulate syngeneic spleen cells [29,30]. Then evidence was obtained that autoreactive T-cells emerge or expand in $HgCl_2$-injected Brown Norway rats. Using limiting dilution analysis, Pelletier et al [submitted for publication] have shown that frequent autoreactive T-cell can be detected in these rats from day four following the first injection of $HgCl_2$. Interestingly some of these autoreactive T-cells, present from day six recognize normal class II antigens on B-cells. Anti-self Ia autoreactive T-cells induce polyclonal activation of B-cells in vitro [31]. Thus, it is tempting to consider that these autoreactive T-cells and among them anti-self Ia T-cell are important in the pathogenesis of the disease. To test this hypothesis, normal Brown Norway rats or T-cell-deprived (BN 'B') rats were infused with various cell populations purified from the spleen of $HgCl_2$-injected rats [Pelletier et al, submitted for publication]. When such T-cells were transferred to BN 'B' rats a full-blown disease developed in the recipients. This included anti-glomerular basement membrane antibody production, an autoimmune glomerulonephritis with heavy proteinuria and an increase in total serum IgE level. However when recipients were normal Brown Norway rats, there was a marked lymphoproliferation that affected mainly $OX8^+$ (suppressor/cytotoxic) T-cells. The disease observed was rather mild but became quite impressive when rats were pretreated with OX8 antibodies to deplete them of T-suppressor cells. Interestingly $OX8^+$ T-cells do not proliferate in $HgCl_2$-injected Brown Norway rats.

These findings, taken together suggest that $HgCl_2$ induces the appearance or the expansion of autoreactive T-cells including anti-self Ia autoreactive T-cells. These cells probably stimulate B cells polyclonally leading to antibody production. In addition, it is likely that the T-suppressor cell function is depressed in mercury-injected rats. It is well known that anti-self Ia T-cells are regulated by T-suppressor/cytotoxic cells [32]. A defect at the T-suppressor cytotoxic level could contribute to the expansion of autoreactive T-cells.

The respective rôles of different sets of autoreactive T-cells, relationships between them, as well as details of the mechanisms leading to these modifications remain to be elucidated. T-cell clone technology will probably be very helpful in that respect.

Spontaneous regulation of mercury-induced autoimmune disease (Table IV)

Another interesting feature of the disease induced in Brown Norway rats is the spontaneous regulation that occurs after two to three weeks even when $HgCl_2$ injections are continued [17]. Bowman et al [33] observed that the disease cannot be induced again in animals that have recovered, and that Brown Norway rats can be rendered tolerant if they are first injected with low doses of $HgCl_2$. This suggests that suppressor cells could be responsible for the spontaneous regulation observed. Spleen cells from convalescent animals were indeed able to transfer resistance when injected into naive syngeneic recipients, unless the cells transferred were depleted in $OX8^+$ (suppressor/cytotoxic) T-cells.

The rôle of auto-anti-idiotypic antibodies has also been investigated. Using an anti-glomerular basement membrane plaque-forming cell assay, Chalopin and Lockwood [34] showed that the serum of $HgCl_2$-injected rats could augment the plaque-forming cell response. This phenomenon is probably due to auto-anti-idiotypic antibodies.

As mentioned previously, Pelletier et al [submitted for publication] have performed limiting dilution analysis at the time when Brown Norway rats recover and have obtained two interesting results. Rare T-suppressor cells with the $OX8^+$ phenotype appear in these rats from day 14. These cells inhibited the proliferation of autoreactive T-cells in the presence of syngeneic spleen cells. They also found a progressive decline in the frequency of autoreactive T-cells. These data could explain the spontaneous autoregulation observed. However, OX8 treatment of $HgCl_2$-injected rats affected only moderately the course of the disease. This suggests that there are other mechanisms besides T-suppressor cells in the autoregulating process. Anti-idiotypic antibodies could be an important additional factor as already inferred by Chalopin and Lockwood.

Mercury-induced glomerulonephritis in other strains of rats

About 30% of outbred Wistar rats develop a membranous glomerulonephritis [35] or mesangial deposits, but the antigen responsible has not been identified. Several inbred strains with the RT1u haplotype have been tested subsequently [22]. Most of them (Wistar AG, LOU) were found to be resistant, but a membranous glomerulonephritis was found in a percentage of inbred Wistar-Furth rats injected with 0.4mg of $HgCl_2$. Several other strains of rats developed an immune complex-type glomerulonephritis (Table V). Antinuclear antibodies have been found by indirect immunofluorescence and anti-ss DNA by the Farr assay in some of these strains. Anti-ss DNA antibodies have been eluted from the

TABLE V. Glomerular lesions in various rat strains after injection of $HgCl_2$

Strain	RT1	Glomerular lesion
Brown Norway	n	Anti-glomerular basement membrane glomerulonephritis Immune complex-type nephritis
PVG/C, AUG	c	Immune complex-type nephritis
AVN, DA	a	Immune complex-type nephritis
BDV	d	Immune complex-type nephritis
BUF	b	Immune complex-type nephritis
OKA	k	Immune complex-type nephritis
AS2	f	Immune complex-type nephritis
Lewis, F 344	l	None
AS, BS	l	None
Wistar AG, LOU	u	None
Wistar-Furth	u	Immune complex-type nephritis

kidneys of PVG/c rats, suggesting that they may be of pathogenic significance [22]. Weening et al [36] have obtained evidence that the disease in PVG/c rats is associated with inhibition of suppressor cell function.

Mercury-induced autoimmune glomerulonephritis in other species

In outbred rabbits $HgCl_2$ induces a disease quite similar to that seen in Brown Norway rats [37]. Rabbits develop anti-glomerular basement membrane antibodies and circulating immune complexes. Linear IgG deposits along the glomerular capillary wall are followed by granular IgG deposits in a subepithelial position in glomeruli and in vessel walls of several organs. Interestingly using ^{203}Hg and autoradiography, mercury was found in the proximal tubular cells, but not within the immune deposits.

Several authors have found that a mesangial glomerulopathy could be induced in BALB/c mice and Swiss mice [38–40]. Granular IgG deposits along the glomerular capillary wall have been reported in BALB/c mice together with the appearance of anti-gp330 antibodies [40]. These mice also develop antinuclear antibodies. Production of antinuclear antibodies is genetically controlled [41]. No anti-glomerular basement membrane antibodies have been observed until now but an increase in total serum IgE level has also been observed [Gleichmann E, personal communication].

Other experimental autoimmune glomerulonephritis induced by drugs and toxins (Table VI)

It has been reported that diones induce the nephrotic syndrome in Wistar rats. Nagi et al [42] showed that a membranous glomerulonephritis occurs as a

TABLE VI. Experimental toxic immune nephropathies

Toxin	Species	Renal lesion
Mercury	Rat	Anti-glomerular basement membrane glomerulonephritis Membranous glomerulonephritis
	Rabbit	Anti-glomerular basement membrane glomerulonephritis Membranous glomerulonephritis
	Mouse	Immune complex glomerulonephritis
Gold	Rat	Membranous glomerulonephritis Immune complex glomerulonephritis
	Guinea pig	Immune complex glomerulonephritis Anti-TBM abs
D-penicillamine	Rat	Membranous glomerulonephritis Anti-glomerular basement membrane glomerulonephritis Immune complex glomerulonephritis
Hydralazine	Mouse	Immune complex glomerulonephritis
Alfalfa sprout	Monkey	Immune complex glomerulonephritis
Cephalothin	Mouse	Acute interstitial nephritis

consequence of gold thiomalate administration in Wistar rats. Ueda et al [43] reported that guinea pigs exposed to gold develop anti-tubular basement membrane antibodies or an immune complex type glomerulonephritis associated with the production of anti-brush border antibodies. Brown Norway rats receiving gold also develop an immune complex type glomerulonephritis while Lewis rats are resistant [44]. Wistar rats fed D-penicillamine develop a membrane glomerulonephritis [45] while Brown Norway rats develop a disease quite similar to that described after injections of $HgCl_2$ [46]. Linear IgG deposits were indeed observed along the glomerular capillary wall and several rats died as a consequence of intravascular coagulation. Lewis rats and Sprague-Dawley rats are resistant. Thus there are striking similarities between diseases observed in Brown Norway rats receiving $HgCl_2$ and D-penicillamine, which suggests similar mechanisms of induction. In contrast, captopril does not induce any detectable autoimmunity in Brown Norway rats [46].

Hydralazine may give rise to antinuclear antibodies, lymphoproliferation, polyclonal Ig increase and also to mesangial IgG deposits. Ajax mice appeared to be more affected than BALB/CJ mice [47]. Another lupus-like syndrome with renal involvement has been induced in monkeys fed alfalfa sprouts and a rôle for L-canavanine a non-protein aminoacid, present in alfalfa sprouts, has been proposed [48].

Experimental immune interstitial nephritis

Except for the production of anti-tubular basement membrane antibodies in guinea pigs receiving gold, no experimental model of drug-induced immune interstitial nephritis is available. However, it has recently been reported that mice immunized with cephalothin-protein conjugates develop an acute interstitial nephritis together with IgG and IgE antibodies [49].

MECHANISMS OF DRUG-INDUCED AUTOIMMUNITY

Modification of autoantigen

Drugs may bind to, and modify autoantigens rendering them immunogenic. Anti-histone antibodies result from binding of hydralazine to desoxyribonucleoprotein [50]. Binding of dimethoxiphenylpenicilloyl (a metabolite of methicillin) to tubular basement membrane may explain the formation of anti-tubular basement membrane antibodies [13].

Release of autoantigens

It has often been speculated that toxic agents (mercury, gold) could induce the release of brush border antigens, but it has never been demonstrated. Curiously, $HgCl_2$ which induces autoimmunity in Brown Norway rats, has an immunosuppressive effect in Lewis rats [51] and is able to prevent the formation of anti-brush border antibodies and consequently of Heymann's nephritis in this strain [52].

Anti-hapten immune response

Drugs could also induce an immune response against themselves. It has been suggested that the metabolite of methicillin binds to tubular basement membrane and behaves as a planted antigen. Anti-hapten antibodies would then bind to the hapten on the basement membrane [53]. A similar mechanism could be involved in mice immunized with cephalothin-protein conjugates [49]. Anti-drug antibodies could also theoretically induce tissue damage if they recognize a cross-reactive epitope on autoantigens.

Direct effect on the immune system

A direct effect on the immune system is a more likely reason when numerous autoantibodies are produced. Drugs may inhibit suppressor T-cells. This has been shown for methyldopa [54] and also in PVG/c rats injected with $HgCl_2$ [36]. A defect at the suppressor T-cell level may play a rôle in $HgCl_2$-injected Brown Norway rats.

Drugs may generate an excess of help from T-cells. This has been reported for procainamide [55] and we have shown that $HgCl_2$ induces autoreactive T-cells in Brown Norway rats.

Chemicals such as TNP may bind to class II molecules [56]. The modified Ia would then be recognized by autologous T-helper cells which consequently stimulate polyclonally B-cells. Diphenylhydantoin probably acts similarly [57] and T-cell proliferation has been reported in mice in response to macrophages haptenized with D-penicillamine [58]. In these situations a graft-versus-host like reaction would ensue [59]. There are many other hypothetical mechanisms such as direct effect on B-cells or on interleukin production. In that respect it is interesting that mercury induces a tremendous IgE increase in Brown Norway rats. This could be explained by preferential Interleukin 4 production which affects mainly IgE production [60].

Genetic factors

It is clear from human and experimental studies that genetic predisposition is essential. MHC-linked genes are clearly involved in gold [4], D-penicillamine [6] and hydralazine-induced [8] autoimmunity in humans. Non-MHC-linked genes such as those governing the acetylator [9] or sulphoxidator [6] status are also important. Experimental data have confirmed the rôle of genes inside and outside the MHC. Brown Norway rats seem to be particularly interesting for immunotoxicological studies since they are susceptible to mercury, gold and D-penicillamine induced autoimmune glomerulonephritis while Lewis rats are resistant. An important goal in the future will be to localize the non-MHC-linked genes involved in autoimmune nephritis in Brown Norway rats.

Conclusion

Many drugs and toxins are responsible for immune nephropathies. Recently developed experimental models have shed some light on possible mechanisms of induction and regulation of autoimmune reactions. A better understanding of these mechanisms will probably increase understanding of 'spontaneous' autoimmunity and lead to the proposed new therapeutic approaches. Furthermore, drug-induced autoimmunity represents a unique situation for the study of factors governing susceptibility which in time could allow identification of patients at risk.

References

1. Fillastre JP, Mery JPH, Druet P. Drug induced glomerulonephritis. In Cameron JS, Glassock RJ, eds. *The Nephrotic Syndrome.* New York: Marcel Dekker. In press
2. Druet P, Jacquot C, Baran D et al. Immunological mediated nephritis induced by toxins and drugs. In *Nephrotoxicity in the Experimental and Clinical Situation.* Lancaster: MTP. In press
3. Shaloub RJ. Pathogenesis of lipoid nephrosis. A disorder of T-cell function. *Lancet 1974; ii:* 556–560
4. Wooley PH, Griffin J, Panayi GS et al. HLA-DR antigens and toxic reaction to sodium aurothimalate and D-penicillamine in patients with rheumatoid arthritis. *N Engl J Med 1980; 303:* 300–302
5. Törnroth T, Skrifvars B. Gold nephropathy prototype of membranous glomerulonephritis. *Am J Pathol 1974; 75:* 573–590
6. Emery P, Panayi GS, Huston G et al. D-penicillamine induced toxicity in rheumatoid arthritis: the role of sulphoxidation status and HLA-DR3. *J Rheumatol 1984; 11:* 626–632
7. Ihle BU, Whitworth JA, Dowling JP, Kincaid-Smith P. Hydralazine and lupus glomerulonephritis. *Clin Nephrol 1984; 22:* 230–238
8. Batchelor JR, Welsh KI, Mansilla-Tinoco R et al. Hydralazine-induced systemic lupus erythematosus: influence of HLA-DR and sex on susceptibility. *Lancet 1984; i:* 1107–1109
9. Woosley RL, Drayer DE, Reidenberg MM et al. Effect of acetylator phenotype on the rate at which procainamide induces antinuclear antibodies and the lupus syndrome. *N Engl J Med 1978; 298:* 1157–1159
10. Polla B, Pirson Y, Cosyns JP, Van Ypersele de Strihou C. Toxic anti-GBM glomerulonephritis. *Clin Nephrol 1983; 19:* 45–47
11. Kleinknecht D, Vanhille PH, Morel-Maroger L et al. Acute interstitial nephritis due to drug hypersensitivity. An up-to-date review with a report of 19 cases. In Grünfeld JP, Maxwell MH, eds. *Advances in Nephrology.* Chicago: Year Book. 1983: 277–308
12. Brazin JH, Katz SM, Schwartz AB, Chinitz JL. Reversible renal failure and nephrotic syndrome associated with nonsteroidal anti-inflammatory drugs. *N Engl J Med 1979; 23:* 1271–1273
13. Border WA, Lehman DH, Egan JD et al. Anti-tubular basement membrane antibodies in methicillin associated interstitial nephritis. *N Engl J Med 1974; 291:* 381–384
14. Mignon F, Mery JPH, Mougenot B et al. Granulomatous interstitial nephritis. In Grünfeld JP, Maxwell MH, eds. *Advances In Nephrology.* Chicago: Year Book. 1984: 219–245
15. Stachura I, Jayakumar S, Bourke E. T and B lymphocytes subsets in fenoprofen nephropathy. *Am J Med 1983; 75:* 9–16
16. Hirsch F, Couderc J, Sapin C et al. Polyclonal effect of $HgCl_2$ in the rat, its possible role in an experimental autoimmune disease. *Eur J Immunol 1982; 12:* 620–625

17 Bellon B, Capron M, Druet E et al. Mercuric chloride induced autoimmune disease in Brown-Norway rats: sequential search for anti-basement membrane antibodies and circulating immune complexes. *Eur J Clin Invest 1982; 12:* 127–133

18 Proovost-Danon A, Abadie A, Sapin C et al. Induction of IgE synthesis and potentiation of anti-ovalbumin IgE antibody response by $HgCl_2$ in the rat. *J Immunol 1981; 126:* 699–702

19 Druet P, Druet E, Potdevin F, Sapin C. Immune type glomerulonephritis induced by $HgCl_2$ in the Brown-Norway rat. *Ann Immunol (Institut Pasteur) 1978; 129C:* 777–792

20 Fukatsu A, Brentjens J, Klinen P et al. Glomerular immune deposits in rats injected with mercuric chloride ($HgCl_2$). *Kidney Int 1987; 31:* 320

21 Druet P, Baran D, Pelletier L et al. Drug-induced experimental autoimmune nephritis. In Cruse JM, Lewis RE, eds. *Concepts of Immunopathology.* Basel: Karger. 1986: 311–330

22 Druet E, Sapin C, Fournie G et al. Genetic control of susceptibility to mercury-induced immune nephritis in various strains of rat. *Clin Immunol Immunopathol 1982; 25:* 203–212

23 Druet E, Sapin C, Gunther E et al. Mercuric chloride induced anti-glomerular basement membrane antibodies in the rat: genetic control. *Eur J Immunol 1977; 7:* 348–351

24 Sapin C, Hirsch F, Delaporte JP et al. Polyclonal IgE increase after $HgCl_2$ injections in BN and LEW rats: a genetic analysis. *Immunogenetics 1984; 20:* 227–236

25 Druet E, Houssin D, Druet P. Mercuric chloride nephritis depends on host rather than kidney strains. *Clin Immunol Immunopathol 1983; 29:* 141–145

26 Sapin C, Druet P, Mandet C. Induction of susceptibility to $HgCl_2$ immune glomerulonephritis in the Lewis rat by immunocompetent cells from susceptible F1 hybrids. *Eur J Immunol 1980; 10:* 371–374

27 Hirsch F, Kuhn J, Ventura M et al. Autoimmunity induced by $HgCl_2$ in Brown-Norway rats. I. Production of monoclonal antibodies. *J Immunol 1986; 136:* 3272–3276

28 Pelletier L, Pasquier R, Vial MC et al. Mercury-induced autoimmune glomerulonephritis: requirement for T-cells. *Nephrol Dial Transplant 1987; 1:* 211–218

29 Pelletier L, Pasquier R, Hirsch F et al. In vivo self reactivity of mononuclear cells to T cells and macrophages exposed to $HgCl_2$. *Eur J Immunol 1985; 15:* 460–465

30 Pelletier L, Pasquier R, Hirsch F et al. Induction of autoreactive T cells in mercury-induced autoimmune disease. *J Immunol 1986; 137:* 2548–2554

31 Finnegan A, Needleman B, Hodes RJ. Activation of B cells by autoreactive T cells: cloned autoreactive T cells activate B cells by two distinct pathways. *J Immunol 1984; 133:* 78–85

32 Sano K, Fujisawa I, Abe R et al. MHC-restricted minimal regulatory circuit initiated by a class II-autoreactive T cell clone. *J Exp Med 1987; 165:* 1284–1295

33 Bowman C, Mason DW, Pusey CD, Lockwood CM. Autoregulation of antibody response in mercuric chloride nephritis in the Brown-Norway rat. I. A role for T suppressor cells. *Eur J Immunol 1984; 14:* 464–470

34 Chalopin JM, Lockwood CM. Autoregulation of autoantibody synthesis in mercuric chloride nephritis in the Brown-Norway rat. II. Presence of antigen augmentable plaque-forming cells in the spleen is associated with humoral factors behaving as auto-anti-idiotypic antibodies. *Eur J Immunol 1984; 14:* 470–475

35 Bariety J, Druet P, Laliberte F, Sapin C. Glomerulonephritis with α and β1C-globulin deposits induced in rats by mercuric chloride. *Am J Path 1971; 65:* 293–302

36 Weening JJ, Hoedemaeker PJ, Bakker WW. Immunoregulation and antinuclear antibodies in mercury-induced glomerulopathy in the rat. *Clin Exp Immunol 1981; 45:* 64–71

37 Roman-Franco AA, Turiello M, Albini B et al. Anti-basement membrane antibodies and antigen-antibody complexes in rabbits injected with mercuric chloride. *Clin Immunol Immunopathol 1978; 9:* 464–481

38 Albini B, Glurich I, Andres GA. Mercuric chloride-induced immunologically mediated diseases in experimental animals. In Porter GA, ed. *Nephrotoxic Mechanisms of Drugs and Environmental Toxins.* New York: Plenum Press. 1982: 413–423
39 Hultman P, Enestrom S. The induction of immune complex deposits in mice by per oral and parenteral administration of mercuric chloride: strain dependent susceptibility. *Clin Exp Immunol 1987; 67:* 283–292
40 Fleuren GJ, de Heer E, Brugers JV et al. Mercuric chloride-induced autoimmune glomerulopathy in Balb/c mice. *Kidney Int 1985; 28:* 702
41 Robinson CJG, Balazs T, Egorov IK. Mercuric chloride, gold sodium thiomalate and D-penicillamine-induced anti-nuclear antibodies in mice. *Toxicol Appl Pharmacol 1986; 86:* 159–169
42 Nagi AH, Alexander F, Barbas AZ. Gold nephropathy in rats. Light and electron microscopic studies. *Exp Molec Pathol 1971; 15:* 354–362
43 Ueda S, Wakashin M, Wakashin Y et al. Experimental gold nephropathy in guinea pigs: detection of autoantibodies to renal tubular antigens. *Kidney Int 1986; 29:* 539–548
44 Balazs T, Robinson C, Abraham A. Drug-induced autoimmunity in rats. *Sixth International Congress of Immunology.* Toronto 1986
45 Seelig HP, Seelig R, Fisher A et al. Immun-komplex-glomerulonephritis nach peroraler Penicillamin applikation bei ratten. *Res Exp Med 1977; 170:* 35–55
46 Donker ABJ, Venuto RC, Vladutiu AO et al. Effects of prolonged administration of D-penicillamine or captopril in various strains of rats. *Clin Immunol Immunopathol 1984; 30:* 142–155
47 Ten Veen JH, Feltkamp-Vroom TM. Studies on drug-induced lupus erythematosus in mice. III. Renal lesions and spenomegaly in drug-induced lupus erythematosus. *Clin Exp Immunol 1973; 15:* 591–600
48 Malinow MR, Bardana EJ, Pirofsky B et al. Systemic lupus erythematosus-like syndrome in monkeys fed alfalfa sprouts: role of nonprotein amino acid. *Science 1982; 216:* 415–417
49 Shibasaki T, Joh K, Watanabe N et al. Drug-induced hypersensitivity nephritis in mice. *Kidney Int 1987; 31:* 330
50 Tan EM. Drug-induced autoimmune disease. *Fed Proc 1974; 33:* 1894–1896
51 Pelletier L, Pasquier R, Rossert J, Druet P. $HgCl_2$ induces nonspecific immunosuppression in Lewis rats. *Eur J Immunol 1987; 17:* 49–54
52 Pelletier L, Galceran M, Pasquier R et al. Down modulation of Heymann's nephritis by mercuric chloride. *Kidney Int 1987; 32:* in press
53 Colvin RB, Burton NE, Hyslop NE. Penicillin associated interstitial nephritis. *Ann Intern Med 1974; 81:* 404–405
54 Kirtland HH, Mohler DN, Horwitz DA. Methyldopa inhibition of suppressor-lymphocyte function. A proposed cause of autoimmune hemolytic anemia. *N Engl J Med 1980; 302:* 825–832
55 Bluestein HG, Weisman MH, Svaifler NJ, Shapiro RF. Lymphocyte alteration by procainamide: relation to drug-induced lupus erythematosus syndrome. *Lancet 1979; ii:* 816–819
56 Eastman AY, Lawrence DA. TNP-modified syngeneic cells enhance immunoregulatory T cell activities similar to allogeneic effects. *J Immunol 1982; 126:* 926–931
57 Gleichmann HIK, Pals ST, Radaszkiewics T. T cell-dependent B-cell proliferation and activation induced by administration of the drug diphenylhydantoin in mice. *Hematol Oncol 1983; 1:* 165–176
58 Nagata N, Hurtenbach U, Gleichmann E. Specific sensitization of lyt-1^+2^- T cells to spleen cells modified by the drug D-penicillamine or a steroisomer. *J Immunol 1986; 136:* 136–142
59 Fleichmann E, Pals ST, Rolink AG et al. Graft-versus-host reactions: clues to the etiopathology of a spectrum of immunological diseases. *Immunol Today 1984; 5:* 324–332
60 Paul WE, Ohara J. B cell-stimulatory factor 1 or interleukin 4. *Ann Rev Immunol 1987; 5:* 419–459

MEDIATORS OF IMMUNOLOGICAL INJURY

THE MEMBRANE ATTACK COMPLEX OF COMPLEMENT IN GLOMERULAR INJURY

D J Salant, A V Cybulsky, R J Quigg, J Badalamenti

The University Hospital, Boston University Medical Center, Boston, Massachusetts, USA

Introduction

In addition to its function in host defence against micro-organisms, the complement system is an important mediator of the inflammatory response. Components of the classical, alternative and terminal complement pathways can be demonstrated in glomeruli of patients with a variety of immunological and non-immunological renal diseases and, through the use of animal models of glomerular diseases, have been shown to be important mediators of certain types of glomerular injury. The best recognized action of complement in tissue injury is its ability to stimulate an influx of leucocytes into an inflammatory focus, as in the heterologous phase of anti-glomerular basement membrane nephritis in rats and rabbits. This action depends on the chemotactic and immune adherent properties of C5a and C3b generated during activation of the classical or alternative pathways. Activation of complement in the immediate vicinity of a cell also leads to assembly of the terminal C5b–9 membrane attack complex and its insertion into the cell plasma membrane. This property of complement has recently been identified as an alternative, leucocyte-independent mechanism of glomerular injury and is the major subject of this review.

The nature of antibody governs whether or not complement-fixation occurs in glomeruli [1], but the site at which immune deposits form within the glomerular capillary wall determines whether or not leucocytes are recruited [2]. Other potentially important properties of complement that may be relevant to immune renal disease are included in Table I but will not be discussed here.

Complement activation and assembly of the membrane attack complex

When antibodies deposit in tissues, classical pathway activation of complement will follow if the antibodies are of complement-fixing subclass and if adjacent molecules are sufficiently closely spaced to be cross-linked by at least two 'arms' of Clq. Clq fixation leads to the activation of Clr and Cls to form Clqrs,

TABLE I. Potential rôles of complement in glomerular injury

PROINFLAMMATORY PROPERTIES	
Leucocyte chemotaxis and immune adherence	C5a and C3b
Release of inflammatory mediators from leucocytes and mast cells	C3 and C5 cleavage products
Direct (leucocyte-independent) tissue injury	C5b–9 complex
IMMUNOREGULATORY PROPERTIES	
Modulation of humoral and cellular immune responses	C3b and C5a
Immune complex lattice modification and dissolution	C1–C3
Immune complex transport and clearance in primates	C3b–CR1
OTHER PROPERTIES	
Binding to laminin and fibronectin	C1q, C3d

followed by the sequential enzymatic cleavage of C4 and C2, and the formation of the C3 and C5 convertases, C4b2a and C4b2a3b, respectively [3,4]. C3 may also be cleaved by a convertase (C3bBb) generated upon activation of the alternative pathway [3].

Activation of the terminal complement pathway [3,4] follows cleavage of C5 by the C5 convertase and leads to the formation of the soluble bimolecular complex C5b6. Upon binding C7 to form C5b–7, the trimolecular complex acquires hydrophobic phospholipid-binding domains and, if formed near a cell surface, it can insert into a cell membrane. By itself, C5b–7 has no deleterious effect on membrane integrity, however, binding of C8 to the complex results in membrane damage, a process that is accelerated by the subsequent binding of C9. Formation of the membrane attack complex concomitantly results in the development of antigenic determinants that are found on the assembled complex of C5b–9 but not on the individual complement molecules. This property of the membrane attack complex has enabled production of antibodies that recognize only the 'neoantigenic' determinants, allowing for immunohistological detection of the membrane attack complex in tissues, or for quantification of the membrane attack complex in biological fluids.

The insertion of the membrane attack complex into a plasma membrane alters transmembrane ion fluxes, collapses electrochemical gradients, and may result in membrane disassembly and cell death. The fully assembled membrane attack complex contains multiple C9 molecules [5] and, by electronmicroscopy, appears as a 'doughnut-shaped' hollow cylinder with an internal diameter of 10nm [6]. Based on this ultrastructural appearance it has been proposed that the membrane attack complex alters membrane permeability by acting as a cylindrical transmembrane conduit for unregulated ion and water flux. It has also been proposed that membrane attack complex insertion leads to diffuse perturbations in the plasma membrane due to disorganization and disruption of the lipid bilayer and release of phospholipids. The arguments for and against these various hypotheses are discussed elsewhere [6–8].

In contrast to erythrocytes in which lysis by complement has been considered a 'one-hit' event, i.e. one C5b–9 lesion suffices for haemolysis, nucleated cells are generally more resistant to complement attack and require multiple 'hits' by the membrane attack complex for lysis to occur [9]. The relative resistance of nucleated cells to complement lysis is probably attributable to their ability to eliminate the membrane attack complex, repair the plasma membrane, and regulate cell volume. Furthermore the membrane attack complex can alter plasma membrane permeability of nucleated cells without causing their death. Such 'sublytic' cytotoxicity can be demonstrated by the presence of membrane permeability to small molecules in the absence of cytolysis. Sublytic doses of complement can also activate nucleated cells to produce various soluble mediators [10–14]. For example, after exposure to C5b–9, synthesis of prostaglandins and thromboxane by rat peritoneal macrophages [10,11], mesangial cells [12], and glomerular epithelial cells [14] is stimulated. Further studies of phospholipid metabolism indicate that C5b–9 induces arachidonic acid release from phosphatidyl choline and phosphatidyl ethanolamine [15]. These findings suggest activation of phospholipase A_2, which results in an increased intracellular free fatty acid pool and increased substrate availability for eicosanoid biosynthesis. Therefore, in sublytic doses the membrane attack complex is not only *cytotoxic*, but may *activate* membrane-associated or cytoplasmic metabolic processes.

Rôle of the membrane attack complex in experimental glomerular injury

Experimental membranous nephropathy

Most evidence implicating the membrane attack complex as an agent of immunological glomerular injury is derived from the study of experimental membranous nephropathy, especially passive Heymann nephritis. Membranous nephropathy in both humans and experimental animals is characterized morphologically by the presence of glomerular immune deposits of IgG and complement in the absence of an inflammatory cell infiltrate. These are associated with injury to the glomerular capillary wall, which manifests primarily as proteinuria

Functional studies. Glomerular injury (assessed by urine protein excretion) in the passive Heymann nephritis model of experimental membranous nephropathy in the rat is complement-mediated but leucocyte-independent [16]. Passive Heymann nephritis is produced in the rat by a single injection of complement-fixing antibody raised to a fraction of rat kidney proximal tubule brush border (Fx1A). This antibody (anti-Fx1A) cross reacts with intrinsic glomerular antigens and forms subepithelial immune deposits in situ [17,18]. The putative nephritogenic antigen (gp330) has been identified in coated pits on proximal tubular cells and glomerular visceral epithelial cells [19]. Anti-Fx1A and anti-gp330 also identify surface antigens on cultured glomerular epithelial cells and induce their redistribution and disappearance from the plasma membrane [20], a process that may be responsible for the formation of subepithelial immune deposits in vivo [21]. Activation of the complement cascade by the subepithelial immune complexes (or by antibody bound to the glomerular epithelial cell membrane) leads to proteinuria 4–5 days after the administration of antibody. In vivo decomplementation of rats with cobra venom factor, prior to the administration of antibody, does not affect glomerular antibody deposition, but prevents the development of glomerular injury [16]. In contrast, administration of anti-neutrophil serum prior to anti-Fx1A does not diminish urine protein excretion. Similar findings are also evident in various active or passive autologous-phase models of passive Heymann nephritis in which complement-fixing host or isologous anti-IgG antibodies react with non-complement-fixing sheep anti-Fx1A IgG planted in the subepithelial space [22].

Observations on the direct mediation of injury by complement were further extended in the rabbit, in a variant model of serum sickness that resembles membranous nephropathy. Groggel et al [23] produced rabbit membranous nephropathy by daily immunization of normal and genetically C6-deficient rabbits with cationized bovine serum albumin (BSA). After 1–2 weeks both normal and C6-deficient rabbits developed subepithelial, electron-dense deposits, and a non-inflammatory glomerular lesion resembling early human membranous nephropathy. Despite equal amounts of glomerular immune IgG, C6-deficient animals failed to develop the proteinuria seen in their complement-replete counterparts, thus implicating the terminal complement pathway.

Definitive functional evidence for the pathogenic rôle of the C5b–9 membrane attack complex in membranous nephropathy was provided by recent studies on the cell-free isolated perfused rat kidney [24,25]. The rationale for these studies was based on the key membranolytic rôle of C8 in the formation of the membrane attack complex, outlined above. Because there are no C8-deficient rat strains and depletion of C8 is difficult to achieve in vivo, a passive-autologous phase model of passive Heymann nephritis was developed in the isolated perfused kidney [24]. Rats were injected with a subnephritogenic dose of the non-complement-fixing γ_2 subclass of sheep anti-Fx1A IgG prior to kidney perfusion ('planted' antigen). Kidneys were isolated and perfused for two hours in vitro with complement-fixing guinea pig anti-sheep IgG and various human plasmas serving as sources of complement. Perfusion with complement-replete normal plasma resulted in a rapidly progressive rise in proteinuria (Table II). In contrast, protein excretion remained at levels of control kidneys when normal plasma was substituted with C8-deficient plasma (Table II). Glomerular antibody deposition was not affected by the absence of C8 [24]. Reconstitution of the C8-deficient plasma with sources of C8 restored proteinuria to levels seen with normal plasma. Similar observations were also made in a heterologous-phase model of passive Heymann nephritis in the isolated perfused rat kidney [25].

TABLE II. Rôle of C5b–9 in the development of proteinuria in a passive autologous-phase model of passive Heymann nephritis in the isolated perfused rat kidney

Group[1]		Subepithelial antigen[2]	Perfusate composition		Urine protein excretion, µg/min[5]	
			Antibody[3]	Complement source[4]	40–60 min	100–120 min
I	(8)	+	+	NHP	1008	4269
II	(6)	+	+	HIP	203	102
III	(6)	–	+	NHP	333	299
IV	(5)	+	+	C8D	302	236
V	(3)	+	+	C8D + C8	4871	4110

1 Number of kidneys studied is in parentheses.
2 Non-complement-fixing γ_2 sheep anti-Fx1A injected three days prior to perfusion.
3 Complement-fixing guinea pig anti-sheep IgG.
4 NHP=normal human plasma; HIP=heat-inactivated human plasma; C8D=C8-deficient human plasma; C8D + C8=reconstituted C8D; all at 50% in bovine albumin-buffer.
5 Only mean values are shown. Groups I and V are significantly greater than the other groups at both time intervals.

Perfusion of kidneys containing complement-fixing γ_1 anti-Fx1A IgG with plasma resulted in increased proteinuria only in the presence of complement-replete plasma but not with C8-deficient human plasma or C6-deficient rabbit serum. Combination of the C8 and C6-deficient reagents, whether simultaneously or in sequence, reproduced the increased proteinuria [25]. Therefore, since C8 is essential for complement-mediated membranolysis and has no other defined rôle, it is reasonable to conclude that injury in rat membranous nephropathy is mediated by the membrane attack complex.

This conclusion is further supported by a recent study in which a rôle for C6 was also demonstrated in passive Heymann nephritis in vivo [26]. Rats were treated with an antibody against rat C6 to reduce serum C6 haemolytic activity to <5%. After the administration of anti-Fx1A, these rats developed subepithelial immune deposits in amounts equal to those in rats given anti-Fx1A alone (without C6 depletion). Proteinuria developed only in the C6-replete group. Subsequently, Ochi et al confirmed a functional rôle for C6 in another in vivo rat model of membranous nephropathy, induced by unilateral renal perfusion with cationized human IgG, followed by passive immunization with anti-IgG [27]. After 24–48 hours, rats developed immune deposits of IgG and proteinuria. Pretreatment of rats with anti-C6 antibody reduced serum concentrations of C6 to <3% of normal and proteinuria by ~50%, without influencing the quantities of antigen or antibody deposited in glomeruli. The residual proteinuria in this 'planted antigen' model may be due to leucocyte-mediated injury [28].

Immunohistological studies. Indirect evidence suggests that in active Heymann nephritis proteinuria is also complement-mediated. This lesion is induced by immunization of Lewis rats, or other susceptible strains with Fx1A. After six weeks, subepithelial immune deposits develop in all rats [29]. Of these, ~60% demonstrate glomerular C3 deposition by immunofluorescence microscopy, and are proteinuric. The remainder do not have C3 deposits and excrete normal levels of protein. Of this subgroup, about 60% will develop glomerular deposits of C3 and proteinuria concurrently, when reimmunized with Fx1A. Furthermore, terminal complement components and membrane attack complex neoantigens have been identified in the glomeruli of rats with Heymann nephritis [30–33], and are distributed in a peripheral granular pattern resembling that of IgG and C3. Thus, the close association of proteinuria with glomerular complement deposits in the absence of inflammatory cells strongly suggests that glomerular injury in Heymann nephritis, as in passive Heymann nephritis, is dependent on the membrane attack complex.

Terminal complement components and membrane attack complex neoantigens have also been demonstrated by direct immunofluorescence and immunoelectron microscopy in kidney biopsy tissue from other experimental animal models of membranous nephropathy, including passive Heymann nephritis and chronic serum sickness in the rat [30,31,34]. Moreover, in passive Heymann nephritis the presence of terminal complement components and the membrane attack complex could be correlated with functional evidence of complement-mediated proteinuria [30,31].

Target of injury. There are several reasons to believe that the visceral glomerular epithelial cell is the initial target of antibody-directed, complement-mediated injury in experimental membranous nephropathy, and that this injury may directly account for proteinuria in membranous nephropathy. Glomerular epithelial cell alterations, including effacement of foot processes, microvillus transformation and displacement of slit diaphragms are found in experimental membranous nephropathy [35], and are accompanied by glomerular epithelial cell dysfunction as demonstrated by the impaired clearance of protamine-heparin aggregates [36]. More direct evidence of glomerular epithelial cell injury in experimental membranous nephropathy was recently obtained in the isolated perfused kidney model of autologous-phase passive Heymann nephritis [24], in which kidneys perfused in vitro with complement-fixing antibodies and C8-deficient human plasma contained glomerular subepithelial electron-dense deposits and normal glomerular epithelial cell morphology. In contrast, kidneys perfused with the same antibody in the presence of complement-replete or C8-reconstituted human plasma suffered severe glomerular epithelial cell injury in the vicinity of subepithelial immune deposits. Extensive effacement of foot processes and villous transformation of the plasma membranes were seen, together with vacuolization, degeneration and focal detachment of epithelial cells. The severity of glomerular epithelial cell damage seen in the perfused kidney model is probably amplified by facilitated delivery of complement to the subepithelial space (due to the intrinsic proteinuric nature of the model) and by the use of heterologous complement components [37]. Nevertheless, these studies conclusively showed that severe glomerular epithelial cell damage is a potential consequence of full assembly of the membrane attack complex when induced by complement-fixing antibodies in the subepithelial space. Moreover, urinary excretion of the membrane attack complex occurs uniquely in passive Heymann nephritis and not in other proteinuric states associated with circulating C5b–9, suggesting that the membrane attack complex is assembled in close proximity to the urinary space on the epithelial cell surface [38].

Localization of the membrane attack complex was studied by immunoelectron microscopy in a rat model of chronic serum sickness [34]. Using a polyclonal antiserum to human C9 and C5b–9, these authors showed that membrane attack complex antigens colocalized with BSA, rat IgG and C3 in subepithelial immune deposits but, more interestingly, membrane attack complex antigens were present on the overlying, partly detached and effaced, podocyte plasma membrane. Failure of acid elution to remove the membrane-associated membrane attack complex antigens suggests that they were inserted into the plasma membrane, probably after diffusion of C5b6 from the site of activation in the subepithelial deposits and subsequent fixation of C7 [34]. Although it is difficult to demonstrate a functional rôle for terminal complement components in chronic serum sickness in the rat, it is possible that glomerular damage is mediated by mechanisms similar to those described in other models in which complement-fixing antibodies bind to a planted, exogenous, subepithelial antigen and induce proteinuria through the action of the terminal complement pathway [23,27].

Pathophysiology of glomerular injury in membranous nephropathy. Functional and morphological observations in the isolated perfused rat kidney model of experimental membranous nephropathy favour a structural defect in the filtration barrier, and suggest that this defect is sufficient to cause proteinuria [24, 25]. Moreover, dextran clearance studies in both passive Heymann nephritis and human membranous nephropathy have disclosed a size-selective sieving defect, the magnitude of which appears to be influenced by haemodynamic factors [39,40], particularly glomerular capillary pressure [39].

The mechanisms by which sublytic glomerular epithelial cell injury contributes to proteinuria are unknown. They might include glomerular epithelial cell shape alterations that are unfavourable to the maintenance of glomerular permselectivity, disordered glomerular basement membrane matrix synthesis, or production of secondary mediators, some of which have been implicated in disorders of glomerular permselectivity. Disordered glomerular basement membrane matrix synthesis might contribute to long-term alterations in glomerular permeability and glomerular basement membrane thickening characteristic of advanced experimental and human membranous nephropathy, but it probably does not account for the rapid onset of complement-mediated proteinuria seen in passive Heymann nephritis, in vivo or in the isolated perfused kidney.

Among the secondary mediators, the rôle of glomerular eicosanoids has been examined most closely in membranous nephropathy. Patients with membranous nephropathy and other forms of nephrotic syndrome, when treated with indomethacin, experience a decline in proteinuria and an increase in the 'selectivity index' [41], an effect that is at least in part secondary to the drug's effect on glomerular haemodynamics [40]. Experiments seeking a direct rôle of eicosanoids in experimental membranous nephropathy have come to variable conclusions. Glomerular thromboxane production is increased in proteinuric rats with passive Heymann nephritis [42,43] and this increase is complement-dependent [42]. Cyclo-oxygenase inhibition with indomethacin reduced proteinuria by 60% in active Heymann nephritis [44] and by 74% in the autologous phase of passive Heymann nephritis [43]; in this latter study, there was a quantitatively similar decrease in urinary thromboxane excretion. The glomerular filtration rate was not substantially altered in either study. In the isolated perfused rat kidney model of passive Heymann nephritis, Cybulsky et al showed that inhibition of thromboxane synthetase with OKY-046, in doses sufficient to suppress renal thromboxane production, reduced complement-dependent proteinuria by 75% without altering glomerular filtration rate or renal vascular resistance [45]. In contrast, in vivo treatment of passive Heymann nephritis rats with the thromboxane synthetase inhibitor UK 38485 inhibited glomerular thromboxane production by ~80% in the heterologous phase [42] and urinary thromboxane excretion by about 50% in the autologous phase [43] but it did not reduce proteinuria in either case. Thus, it appears that complement-mediated glomerular injury can induce endogenous glomerular cells to increase their production of eicosanoids (particularly thromboxane A_2), but the pathophysiological consequences of this phenomenon are, as yet, incompletely understood.

Other models of experimental glomerulonephritis

Anti-glomerular basement membrane antibodies are able to induce glomerular capillary wall injury and proteinuria through the action of several mediator systems [46]. Recently, a direct rôle for C5b–9 in anti-glomerular basement membrane nephritis has been demonstrated too. In the cell-free, isolated perfused rat kidney, perfusion with anti-glomerular basement membrane antibody and complement-replete plasma resulted in proteinuria, whereas a major reduction in proteinuria was observed when plasma was decomplemented [47]. In rabbit anti-glomerular basement membrane nephritis in vivo, heterologous-phase proteinuria was substantially lower and renal function better preserved in C6-deficient rabbits than in their normal counterparts, despite identical amounts of glomerular-bound antibody [48], indicating a major contribution by the terminal complement pathway. The primary target of injury by complement has not been defined in anti-glomerular basement membrane nephritis, but it is likely that glomerular cells are damaged by the membrane attack complex. This could arise either by diffusion of C5b6 from adjacent immune complexes in the glomerular basement membrane to the glomerular epithelial cells where the membrane attack complex is completed by addition of C7–C9, or from the activation of complement at the cell membrane by cell-specific antibodies contained in the polyspecific anti-glomerular basement membrane antiserum.

Another model in which C5b–9 may produce cytotoxicity of intrinsic glomerular cells is that induced in rats by injecting heterologous, complement-fixing, anti-thymocyte antiserum or monoclonal antibodies with specificity for the Thy 1 antigen. Thy 1 is a thymocyte antigen that is also expressed by certain parenchymal cells including mesangial cells [49,50]. Mesangial cell lysis is visible within one hour of a single dose of antibody, is accompanied by mesangial deposits of C3, C9, and membrane attack complex neo-antigens [51,52], and can be prevented by depletion of complement but not depletion of leucocytes [52]. Mesangiolysis may also be accompanied by transient, heavy proteinuria [51] but it has not been established that proteinuria is complement-dependent.

The membrane attack complex in human renal disease

Evidence that the membrane attack complex may be involved in mediating tissue injury in human renal disease is inferred from immunohistological studies demonstrating terminal complement components and membrane attack complex neoantigens at the site of disease. These components have been visualized in association with IgG and C3 in several glomerular diseases believed to be caused by humoral immune mechanisms including lupus nephritis, idiopathic membranous nephropathy, de novo membranous nephropathy in renal allografts, anti-glomerular basement membrane nephritis, membranoproliferative glomerulonephritis (Types I and II), IgA nephropathy, Henoch-Schönlein nephritis and post-streptococcal glomerulonephritis [53–60]. Although the colocalization of terminal complement components and IgG and/or C3 in these diseases tends to implicate the membrane attack complex in their immunopathogenesis, it is important to recognize the possibility of an epiphenomenon. For instance, in certain immune complex glomerular diseases, small amounts of membrane attack complex antigens may be found at sites remote from immunoglobulin deposits; in other 'non-immune' diseases such as diabetes, hypertension, amyloidosis, obstructive uropathy, dysplasia and other chronic nephritides, membrane attack complex deposits are present in areas of sclerosis [55,56]. These deposits may simply represent macromolecules 'trapped' in sclerosing lesions, or they may be an inevitable consequence of cellular injury leading to antibody-independent complement activation via the alternate pathway [61].

Furthermore, mesangial clusters of membrane attack complex antigens have even been detected in patients with minimal change disease, and in normal kidneys [55,56]. On the other hand, several observations are consistent with glomerular epithelial cell injury and a rôle for the membrane attack complex in human membranous nephropathy.

Complement components (especially C3) codistribute with IgG in a granular immunofluorescence pattern in the glomeruli of a high proportion of patients with idiopathic membranous nephropathy [62], and several recent studies have shown concordance between granular glomerular capillary wall staining for poly C9, membrane attack complex neoantigens and terminal complement components and IgG and C3 in idiopathic membranous nephropathy [54–57,59]. Focal glomerular epithelial cell abnormalities resembling those described in the isolated rat kidney model of membranous nephropathy [24] and in Heymann nephritis [35], have also been noted in some cases of human membranous nephropathy. In addition, functional evidence for the presence of focal defects in the glomerular filtration barrier in human membranous nephropathy was recently obtained by Shemesh et al using macromolecular clearance techniques [40], which suggests that the pathogenesis of proteinuria might be similar to that defined in experimental membranous nephropathy.

Complement induced injury of cultured glomerular cells

Epithelial cells. With the knowledge that anti-Fx1A and anti-gp330 [20,63] bind directly to the plasma membrane of cultured rat glomerular epithelial cells, we assessed the ability of a nephritogenic preparation of anti-Fx1A to induce cellular damage of primary and long-term cultured rat glomerular epithelial cells [64]. Glomerular epithelial cells were sensitized with the complement-fixing γ_1 subclass of sheep anti-Fx1A IgG and exposed to various sera serving as sources of complement. Incubation of antibody-sensitized glomerular epithelial cells in normal human serum resulted in a sigmoidal relationship between cytotoxicity (release of cellular LDH) and complement dose, consistent with the multi-hit requirement for cytolysis observed in other nucleated cell types [9]. Cytolysis was evident with anti-Fx1A and normal serum, but was not evident if non-immune IgG was used in place of antibody, or if C8-deficient plasma was substituted for normal serum. Reconstitution of C8-deficient plasma with purified rat C8 restored cytolysis. Therefore, the nephritogenic antibody of passive Heymann nephritis directs insertion of the membrane attack complex into the glomerular epithelial cell plasma membrane, resulting in cytotoxicity. Sublytic injury (of particular relevance to membranous nephropathy) was assessed using antibody-sensitized glomerular epithelial cells that were preloaded with biscarboxyethyl carboxyfluorescein (BCECF; MW ~520 daltons), a low molecular weight molecule that is largely retained by non-permeabilized cells. When subsequently incubated with a series of limiting doses of complement, BCECF was released at doses that did not cause release of LDH, thus demonstrating cell membrane perturbation in the absence of cell death [64].

As discussed earlier in this review, sublytic doses of complement, in addition to altering cell membrane integrity and morphology, can stimulate nucleated cells to release various soluble mediators. In recent studies using glomerular epithelial cell outgrowths from explanted glomeruli, Hänsch et al showed that C5b–9 stimulated a dose-dependent release of prostaglandin E and thromboxane B_2 within 5 to 10 minutes [14]. Prostaglandin E release was inhibited by both cyclo-oxygenase and phospholipase A_2 inhibitors. These findings are consistent with a complement-mediated increase in membrane phospholipid turnover in glomerular epithelial cells and concur with observations of stimulated glomerular prostanoid production in passive Heymann nephritis. Thus, cell culture experiments have confirmed that glomerular epithelial cells can be a target for sublytic complement-mediated injury, and are beginning to provide information on the alterations in cell function induced by such injury.

Mesangial cells. In keeping with the complement-dependent mesangiolysis observed in vivo in rats injected with anti-Thy 1 [50,51], cultured mesangial cells that are sensitized with anti-Thy 1 in vitro undergo lysis when exposed to complement [65]. Moreover, exposing cultured mesangial cells to sublytic doses of complement induces them to release reactive oxygen species [13], prostanoids [12] and interleukin 1 [12]. Although, in vivo, complement has been found to produce functional derangements only in the anti-Thy 1 model of mesangial injury, the potential clearly exists for mesangial cells to produce a variety of inflammatory mediators in response to antibody- or immune complex-mediated complement activation.

Summary

From the information presented in this review, it can now be concluded that glomerular injury in experimental membranous nephropathy is dependent on the assembly of the membrane attack complex. We have also presented evidence that allows us to propose that the glomerular epithelial cell is the site of injury in membranous nephropathy, and that complement exerts its cytotoxic effect in the absence of cell lysis. These sublytic effects appear to include plasma membrane-associated metabolic processes and production of secondary mediators that may contribute to, or aggravate, the abnormality in glomerular capillary wall permeability. There is also increasing experimental and clinical evidence that this novel mediator of parenchymal cell damage may be responsible for other forms of glomerular and non renal disease [4,66] in which complement-fixing antibodies are directed at cell-associated antigens, or in which immune complexes form in close proximity to cell membranes.

Acknowledgments

Portions of this work were supported by research grant DK30932 and National Research Service Award DK07730 (Dr Quigg) from the United States Public Health Service, and a Grant-in-Aid from the American Heart Association, Massachusetts Affiliate. Dr Cybulsky is a fellow of the Medical Research Council of Canada. Dr Salant is an Established Investigator of the American Heart Association.

References

1 Lewis EJ, Busch GJ, Schur PH. Gamma G globulin subgroup composition of the glomerular deposits in human renal diseases. *J Clin Invest 1970; 49:* 1103–1113

2 Salant DJ, Adler S, Darby C et al. Influence of antigen distribution on the mediation of immunological glomerular injury. *Kidney Int 1985; 27:* 938–950

3 Schreiber RD, Müller-Eberhard HJ. Complement and renal disease. *Contemp Issues Nephrol 1979; 3:* 67–105

4 Couser WG, Baker PJ, Adler S. Complement and the direct mediation of immune glomerular injury: a new perspective. *Kidney Int 1985; 28:* 879–890

5 Podack ER, Tschopp J, Müller-Eberhard HJ. Molecular organization of C9 within the membrane attack complex of complement. Induction of circular C9 polymerization by the C5b–8 assembly. *J Exp Med 1982; 156:* 268–282

6 Bhakdi S, Tranum-Jensen J. Membrane damage by complement. *Biochim Biophys Acta 1983; 737:* 343–371

7 Mayer MM, Michaels DW, Ramm LE et al. Membrane damage by complement. *Crit Rev Immunol 1981; 2:* 133–166

8 Müller-Eberhard HJ. The membrane attack complex. In Müller-Eberhard HJ, Miescher PA, eds. *Complement.* Berlin: Springer-Verlag. 1984: 227–275

9 Koski CL, Ramm LE, Hammer CH et al. Cytolysis of nucleated cells by complement: cell death displays multi-hit characteristics. *Proc Natl Acad Sci USA 1983; 60:* 3816–3820

10 Imagawa DK, Osifchin NE, Paznekas WA et al. Consequences of cell membrane attack by complement: release of arachidonate and formation of inflammatory derivatives. *Proc Natl Acad Sci USA 1983; 80:* 6647–6651

11 Hänsch GM, Seitz M, Martinotti G et al. Macrophages release arachidonic acid, prostaglandin E_2, and thromboxane in response to late complement components. *J Immunol 1984; 133:* 2145–2150

12 Lovett DH, Haensch GM, Goppelt M et al. Activation of glomerular mesangial cells by the terminal membrane attack complex of complement. *J Immunol 1987; 138:* 2473–2480

13 Adler S, Baker PJ, Johnson RJ et al. Complement membrane attack complex stimulates production of reactive oxygen metabolites by cultured rat mesangial cells. *J Clin Invest 1986; 77:* 762–767

14 Hänsch GM, Betz M, Günther J et al. The complement membrane attack complex stimulates the prostanoid production of cultured glomerular epithelial cells. *Int Arch Appl Immunol 1987; 4:* in press

15 Betz M, Hansch GM. Release of arachidonic acid: a new function of the late complement components. *Immunobiol 1984; 166:* 473–483

16 Salant DJ, Belok S, Madaio MP, Couser WG. A new role for complement in experimental membranous nephropathy in rats. *J Clin Invest 1980; 66:* 1339–1350

17 Couser WG, Steinmuller DR, Stilmant MM et al. Experimental glomerulonephritis in the isolated perfused rat kidney. *J Clin Invest 1978; 62:* 1275–1287

18 Van Damme BJC, Fleuren GJ, Bakker WW et al. Experimental glomerulonephritis in the rat induced by antibodies directed against tubular antigens. V. Fixed glomerular antigens in the pathogenesis of heterologous immune complex glomerulonephritis. *Lab Invest 1978; 38:* 502–510

19 Kerjaschki D, Farquhar MG. Immunocytochemical localization of the Heymann nephritis antigen (gp330) in glomerular epithelial cells of normal Lewis rats. *J Exp Med 1983; 157:* 667–686

20 Camussi G, Brentjens JR, Noble B et al. Antibody-induced redistribution of Heymann's antigen on the surface of cultured glomerular visceral epithelial cells: possible role in the pathogenesis of Heymann glomerulonephritis. *J Immunol 1985; 135:* 2409–2416

21 Andres G, Brentjens JR, Caldwell PRB et al. Formation of immune deposits and disease. *Lab Invest 1986; 55:* 510–516

22 Adler S, Salant DJ, Dittmer JE et al. Mediation of proteinuria in membranous nephropathy due to a planted glomerular antigen. *Kidney Int 1983; 23:* 807–815

23 Groggel GC, Adler S, Rennke HG et al. Role of the terminal complement pathway in experimental membranous nephropathy in the rabbit. *J Clin Invest 1983; 72:* 1948–1957
24 Cybulsky AV, Rennke HG, Feintzeig ID, Salant DJ. Complement-induced glomerular epithelial cell injury. Role of the membrane attack complex in rat membranous nephropathy. *J Clin Invest 1986; 77:* 1096–1107
25 Cybulsky AV, Quigg RJ, Salant DJ. The membrane attack complex in complement-mediated glomerular epithelial cell injury: formation and stability of C5b–9 and C5b–7 in rat membranous nephropathy. *J Immunol 1986; 137:* 1511–1516
26 Baker PJ, Ochi RF, Adler S et al. C6 depletion abolishes proteinuria in experimental membranous nephropathy. *Clin Res 1985; 33 (Abstract):* 475A
27 Ochi RF, Johnson RJ, Baker PJ et al. C6 depletion diminishes proteinuria in experimental membranous nephropathy induced by an exogenous antigen. *Kidney Int 1986; 29 (Abstract):* 287
28 Thaiss F, Batsford S, Mihatsch MJ et al. Mediator systems in a passive model of in situ immune complex glomerulonephritis. Role for complement, polymorphonuclear granulocytes and monocytes. *Lab Invest 1986; 54:* 624–635
29 Noble B, Van Liew JB, Andres GA, Brentjens JR. Factors influencing susceptibility of LEW rats to Heymann nephritis. *Clin Immunol Immunopathol 1984; 30:* 241–254
30 Adler S, Baker PJ, Pritzl P, Couser WG. Detection of terminal complement components in experimental immune glomerular injury. *Kidney Int 1984; 26:* 830–837
31 Perkinson DT, Baker PJ, Couser WG et al. Membrane attack complex deposition in experimental glomerular injury. *Am J Pathol 1985; 120:* 121–128
32 Biesecker G, Noble B, Andres GA, Koffler D. Immunopathogenesis of Heymann's nephritis. *Clin Immunol Immunopathol 1984; 33:* 333–338
33 De Heer E, Daha MR, Bhakdi S et al. Possible involvement of terminal complement complex in active Heymann nephritis. *Kidney Int 1985; 27:* 388–393
34 Koffler D, Biesecker G, Noble B et al. Localization of the membrane attack complex (MAC) in experimental immune complex glomerulonephritis. *J Exp Med 1983; 157:* 1885–1905
35 Schneeberger EE, Grupe WE. The ultrastructure of the glomerular slit diaphragm in autologous immune complex nephritis. *Lab Invest 1976; 34:* 298–305
36 Sharon Z, Schwartz MM, Pauli BU, Lewis EJ. Impairment of glomerular clearance of macroaggregates in immune complex glomerulonephritis. *Kidney Int 1982; 22:* 8–12
37 Hänsch GM, Hammer CH, Vanguri P, Shin ML. Homologous species restriction in lysis of erythrocytes by terminal complement proteins. *Proc Natl Acad Sci USA 1981; 78:* 5118–5121
38 Schulze M, Baker PJ, Ochi R et al. Urinary excretion of complement C5b–9 in experimental membranous nephropathy. *Kidney Int 1987; 31 (Abstract):* 329
39 Yoshioka T, Rennke HG, Salant DJ et al. Role of abnormally high transmural pressure in the permselectivity defect of glomerular capillary wall: a study in early passive Heymann nephritis. *Circ Res 1987:* in press
40 Shemesh O, Ross JC, Deen WM et al. Nature of the glomerular capillary injury in human membranous glomerulopathy. *J Clin Invest 1986; 77:* 868–877
41 Arisz L, Donker AJM, Brentjens JRH, van der Hem GK. The effect of indomethacin on proteinuria and kidney function in the nephrotic syndrome. *Acta Med Scand 1976; 199:* 121–125
42 Stahl RAK, Adler S, Baker PJ et al. Enhanced glomerular prostaglandin formation in experimental membranous nephropathy. *Kidney Int 1987; 31:* 1126–1131
43 Zoja C, Benigni A, Verroust P et al. Indomethacin reduces proteinuria in passive Heymann nephritis in rats. *Kidney Int 1987; 31:* 1335–1343
44 Kirschenbaum MA, Liebross BA, Serros ER. Effect of indomethacin on proteinuria in rats with autologous immune complex nephropathy. *Prostaglandins 1985; 30:* 295–303
45 Cybulsky AV, Lieberthal W, Quigg RJ et al. A role for thromboxane in complement-mediated glomerular injury. *Am J Pathol 1987; 128:* in press
46 Couser WG, Salant DJ, Immunopathogenesis of glomerular capillary wall injury in nephrotic states. *Contemp Issues Nephrol 1982; 9:* 47–83

47 Boyce NW, Holdsworth SR. Anti-glomerular basement membrane antibody-induced experimental glomerulonephritis: evidence for dose-dependent, direct antibody and complement-induced, cell-independent injury. *J Immunol 1985; 135:* 3918–3921

48 Groggel GC, Salant DJ, Darby C et al. Role of terminal complement pathway in the heterologous phase of antiglomerular basement membrane nephritis in the rabbit. *Kidney Int 1985; 27:* 643–651

49 Ishizaki M, Sato S, Sano J et al. The presence of Thy 1.1 antigen in rat glomerular mesangial cells. *Biomed Res 1980; 1:* 438–442

50 Yamamoto T, Yamamoto K, Kawasaki K et al. Immunoelectron microscopic demonstration of thy-1 antigen on the surfaces of mesangial cells in the rat glomerulus. *Nephron 1986; 43:* 293–298

51 Bagchus WM, Hoedemaeker PhJ, Rozing J, Bakker WW. Glomerulonephritis induced by monoclonal anti-Thy 1.1 antibodies. *Lab Invest 1986; 55:* 680–687

52 Yamamoto T, Wilson CB. Complement dependence of antibody-induced mesangial cell injury in the rat. *J Immunol 1987; 138:* 3758–3765

53 Biesecker G, Katz S, Koffler D. Renal localization of the membrane attack complex in systemic lupus erythematosus nephritis. *J Exp Med 1981; 151:* 1779–1794

54 Cosyns JP, Kazatchkine MD, Bhakdi S et al. Immunohistochemical analysis of C3 cleavage fragments, factor H, and the C5b–9 terminal complex of complement in de novo membranous glomerulonephritis occurring in patients with renal transplant. *Clin Nephrol 1986; 26:* 203–208

55 Hinglais N, Kazatchkine MD, Bakdi S et al. Immunohistochemical study of the C5b–9 complex of complement in human kidneys. *Kidney Int 1986; 30:* 399–410

56 Falk RJ, Dalmasso AP, Kim Y et al. Neoantigen of the polymerized ninth component of complement. Characterization of a monoclonal antibody and immunohistochemical localization in renal tissue. *J Clin Invest 1983; 72:* 560–573

57 Rauterberg EW, Gehrig T, Lieberknecht M. C5–9 neoantigen detection indicates a complete complement activation in various types of glomerulonephritis. *Mol Immunol 1982; 19 (Abstract):* 1398

58 Rauterberg EW, Lieberknecht H-M, Wingen A-M, Ritz E. Complement membrane attack (MAC) in idiopathic IgA-glomerulonephritis. *Kidney Int 1987; 31:* 820–829

59 Rus HG, Niculescu F, Nanulescu M et al. Immunohistochemical detection of the terminal C5b–9 complement complex in children with glomerular diseases. *Clin Exp Immunol 1986; 65:* 66–72

60 Parra G, Platt JL, Falk RJ et al. Cell populations and membrane attack complex in glomeruli of patients with post-streptococcal glomerulonephritis: identification using monoclonal antibodies by indirect immunofluorescence. *Clin Immunol Immunopathol 1984; 33:* 324–332

61 Baker PJ, Adler S, Yang Y, Couser WG. Complement activation by heat-killed human kidney cells: formation, activity and stabilization of cell bound C3 convertases. *J Immunol 1984; 133:* 877–881

62 Verroust PJ, Wilson CB, Cooper NR et al. Glomerular complement components in human glomerulonephritis. *J Clin Invest 1974; 53:* 77–84

63 Bertani T, Nolin L, Foidart J et al. The effect of puromycin on subepithelial deposits induced by antibodies directed against tubular antigens: a quantitative study. *Eur J Clin Invest 1979; 9:* 465–472

64 Quigg RJ, Cybulsky AV, Salant DJ. Passive Heymann nephritis antibody produces complement-dependent cytotoxicity of cultured rat glomerular epithelial cells. *Kidney Int 1987; 31 (Abstract):* 328

65 Yamamoto T, Wilson CB. Mesangial cell injury and proliferation produced by antibody: a role for the membrane attack complex. *Kidney Int 1987; 31 (Abstract):* 333

66 Biesecker G. Membrane attack complex of complement as a pathologic mediator. *Lab Invest 1983; 49:* 237–249

NEW MECHANISMS OF OXIDANT-INDUCED GLOMERULAR INJURY*

W G Couser, R J Johnson, S J Klebanoff

University of Washington, Seattle, Washington, USA

Introduction

Both proliferative and exudative glomerulonephritis may be associated with a rapid decline in renal function, and can be marked by an infiltration with neutrophils and macrophages. Studies in experimental models document that infiltrating neutrophils (PMNs) and monocytes can mediate glomerular injury. A major mechanism of PMN-induced damage to the glomerular capillary wall is extracellular release of proteases that can degrade glomerular basement membrane [1]. However, PMNs can also generate highly toxic oxidants termed reactive oxygen species which are derived from the stepwise reduction of oxygen [reviewed in 2,3]. Reactive oxygen species have recently been incriminated in the pathogenesis of several forms of PMN-mediated glomerular injury [4–6]. Monocytes, which also produce reactive oxygen species, may also cause glomerular injury via this mechanism. The demonstration that both glomeruli [7] and resident glomerular cells [8,9] can also produce reactive oxygen species raises the possibility that oxidants may mediate glomerular injury independent of circulating leucocytes [10–12]. In this paper we will focus on new data related to mechanisms of PMN-induced glomerular oxidant injury.

Rôle for neutrophils in human glomerulonephritis

Certain types of glomerulonephritis in man are often associated with glomerular infiltration by PMNs. These include glomerulonephritis associated with subendothelial deposits such as systemic lupus erythematosus [131], and essential mixed cryoglobulinaemia [14], and anti-glomerular basement membrane nephritis

* Portions of the text of this article have been adapted with permission from Johnson RJ, Klebanoff SJ, Couser WG. Oxidants in glomerular injury. In Wilson C, Bremmer BM, Stein J, eds. *Immunopathology of Renal Disease.* New York: Churchill Livingstone. 1988: in press

[15]. In anti-glomerular basement membrane nephritis, PMNs may be seen juxtaposed to normal and damaged glomerular basement membranes [15]. PMNs are not seen in membranous nephropathy, perhaps due to the relative inaccessibility of the subepithelial immune complexes and chemotactic factors to circulating leucocytes [16]. PMNs are common in post-streptococcal glomerulonephritis, which has characteristic subepithelial deposits ('humps'). The PMNs are probably due to the coexistence of deposits in mesangial and occasionally subendothelial locations [17,18].

Experimental models of glomerulonephritis

PMNs have been implicated in causing glomerular injury in various animal models of glomerulonephritis, primarily by showing that PMN depletion ameliorates the disease. The initial (heterologous) phase of anti-glomerular basement membrane nephritis is the classic model of PMN-mediated injury [4,19–23]. In nephrotoxic nephritis, PMNs localize in the glomerulus from one to six hours after antibody deposition and correlate with an increase in glomerular permeability [22]. The quantity of proteinuria varies with the number of infiltrating PMNs [19,21]. Depletion of PMNs in experimental anti-glomerular basement membrane nephritis prevents or decreases proteinuria [4,19], which can be partially restored when exogenous PMNs are supplied [20]. Not all anti-glomerular basement membrane antibodies result in a PMN-dependent lesion [19,24,25]. This may relate to species [24], antibody dose [19], or the arrangement of the immune deposits formed and ability to fix complement [19,24]. Anti-glomerular basement membrane antibodies may also produce proteinuria in the absence of cells and complement [24,25].

Mechanisms of PMN localization in glomeruli

The initial formation of an immune complex in the glomerulus usually results in complement activation and release of potent chemotactic factors, principally C5a. Damaged endothelial and mesangial cells, platelets and monocytes, as well as the PMN itself, may also release chemotactic factors. Some of these factors include platelet activating factor, platelet-derived growth factor, leukotriene B4, and other lipoxygenase products [26–29].

Once localized in glomeruli, several receptors modulate PMN adherence including the F_c receptor, C3b (CR1) receptor, and the recently described LFA-1, Mac-1 glycoprotein family (also called CDw18) which includes the receptor for C3bi (CR3) [30]. Other substances including damaged fibronectin [31], platelet activating factor [26], thromboxane A_2 [32], interleukin I [33], C5a [34], leukotriene B4 [35] and tumour necrosis factor [36] also promote PMN adherence. Some of these inflammatory stimuli may also have direct effects on endothelium that results in increased PMN adherence [35–37].

Some studies on PMN localization in glomerulonephritis have suggested that immune adherence to immune complexes is both F_c and complement dependent

[19,38]. The importance of complement is most easily demonstrated in the heterologous phase of anti-glomerular basement membrane glomerulonephritis in which complement depletion can prevent both PMN infiltration and proteinuria in some models [19]. Whether this occurs due to the blocking of C3b (or C3bi) adherence or diminished C5a formation is unknown. The importance of F_c receptor binding has also been demonstrated in a complement-independent model of anti-glomerular basement membrane disease in rabbits [38].

Evidence for proteases as mediators of PMN-induced glomerulonephritis

Neutrophils (and monocytes) can release many toxic and vasoactive substances including proteases, toxic oxidants, prostaglandins, leukotrienes and platelet activating factor [39–41]. Neutrophils contain two major populations of granules which can degranulate. The azurophil (primary) granule contains the neutral serine proteases (elastase and cathepsin G), the acid hydrolases, myeloperoxidase (MPO), lysozyme, and other cationic proteins. The specific (secondary) granule contains a specific collagenase, lysozyme, lactoferrin and vitamin B12 binding protein. In addition, 'C' particles have been described which contain gelatinase, proteinase 3 and acid hydrolases which can undergo exocytosis [40].

Although acidic proteases [42,43] and metalloenzyme proteases [44] can digest glomerular basement membrane, most studies have suggested that the neutral serine proteases (elastase and cathepsin G) [43–47] are the major proteases capable of degrading whole glomerular basement membrane and type IV collagen in vitro [43–47]. For example, when PMNs are incubated with glomerular basement membrane and anti-glomerular basement membrane antibody [48], glomerular basement membrane breakdown as measured by hydroxyproline release can be prevented by inhibitors of neutral serine proteases. Neutrophil-mediated endothelial cell detachment may also be dependent on neutral proteases [49], or be mediated by reactive oxygen species [50,51]. Proteases and glomerular basement membrane fragments, including type IV collagen and laminin, are also present in the urine of animals and man with PMN-mediated glomerulonephritis [52–54].

Despite the accumulation of in vitro and epidemiological data suggesting that proteases mediate tissue injury, several in vivo studies in disease models have failed to verify their importance [55–58]. Recently, however, there have been two preliminary reports that the administration of the antiprotease bis (5-amidino-2-benzimidazolyl) methane (BABIM) lessened 'glomerular necrosis' and renal insufficiency in mice with chronic immune complex glomerulonephritis induced with repeated injections of horse apoferritin [59,60].

Reactive oxygen species

Release of reactive oxygen species is now believed to be of equal or greater importance than proteases in PMN-mediated tissue injury [55,61]. Neutrophils become activated by a variety of stimuli (including immune complexes and C5a)

[62–64] and undergo a 'respiratory burst' characterized by increased oxygen consumption, increased utilization of glucose by the hexose monophosphate shunt and formation of reduced or excited products of oxygen which can function as powerful oxidants [2,3,65]. Superoxide anion (O_2^-) is formed by the univalent reduction of oxygen by a membrane-bound oxidase, which utilizes reduced nicotinamide adenine dinucleotide phosphate (NADPH) as a substrate:

$$O_2 + NADPH \xrightarrow{\text{oxidase}} O_2^- + H^+ + NADP$$

Superoxide anion (O_2^-) can then dismutate either spontaneously (particularly in the acidic environment of the PMN phagosome) or by catalysis by the enzyme superoxide dismutase (SOD) to form hydrogen peroxide (H_2O_2):

$$2O_2^- + 2H^+ \longrightarrow O_2 + H_2O_2$$

Hydrogen peroxide is a relatively weak oxidant but its toxicity is enhanced by further reduction to form the hydroxyl radical (•OH). This reaction is now believed to result from the reduction of H_2O_2 by Fe^{2+} (ferrous ion) (Fenton's reagent). The regeneration of Fe^{2+} from the ferric iron (Fe^{3+}) formed is accomplished by reaction with O_2^-. This two step reaction for the reduction of H_2O_2 by O_2^- using iron as a catalyst is called the Haber-Weiss reaction [2,3]:

$$\begin{aligned} Fe^{2+} + H_2O_2 &\longrightarrow Fe^{3+} + \cdot OH + OH^- \\ O_2^- + Fe^{3+} &\longrightarrow O_2 + Fe^{2+} \\ O_2^- + H_2O_2 &\longrightarrow O_2 + \cdot OH + OH^- \end{aligned}$$

Hydroxyl radical-mediated toxicity can be ameliorated by substances that scavenge •OH directly (dimethylthiourea (DMTU), dimethylsulfoxide (DMSO), mannitol, ethanol), or by agents which limit its formation by iron chelation (desferrioxamine, DFO), degradation of H_2O_2 (catalase), or scavenging of O_2^- (SOD).

Hydrogen peroxide toxicity can also be enhanced by its reaction with halides in the presence of the PMN enzyme myeloperoxidase (MPO) to form toxic hypohalous acids:

$$H_2O_2 + Cl^- + H^+ \xrightarrow{\text{MPO}} H^2O + HOCl$$

The hypohalous acids can then react with halides to form halogens such as chlorine:

$$HOCl + Cl^- \longrightarrow Cl_2 + OH^-$$

Finally, singlet oxygen ($^1O_2$) has been proposed as a product of the respiratory burst of PMNs [2]. Its formation by PMNs, however, has not been definitively demonstrated and its rôle in tissue injury is therefore uncertain.

Rôle of reactive oxygen species in glomerulonephritis

Evaluation of the rôle of reactive oxygen species in tissue injury such as the reverse passive Arthus reaction in the skin and lungs, and the lung injury associated with systemic complement activation suggest a major rôle for reactive oxygen species [57,66–70]. There is now evidence for reactive oxygen species participation in glomerular disease. McCord et al first studied mice with glomerulonephritis resulting from the injection of albumin–anti-albumin immune complexes [71,72], and reported that superoxide dismutase administration was associated with reduced severity of histological injury, thus suggesting that the injury was mediated by O_2^- [71,72]. Superoxide anion has also been reported to participate in the autologous phase of anti-glomerular basement membrane nephritis in rats [73], although this has not been confirmed by others [74]. However, most inhibitor studies have not excluded potential non-enzymatic effects of these agents on antibody deposition or renal function that may partially explain the results observed [71–73]. For example, chronic SOD administration is known to decrease autoantibody production and glomerular antibody deposition in NZB mice with a lupus-like syndrome [75].

A series of studies by Rehan, Wiggins and Johnson has provided more compelling evidence for the importance of reactive oxygen species in PMN-mediated glomerular injury [4–6]. They first perfused the renal artery of rats with phorbol myristate acetate (PMA), a potent stimulant to reactive oxygen species production by the PMN. The proteinuria and histological injury which resulted was documented to be PMN-mediated, and could be prevented by the administration of catalase (which degrades H_2O_2) but not by SOD [5]. The mechanism of H_2O_2 action was not further elucidated.

Subsequent studies included infusion of cobra venom factor (CVF) into the renal artery of rats, which also causes a PMN-mediated proteinuria that is inhibited by catalase, but not SOD, again implicating H_2O_2 in its pathogenesis [6]. Unlike CVF-induced lung injury, which is •OH radical mediated [70], the infusion of the •OH scavengers DFO and DMSO were not protective in the renal model [6].

Reactive oxygen species scavengers have also been given in the PMN-dependent heterologous phase of anti-glomerular basement membrane nephritis in rats [4,76]. This lesion was shown to be H_2O_2-dependent but not •OH dependent because DMSO was not protective [4]. Another study of this model in rabbits suggested a rôle for •OH because both DMTU and DFO reduced injury without affecting antibody binding, renal function, complement activity or PMN levels [76].

Finally, there are recent reports that reactive oxygen species may mediate glomerular injury that is independent of neutrophils and monocytes [10–12]. The nephrosis induced in rats with the aminonucleoside of puromycin may result from O_2^- production, presumably by glomerular epithelial cells, and the administration of SOD at the time of aminonucleoside injection decreases injury [10]. Also provocative is the preliminary report by Shah that a C5b-9 dependent, inflammatory cell-independent, model of membranous nephropathy in rats, passive Heymann nephritis, may be mediated in part by •OH, as evidenced by the protective effects of DMTU [12]. This is especially interesting in light of the observation that the C5b-9, or membrane attack complex of complement, which mediates the proteinuria in passive Heymann nephritis [77], can cause the release of reactive oxygen species from resident glomerular mesangial cells [9].

Although studies which rely exclusively on inhibitors given in vivo to define a particular pathogenetic mechanism must always be interpreted with caution because of the multiple non-specific effects of these agents which may interfere with several components of the disease mechanism, taken together these data provide strong evidence that reactive oxygen species, and primarily H_2O_2, are important mediators of PMN-induced glomerular injury.

The MPO-H_2O_2-halide system

The hypothesis that H_2O_2-dependent injury by PMNs might involve the MPO-H_2O_2-halide system has been studied in detail recently by us [78,79]. MPO is a potent cationic enzyme present in the azurophil (primary) granules of PMNs and monocytes [2,65]. In the presence of H_2O_2, which could be provided by the respiratory burst of PMNs and monocytes [2,3], and also by mesangial cells [8,9], the MPO system can lead to production of hypohalous acids and halogens that oxidize and halogenate tissue [2,78]. Due to the extracellular release of MPO, H_2O_2 and their toxic products, the system is also capable of injuring neighbouring cells [2,65].

Glomerular injury induced by the MPO system

To test the hypothesis that the MPO-H_2O_2-halide system may cause direct glomerular injury, we infused the isolated components of this system into the renal artery of rats [79]. Because MPO is cationic (pI>10) [80] it will bind to the anionic sites in the capillary wall [81] as has been reported for other PMN and platelet-derived cationic proteins [82,83]. Subsequent infusion of H_2O_2 and halides might then result in the production of hypochlorous acid and other oxidants at the filtration barrier and thus potentially mimic the effects of a degranulating PMN on glomerular basement membrane in vivo.

The left renal artery of rats was perfused with purified canine MPO (108μg, 9 units) followed by H_2O_2 in phosphate buffered saline (PBS) using a perfusion pump [79]. Controls received either PBS, MPO or H_2O_2 alone. Urine protein excretion was measured, and serial biopsies were obtained for light and electron microscopic study. Localization of MPO to the glomerular capillary wall was confirmed using a modified version of the diaminobenzidine method of Graham and Karnovsky [81]. Halogenation of isolated whole glomeruli was also documented in separate experiments by adding ^{125}I to the perfusate. Localization of the iodination was determined by electron microscopic autoradiography.

The perfusion of the renal artery with MPO resulted in immediate binding of MPO to glomerular anionic sites, particularly in the subepithelial space [79]. When MPO was extracted from glomeruli isolated immediately following perfusion [84], only 0.3% of the injected MPO was bound. This corresponds to less than that which can be extracted from a single rat PMN, thus suggesting that the amount of MPO present in the glomeruli in these studies could easily be achievable in vivo in glomerulonephritis.

The infusion of MPO-H_2O_2 and a halide resulted in significant proteinuria not seen in controls. Iodination, a reflection of MPO action [65,85] was also produced. By electronmicroscopic autoradiography iodination was present on endothelial, mesangial and epithelial cells and in peripheral capillary loops centred on the glomerular basement membrane [84].

The natural history of the MPO-H_2O_2-halide induced lesion has been studied over 21 days [86]. Acutely (10 minutes), rats perfused with MPO, H_2O_2 and chloride had obvious glomerular injury primarily of the endothelial (and mesangial) cells with swelling and detachment. A prominent platelet influx was also noted, with many of the 'activated' platelets adherent to bare glomerular basement membrane where they appeared to be degranulated [79]. Fibrin accumulation was also noted within 24 hours.

By four days platelet infiltrates had disappeared, and a marked proliferation of resident glomerular cells developed [79]. The proliferative endocapillary lesion was not unlike that seen in post-infectious glomerulonephritis. By 21 days after perfusion, however, the glomeruli appeared essentially normal.

Evidence for participation of the MPO system in immune complex glomerulonephritis

We next sought to document activation of the MPO-H_2O_2-halide system in a model of immune complex glomerulonephritis in vivo. Since iodination in the presence of PMNs, and in tissue lacking endogenous peroxidase activity, can be taken as an index of the action of the MPO-H_2O_2-halide system [65,85], we measured glomerular iodination in glomerulonephritis [78]. (Although some iodination can be produced by •OH that is independent of MPO [87], there is no evidence that this is a major iodination mechanism in neutrophils.)

Immune complex glomerulonephritis was produced in rats by intrarenal perfusion of concanavalin A (con A) followed by anti-concanavalin A antibody (anticon A) [78] as originally described by Golbus and Wilson [88]. Con A, a lectin, binds to the glucose and mannose residues in glomerular basement membrane in a subendothelial distribution thus serving as a planted antigen [89]. Antibody deposition results in in-situ subendothelial immune complex formation [78,88]. Controls were rats perfused with con A followed by nonspecific rabbit IgG. To document the rôle of PMNs in mediating disease in this model, a third group was rendered neutropenic before disease induction with a specific rabbit anti-PMN antibody which maintained PMNs at $<250/mm^3$ throughout the study. Parameters measured in these groups included urine protein excretion (24 to 48hr period), serum creatinine (48hr) and renal morphology by light, immunofluorescence and electron microscopy. In some rats in each group free ^{125}I was given three and six hours after disease induction and glomeruli and glomerular basement membrane were isolated at 48 hours for measurement of iodination.

Marked proteinuria occurred in con A-anticon A rats and was significantly inhibited by PMN depletion. Con A-anticon A rats had a proliferative glomerulonephritis with a marked glomerular PMN infiltrate at 24 hours. Controls had minimal evidence of histological injury. Of greatest interest was the demonstration that substantial iodination (1200cpm/total glomeruli) could be documented in the isolated whole glomeruli and purified glomerular basement membrane of the diseased rats but did not occur in control rats (45cpm) or in neutropenic rats with conA-anticon A glomerulonephritis (88cpm). Thus the MPO system is apparently activated in this PMN-mediated model of glomerulonephritis and produces halogenation of glomerular structural proteins.

Mechanisms of reactive oxygen species-mediated glomerular injury

The mechanisms by which reactive oxygen species result in an increase in glomerular permeability remain poorly defined but may involve both direct oxidant injury to resident cells or indirect effects including the activation and potentiation of proteases.

Most cells are susceptible to direct oxidant injury, presumably due to lipid peroxidation, oxidative decarboxylation of aminoacids, oxidation of sulphydryl and sulphur-ether groups, oxidation of iron-sulphur centres, and the generation of toxic aldehydes and chloramines [2,3]. Prior to death, cells undergo swelling of the cytoplasm with loss of ATP, oxidation of intracellular glutathione and an increase in F actin content [90–92].

Although glomerular endothelial cells have not been studied, non-glomerular endothelial cells are susceptible to H_2O_2-dependent killing [50,51]. Sublethal oxidant injury can produce altered release of vasoactive substances such as prostacyclin [93–96]. Reactive oxygen species have been reported to cause both a stimulation [97] and a biphasic response [98] of prostaglandin release by mesangial cells. Mesangial cells can also be killed by the MPO system in the presence of non-toxic concentrations of H_2O_2 [unpublished data].

Another mechanism for reactive oxygen species action may be injury to the glomerular basement membrane, either directly or indirectly by the activation or potentiation of protease action. Neutrophils in the presence of antibody bound to glomerular basement membrane produce chemiluminescence (a marker for reactive oxygen species production) [48,99] and reactive oxygen species

[100]. Oxygen-derived free radicals can also directly degrade collagen [101] and collagen proteoglycans [102]. However, hydroxyproline release as a reflection of type IV collagen breakdown in glomerular basement membrane by stimulated PMNs appears to involve proteases [44,103]. Vissers has reported that hydroxyproline release by PMNs stimulated with glomerular basement membrane-aggregated IgG can be inhibited with the neutral serine proteinase inhibitor phenylmethyl sulphonyl fluoride (PMSF) [103], whereas in the studies by Shah a metalloproteinase released by PMA-stimulated PMNs appeared primarily responsible for glomerular basement membrane breakdown [44]. However, in both studies the use of reactive oxygen species inhibitors suggested that reactive oxygen species, and particularly the MPO-H_2O_2-halide system, facilitated protease action [44,102]. This may reflect the ability of reactive oxygen species to render the glomerular basement membrane more susceptible to proteolytic attack as has previously been shown for collagen [101] and other proteins [104]. Other studies suggest that the MPO system activates a latent metalloenzyme protease [44], as has been reported previously with PMN-derived collagenase (a metalloproteinase) [105]. Protease action could also be produced by the MPO system through its ability to inactivate the antiprotease α-1-proteinase inhibitor (α_1-anti-trypsin) [106].

Despite these studies of reactive oxygen species-protease interaction, our finding that perfusion of the MPO system alone into the renal artery of rats results in significant glomerular injury documents the potential for direct oxidant-mediated injury in glomerulonephritis [79].

Conclusion

PMN-mediated glomerulonephritis can no longer be attributed solely to the release of proteases. Rather, reactive oxygen species, and particularly H_2O_2, also appear to mediate an increase in glomerular permeability. H_2O_2 is not a particularly potent oxidant in itself, and evidence has been provided to support participation of the MPO-H_2O_2-halide system in PMN-mediated glomerulonephritis. A rôle for other reactive oxygen species, especially $\cdot OH$ and O_2^-, in non-PMN mediated glomerulonephritis is also emerging. The relative contributions of direct oxidant injury and oxidant-protease interactions in glomerular injury requires further study.

Acknowledgments

Portions of this work were supported by United States Public Health Service research grants AM32051, AI07763, AM34198, AM07467, AI07044 and a research grant from the Northwest Kidney Foundation. While conducting some of the studies reported, Dr Johnson was the recipient of an American Society of Nephrology/Hoffman La Roche Fellowship from the National Kidney Foundation.

References

1 Cochrane CG. Immunologic tissue injury mediated by neutrophilic leukocytes. *Adv Immunol 1968; 9:* 99–162

2 Klebanoff SJ. Oxygen metabolism and the toxic properties of phagocytes. *Ann Int Med 1980; 93:* 480–489

3 Root RK, Cohen MS. The microbicidal mechanisms of human neutrophils and eosinophils. *Rev Inf Dis 1981; 3:* 565–598

4 Rehan A, Johnson KJ, Wiggins RC et al. Evidence for the role of oxygen radicals in acute nephrotoxic nephritis. *Lab Invest 1984; 51:* 396–403

5 Rehan A, Johnson KJ, Kunkel RC, Wiggins RC. Role of oxygen radicals in phorbol myristate acetate-induced glomerular injury. *Kidney Int 1985; 27:* 503–511

6 Rehan A, Wiggins RC, Kunkel RG et al. Glomerular injury and proteinuria in rats after intrarenal injection of cobra venom factor. *Am J Pathol 1986; 123:* 57–66

7 Shah SV. Light emission by isolated rat glomeruli in response to phorbol myristate acetate. *J Lab Clin Med 1981; 98:* 46–57

8 Baud L, Hagege J, Sraer J et al. Reactive oxygen production by cultured rat glomerular mesangial cells during phagocytosis is associated with stimulation of lipoxygenase activity. *J Exp Med 1983; 158:* 1836–1852

9 Adler S, Baker PJ, Johnson RJ et al. Complement membrane attack complex stimulates production of reactive oxygen metabolites by cultured rat mesangial cells. *J Clin Invest 1986; 77:* 762–767

10 Diamond JR, Bonventre JV, Karnovsky MJ. A role for oxygen free radicals in aminonucleoside nephrosis. *Kidney Int 1986; 29:* 478–483

11 Lotan D, Kaplan BS, Fong JSC et al. Reduction of protein excretion by dimethyl sulfoxide in rats with passive Heymann nephritis. *Kidney Int 1984; 25:* 778–788

12 Shah SV, Baricos WH, Schwartz S, Walker PP. Dimethylthiourea (DMTU), hydroxyl radical scavenger, reduces proteinuria in passive Heymann nephritis (PHN) in rats. *Kidney Int 1987; 31 (Abstract):* 330

13 Appel GB, Silva FG, Pirani CL et al. Renal involvement in systemic lupus erythematosus: a study of 56 patients emphasizing histologic classification. *Medicine 1978; 57:* 371–412

14 Tarantino A, DeVecchi A, Montagnino G et al. Renal disease in essential mixed cryoglobulinemia. *Q J Med 1981; 197:* 1–30

15 Min KW, Gyorkey F, Gyorkey P et al. The morphogenesis of glomerular crescents in rapidly progressive glomerulonephritis. *Kidney Int 1974; 5:* 47–56

16 Salant DJ, Adler S, Darby C et al. Influence of antigen distribution on the mediation of immunological glomerular injury. *Kidney Int 1985; 27:* 938–950

17 Lewy JE, Salinas-Madrigal L, Herdson PB et al. Clinico-pathologic correlations in acute poststreptococcal glomerulonephritis. *Medicine 1971; 50:* 453–502

18 Sorger K, Gessler U, Hubner FK et al. Subtypes of acute postinfectious glomerulonephritis. Synopsis of clinical and pathological features. *Clin Nephrol 1982; 17:* 114–128

19 Cochrane CG, Unanue ER, Dixon FJ. A role of polymorphonuclear leukocytes and complement in nephrotoxic nephritis. *J Exp Med 1965; 122:* 95–110

20 Henson PM. Pathologic mechanisms in neutrophil mediated injury. *Am J Pathol 1972: 68:* 593–612

21 Hawkins D, Cochrane CG. Glomerular basement membrane damage in immunological glomerulonephritis. *Immunology 1968; 14:* 665–680

22 Gang NF, Mautner W, Kalant N. Nephrotoxic serum nephritis. II Chemical, morphologic, and functional correlates of glomerular basement membrane at the onset of proteinuria. *Lab Invest 1970; 23:* 150–157

23 Kuhn K, Ryan GB, Hein SJ et al. An ultrastructural study of the mechanisms of proteinuria in rat nephrotoxic nephritis. *Lab Invest 1977; 36:* 375–387

24 Couser WG, Stilmant MM, Jermanovich NB. Complement-independent nephrotoxic nephritis in the guinea pig. *Kidney Int 1977; 11:* 170–180

25 Couser WG, Darby C, Salant DJ et al. AntiGBM antibody-induced proteinuria in isolated perfused rat kidney. *Am J Physiol 1985; 18:* F241–F250

26 Camussi G. Potential role of platelet-activating factor in renal pathophysiology. *Kidney Int 1986; 29:* 469–477
27 Deuel TF, Senior RM, Huang JS, Griffin GL. Chemotaxis of monocytes and neutrophils to platelet-derived growth factor. *J Clin Invest 1982; 69:* 1046–1049
28 Lewis RA, Austen KF. The biologically active leukotrines – biosynthesis, metabolism, receptors, functions and pharmacology. *J Clin Invest 1984; 73:* 889–897
29 Kuehl FA, Egan RW. Prostaglandins, arachidonic acid and inflammation. *Science 1980; 210:* 978–984
30 Springer TA. The LFA-1, Mac-1 glycoprotein family and its deficiency in an inherited disease. *Fed Proc 1985; 44:* 2660–2663
31 Vercellotti GM, McCarthy J, Furcht LT et al. Inflamed fibronectin: an altered fibronectin enhances neutrophil adhesion. *Blood 1983; 62:* 1063–1069
32 Spagnuolo PJ, Ellner JL, Hassid A, Dunn MJ. Thromboxane A_2 mediates augmented polymorphonuclear adhesiveness. *J Clin Invest 1980; 66:* 406–414
33 Bevilacqua MP, Pober JS, Wheeler ME et al. Interleukin I activation of vascular endothelium. Effects of procoagulant activity and leukocyte adhesion. *Am J Pathol 1985; 121:* 393–403
34 Tonnesen MG, Smedly A, Henson PM. Neutrophil-endothelial cell interactions; modulation of neutrophil adhesiveness induced by complement fragments C5a and C5a des arg and formylmethionyl-leucyl-phenylalanine in vitro. *J Clin Invest 1984; 74:* 1581–1592
35 Hoover RL, Karnovsky MJ, Austen KF et al. Leukotriene B4 action on endothelium mediates augmented neutrophil/endothelial adhesion. *Proc Natl Acad Sci USA 1984; 81:* 2191–2193
36 Gamble JR, Harlan JM, Klebanoff SJ, Vadas MA. Stimulation of the adherence of neutrophils to umbilical vein endothelium by human recombinant tumor necrosis factor. *Proc Natl Acad Sci USA 1985; 82:* 8667–8671
37 Schleimer RP, Rutledge BK. Cultured human vascular endothelial cells acquire adhesiveness for neutrophils after stimulation with interleukin I, endotoxin, and tumor-promoting phorbol diesters. *J Immun 1986; 136:* 649–654
38 Sindrey M, Naish P. The mediation of the localization of polymorphonuclear leukocytes in glomeruli during the autologous phase of nephrotoxic nephritis. *Clin Exp Immunol 1979; 35:* 350–355
39 Weissman G, Smolen JE, Korchak HM. Release of inflammatory mediators from stimulated neutrophils. *N Engl J Med 1980; 303:* 27–34
40 Baggiolini M, Dewald B. Regulation of leukocyte function. In Snydermen R, ed. *Contemporary Topics in Immunobiology*. New York: Plenum Press. 1984: 221–246
41 Camussi G, Tetta C, Bussolino F et al. Mediation of immune-complex-induced aggregation of polymorphonuclear neutrophils. *Int Arch Allergy Appl Immunol 1981; 64:* 25–41
42 Cochrane CG, Aikin BS. Polymorphonuclear leukocytes in immunologic reactions. *J Exp Med 1966; 124:* 733–752
43 Davies M, Barrett J, Travis J et al. The degradation of human glomerular basement membrane with purified lysosomal proteinases. Evidence for the pathogenic role of the polymorphonuclear leukocyte in glomerulonephritis. *Clin Sci Mol Med 1978; 54:* 233–240
44 Shah SV, Baricos WH, Basci A. Degradation of human glomerular basement membrane by stimulated neutrophils. *J Clin Invest 1987; 79:* 25–31
45 Vissers MCM, Winterbourn CC, Hunt JS. Degradation of glomerular basement membrane by human neutrophils in vivo. *Biochim Biophys Acta 1984; 804:* 154–160
46 Davies M, Coles GA, Hughes KT. Glomerular basement membrane injury by neutrophil and monocyte neutral proteinases. *Renal Physiol 1980; 3:* 106–111
47 Uitto V-J, Schwartz D, Veis A. Degradation of basement-membrane collagen by neutral proteases from human leukocytes. *Eur J Biochem 1980; 105:* 409–417
48 Davies M, Coles GA, Harber MJ. Effect of glomerular basement membrane on the initiation of chemiluminescence and lysosomal enzyme release in human polymorphonuclear leukocytes, an in vitro model of glomerular disease. *Immunology 1984; 52:* 151–159

49 Harlan JM, Killen DD, Harker LA et al. Neutrophil-mediated endothelial injury in vitro. *J Clin Invest 1981; 68:* 1394–1400

50 Sacks T, Moldow CF, Craddock PR et al. Oxygen radicals mediate endothelial cell damage by complement-stimulated granulocytes. *J Clin Invest 1978; 61:* 1161–1167

51 Martin WJ. Neutrophils kill pulmonary endothelial cells by a hydrogen-peroxide-dependent pathway. *Am Rev Resp Dis 1984; 130:* 209–213

52 Davin J-C, Davies M, Foidart J-M et al. Urinary excretion of neutral proteases in nephrotic rats with a glomerular disease. *Kidney Int 1987; 31:* 32–40

53 Davies M, Sanders E, Coles GA, Hughes KT. The isolation of a neutral protease from the urine of a patient with Goodpasture's syndrome. *Biochem Soc Trans 1978; 6:* 947–949

54 Sanders E, Davies M, Coles GA. On the pathogenesis of glomerulonephritis – a clinico-pathological study indicating that neutrophils attack and degrade glomerular basement membrane. *Renal Physiol 1980; 3:* 355–359

55 Johnson KT, Ward PA. Newer concepts in the pathogenesis of immune complex-induced tissue injury. *Lab Invest 1982; 47:* 218–226

56 Janoff A, Sloan B, Weinbaum G et al. Experimental emphysema induced with purified human neutrophil elastase: tissue localization of the instilled protease. *Am Rev Resp Dis 1977: 115:* 461–477

57 Johnson KJ, Ward PA. Role of oxygen metabolites in immune complex injury of lung. *J Immunol 1981; 126:* 2365–2369

58 Johnson KJ, Varani J, Oliver J, Ward PA. Immunologic vasculitis in beige mice with deficiency of leukocytic neutral protease. *J Immunol 1979; 122:* 1807–1811

59 Falk RJ, Tidwell R, Geratz D, Jennette JC. Amelioration of immune complex mediated murine glomerulonephritis by a synthetic protease inhibitor. *Kidney Int 1987; 31 (Abstract):* 318

60 Gidlespie GY, Jennette JC, Tidwell RR et al. Protease inhibitor amelioration of immune complex mediated necrotizing glomerulonephritis. *Kidney Int 1986; 29 (Abstract):* 275

61 Fantone JC, Ward PA. Role of oxygen-derived free radicals and metabolites in leukocyte-dependent inflammatory reactions. *Am J Path 1982; 107:* 397–418

62 Weiss SJ, Ward PA. Immune complex induced generation of oxygen metabolites by human neutrophils. *J Immunol 1982; 129:* 309–313

63 Ward PA, Duque RE, Sulavik MC, Johnson KJ. In vitro and in vivo stimulation of rat neutrophils and alveolar macrophages by immune complexes. *Am J Pathol 1983; 110:* 297–309

64 Goldstein IM, Roos D, Kaplan HB, Weissmann G. Complement and immunoglobulins stimulate superoxide production by human leukocytes independently of phagocytosis. *J Clin Invest 1975; 56:* 1155–1163

65 Klebanoff SJ. Oxygen-dependent cytotoxic mechanisms of phagocytes. In Gallin JI, Fauci AS, eds. *Advances in Host Defense Mechanisms, Volume 1.* New York: Raven Press. 1982: 111–162

66 McCord JM, Wong K. *Phagocyte-produced Free Radicals: Roles in Cytotoxicity and Inflammation. CIBA Foundation Symposium 65.* Amsterdam: Excerpta Medica. 1979: 343–360

67 McCormick JR, Harkin MM, Johnson KJ, Ward PA. Suppression by superoxide dismutase of immune complex induced pulmonary alveolitis and dermal inflammation. *Am J Pathol 1981; 102:* 55–61

68 Till G, Beauchamp C, Menapace D et al. Oxygen radical dependent lung damage following thermal injury of rat skin. *J Trauma 1983; 23:* 269–277

69 Till G, Johnson KJ, Kunkel R, Ward PA. Intravascular activation of complement and acute lung injury. *J Clin Invest 1982; 69:* 1126–1135

70 Ward PA, Till G, Kunkel R, Beauchamp C. Evidence for role of hydroxyl radical in complement and neutrophil-dependent tissue-injury. *J Clin Invest 1983; 72:* 789–801

71 Stokes SH, McCord JM. Prevention of immune-complex induced glomerulonephritis by superoxide dismutase. *Ala J Med Sci 1979; 16:* 33

72 McCord JM, Stokes SH, Wong K. Superoxide radical as a phagocyte-produced chemical mediator of inflammation. In Weissmann G et al, eds. *Advances in Inflammation Research Volume 1.* New York: Raven Press. 1979: 273–280
73 Adachi T, Fukuta M, Ito Y et al. Effect of superoxide dismutase on glomerular nephritis. *Biochem Pharmacol 1986; 35:* 341–345
74 Webb DB, MacKenzie R, Zoob N, Rees AJ. Evidence against a role for superoxide anions in the injury of nephrotoxic nephritis in rats. *Clin Science 1985; 69:* 687–689
75 Huber W, Saifer MGP. Orgotein, the drug version of bovine Cu-Zn superoxide dismutase. A summary account of safety and pharmacology in laboratory animals. In Michelson AM, McCord JM, Fridovich I, eds. *Superoxide and Superoxide Dismutases.* New York: Academic Press. 1979: 517–534
76 Boyce NW, Holdsworth SR. Hydroxyl radical mediation of immune renal injury by desferrioxamine. *Kidney Int 1986; 30:* 813–817
77 Couser WG, Baker PJ, Adler S. Complement and the direct mediation of immune glomerular injury: a new perspective (editorial review). *Kidney Int 1985; 28:* 879–890
78 Johnson RJ, Klebanoff SJ, Ochi RF et al. Participation of the myeloperoxidase-H_2O_2-halide system in immune complex nephritis. *Kidney Int; 1987:* in press
79 Johnson RJ, Couser WG, Chi EY et al. A new mechanism for glomerular injury: the myeloperoxidase-hydrogen-peroxide-halide system. *J Clin Invest 1987; 79:* in press
80 Agner K. Verdoperoxidase. A ferment isolated from leukocytes. *Acta Physiol Scand 1941; 2 (Suppl 8):* 1–62
81 Graham RC, Karnovsky MJ. Glomerular permeability. Ultrastructural cytochemical studies using peroxidases as protein tracers. *J Exp Med 1966; 124:* 1123–1131
82 Camussi G, Tetta C, Segoloni G et al. Localization of neutrophil cationic proteins and loss of anionic changes in glomeruli of patients with systemic lupus erythematosus glomerulonephritis. *Clin Immunol Immunopath 1982; 24:* 299–314
83 Barnes JL, Levine SP, Venkatachalam MA. Binding of platelet factor 4 to glomerular polyanion. *Kidney Int 1984; 25:* 759–765
84 Patriarca P, Cramer R, Marussi M et al. Mode of activation of granule-bound NADPH oxidase in leukocytes during phagocytosis. *Biochim Biophys Acta 1971; 237:* 335–338
85 Klebanoff SJ. Iodination of bacteria: a bactericidal mechanism. *J Exp Med 1967; 126:* 1063–1078
86 Johnson RJ, Guggenheim S, Klebanoff SJ et al. Pathological studies of the glomerulonephritis induced by the myeloperoxidase-hydrogen peroxide-halide system of neutrophils: submitted for publication
87 Klebanoff S. Iodination catalyzed by the xanthine oxidase system: role of hydroxyl radicals. *Biochem 1982; 21:* 4110–4116
88 Golbus SM, Wilson CB. Experimental glomerulonephritis induced by in situ formation of immune complexes in glomerular capillary wall. *Kidney Int 1979; 16:* 148–157
89 Bretton R, Bariety J. Ultrastructural localization of concanavalin A in normal rat kidney – glomeruli and arterioles. *J Ultrastruc Research 1974, 48:* 396–403
90 Spragg RG, Hinshaw DB, Hyslop PA et al. Alterations in adenosine triphosphate and energy change in cultured endothelial and P388D_1 cells following oxidant injury. *J Clin Invest 1985; 76:* 1471–1476
91 Schraufstatter IU, Hinshaw DB, Hyslop PA et al. Glutathione cycle activity and pyridine nucleotide levels in oxidant induced injury of cells. *J Clin Invest 1985; 76:* 1131–1139
92 Hinshaw DB, Sklar LA, Bohl B et al. Cytoskeletal and morphologic impact of cellular oxidant injury. *Am J Pathol 1986; 123:* 454–464
93 Ager A, Gordan JL. Differential effects of hydrogen peroxide on indices of endothelial cell function. *J Exp Med 1984; 159:* 592–603
94 Harlan JM, Callahan KS. Role of hydrogen peroxide in the neutrophil-mediated release of prostacyclin from cultured endothelial cells. *J Clin Invest 1984; 74:* 442–448

95 Whorton AR, Montgomery ME, Kent RS. Effect of hydrogen peroxide on prostaglandin production and cellular integrity in cultured porcine aortic endothelial cells. *J Clin Invest 1985; 76:* 295–302

96 Setty BNY, Jurek E, Ganley C, Stuart MJ. Effects of hydrogen peroxide on vascular arachidonic acid metabolism. *Prostaglandins Med 1985; 14:* 205–213

97 Sedor JR, Abboud HE. Hydrogen peroxide stimulates PGE_2 synthesis by cultured rat mesangial cell. *Kidney Int 1986; 29 (Abstract):* 291

98 Adler S, Stahl RAK, Baker PJ et al. Biphasic effect of oxygen radicals on prostaglandin production by rat mesangial cells. *Am J Physiol; 1987:* in press

99 Mossman H, Hoyer B, Walz W et al. Antibody-dependent cellular cytotoxicity and chemiluminescence as a tool for studying the mechanism of anti-glomerular basement membrane nephritis. The role of the cytotoxic potential of polymorphonuclear granulocytes and monocytes. *Immunol 1984; 53:* 545–552

100 Vissers MCM, Day WA, Winterbourn CC. Neutrophils adherent to a non-phagocytosable surface (glomerular basement membrane) produce oxidants only at the site of attachment. *Blood 1985; 66:* 161–166

101 Curran SF, Amoruso MA, Goldstein BD, Berg RA. Degradation of soluble collagen by ozone or hydroxyl radicals. *FEBS Lett 1984; 176:* 155–160

102 Bates EJ, Harper GS, Lowther DA, Preston BN. Effect of oxygen-derived reactive species on cartilage proteoglycan-hyaluronate aggregates. *Biochem Int 1984; 8:* 629–637

103 Vissers MCM, Winterbourn CC. The effect of oxidants on neutrophil-mediated degradation of glomerular basement membrane collagen. *Biochim Biophys Acta 1987:* in press

104 Fligiel SE, Lee EC, McCoy JP et al. Protein degradation following treatment with hydrogen peroxide. *Am J Pathol 1984; 115:* 418–425

105 Weiss SJ, Peppin G, Ortiz X et al. Oxidative autoactivation of latent collagenase by human neutrophils. *Science 1985; 227:* 747–749

106 Clark RA. Extracellular effects of the myeloperoxidase-hydrogen peroxide-halide system. *Adv Inflamm Res 1983; 5:* 107–146

SELECTIVE GLOMERULAR CELL IMMUNE INJURY – ANTI-MESANGIAL CELL ANTIBODIES

C B Wilson, T Yamamoto, P Moullier, *R C Blantz

Research Institute of Scripps Clinic, La Jolla, California,
**University of California, San Diego School of Medicine and Veterans Administration Medical Center, San Diego, California, USA*

The basic tenets of antibody-associated immune deposit forms of glomerular injury which were well established 25 years ago have been continuously subjected to refinement and expansion based largely on studies in model systems (Table I) [reviewed in 1]. Extension of the modified concepts from these models to human glomerular disease, unfortunately, remains slow. In immune deposit forms of injury, antibody can become fixed in the glomerulus by active or passive means. The active pathway results from antibody binding to either native or trapped glomerular antigens. The passive pathway is represented by the glomerular accumulation of immune complexes originating from the circulation. The phlogogenic antibody-rich deposits generated by either the direct or passive pathways in turn lead to recruitment of humoral and cellular mediators to cause inflammatory injury in the vicinity of the deposit. These mediator pathways have been the subject of intense study with considerable molecular definition of their interactions [1–3].

Immune deposit forms of glomerular injury

The 'passive' immune complex mechanism of injury has been shown to include the local and dynamic interaction of extrarenal antigen and the corresponding antibody components of the complex. The immune complex deposit cannot be thought of as a static element, but must instead be viewed as a site that can be reshaped relative to the fluctuations of free antigen and antibody in its immediate environment [1,4]. These fluctuations are governed in part by blood flow, location of the deposit, degree of inflammatory response, and extrarenal features which influence rates of antibody production, antigen release, and immune complex clearance. The reshaping is also affected, in part, by the epitope diversity of the antigen involved in the immune reaction as well as the quantities of different antibodies present and the qualitative features of each individual antibody's binding characteristics. The latter interactions can be modified by

TABLE I. Humoral mechanisms of immune glomerular injury

Antibody reactions leading to phlogogenic immune deposit formation

Active antibody binding

  Antibodies reactive with structural antigens (eluted antibody reacts with normal glomerular structures)

    Glomerular basement membrane-associated antigens, ?Fx1A-associated antigens, etc.

  Antibodies reactive with trapped antigens (eluted antibodies will react with glomeruli only if antigen is first trapped)

    Idiotypes, charged or lectin-like materials, ?DNA, ?bacterial products, etc.

Passive antibody accumulations

  Antibodies reactive with antigens in dynamic equilibrium forming immune complexes (eluted antibodies will not react with normal glomeruli)

    Exogenous antigens – a wide variety of infectious agents, drugs, etc.

    Endogenous antigens – nuclear antigens, thyroglobulins, tumour antigens, etc.

Antibody reactions leading to selective injury to glomerular cells

  Antibodies reactive with native cell surface antigens

    Thy-1.1, Fx1A-associated antigens, angiotensin converting enzyme, ?other

  Antibodies reactive with other cell or cell-associated antigens, phagocytosed materials, trapped or adherent materials, etc.

---

secondary immune responses producing antibodies such as those reactive with idiotypic differences present on the primary antibody populations [5,6]. Mediator activation, particularly formation of C3b and interaction with complement receptors, also modifies the handling and fate of immune complex material [7,8]. Selective localization of the antigen (or antibody) portion of the immune complex related to its physicochemical interaction with the glomerular capillary wall would be expected to alter free interchange within the immune complex and thereby affect the dynamic equilibrium. In this way the passive immune complex mechanism and the trapped antigen mechanism of active antibody binding may overlap.

Active binding of antibody to antigens within the glomerulus as a nephritogenic stimulus has expanded from the classic example of glomerular basement membrane antigens to include a number of additional endogenous structural or exogenous trapped antigenic epitopes in model systems (Table I) [1]. This list can be expected to continue to grow. The direct antibody mechanism can now be broadened and subdivided with the recent observations that antibody reactions with glomerular cell surface antigens may lead to selective glomerular cell binding of antibody with antigen shedding as an immune deposit and/or cellular damage. This selective cellular damage contrasts with the rather nonselective phlogogenic effects generated by an immune deposit focus with its nephritogenic potential to neighbouring structures governed via the magnitude and duration of activation of the various mediator pathways.

Antibody reactions with selective glomerular cell populations

Recognizing the potential of selective glomerular cell attack via direct antibody reactions in model systems adds a new dimension to understanding nephritogenic antibody mechanisms. The concept now needs exploration as a possible cause of glomerulonephritis in humans. In addition, when the antibody reaction leads to selective cell destruction, it may provide a model to address questions regarding the normal and pathophysiological functions of the particular glomerular cell type involved.

The direct reaction of antibody with cell surface antigens can have at least two consequences. First, the immune reaction can lead to the formation of immune deposits apparently by the reaction of antibody with cell surface antigens, followed by capping and shedding of the antigen-antibody complex [9]. Recently, this concept has been described in antibody reactions with glomerular epithelial or endothelial cell surface antigens (see below). Second, the antibody reaction may lead to the rapid destruction of the targetted cell. This latter mechanism occurs with antibodies reactive with the mesangial cell [10] to be described herein. In this particular case there is only short-term antibody binding with complement fixation but no long-lasting immune deposit formation.

Antibody-induced injury to epithelial cells

Heymann's nephritis is induced typically by immunization with a crude homologous renal tubular fraction designated Fx1A [11]. Reaction of antibody with glomerular antigens was found in both passive [12,13] and active Heymann's nephritis [14,15]. Membrane antigens on glomerular epithelial cells appear to be involved in direct antibody attack in the Heymann's nephritis model. One such antigen has been defined as a glycoprotein (gp330) which is located in the coated pits of the glomerular epithelial cells [16,17]. A number of other antigens have been suggested in this model as well, including some in the endothelial region and on T-cells as well as idiotypic antigens [18–24]. The full blown disease is clearly easier to induce with the crude nephritogenic tubular antigen fraction, Fx1A, than with any of the single purified reactive molecules, suggesting that more than one antigen or mechanism may be involved. Recent studies indicate that the reactive glomerular epithelial cell surface antigens are cross-linked and capped by the antibody reaction, leading to shedding of the antigen-antibody complex as an immune deposit along the subepithelial aspect of the glomerular basement membrane [25–27]. Loss of epithelial cells does not appear to be an important feature of the lesion although the degree of effacement of epithelial cell foot processes which increases slowly (between 3–5 days) is; the degree of effacement relates to the amount of immune deposit formation [28].

The development of proteinuria within five days of administration of anti-Fx1A antibodies in the passive Heymann's nephritis lesion has been shown to be complement dependent and to involve elements of the membrane attack complex of the terminal complement components [29–31]. Complement mediated lysis of anti-Fx1A antibody sensitized cultured glomerular epithelial cells has recently been reported [32]. Complement depletion, however, does not prevent all effects of anti-Fx1A antibody binding as measured by glomerular micropuncture [33].

Antibody-induced endothelial cell injury
The rabbit glomerular endothelial cell also has been suggested to be a focus for nephritogenic antibody attack. As in the ovary and lung [9,34], antibodies can react with the glomerular endothelial cell surface angiotensin-converting enzyme [35]. Heterologous anti-angiotensin-converting enzyme reactive with the endothelial cell surface can lead to subsequent subepithelial immune deposits containing the heterologous Ig, rabbit Ig, and C3. The endothelial cells themselves become swollen and contain numerous blebs. This morphological change is most severe three days after the antibody injection. The relationship between the endothelial reaction, the immune deposit formation, and the morphological changes seen in the endothelial cells has not been completely defined.

Antibody-induced mesangial cell injury
The third glomerular cell type, the mesangial cell (a smooth muscle-like cell), is located in a central supporting position between the glomerular capillary loops and is in contact with the capillary lumen and vascular compartment through the fenestrated glomerular endothelium [36,37]. The mesangial stalk area normally also contains a few leucocyte common antigen and Ia-positive mononuclear phagocytes [38–40]. The mesangium has a number of potential physiological and possible phlogogenic functions that may contribute to nephritogenic immune processes [41,42]. The mesangium is a focus for accumulation of immune deposits in many forms of experimental and human glomerulonephritis. Mesangial hypercellularity is a frequent early finding in immune renal injury and increased production of mesangial matrix and sclerosis are frequent sequelae. The mesangial cell itself appears to have only a limited rôle in clearing aggregates from the glomerular capillary lumen. The phagocytic function of the mononuclear phagocytes in the mesangium as well as transport through mesangial channels are probably the major means of handling immune aggregates [41–45]. Immune related stimuli such as the membrane attack complex [46] can cause mesangial cells to produce or release a number of products including enzymes, arachidonic acid metabolites, and interleukin 1-like materials which could influence the course of glomerular injury [36,47–49]. The mesangial cell also has angiotensin II receptors and could possibly respond to this stimulus [50,51], suggesting a rôle for the cell in maintaining glomerular haemodynamics.

Better definition of the many possible contributions of the mesangial cell both as a target and as an active contributor in immune glomerular injury remains an important goal. We have sought to study the consequences of immune mesangial cell injury and also have been interested in determining the consequences of selective mesangial cell loss as one means of studying this cell's contributions to normal glomerular function [10,52]. Previously the mesangial cell had been relatively hard to injure selectively. Habu snake venom produces injury and a proliferative mesangial response sensitive to anticoagulant heparin [53–55]. Antibodies cause an inflammatory mesangial lesion when they react with materials taken up by the mesangium [56]. Antibodies reactive with rat mesangium have been induced with porcine lung [57] and anti-Forssman antibody can bind to guinea pig mesangium producing increased cellularity [58]. Monoclonal antibodies reactive in vivo with the mesangial matrix have also been reported [59]. Recently, antibodies reactive with Thy 1.1-like antigens associated with the mesangial cell membrane have been shown to induce acute mesangial injury [10,52,60–64].

Thy 1 is a glycoprotein with a relative molecular mass of 18,000, one-third of which is carbohydrate located on the cell surface of certain cells, particularly thymus and brain. Its cDNA indicates a molecule of 143 aminoacids with a hydrophobic domain for insertion in the cell membrane [65,66]. In the rat, anti-Thy 1.1 antibodies have been reported to react with brain, thymocytes, B-cell precursors, bone marrow cells, fibroblasts, and kidney [reviewed in 67]. Thy 1.1 reactivity has been demonstrated in the rat glomerulus using monoclonal anti-Thy 1.1 antibody or heterologous anti-rat thymocyte antibody [68–71]. The Thy 1-like antigen has been localized on the surface of mesangial cells by electron microscopy [60,72]. We were interested in using this antigenic site as a possible target for selective antibody-induced mesangial cell destruction. Bagchus et al have employed monoclonal anti-thymocyte antibodies for a similar purpose [63,64].

Anti-rat thymocyte antibodies were prepared in rabbits and were shown to react with rat mesangium in vivo and mesangial cell surface antigens in vitro [10,52,61,62]. The mesangial reaction could be blocked by prior absorption of the antibody with thymus or brain. The predominant antigen appeared to be Thy 1.1-like based on absorption studies and selective inhibition of anti-thymocyte serum fixation with monoclonal Thy 1.1 antibody OX7, but not OX2, another monoclonal antibody reactive with a rat thymus glycoprotein also present in rat glomeruli. It is not yet clear if the cross-reactivity represents the presence of the same molecule or rather a sharing of epitopes by dissimilar molecules. Studies in progress suggest that messenger RNA recovered from glomeruli will hybridize to some extent with a rat Thy 1.1 cDNA probe.

Using the anti-thymocyte serum antibody, a dose dependent lytic lesion of glomerular mesangial cells could be induced within one hour of antibody administration in Lewis rats. The lesion was typified by karyorrhexis and pyknosis of mesangial nuclei (Figure 1A) and a decrease in total glomerular nuclear counts from a normal mean of 48.6 to 39.8 and 37.4 at one and four hours respectively ($p<0.001$). This could be interpreted to mean that 72–92% of the mesangial cells, estimated to comprise about 25% of glomerular cells [73] were damaged. Occasional polymorphonuclear leucocytes (mean 2.4 compared to 0.2/glom

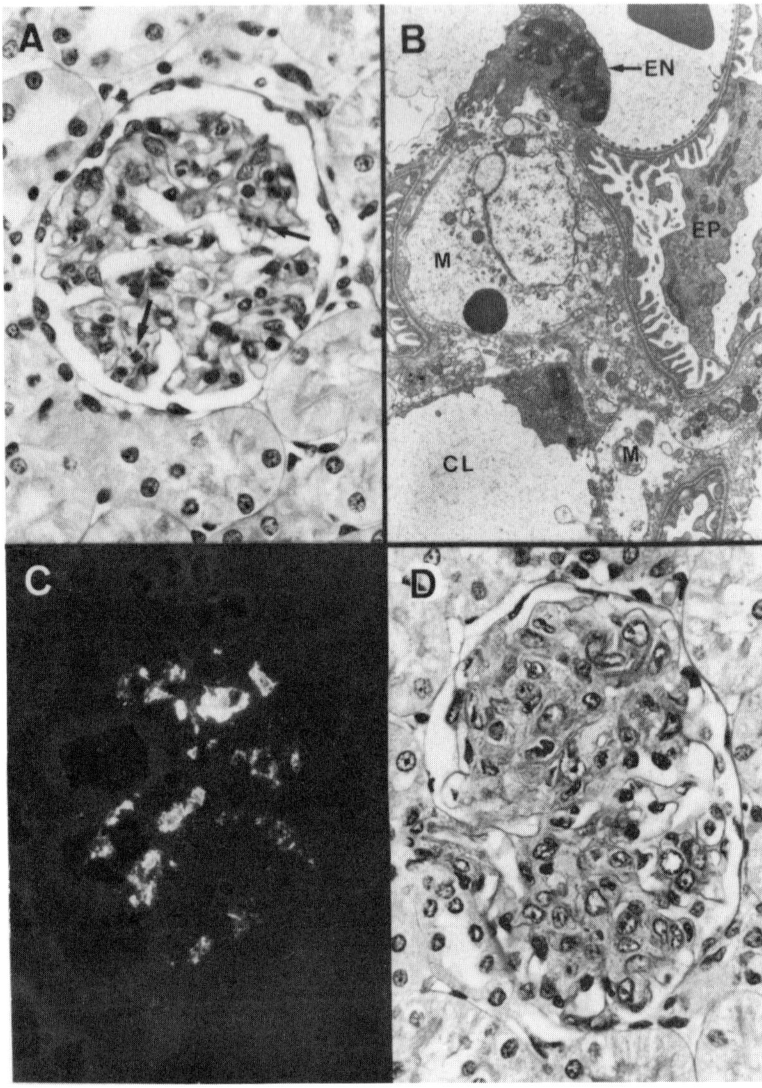

Figure 1. A) Fragments of degenerating mesangial cell nuclei (arrows) are observed in the glomerulus of a Lewis rat one hour after administration of 0.5ml anti-thymocyte serum/ 100g body weight. B) At the electronmicroscopic level, the degenerative changes in mesangial cells (M) at one hour after anti-thymocyte serum administration can be seen. Both endothelial (EN) and epithelial (EP) cells appear well preserved. Additional abbreviation: CL=capillary lumen. C) Deposits of rabbit IgG accompanied by C3, C5, C6, C7, C9 and membrane attack complex neoantigens were observed at one hour after administration of the dose of antibody used in Figure 1A. D) A glomerulus at four days demonstrates hypercellularity largely confined to mesangial areas. This change began at two to three days after administration of anti-thymocyte serum in the dose used in Figure 1A

cross section in controls) were identified at one hour in the mesangial areas. By electronmicroscopy, the degeneration of glomerular mesangial cells was striking with intact endothelial and epithelial cell structures (Figure 1B). Heterologous IgG and rat C3 were found in the mesangial areas one hour after antibody administration (Figure 1C). These immune reactants resolved over the next four days.

The degree of initial lysis was found to be dose dependent and occurred with fixation of relatively small amounts of antibody ($11.6\mu g/7x10^4$ glomeruli). This amount of antibody is considerably less than that required for the induction of immune deposit forms of glomerular injury such as that associated with anti-glomerular basement membrane antibodies or planted antigen mechanisms such as those utilizing the lectin concanavalin A [74,75], which require a fixation of 150–170μg antibody per two kidneys. Glomerular binding (67% of maximum) was observed after only 15 minutes, and the binding was maximal at one hour, receding thereafter corresponding to the disappearance noted by immunofluorescence. Binding of radiolabelled anti-thymocyte serum/gram of dry weight reached 0.38μg/g dry weight in liver at six hours. Binding to other organs was absent or only minimal in lung, brain, heart, spleen, or thymus of the rats 1, 6, 24 or 96 hours after administration. Maximum binding was found in spleen (0.1μg/g dry weight at 24 hours). Maximum uptake in thymus was 0.01μg/g dry weight also at 24 hours [62].

Depending on the degree of initial injury, the lytic lesion was replaced beginning in 2–3 days by glomerular hypercellularity (Figure 1D) with slow resolution over the next 4–6 weeks. A mild residual mesangial matrix increase and sclerosis persisted at three months.

The morphological lesion in the Lewis rat is not accompanied by increased proteinuria; however, in the Munich Wistar rat similar amounts of this anti-thymocyte serum did result in a proteinuric glomerular lesion, as has been reported with the use of monoclonal anti-Thy 1.1 antibody in Wistar rats [63, 64]. Serum creatinine increased slightly but uniformly in the Lewis rat from a mean of 0.53 to 0.72mg/dl at four days after anti-thymocyte serum injection ($p<0.05$).

Glomerular haemodynamics at 24 hours after anti-thymocyte serum administration reveal that the glomerular capillary pressure tends to rise significantly, but so does Bowman's space pressure, resulting in only a modest elevation in the hydrostatic pressure gradient. The single nephron filtration rate does fall, however, compared to normal animals primarily, if not solely, as a result of a large decrease in the glomerular ultrafiltration coefficient to approximately 40% of the normal value. The glomerular capillary pressure was easily obtained, suggesting that the luminal diameter of the capillary was increased or the 'capillary tone' provided by the mesangial cell diminished as a result of the cell's injury. Studies in progress to assess the effects of anti-thymocyte serum on mesangial cell angiotensin II receptors should provide useful information regarding one mechanism that might contribute to this observation. The morphological findings described above, including the ballooning of some capillary loops, probably also play a rôle.

The initial lytic mesangial lesion was associated with rat C3 fixation. When studied in more detail, complement components of the terminal complement sequence were detected using human anti-C5, C6, C7, C9, and membrane attack complex neoantigen antibodies [61]. This finding suggested that the membrane attack complex might be contributing to the lytic lesion. Indeed the one-hour lytic lesion was found to be complement dependent using rats which had been depleted of >95% of their C3 using cobra venom factor [61]. The effects of any residual phospholipase A2 in the cobra venom factor were excluded by its pretreatment with p-bromophenacyl bromide, which gave results identical to the native cobra venom factor. The complement depletion of cobra venom factor did not affect the amount of anti-thymocyte serum bound in the glomeruli as determined by immunofluorescence staining or paired label isotope quantitation. No nuclear loss was detected at one hour in the anti-thymocyte serum plus cobra venom factor group and was indistinguishable from the saline treated control rats by light microscopy (mean 51.5 versus 50.6 nuclei/glomerular cross section). The anti-thymocyte serum plus saline positive control group has the typical loss of nuclei (mean 40.6/glomerular cross section). The glomerular electronmicroscopic changes of mesangial cell lysis observed in control rats were also completely prevented by C3 depletion with cobra venon factor. When studied by immunofluorescence, well defined mesangial deposits of C3 were observed in the complement replete saline treated controls; however, C3 deposits were not observed in the cobra venom factor-treated rats. The complement dependence of the mesangial cell injury is also supported by the absence of lesions after administration of a non-complement-fixing monoclonal anti-thymocyte antibody [63]. The blockade of the acute necrotic lesion by cobra venom factor prevented the hypercellular lesion typically observed at day four with the dose of anti-thymocyte serum used [61].

Because a small number of polymorphonuclear leucocytes were observed in the one hour lesion, polymorphonuclear leucocyte depletion (<40/mm^3) using anti-polymorphonuclear antibody or leucocyte depletion (<500/mm^3) using whole body irradiation with splenectomy and kidney shielding were done to determine the relative importance of leucocytes in generating the initial lytic lesion [61]. This treatment had no effect on the one hour lytic lesion with nuclear counts falling to levels indistinguishable from controls (39.5,38.2, and 40.6 nuclei/glomerular cross section for the irradiation, anti-polymorphonuclear antibody, and saline plus anti-thymocyte serum control groups respectively). Of interest, total leucocyte depletion did appear to reduce somewhat the magnitude of the four-day hypercellular response (55.5 versus 64.3 nuclei/glomerular cross section for irradiated and control groups, respectively).

To further investigate the rôle of complement as evidenced by cobra venom factor depletion and the presence of early- and late-acting complement components in the glomerular lesion, cultured glomerular mesangial cells were subjected to anti-thymocyte serum treatment in vitro. This treatment resulted in ^{51}Cr release during the first 30–120 minutes in the presence, but not the absence, of a complement source.

The direct effect of complement on anti-thymocyte serum treated cultured mesangial cells was studied using electronmicroscopy with negative staining [52]. Doughnut-shaped lesions of about 90Å were found typical of those associated with membrane attack complex lesions in nucleated cells [76–79]. The size of the doughnut-like channel lesion of the membrane attack complex, which may vary somewhat depending on the cell type and complement source, appears to relate in part to the number of C9 molecules in the complex [80,81]. The lytic effect is felt to relate to the ability of the cell to shed the membrane attack complex and repair any membrane damage [78,79]. Studies in progress using anti-thymocyte serum in the isolated perfused kidney with controlled complement sources should provide more direct evidence for the rôle of the membrane attack complex in damaging the mesangial cells in vivo.

The immediate anti-thymocyte serum induced, complement mediated mesangial cell lysis was followed after about 48 hours by an increase in glomerular cellularity with mean glomerular nuclear counts of 55–65 between days 4–14 (control 49 nuclei/glomerular cross section). A minimal increase in mean glomerular polymorphonuclear leucocyte counts was found after four days. The hypercellularity occurred after the IgG and C3 deposits diminished or disappeared. In areas, ballooning of the glomerular capillary loops was evident, producing small aneurysmal dilatations which were involved in the hypercellular response. In some of these dilatations, polymorphonuclear leucocytes were frequent. By electronmicroscopy, the hypercellularity was characterized by two morphologically different cell types present in the expanded mesangial areas [62]. A major cell type had a large nucleus, a single nucleolus, relatively scant cytoplasm, with a smooth cell surface and scant organelles other than rough endoplasmic reticulum. The other cell type had pseudopods on the surface and plentiful cell organelles, including phagosomes.

The phenotypic characterization of the majority of the cells in the hypercellular lesions revealed cells that were mesangial in nature reacting with the anti-thymocyte serum and monoclonal Thy 1.1 antibodies as well as anti-desmin antisera, but not with anti-von Willebrand factor antibody. A small increase in cells reacting with anti-leucocyte common antigen or anti-Ia monoclonal antibodies was also found. In addition, mitotic figures were seen in the hypercellular glomeruli and a mean of 5–6 cells per glomerulus reacted with an antibody reactive with antigens in proliferating cell nuclei [82]. All of these findings suggested that the major contributor to the hypercellularity was the glomerular mesangial cell. Leucocyte depletion using whole body irradiation or anti-polymorphonuclear antibody, as noted earlier, also produced a limited suppressive effect on the glomerular hypercellular response, suggesting that leucocytes were not an essential feature in the hypercellular reaction.

The mesangial nature of the hypercellularity was also supported by in vitro studies using culture of glomeruli treated in vivo with anti-thymocyte serum. In these glomeruli increased uptake of ^{3}H-thymidine was not suppressed by the glomerular epithelial cell toxin, aminonucleoside of puromycin [52]. Electron-microscopy of these glomeruli also revealed that the increase in cells was endocapillary rather than epithelial in position.

In studies using much larger doses of anti-thymocyte serum, the subsequent hypercellularity was prevented or delayed presumably related to more complete initial killing of these cells. Readministration of anti-thymocyte serum during the hypercellular response had only a partial acute lytic effect with some reduction in glomerular cell nuclear counts. The apparent density of reactive epitopes on the proliferating glomerular cells appeared to be somewhat less than on native cells as judged by the intensity of indirect immunofluorescence staining in vitro. In vivo, the anti-thymocyte serum may also have had difficulty reaching available epitopes due to the density of cells packed in the lesions.

To use the anti-thymocyte serum induced mesangial cell injury to examine mesangial cell function, we evaluated the effects of anti-thymocyte serum treatment on glomerular uptake and disappearance of aggregated test molecules or preformed immune complexes [62]. A small increase (three times control) in glomerular uptake was noted when anti-thymocyte serum was administered simultaneously with the test aggregate. When the test aggregate was given four hours after anti-thymocyte serum, the glomerular uptake increased 48 times the control value. The values then fell to 14, 13, and 6 times when the anti-thymocyte serum preceded the test aggregate by one, three, and seven days, respectively. The disappearance of the test aggregate from the serum or its handling by other organs was unaffected by anti-thymocyte serum. The aggregate was found in the glomerular mesangial region by immunofluorescence and immunoelectron-microscopy at one and four hours after administration, but had largely disappeared by 24 hours. Findings with aggregated bovine serum albumin and preformed immune complexes were similar except that the bovine serum albumin was cleared from the mesangial areas somewhat more slowly. The findings suggest that mesangial uptake of macromolecules increases remarkably when the mesangial cell is injured; however, the cell itself does not seem essential for the removal of trapped macromolecules.

Summary

The antibody and complement related anti-mesangial cell lysis in this model represents a striking example of selective antibody induced glomerular cell injury. The recognition of antibody's ability to selectively injure one or another glomerular cell type adds a finer level of specificity to our understanding of humoral immune mechanisms responsible for glomerular damage. Models of selective glomerular cell injury should provide a way to study the functional rôles of the different glomerular cell populations. The infrequent suggestions in the literature of anti-mesangial cell antibodies in patients with IgA nephropathy [83] may deserve a closer look in view of the findings reported herein.

Acknowledgments
This is publication No 4941-IMM from the Department of Immunology, Research Institute of Scripps Clinic, La Jolla, California. This work was supported in part by United States Public Health Service Grants AI-07007, AG-04342, DK-20043, DK-28602, DK-33692; funds provided by the Research Service of the Veterans Administration; and Biomedical Research Support Grant RRO-5514.

References

1 Wilson CB, Dixon FJ. The renal response to immunological injury. In Brenner BM, Rector FC Jr, eds. *The Kidney, 3rd Edition.* Philadelphia: W B Saunders. 1986: 800–889
2 Couser WG, Baker PJ, Adler S. Complement and the direct mediation of immune glomerular injury: a new perspective. *Kidney Int 1985; 28:* 879–890
3 Johnson RJ, Couser WG, Chi EY et al. New mechanism for glomerular injury. Myeloperoxidase-hydrogen peroxide-halide system. *J Clin Invest 1987; 79:* 1379–1387
4 Ward DH, Lee S, Wilson CB. Direct antigen binding to glomerular immune complex deposits. *Kidney Int 1986; 30:* 706–711
5 Goldman M, Rose LM, Hochmann A et al. Deposition of idiotype-anti-idiotype immune complexes in renal glomeruli after polyclonal B cell activation. *J Exp Med 1982; 156:* 1385–1399
6 Zanetti M, Wilson CB. Participation of auto-anti-idiotypes in immune complex glomerulonephritis in rabbits. *J Immunol 1983; 131:* 2781–2783
7 Miller GW, Nussenzweig V. A new complement function: solubilization of antigen-antibody aggregates. *Proc Natl Acad Sci USA 1975; 72:* 418–422
8 Iida K, Nussenzweig V. Functional properties of membrane-associated complement receptor CR1. *J Immunol 1983; 130:* 1876–1880
9 Matsuo S, Caldwell PRB, Brentjens JR, Andres G. In vivo interaction of antibodies with cell surface antigens: a mechanism responsible for in situ formation of immune deposits in the zona pellucida of rabbit oocytes. *J Clin Invest 1985; 75:* 1369–1380
10 Yamamoto T, Wilson CB. Antibody-induced mesangial cell damage: the model, functional alterations, and effects of complement. *Kidney Int 1986; 29 (Abstract):* 296
11 Edgington TS, Glassock RJ, Dixon FJ. Autologous immune complex nephritis induced with renal tubular antigen. I. Identification and isolation of the pathogenetic antigen. *J Exp Med 1968, 127:* 555–572
12 Couser WG, Steinmuller DR, Stilmant MM et al. Experimental glomerulonephritis in the isolated perfused rat kidney. *J Clin Invest 1978; 62:* 1275–1287
13 Van Damme BJC, Fleuren GJ, Bakker WW et al. Experimental glomerulonephritis in the rat induced by antibodies directed against tubular antigens. V. Fixed glomerular antigens in the pathogenesis of heterologous immune complex glomerulonephritis. *Lab Invest 1978; 38:* 502–510
14 Neale JT, Wilson CB. Glomerular antigens in Heymann's nephritis: reactivity of eluted and circulating antibody. *J Immunol 1982; 128:* 323–330
15 Neale JT, Couser WG, Salant DJ et al. Specific uptake of Heymann's nephritic kidney eluate by rat kidney. *Lab Invest 1982; 46:* 450–453
16 Kerjaschki D, Farquhar MG. Immunocytochemical localization of the Heymann nephritis antigen (gp330) in glomerular epithelial cells of normal Lewis rats. *J Exp Med 1983; 157:* 667–686

17 Ronco P, Neale TJ, Wilson CB et al. An immunopathologic study of a 330-kD protein defined by monoclonal antibodies and reactive with anti-RTE-alpha-5 antibodies and kidney eluates from active Heymann nephritis. *J Immunol 1986; 136:* 125–130

18 Makker SP, Singh AK. Characterization of the antigen (gp600) of Heymann nephritis. *Lab Invest 1984; 50:* 287–293

19 Jeraj K, Vernier RL, Sisson SP, Michael AF. A new glomerular antigen in passive Heymann's nephritis. *Br J Exp Path 1984; 65:* 485–498

20 Kamata K, Baird ME, Erikson ME et al. Characterization of antigens and antibody specificities involved in Heymann nephritis. *J Immunol 1985; 135:* 2400–2408

21 Bagchus WM, Vos JTWM, Hoedemaeker J, Bakker WW. The specificity of nephritogenic antibodies. III. Binding of anti-Fx1A antibodies in glomeruli is dependent on dual specificity. *Clin Exp Immunol 1986; 63:* 639–647

22 Abrass CK. Evaluation of sequential glomerular eluates from rats with Heymann nephritis. *J Immunol 1986; 137:* 530–535

23 Natori Y, Hayakawa I, Shibata S. Passive Heymann nephritis with acute and severe proteinuria induced by heterologous antibody against renal tubular brush border glycoprotein gp108. *Lab Invest 1986; 55:* 63–70

24 Chatelet F, Brianti E, Ronco P et al. Ultrastructural localization by monoclonal antibodies of brush border antigens expressed by glomeruli. I. Renal distribution. *Am J Pathol 1986; 122:* 500–511

25 Camussi G, Brentjens JR, Noble B et al. Antibody-induced redistribution of Heymann antigen on the surface of cultured glomerular visceral epithelial cell: possible role in the pathogenesis of Heymann glomerulonephritis. *J Immunol 1985; 135:* 2409–2416

26 Allegri L, Brianti E, Chatelat F et al. Polyvalent antigen-antibody interactions are required for the formation of electron-dense immune deposits in passive Heymann's nephritis. *Am J Pathol 1986; 125:* 1–6

27 Camussi G, Noble B, Van Liew J et al. Pathogenesis of passive Heymann glomerulonephritis: chlorpromazine inhibits antibody mediated redistribution of cell surface antigens and prevents development of the disease. *J Immunol 1986; 136:* 2127–2135

28 Gabbai FB, Gushwa LC, Wilson CB, Blantz RC. An evaluation of the development of experimental membranous nephropathy. *Kidney Int 1987; 31:* 1267–1278

29 Salant DJ, Belok S, Madaio MP, Couser WG. A new role for complement in experimental membranous nephropathy in rats. *J Clin Invest 1980; 66:* 1339–1350

30 Cybulsky AV, Quigg RJ, Salant DJ. The membrane attack complex in complement mediated glomerular epithelial cell injury: formation and stability of C5b-9 and C5b-7 in rat membranous nephropathy. *J Immunol 1986; 137:* 1511–1516

31 Cybulsky AV, Rennke HG, Feintzeig ID, Salant DJ. Complement-induced glomerular epithelial cell injury. Role of the membrane attack complex in rat membranous nephropathy. *J Clin Invest 1986; 77:* 1096–1107

32 Quigg RJ, Cybulsky AV, Salant DJ. The nephritogenic antibody (AB) of passive Heymann nephritis (PHN) directs complement (C)-mediated cytotoxicity of cultured glomerular visceral epithelial cell (GEC). *Kidney Int 1987; 31 (Abstract):* 328

33 Blantz RC, Gabbai F, Mundy C, Wilson CB. Changes in glomerular hemodynamics (GH) induced by complement depletion (CD) in passive Heymann's nephritis (PHN). *Kidney Int 1986; 29 (Abstract):* 380

34 Barba LM, Caldwell PRB, Downie GH et al. Lung injury mediated by antibodies to endothelium. I. In the rabbit a repeated interaction of heterologous anti-angiotensin-converting enzyme antibodies with alveolar endothelium results in resistance to immune injury through antigenic modulation. *J Exp Med 1983; 158:* 2141–2158

35 Matsuo S, Fukatsu A, Taub ML et al. Glomerulonephritis induced in the rabbit by antiendothelial antibodies. *J Clin Invest 1987; 79:* 1798–1811

36 Striker GE, Striker LJ. Biology of disease. Glomerular cell culture. *Lab Invest 1985; 53:* 122–131

37 Kashgarian M. Editorial. Mesangium and glomerular disease. *Lab Invest 1985; 52:* 569–571

38 Schreiner GF, Kiely J-M, Cotran RS, Unanue ER. Characterization of resident glomerular cells in the rat expressing Ia determinants and manifesting genetically restricted interactions with lymphocytes. *J Clin Invest 1981; 68:* 920–931

39 Schreiner GF, Unanue ER. Origin of the rat mesangial phagocyte and its expression of the leukocyte common antigen. *Lab Invest 1984; 51:* 515–523

40 Schreiner GF, Cotran RS, Unanue ER. Modulation of Ia and leukocyte common antigen expression in rat glomeruli during the course of glomerulonephritis and aminonucleoside nephrosis. *Lab Invest 1984; 51:* 524–533

41 Michael AF, Keane WF, Raij L et al. The glomerular mesangium. *Kidney Int 1980; 17:* 141–154

42 Sterzel RB, Lovett DH. Interactions of inflammatory and glomerular cells in the response to glomerular injury. In Brenner BM, Stein JH, eds; Wilson CB, guest ed. *Contemporary Issues in Nephrology.* New York: Churchill Livingstone. 1987: in press

43 Keane WF, Raij L. Impaired mesangial clearance of macromolecules in rats with chronic mesangial ferritin-antiferritin immune complex deposition. *Lab Invest 1980; 43:* 500–508

44 Mancilla-Jimenez R, Bellon B, Kuhn J et al. Phagocytosis of heat-aggregated immunoglobulins by mesangial cells. An immunoperoxidase and acid phosphatase study. *Lab Invest 1982; 46:* 243–253

45 Latta H, Fligiel S. Mesangial fenestrations, sieving, filtration, and flow. *Lab Invest 1985; 52:* 591–598

46 Lovett DH, Haensch G-M, Goppelt M et al. Activation of glomerular mesangial cells by the terminal membrane attack complex of complement. *J Immunol 1987; 138:* 2473–2480

47 Lovett DH, Ryan JL, Sterzel RB. A thymocyte-activating factor derived from glomerular mesangial cells. *J Immunol 1983; 130:* 1796–1801

48 MacCarthy EP, Hsu A, Ooi YM, Ooi BS. Evidence for a mouse mesangial cell-derived factor that stimulates lymphocyte proliferation. *J Clin Invest 1985; 76:* 426–430

49 Lovett DH, Szamel M, Ryan JL et al. Interleukin 1 and the glomerular mesangium. I. Purification and characterization of a mesangial cell-derived autogrowth factor. *J Immunol 1986; 136:* 3700–3705

50 Ausiello DA, Kreisberg JI, Roy C, Karnovsky MJ. Contraction of cultured rat glomerular cells of apparent mesangial origin after stimulation with angiotensin II and arginine vasopressin. *J Clin Invest 1980; 65:* 754–760

51 Raij L, Keane WF. Glomerular mesangium: its function and relationship to angiotensin II. *Am J Med 1985; 79 (Suppl 3C):* 24–30

52 Yamamoto T, Wilson CB. Mesangial cell (MC) injury and proliferation produced by antibody: a role for the membrane attack complex (MAC). *Kidney Int 1987; 31 (Abstract).* 333

53 Cattell V, Bradfield JWB. Focal mesangial proliferative glomerulonephritis in the rat caused by Habu snake venom. A morphologic study. *Am J Pathol 1977; 87:* 511–524

54 Morita T, Kihara I, Oite T et al. Mesangiolysis. Sequential ultrastructural study of Habu venom-induced glomerular lesions. *Lab Invest 1978; 38:* 94–102

55 Coffey AK, Karnovsky MJ. Heparin inhibits mesangial cell proliferation in Habu-venom-induced glomerular injury. *Am J Pathol 1985; 120:* 248–255

56 Mauer SM, Sutherland DER, Howard RJ et al. The glomerular mesangium. III. Acute immune mesangial injury: a new model of glomerulonephritis. *J Exp Med 1973; 137:* 553–570

57 Seelig HP, Seelig R, Roth E, Roth E. Antibodies reacting with the glomerular mesangium. Isolation and immunopathology. *Virchows Arch [A] 1975; 366:* 313–330

58 Barbosa JE, Rossi MA, Mello de Oliveira JA, Sarti W. Nephropathy produced by Forssman antibody in guinea pigs: an experimental model of mesangial injury. *Res Exp Med 1985; 185:* 283–290

59 Mendrick DL, Rennke HG. Immune deposits formed in situ by a monoclonal antibody recognizing a new intrinsic rat mesangial matrix antigen. *J Immunol 1986; 137:* 1517–1526

60 Yamamoto T, Yamamoto K, Kawasaki K et al. Immunoelectron microscopic demonstration of Thy-1 antigen on the surfaces of mesangial cells in the rat glomerulus. *Nephron 1986; 43:* 293–298
61 Yamamoto T, Wilson CB. Complement dependence of antibody-induced mesangial cell injury in the rat. *J Immunol 1987; 138:* 3758–3765
62 Yamamoto T, Wilson CB. Quantitative and qualitative studies of antibody-induced mesangial cell damage in the rat. *Kidney Int 1987:* in press
63 Bagchus WM, Hoedemaeker PJ, Rozing J, Bakker WW. Acute glomerulonephritis after intravenous injection of monoclonal anti-thymocyte antibodies in the rat. *Immunol Lett 1986; 12:* 109–113
64 Bagchus WM, Hoedemaeker PJ, Rozing J, Bakker WW. Glomerulonephritis induced by monoclonal anti-Thy 1.1 antibodies. A sequential histological and ultrastructural study in the rat. *Lab Invest 1971; 55:* 680–687
65 Seki T, Chang H-C, Moriuchi T et al. A hydrophobic transmembrane segment at the carboxyl terminus of Thy-1. *Science 1985; 227:* 649–651
66 Seki T, Moriuchi T, Chang H-C et al. Structural organization of the rat Thy-1 gene. *Nature 1985; 313:* 485–487
67 Crawford JM, Barton RW. Biology of disease. Thy-1 glycoprotein: structure, distribution, and ontogeny. *Lab Invest 1986; 54:* 122–135
68 Ishizaki M, Sato S, Sano J et al. The presence of Thy-1.1 antigen in rat glomerular mesangial cells. *Biomed Res 1980; 1:* 438–442
69 Barclay AN. Different reticular elements in rat lymphoid tissue identified by localization of Ia, Thy-1 and MRC OX 2 antigens. *Immunology 1981; 44:* 727–736
70 Harada K, Yamamoto T, Hara M, Kihara I. Antigenic association between kidney and thymocyte. *Acta Pathol Jpn 1982; 32:* 483–489
71 Morris RJ, Ritter MA. Association of Thy-1 cell surface differentiation antigen with certain connective tissues in vivo. *Cell Tissue Res 1980; 206:* 459–475
72 Paul LC, Rennke HG, Milford EL, Carpenter CB. Thy-1.1 in glomeruli of rat kidneys. *Kidney Int 1984; 25:* 771–777
73 Iidaka K, McCoy J, Kimmelstiel P. The glomerular mesangium. A quantitative analysis. *Lab Invest 1968; 19:* 573–579
74 Unanue ER, Dixon FJ. Experimental glomerulonephritis. V. Studies on the interaction of nephrotoxic antibodies with tissues of the rat. *J Exp Med 1965; 121:* 697–714
75 Golbus SM, Wilson CB. Experimental glomerulonephritis induced by in situ formation of immune complexes in glomerular capillary wall. *Kidney Int 1979; 16:* 148–157
76 Schreiber RD, Pangburn MK, Medicus RG, Muller-Eberhard HJ. Raji cell injury and subsequent lysis by the purified cytolytic alternative pathway of human complement. *Clin Immunol Immunopathol 1980; 15:* 384–396
77 Koski CL, Ramm LE, Hammer CH et al. Cytolysis of nucleated cells by complement: cell death displays multi-hit characteristics. *Proc Natl Acad Sci USA 1983; 80:* 3816–3820
78 Ramm LE, Whitlow MB, Mayer MM. Complement lysis of nucleated cells: effect of temperature and puromycin on the number of channels required for cytolysis. *Mol Immunol 1984; 21:* 1015–1021
79 Carney DF, Koski CL, Shin ML. Elimination of terminal complement intermediates from the plasma membrane of nucleated cells: the rate of disappearance differs for cells carrying C5b-7 or C5b-8 or a mixture of C5b-8 with a limited number of C5b-9. *J Immunol 1985; 134:* 1804–1809
80 Bhakdi S. Traumm-Jensen J. On the cause and nature of C9-related heterogeneity of terminal complement complexes generated on target erythrocytes through the action of whole serum. *J Immunol 1984; 133:* 1453–1463
81 Ramm LE, Whitlow MB, Mayer MM. The relationship between channel size and the number of C9 molecules in the C5b-9 complex. *J Immunol 1985; 134:* 2594–2599
82 Miyachi K, Fritzler MJ, Tan EM. Autoantibody to a nuclear antigen in proliferating cells. *J Immunol 1978; 121:* 2228–2234
83 Lowance DC, Mullins JD, McPhaul JJ Jr. Immunoglobulin A (IgA) associated glomerulonephritis. *Kidney Int 1973; 3:* 167–176

THE ROLE OF MONONUCLEAR LEUCOCYTES IN GLOMERULONEPHRITIS

S R Holdsworth, N W Boyce, P G Tipping

Monash University, Prince Henry's Hospital, Melbourne, Australia

Mononuclear leucocyte participation in glomerulonephritis

Recognition of the involvement of mononuclear inflammatory cells (macrophages and lymphocytes) in nephritic glomeruli has stimulated new interest into the cellular mechanisms of injury in glomerulonephritis. The presence of these cells went unrecognized until recently because of their lack of characteristic and unique morphological features. Their recognition has awaited the application of techniques exploiting their functional, metabolic or antigenic characteristics. These techniques have included histochemical staining [1], glomerular cell culture [2], recognition of unique ultrastructural features [3] and unique surface antigens by monoclonal antibodies [4].

The mononuclear inflammatory cell most widely recognized in human and experimental glomerulonephritis is the macrophage. These cells have now been demonstrated repeatedly in glomeruli of patients with proliferative and crescentic glomerulonephritis [5,6]. Their involvement in non-proliferative glomerulonephritis is much less common. Macrophages have also been recognized to be prominent participants in proliferative experimental glomerulonephritis initiated by a number of pathogenic mechanisms including anti-glomerular basement membrane antibodies, immune complexes and planted glomerular antigens [7] in a variety of species.

The presence of lymphocytes within glomeruli in glomerulonephritis has been suggested by electron microscopic observations [8]. Confirmation of their participation was provided by immunohistochemical localization studies using specific monoclonal antilymphocyte antibodies [9]. In proliferative anti-glomerular basement membrane antibody initiated glomerulonephritis in rats, a lymphocyte influx preceding macrophage accumulation has been observed. Two studies have now confirmed that lymphocytes also participate in a variety of types of proliferative human glomerulonephritis [11,12]. The participation of both lymphocytes and monocytes provides the basis for the potential involvement of cell mediated immunity in glomerulonephritis.

The rôle of macrophages in glomerulonephritis

Macrophages can subserve affector, regulatory and effector rôles in immunological responses.

Affector rôle

In the affector phase of the immune response, macrophages act as important antigen processing and immune initiating cells. The observation of a resident population of Ia-positive bone marrow derived mononuclear cells with characteristics of macrophages in the rat has suggested that they may play a rôle at a local glomerular level. Subsequent studies have confirmed in vitro that these cells can process antigen and initiate immune responses in a genetically restricted manner [12]. This affector rôle of resident glomerular macrophages has not received wide attention as their presence has not yet been confirmed in other species including man.

Effector cell rôle

The most widely studied rôle of macrophages in glomerular injury is as an effector cell. Macrophages express a vast array of effector functions. Most attention has been focused on their effector rôle in tumour or microbial immune responses. However, many of the functions initially illustrated in these systems are potentially relevant to inflammatory injury in the glomerulus. Macrophages produce a wide array of inflammatory mediators that are injurious to tissues. Synthesis and release of lysosomal hydrolases is well-known and the capacity of these hydrolases to denature glomerular basement membrane has been confirmed [13]. Macrophages also release a number of neutral proteases including collagenase and plasminogen activator which may profoundly alter events in glomerular inflammation. The release and production of cytolytic proteinase confirmed in tumour cell lysis may be relevant to the rôle of these cells in effecting glomerular injury. The generation of reactive oxygen species by phagocytic cells is another important mechanism of immune defence and tissue injury in inflammation. Glomerular injury induced by neutrophil derived hydroxyl ions and hydrogen peroxide has recently been confirmed [14,15]. Macrophages also have the capacity to produce such reactive oxygen species. However the potential for macrophage derived reactive oxygen species to initiate glomerular injury has not yet been assessed.

Macrophages produce a wide variety of cytokines that may potentially influence glomerular injury [16]. These include arachidonic acid metabolites, interleukin 1, platelet activating factor, platelet derived growth factor, interferon and tissue necrosis factor. They also secrete complement components which may be involved in glomerular injury. Macrophages may play a phagocytic rôle in glomerulonephritis and maybe initiate coagulation by the membrane expression of procoagulant activity. Little is currently known of the functions expressed by glomerular macrophages in glomerulonephritis.

The potential for macrophages to induce glomerular injury has been confirmed in studies of experimental glomerulonephritis. Macrophage depletion experiments have shown that glomerular injury (proteinuria, histological appearances of proliferation and reduction in glomerular filtration rate) can be induced by macrophages [7,17]. We have shown, by cell transfer study, that macrophages can induce significant proliferative responses in intrinsic glomerular cells [18]. These findings have been confirmed in vitro [19]. Macrophages play a rôle in the uptake and processing of deposited immune complexes. This has been confirmed by studies in the isolated perfused kidney [20] and by ultrastructural observations [3]. Macrophages have been shown to participate in the formation of glomerular crescents [21,22] although functional studies (adoptive transfer experiments) to more precisely determine their rôle have not been performed.

Recent studies have suggested that macrophages can initiate glomerular fibrin deposition. Fibrin is a major mediator of renal failure in experimental glomerulonephritis and a potent stimulus for crescent formation. Both depletion and transfer experiments have confirmed that fibrin deposition can be induced by the glomerular accumulation of monocytes [23]. Further experiments have suggested that this is likely to be induced by the expression of monocyte procoagulant activity [24]. Nephritic glomeruli isolated from animals with experimental fibrin-related glomerulonephritis have vastly augmented levels of procoagulant activity with the functional characteristics of tissue factor. This glomerular procoagulant activity can be both reduced by macrophage depletion, and augmented by macrophage repletion in experimental glomerulonephritis [23].

Studies of glomeruli isolated from patients with fibrin related proliferative glomerulitis have suggested that these mechanisms also apply in human glomerulonephritis. Glomeruli isolated from such patients have vastly augmented levels of procoagulant activity when compared with normal human glomeruli [25] (Figure 1). This procoagulant has identical functional characteristics to macrophage procoagulant activity. Monoclonal antihuman tissue factor antibodies are able to specifically block this augmented procoagulant activity. Other studies have shown a close correlation between glomerular fibrin deposition and the presence of glomerular macrophages expressing tissue factor [26]. The traditionally held view suggests glomerular fibrin deposition is initiated by the intrinsic coagulation pathway after contact with damaged endothelial cells. This process would involve factor VIII but two studies have failed to confirm local deposition of this factor in human fibrin-related glomerulonephritis [25, 28]. In experimental glomerulonephritis we have been able to demonstrate glomerular deposition of factor VIII. However, this occurred after the onset of glomerular fibrin deposition. Macrophage accumulation coincided with the onset of fibrin deposition [27].

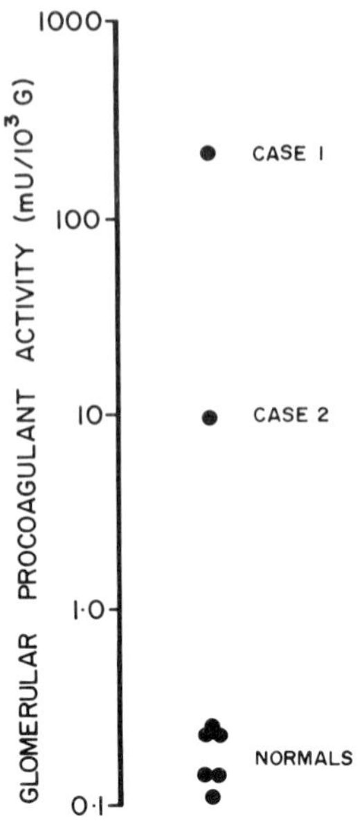

Figure 1. The expression of glomerular procoagulant activity by lysates of glomeruli from two patients (Cases 1 and 2) with crescentic glomerulonephritis with prominent glomerular fibrin deposition and macrophage accumulation compared with the levels in six normal controls

Regulatory rôles

A number of recent studies have shown that intrinsic glomerular cells may also act as modulators of the local glomerular inflammatory response. Mesangial cells have been shown in vitro to produce reactive oxygen species and to synthesize platelet activating factor and eicosanoids. These cells have also been demonstrated to be capable of producing interleukin 1 and platelet derived growth factor [29]. Mononuclear inflammatory cells (at least in vitro) can interact with intrinsic glomerular cells to modulate these functions. Macrophages via their synthesis of interleukin 1 are capable of stimulating mesangial cell proliferation [30]. A number of other macrophage cytokines are capable of stimulating a proliferative response by intrinsic glomerular cells in vitro. Most attention has been focused on the capacity of monocytes to induce acute inflammatory injury. This may occur either directly or indirectly through their interaction with intrinsic glomerular cells. Macrophages also play an important rôle in chronic inflammation. Monocytes can potentially stimulate glomerular fibrosis and sclerosis. Macrophages have been shown to stimulate glomerular cell synthesis of both collagen and collagenase [31] via their production of interleukin 1.

Mechanisms of glomerular macrophage recruitment and activation

Macrophage functions are regulated by a number of influences. It is clear that these cells require direction to acquire the functions that they express in glomerulonephritis. Increasing attention is now being paid to the mechanisms of recruitment and activation of macrophages.

Glomerular macrophage recruitment

A number of studies have addressed the means by which macrophages accumulate in glomeruli. Initial studies addressing these questions looked at the rôle of humoral factors as chemotactic attractants for monocytes. The prominence of complement in the glomeruli of patients and experimental animals with macrophage related proliferative nephritis led to speculation that complement fragments may account for this accumulation. These complement components are known from in vitro studies to be chemotactic for macrophages. However, a number of experimental studies have now clearly demonstrated that complement depletion has no significant effect on monocyte accumulation [7,32]. This does not completely negate a rôle for complement as a monocyte chemoattractant, but may suggest that other factors acting in addition to complement may also be capable of inducing monocyte localization.

The first mechanism shown to account for monocyte localization within glomeruli has been interaction with Fc receptors on immunoglobulin fixed in the kidney. In a passive model of experimental anti-glomerular basement membrane antibody induced glomerulonephritis, it was shown that Fc cleaved immunoglobulin was incapable of attracting a mononuclear cell infiltration [33]. In subsequent studies we have shown that the affinity of the Fc receptor for macrophages is a significant determinant of monocyte accumulation [34]. The capacity for antibody to initiate monocyte mediated glomerular injury could best be described as antibody dependent cell mediated cytotoxicity (ADCC).

The demonstration of lymphocyte participation particularly preceding monocyte accumulation [9] raises the likely involvement of delayed hypersensitivity mechanisms in glomerulonephritis. A number of studies support this hypothesis. We were able to show that lymphocytes accumulating prior to mononuclear cell infiltration secrete migration inhibition factor [35]. Thus these lymphocytes are locally activated sensitized cells producing lymphokines capable of inducing monocyte accumulation and activation. This is in keeping with observations of classical delayed hypersensitivity in the skin. A number of experiments in vivo further support the involvement of cell mediated immunity in glomerulonephritis. Adoptive transfer of lymphocytes sensitized to glomerular antigens was shown to be capable of causing a macrophage accumulation within glomeruli [36]. Although in these studies proteinuria did not occur, the potential for cell mediated immunity was thus suggested. Studies in the bursectomized chicken have shown that immunization can lead to a macrophage associated glomerular lesion in the absence of humoral immunity [37]. Support for these experimental observations comes from recent studies in humans showing a significant accumulation of lymphocytes within the glomeruli of patients with a variety of proliferative types of glomerulonephritis [11,12].

Mechanisms of glomerular macrophage activation

The macrophages infiltrating diseased glomeruli are derived from the circulation. This accumulation is likely to be associated with many changes in the metabolism of these monocytes. As in inflammatory foci elsewhere, it has been assumed that monocytes transform into inflammatory glomerular macrophages, although this hypothesis has not been tested until recently.

Studies now classical in immunology have demonstrated that effector macrophages have greatly enhanced capacity to mediate antitumour and antimicrobial effects. This transition was termed 'activation' [38]. It has been shown subsequently that mononuclear phagocytes show great variety in their capacity to alter their functional characteristics. These functions can be enhanced and repressed independently. The term 'activation' has been applied to any transformation in macrophage function and its use has become somewhat controversial. However, if glomerular macrophages can be shown to have enhanced capacities to mediate tissue injury or stimulate proliferative responses in intrinsic glomerular cells then the acquisition of these functions should appropriately be termed activation.

We have developed a technique for isolating glomerular macrophages from kidneys of animals with experimental glomerulonephritis within an hour of sacrifice [39]. Several functional capacities relevant to the mediation of injury have been assessed. Comparison with circulating blood monocytes and tissue macrophages from the same animals and normal animals isolated under the same conditions allows assessment of the activation status of these glomerular macrophages. The generation of reactive oxygen species (including superoxide and hydroxyl ions), the expression of procoagulant activity and the synthesis of interleukin 1 were measured.

These studies demonstrated that glomerular macrophages had significant augmentation of procoagulant activity expression compared with circulating

TABLE I. The expression of procoagulant and generation of hydroxyl ions and superoxide radicals by macrophages isolated from glomerulonephritic glomeruli compared with control tissue macrophages from the circulation (circulation monocytes) and tissue macrophages (bronchoalveolar macrophages) from the same animals

	Glomerular macrophages	Blood monocytes	Bronchoalveolar macrophages
Procoagulant activity $\mu m/10^3$ cells	2.80±0.74	0.05±0.02	0.09±0.02
Hydroxyl ion generation units/hr/10^6 cells	57.8±4.7	9.9±1.2	11.0±1.8
Superoxide generation nmol/hr/10^6 cells	48.9±5.5	8.6±1.4	9.8±2.0

monocytes and tissue macrophages (Table I). The capacity of glomerular macrophages to generate reactive oxygen species was also significantly enhanced (Table I) and preliminary studies show that their interleukin 1 synthesis is also increased. These results show that glomerular macrophages have enhanced functional capacities warranting the term 'activation', and that this activation occurs within the glomeruli. Support for the concept of local activation of glomerular macrophages comes from the work of Schreiner et al [32] who observed in a rat model of glomerulonephritis that intraluminal monocytes were Ia negative whereas macrophages within the mesangium and in subendothelial positions were Ia positive. These findings would be consistent with activation of recruited circulating monocytes within diseased glomeruli.

The factors determining regulation of glomerular macrophage activation are of potential importance in directing the outcome of macrophage induced injury.

It is known that a variety of stimuli can induce or enhance the functions of macrophages [30]. The most widely studied stimulus is sensitized lymphocyte instruction (delayed hypersensitivity). Several new lines of evidence would suggest such mechanisms may operate in glomerulonephritis. These include the demonstration of T-lymphocytes in diseased glomeruli in association with macrophages in patients and animal models of proliferative glomerulonephritis [9–11]; the demonstration of lymphokine secretion by these lymphocytes [35]; the adoptive transfer experiments of Bhan [36] and the bursectomized chicken model studied by Bolton [37].

The potential for lymphocyte independent glomerular macrophage activation also exists. Macrophages accumulate within glomeruli with prominent immunoglobulin deposition and complement activation. Monocyte Fc receptor/immunoglobulin interaction is known to induce macrophage activation. A rôle for monocyte/IgG Fc interaction in animals decomplemented with Cobra venom factor has been confirmed [33,34]. Several studies have shown the capacity for macrophage activation by a variety of complement factors. The potential for lymphocyte independent glomerular macrophage activation may be assessed by studying the 'activation status' of glomerular macrophages from animals with proliferative glomerulonephritis induced by passive antibody.

Thus several potential pathways for glomerular macrophage activation exist. It is possible that differing stimuli operate in different situations. It is also likely that macrophages express different capacities in different types of glomerulonephritis or at different times in the course of disease. Different populations of glomerular macrophages (macrophage heterogeneity) may co-exist. The demonstration of the greatly enhanced functional capacities of glomerular macrophages highlights the importance of elucidating the factors determining glomerular macrophage activation. This knowledge broadens our perspective of the immunobiology of glomerulonephritis and may offer the potential for therapeutic intervention.

References

1 Holdsworth SR, Allen D, Thomson NM et al. Histochemistry of glomerular cells in animal models of crescentic glomerulonephritis. *Pathology 1980; 12:* 339–346

2 Holdsworth SR, Thomson NM, Glasgow EF et al. Tissue culture of isolated glomeruli in experimental crescentic glomerulonephritis. *J Exp Med 1978; 147:* 89–109

3 Striker GE, Mannik M, Tung MY. Role of marrow-derived monocytes and mesangial cells in removal of immune complexes from renal glomeruli. *J Exp Med 1979; 149:* 127–136

4 Hooke DH, Hancock WW, Gee DC et al. Monoclonal antibody analysis of glomerular hypercellularity in human glomerulonephritis. *Clin Nephrol 1984; 22:* 163–168

5 Atkins RC, Glasgow EF, Holdsworth SR et al. Tissue culture of isolated glomeruli from patients with glomerulonephritis. *Kidney Int 1980; 17:* 515–527

6 Magil AB, Wadsworth LD, Loewen M. Monocytes and human renal glomerular disease: a quantitative evaluation. *Lab Invest 1981; 44:* 23–33

7 Holdsworth SR, Neale TJ, Wilson CB. Abrogation of macrophage-dependent injury in experimental glomerulonephritis in the rabbit. Use of an antimacrophage serum. *J Clin Invest 1981; 58:* 686–698

8 Kreisberg JI, Wayne DB, Karnovsky MJ. Rapid focal loss of negative charge associated with mononuclear cell infiltration early in nephrotoxic serum nephritis. *Kidney Int 1979; 16:* 290–300

9 Tipping PG, Neale TJ, Holdsworth SR. T lymphocyte participation in anti-GBM antibody induced experimental glomerulonephritis. *Kidney Int 1985; 27:* 530–537

10 Stachura I, Si L, Whiteside TL. Mononuclear-cell subsets in human idiopathic crescentic glomerulonephritis (IC glomerulonephritis): analysis in tissue sections with monoclonal antibodies. *J Clin Immunol 1984; 4:* 202–208

11 Nolasco EB, Cameron JS, Hartley B et al. Intraglomerular T cells and monocytes in nephritis. *Kidney Int 1987; 31:* 1160–1166

12 Schreiner GF, Kiely JM, Cotran RS, Unanue ER. Characterization of resident glomerular cells in the rat expressing Ia-determinants and manifesting genetically restricted interactions with lymphocytes. *J Clin Invest 1981; 68:* 920–931

13 Davies M, Barrett AJ, Trouis J et al. The degradation of human glomerular basement membrane with purified lysosomal proteinases. *Clin Sci Mol Med 1978; 54:* 233–240

14 Rehan A, Johnson KJ, Wiggins RC et al. Evidence for the role of oxygen radicals in acute nephrotoxic nephritis. *Lab Invest 1982; 47:* 412–426

15 Boyce NW, Holdsworth SR. Hydroxyl radical mediation of immune renal injury by desferrioxamine. *Kidney Int 1986; 30:* 813–817

16 Nathan CF. Secretory products of macrophages. *J Clin Invest 1987; 79:* 319–326

17 Schreiner GF, Cotran RS, Pardo V, Unanue FR. A mononuclear cell component in experimental immunological glomerulonephritis. *J Exp Med 1978; 147:* 369–384

18 Holdsworth SR, Neale TJ. Macrophage induced glomerular injury: cell transfer studies. *Lab Invest 1984; 51:* 172–179

19 Dubois CH, Foidart JB, Hautier MB et al. Proliferative glomerulonephritis in rats: evidence that mononuclear phagocytes infiltrating the glomeruli stimulate the proliferation of endothelial and mesangial cells. *Eur J Clin Invest 1981; 11:* 91–104

20 Boyce NW, Holdsworth SR. Quantitation of intrarenal uptake of immune complexes by macrophages in diffuse proliferative glomerulonephritis. *Clin Exp Immunol 1986; 64:* 638–645

21 Thomson NM, Holdsworth SR, Glasgow EF, Atkins RC. The macrophage in the development of experimental crescentic glomerulonephritis. *Am J Pathol 1979; 94:* 223–240

22 Cattell V, Aldridge S. The origin of proliferating cells in the glomerulus and Bowman's capsule in nephrotoxic serum nephritis: effects of unilateral renal irradiation. *Br J Exp Path 1981; 62:* 669–675

23 Holdsworth SR, Tipping PG. Macrophage induced glomerular fibrin deposition in experimental glomerulonephritis in the rabbit. *J Clin Invest 1985; 76:* 1367–1372

24 Tipping PG, Worthington LA, Holdsworth SR. Quantitation and characterization of glomerular procoagulant activity in experimental glomerulonephritis. *Lab Invest 1987; 56:* 155–159

25 Tipping PG, Holdsworth SR. Glomerular procoagulant activity in human proliferative glomerulonephritis. *J Clin Invest:* submitted for publication

26 Hancock WW, Atkins RC. Activation of coagulation pathways and fibrin deposition in human glomerulonephritis. *Semin Nephrol 1985; V:* 69–75

27 Tipping PG, Holdsworth SR. The participation of macrophages, glomerular procoagulant activity and Factor VIII in glomerular fibrin deposition. Studies in anti-GBM antibody induced glomerulonephritis in rabbits. *Am J Path 1986; 124:* 10–16

28 Hoyer JR, Michael AF, Hoyer LW. Immunofluorescent localisation of antihemophilic factor antigen and fibrinogen in human renal disease. *J Clin Invest 1974; 53:* 1375–1384

29 Lovett DH, Sterzel RB. Cell culture approaches to the analysis of glomerular inflammation. *Kidney Int 1986; 30:* 246–254

30 Lovett DH, Ryan JL, Sterzl RB. Stimulation of rat mesangial cell proliferation by macrophage interleukin 1. *J Immunol 1983; 131:* 2830–2836

31 Melcion C, Lachman L, Killen PD et al. Mesangial cells, effect of monocyte products on proliferation and matrix synthesis. *Transplant Proc 1982; 141:* 559–564

32 Schreiner GF, Unanue ER, Cotran RS. Glomerular injury: functional and phenotypic characteristics of resident and infiltrating macrophages. In Van Furrh R, ed. *Mononuclear Phagocytes – Characteristics, Physiology and Function.* New York: Martinus Nijhoff. 1985: 785–793

33 Holdsworth SR. Fc dependence of macrophage accumulation and subsequent injury in experimental glomerulonephritis. *J Immunol 1983; 130:* 735–739

34 Boyce NW, Holdsworth SR. A role for macrophage Fc-receptor affinity in determining the cellular mediation of antibody initiated glomerulonephritis in the rabbit. Submitted for publication

35 Boyce NW, Tipping PG, Holdsworth SR. Lymphokine (MIF) production by glomerular T-lymphocytes in experimental glomerulonephritis. *Kidney Int 1986; 30:* 673–677

36 Bhan AK, Schneeberger EE, Collins AB, McCluskey RT. Evidence for a pathogenic role of a cell-mediated immune mechanism in experimental glomerulonephritis. *J Exp Med 1978; 148:* 246–260

37 Bolton WK, Tucker FL, Sturgill BC. A new avaian model of experimental glomerulonephritis consistent with mediation by cellular immunity. *J Clin Invest 1984; 73:* 1263–1276

38 Mackaness GB. The monocyte and cellular immunity. *Semin Haematol 1970; 7:* 172–184

39 Tipping PG, Holdsworth SR. Glomerular macrophages express augmented procoagulant activity in experimental fibrin related glomerulonephritis in rabbits. *J Clin Invest:* submitted for publication

40 Adams DO, Hamilton TA. The cell biology of macrophage activation. *Ann Rev Immunol 1984; 2:* 283–318

INFLAMMATION TO SCLEROSIS. HOW LONG DOES IT TAKE? IMPLICATIONS FOR THERAPEUTIC APPROACHES IN INFLAMMATORY RENAL DISEASE

R Wiggins, G Downer, S Phan

University of Michigan, Ann Arbor, Michigan, USA

Figure 1 emphasizes the critical rôle of the macrophage and T-cell in the induction of the sclerotic response to injury. Thus inflammation in which these cells and/or platelets are involved may go on to sclerosis [1].

In designing rational therapeutic approaches to immunological glomerular injury it is necessary to know the length of time between an inflammatory event and the irreversible scarring (sclerosis) which may occur as a consequence of that event. This is not only true of 'one hit' types of event (e.g. anti-glomerular basement membrane disease) but also of 'multiple hit' events (e.g. lupus nephritis). It is clear that the time taken between the 'hit' and sclerosis will dictate the urgency of therapeutic intervention. In 'multiple hit' events if the time between 'hit' and scar formation is very short then there may not be sufficient time to intervene successfully after a 'hit'. If that were true, then more emphasis must be placed on prevention. On the other hand, if the time lag is long, then it may be appropriate to treat each event as it occurs (e.g. as is commonly done in treating 'flares' of lupus nephritis). Finally, we must distinguish between 'synchronous' hits where all glomeruli appear to be at the same phase of injury at any one time and 'asynchronous' hits where glomeruli are at all stages of progression to sclerosis at one point in time. In the latter, poor renal function at presentation is usually an indicator of irreversible disease (widespread scarring), while in the former, inflammation is often reversible (little scarring) in spite of poor renal function at presentation. With these concepts in mind we examined the time course of progression to sclerosis in a synchronous one-hit rabbit model of anti-glomerular basement membrane disease.

In this model rabbits are preimmunized against guinea pig IgG (day minus 5) and then, as they begin to mount an immune response, guinea pig anti-rabbit glomerular basement membrane IgG is injected intravenously (day 0). The guinea pig IgG binds in the glomerulus and forms the target which the rabbit immune system attacks. The functional changes which occur in this model are shown in

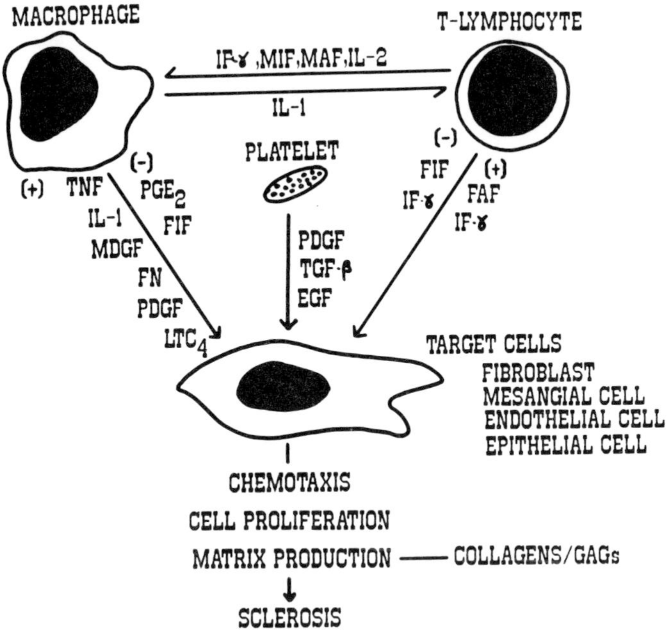

Figure 1. Diagrammatic representation of potential mediators of sclerosis in the glomerulus. The diagram emphasizes the critical rôle played by the macrophages and T-cells, and indicates some of the mediators which may be important from both cell types. These include Tumour Necrosis Factor alpha (TNF), Interleukin-I (IL-I), Macrophage Derived Growth Factor (MDGF), Fibronectin (FN), Thrombospondin (TSP), Platelet-Derived Growth Factor (PDGF), Leukotriene C_4 (LTC_4), Prostaglandin E_2 (PGE_2), Fibroblast Inhibitory Factor (FIF), Interferon gamma (IF-γ), and Fibroblast Activating Factor (FAF). Some interactions between macrophages and T-cells are also indicated by Migration Inhibitory Factor (MIF), Macrophage Activating Factor (MAF), and Interleukin-2 (IL-2). Finally, platelet products that may be important include PDGF, Transforming Growth Factor beta (TGF-β), and Epidermal Growth Factor (EGF). This list is not meant to be exhaustive.

Target cells for these mediators include fibroblasts and mesangial cells. The precise role of glomerular epithelial and endothelial cells in response to these mediators is not well defined at present.

The result of mediator action on target cells is to modify cell behaviour. This includes chemotactic effects, cell division, and the production of matrix. It is the combination of these factors that is responsible for the sclerotic response to injury.

Figure 2, upper panel. Increased protein excretion is first detectable on day 4. Oliguria is seen on days 6 and 7 (not shown), at which time the serum creatinine begins to rise. Abnormal renal function peaks at days 14–21 and then slowly improves.

The time course of histological events is shown in Figure 3. Over the 7–14 day period most (about 90%) glomeruli are obviously involved in the inflammatory event (increase in cells and proteinaceous material in glomeruli). Glomerular scarring as shown by Masson trichrome staining is detectable in some glomeruli

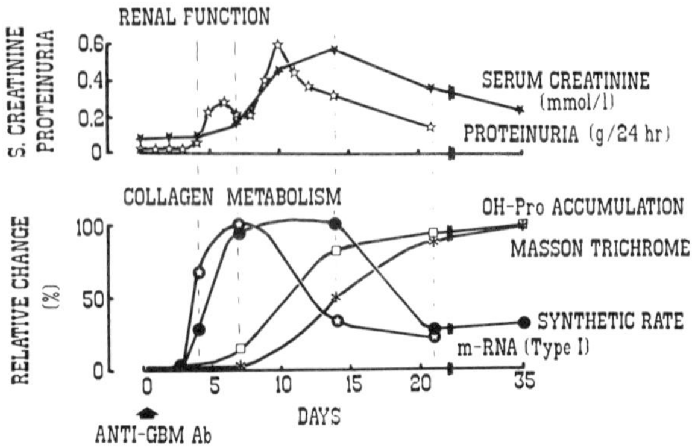

Figure 2. *Upper panel:* renal functional changes in the anti-glomerular basement membrane model as assessed by protein excretion and serum creatinine.

Lower panel: Collagen metabolism in the anti-glomerular basement membrane model at various times as assessed by Masson trichrome stained sections, hydroxyproline accumulation per dry weight of renal cortex, ^{3}H-proline incorporation into cortical slices, and mRNA for type 1 collagen from slot-blot analysis of whole RNA extracted from renal cortex.

Note that on day 4 when serum creatinine is normal and protein excretion is only slightly increased above baseline, the mRNA (type 1) and collagen synthetic rate are already significantly raised (statistics not shown). Monocyte and T-cell influx occur at three days (not shown). By day seven when serum creatinine is elevated collagen synthetic rate has reached maximal levels, but collagen has not begun to accumulate. By day 14 collagen accumulation has occurred, but Masson trichrome staining for collagen is not strongly positive. By day 21 Masson trichrome staining is strongly positive in spite of little increase in collagen content. The serum creatinine falls as the Masson trichrome staining (cross-linked collagen) progresses.

These results emphasize that collagen synthesis occurs very early in the sequence of events in this model. Accumulation of collagen is delayed about seven days behind the collagen synthetic rate increase. Masson trichrome staining is not a good indicator of early collagen synthesis

by day 14 and continues to increase so that by day 50 about half the glomeruli are scarred. Not shown is the fact that the first histological abnormality seen (monocyte and T-cell accumulation in glomeruli) is detectable on day 3 and periglomerular accumulation of cells progressing to interstitial inflammation and scarring begins on days 4–5 and progresses thereafter [2,3].

Glomeruli can be isolated from this model. However, the isolation procedure is skewed towards isolation of more normal glomeruli by day 14 [4]. In spite of this, day 14 glomeruli contain significantly more hydroxyproline per glomerulus (2.4±0.6ng/glomerulus) than do the day seven or control glomeruli (0.8±0.1 and 0.7±0.1, $p<0.05$). A similar result is found if whole cortex is used (Figure 2, lower panel). There is a continued rise in cortical hydroxyproline content through day 35.

When does collagen synthesis start? We have looked at this in two ways. The appearance of mRNA for type I collagen as assessed by slot-blot hybridization

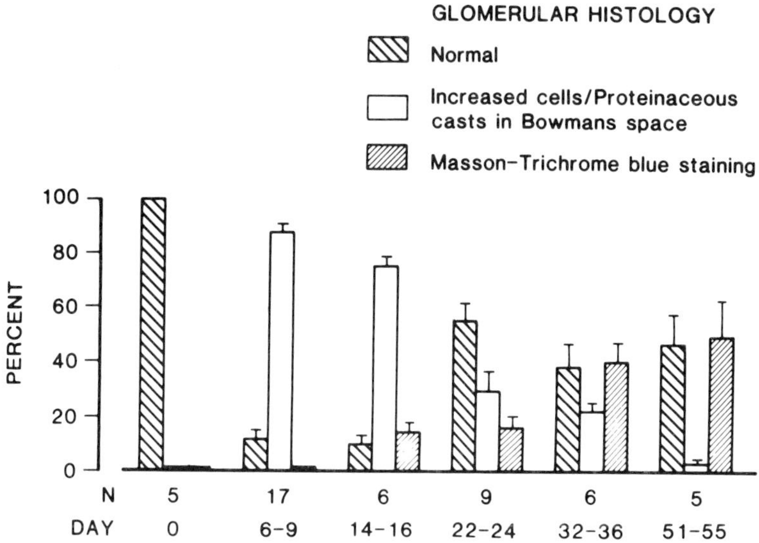

Figure 3. Time course of inflammation and sclerosis in the rabbit anti-glomerular basement membrane model of crescentic nephritis. Note that 90% of glomeruli are involved with an obvious increase in number of cells and proteinaceous material, but by day 50 these changes have disappeared leaving half of the glomeruli normal and half sclerosed. This model has a major interstitial component of sclerosis which parallels the glomerular component

studies using a cDNA probe for type I collagen indicates a significant increase by day 4 (Figure 2, lower panel). ^{3}H-proline incorporation studies in cortical slices also show that by days 3–4 there is significant ^{3}H-proline incorporation to OH-proline (Figure 2, lower panel). Thus, collagen synthesis to form interstitial-type collagen begins on the same day that protein is first detected in the urine, within a day of blood monocytes being first detected in glomeruli and before a detectable rise in serum creatinine has occurred. Collagen synthesis rate peaks by days 7–14 and then falls to lower levels at later time points. Thus by the time serum creatinine was noticeably elevated, collagen synthesis rate had peaked and collagen had significantly accumulated in glomeruli and cortex, although Masson trichrome staining showed only minimal blue-stained material.

Immunofluorescence studies for type I/III and type IV collagen also show an increase in both within glomeruli by day seven. By day 14 there were sheets of type IV collagen within glomeruli. By this time point most of the type I/III staining was outside the glomerulus, but anti-type I/III staining was also present within some glomeruli. The implication of these structural studies is that there are major structural changes (focal or global sclerosis) by day 14 while at day seven there is a general increase in detectable collagen of all types without major structural change.

We can therefore put together the collagen metabolism data and relate them to the renal function data (Figure 2, upper and lower panels). It can be seen that by day four when the collagen synthesis rate is markedly increased the only measurable change in renal function is a small increase in protein excretion. By day seven when the serum creatinine has begun to rise collagen synthesis rate is reaching a peak, although collagen accumulation has not significantly increased. By day 14 when renal function is obviously abnormal collagen synthesis rate is maximal, collagen is accumulating, but Masson trichrome staining shows only minimal blue-stained bands of cross-linked collagen, while fluorescence microscopy for collagen shows obvious abnormalities of glomerular structure. By day 21 when renal function is improving the collagen synthesis rate is reduced towards baseline, collagen accumulation is levelling off and Masson trichrome staining shows clear-cut cross-banded collagen. Renal function continues to improve by day 35 when further collagen accumulation and Masson trichrome staining are present. These results (a) indicate that Masson trichrome is not a sensitive indicator of early collagen synthesis; (b) emphasize the discrepancy between renal function and scar formation; and (c) indicate how soon after initiation of injury collagen synthesis begins and how rapidly collagen accumulates.

What are the implications for management of patients with glomerular inflammation? It is clear that early intervention is necessary if we are to minimize collagen synthesis and that days count, although hours probably do not. 'Time' is likely to be the most important changeable ingredient in the management of our patients with one 'hit' disease and may be more important than the type of anti-inflammatory regimen used. Our efforts should therefore probably focus on early identification and diagnosis in individuals with rapidly progressive glomerulonephritis (i.e. shortening both the interval between the presentation to the first-line physician and referral to the nephrology – PR interval – and the time interval between referral to the nephrologist and the institution of treatment – RT interval). The results of published studies in anti-glomerular basement membrane disease would support this concept [5,6]. The finding that in vasculitis and idiopathic crescentic nephritis severe abnormalities of renal function at presentation do not carry quite the same bad prognosis for long-term renal function [7] is probably a reflection of the 'synchronicity' of these forms of glomerular injury (all glomeruli tend to march through the 'stages' [8] of crescent formation together), and therefore these individuals present early in the sequence of events (perhaps equivalent to day 10 of the model) when collagen synthesis has been initiated but collagen accumulation has not yet occurred and is still largely reversible. In contrast, in anti-glomerular basement membrane disease the disease is often asynchronous, so that many glomeruli are irreversibly scarred at the time of presentation.

What are the implications of the above findings for 'multiple hit' diseases such as lupus nephritis? Our interpretation of these results is that they emphasize the need for prevention of the 'hit', because by the time the 'hit' has occurred and renal function has become abnormal signalling the need for therapeutic intervention, collagen synthesis and accumulation have already taken place. This, then, would provide theoretical support for a therapeutic approach that prevents lupus flares (i.e. immunosuppressive drugs) rather than one that treats inflammation (i.e. glucocorticoids) in those individuals who have a tendency to scar, as has been advocated by the NIH group [9]. An alternative approach might be very early treatment with anti-inflammatory agents, perhaps by self-medication.

Finally, since there is a short window of opportunity between functional renal changes and cross-linking of collagen to form the permanent scar (sclerosis), other agents which specifically interfere with individual mediators released by macrophages or T-cells, or which inhibit collagen synthesis or cross-linking (see Figure 1) may turn out to be useful in some patients. However, this will be true only if patients are identified early in the sequence of events, and in whom early signs of collagen synthesis and accumulation can be detected. Such approaches could use immunofluorescence against particular collagen types, ^{3}H-proline incorporation studies or analysis of mRNA for particular collagen types. The latter approach may be the most sensitive and simple.

In summary, although we tend to think of scarring as associated with 'chronicity' = chronic = long-term, we should realize that while the consequences of scar formation are long-term the time taken to form a scar is short (7–10 days). It is worth keeping these facts in mind when managing individuals with inflammatory renal disease.

References

1 Phan SM. Fibrotic mechanisms in lung diseases. In Ward P, ed. *Handbook of Inflammation, Volume 4.* 1983: 121

2 Wiggins RC, Eldredge C. Monocyte/macrophage heterogeneity and migration into Bowman's space early in crescentic nephritis in the rabbit. *Kidney Int 1987; 31:* 333

3 Eldredge C, Wiggins RC. T cells in the glomerulus, periglomerular region and around venules early in crescentic nephritis in the rabbit. Evidence for glomerulointerstitial signals. *Kidney Int 1987; 31:* 318

4 Wiggins RC, Eldredge C, Kunkel S. Interleukin I production by glomeruli at different stages of crescent formation in the rabbit. *Fed Proc 1987; 46:* 1329

5 Peters DK, Rees AJ, Lockwood CM, Pusey CD. Treatment and prognosis in anti-basement membrane antibody-mediated nephritis. *Transplant Proc 1982; 14:* 513–521

6 Johnson JP, Moore J, Austin HA III et al. Therapy of antiglomerular basement membrane antibody disease: analysis of prognostic significance of clinical pathologic and treatment factors. *Medicine 1985; 64:* 219–227

7 Bolton WK. The case for aggressive use of high dose steroids. In Narins R, ed. *Controversies in Nephrology and Hypertension.* New York: Churchill Livingstone. 1984: 421

8 Wiggins RC, Glatfelter A, Brukman J. Procoagulant activity in glomeruli and urine of rabbits with nephrotoxic nephritis. *Lab Invest 1985; 53:* 156–165

9 Balow JE. Lupus nephritis. *Ann Int Med 1987; 106:* 79–94

MESANGIAL PATHOPHYSIOLOGY

CALCIUM-ACTIVATED CHLORIDE CONDUCTANCE IN MESANGIAL CELLS: ITS REGULATION BY VASOACTIVE PEPTIDES AND GROWTH PROMOTING FACTORS

K Kurokawa, T Okuda, H Matsunaga, H Chang, N Yamashita

The University of Tokyo School of Medicine, Tokyo, Japan

Introduction

Mesangial cells reside in the intercapillary space of the glomerulus and have numerous contractile fibres similar to smooth muscle cells. These characteristics of mesangial cells suggest that they may participate through contraction in the regulation of intraglomerular haemodynamics and thus glomerular filtration rate [1]. It has been reported that a variety of hormones directly act and regulate mesangial cell functions. Of these hormones, the effects of angiotensin II and arginine vasopressin have been examined most extensively. Accordingly, it has been shown that these vasoactive peptides cause mesangial cell contraction [2] and they decrease ultrafiltration, Kf, thus affecting glomerular filtration [1]. These observations support the notion that mesangial cell contraction may underlie the regulation of glomerular haemodynamics and ultrafiltration [1].

Mesangial cell proliferation and mesangial matrix accumulation are most characteristic features of a variety of glomerulonephritis. It has been widely accepted that immunological mechanisms are importantly involved as an initiating event in the pathogenesis of many types of glomerulonephritis, though it is not clear how the immunological events lead to mesangial cell proliferation and accumulation of mesangial matrix. Recent observations indicate that there are certain substances which regulate mesangial cell proliferation [3,4].

Despite the importance of mesangial cells in the regulation of glomerular function in health and disease, our understanding of the mechanisms of action of angiotensin II and arginine vasopressin and of mesangial cell proliferation is very much limited partly because of the paucity of knowledge on the physiological properties of the mesangial cell. We have used cultured (mostly primary culture) mesangial cells, obtained from isolated rat glomeruli to study physiological properties. The details of some of our studies and preliminary results have been published elsewhere [5–12].

Results and discussion

Effects of angiotensin II on mesangial cell contraction and membrane potential [5,6,11]

In response to a brief exposure to angiotensin II by a glass capillary to the proximity of the mesangial cell layer, the membrane potential immediately and transiently depolarized with a decrease in input resistance. Membrane potential changes in a typical experiment are shown in Figure 1. The contraction of

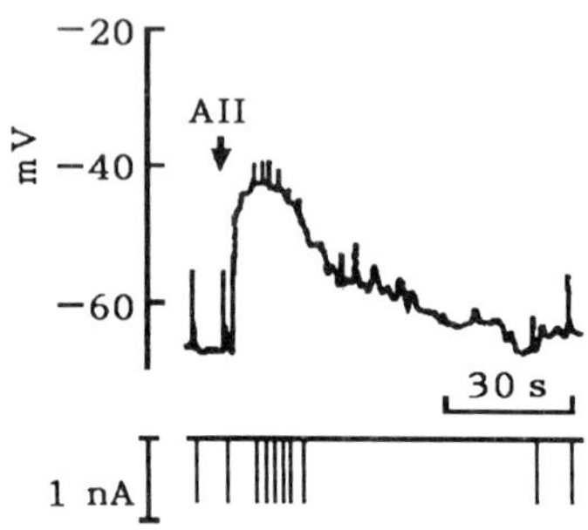

Figure 1. A representative experiment of the membrane potential change in response to 100nM angiotensin II (AII). A mesangial cell incubated in the standard solution was impaled with a glass electrode containing 4.0M K-acetate with a resistance of 30–50MΩ, and current pulses of 600msec duration with constant amplitudes were applied. The membrane potential depolarized by approximately 18mV and the input resistance decreased in response to angiotensin II (an arrow), suggesting an increased permeability to some ions. Reproduced from [5] with permission

mesangial cells began within a minute of angiotensin II delivery, that is following membrane depolarization. This visible cell contraction continued for several minutes. A decrease in input resistance in response to angiotensin II indicates an increase in membrane permeability to some ions. To examine this phenomenon further, the reversal potential (Vr) of the response to angiotensin II was analysed. The Vr determined from the current-voltage (I-V) relation prior to and at the peak of the angiotensin II-induced depolarization was -29 ± 3mV. Similar mesangial cell responses, i.e. cell contraction and membrane potential depolarizations were observed with arginine vasopressin, suggesting that both angiotensin II and arginine vasopressin exert similar effects on mesangial cells. The Vr of the responses to arginine vasopressin was -25 ± 7mV. In the discussion to follow, we will not mention the results with arginine vasopressin since they are almost identical with results obtained with angiotensin II.

The presence of Cl^- channels with an equilibrium potential of about -20 to -30mV have been reported in pancreatic acinar cells and Xenopus oocytes [12,13]. The values of Vr in our study strongly suggest that the opening of Cl^- channels may account for the membrane depolarization evoked by angiotensin II and arginine vasopressin. Consistent with this interpretation was our data that reduction in Cl^- concentration in the incubation medium ($[Cl^-]^o$) was associated with less negative Vr of the membrane depolarization by angiotensin II; in 10mM $[Cl^-]^o$, the Vr became even positive. However, the Vr thus determined deviated slightly from the theoretical equilibrium potential of Cl^- calculated from the Nernst equation, indicating that permeability changes to some other ions may also participate in the membrane depolarization. Indeed, recent observations from our laboratory using patch-clamp techniques have revealed angiotensin II activation of probably non-selective cation channels.

Cell calcium ions in response to angiotensin II [5–7]

The effects of angiotensin II and arginine vasopressin on mesangial cells are thought to be mediated by an increase in the concentration of intracellular Ca^{++} ions ($[Ca^{++}]^i$) by formation of inositol triphosphate and activation of protein kinase C [15–17]. In accordance with these postulates, we have found that a calcium ionophore, A23187, evoked mesangial cell contraction and the membrane potential depolarization with an increased membrane conductance, responses similar to those induced by angiotensin II. The Vr in response to A23187 in the standard medium was -26 ± 7mV, a value identical with that obtained with angiotensin II. Moreover, changes in the Vr in response to A23187 with varying $[Cl^-]^o$ were exactly the same as those in the presence of angiotensin II. These data strongly suggest that the increased Cl^- conductance induced by angiotensin II was mediated by an increase in $[Ca^{++}]^i$, i.e. the presence of Ca^{++}-activated Cl^- conductance in the mesangial cell.

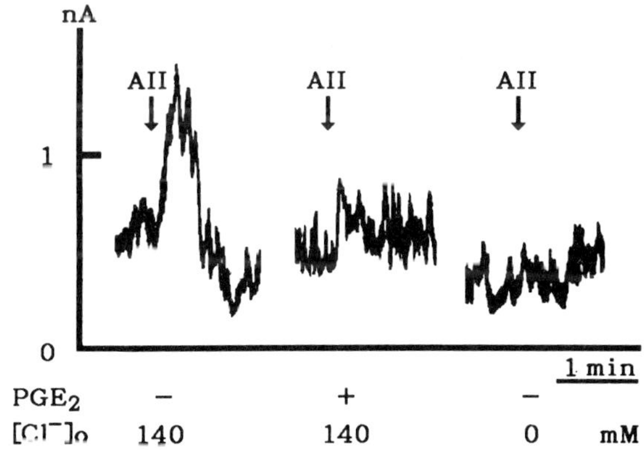

Figure 2. Calcium transients in response to angiotensin II and their modifications by PGE_2 and deletion of Cl^- in the incubation medium. Cultured mesangial cells were loaded with aequorin by the method described from our laboratory [18]. Note the presence of an immediate and transient increase in aequorin luminescence, reflecting a Ca^{++} transient, in response to 100nM angiotensin II. The Ca^{++} transient was suppressed by 5μM PGE_2 and by deletion of Cl^- in the incubation. Separate aliquots of the same preparation of aequorin-loaded mesangial cells were used for each experiment

We next determined changes in luminescence signals from cultured mesangial cells loaded with aequorin, a calcium-sensitive protein which emits light upon binding Ca^{++}. As shown in Figure 2, addition of angiotensin II resulted in an immediate and transient increase in fluorescence intensity, an observation consistent with an increase in $[Ca^{++}]^{i}$.

Rôle of extracellular calcium ions [5–7]

There have been controversies as to whether the effects of angiotensin II on mesangial cells are mediated by Ca^{++} influx from outside the cell or by Ca^{++} released from the intracellular organellae [16,17]. We have found that both mesangial cell contraction and membrane depolarization were clearly detected in response to angiotensin II even in Ca^{++}-free incubation medium containing

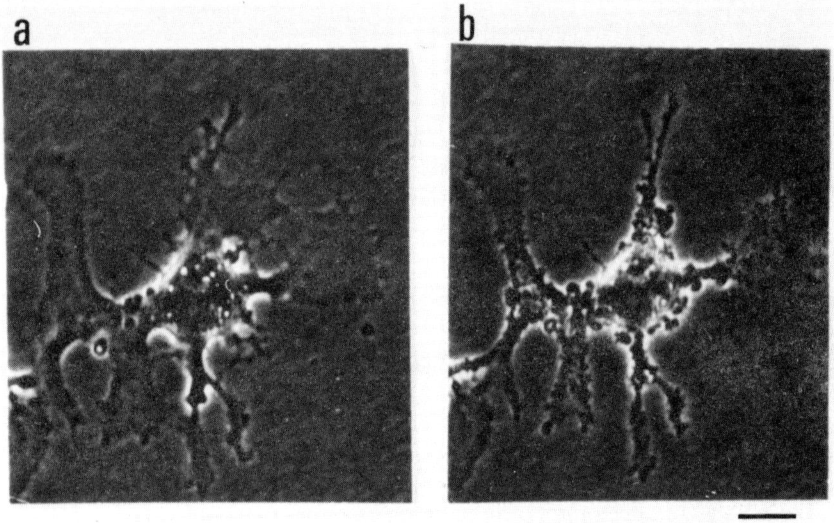

Figure 3. Characteristic morphological changes of mesangial cells under phase contrast stereomicroscope caused by angiotensin II. Cultured mesangial cells were treated for about 10 minutes in Ca^{++}-free phosphate buffered saline containing 0.54mM EDTA, then incubated again for 30 minutes in minimal essential medium containing 18% fetal calf serum. This procedure allows cells to partially detach from the floor of the culture dish and mostly to separate from each other. Then the medium was changed to the appropriate experimental solution and the cells were incubated for another 20–30 minutes. This procedure allows the contraction of individual mesangial cells readily identifiable under microscope. Photographs of several randomly selected areas each containing 15–40 cells were taken before (a) and about one minute after (b) the addition of angiotensin II (or other test agents as appropriate) and each cell was compared before and after hormone addition for the presence of contraction characterized by changes in both cell contour and an appearance of cytoplasmic densities as shown in this figure. The presence and absence of cell contraction was evaluated without knowledge of experimental protocols and the percentage of cell showing contraction was calculated. The bar indicates 25μm

0.5mM EDTA, in which Ca^{++} influx should be virtually absent. Using a technique to semi-quantitatively estimate cell contraction (Figure 3) which is similar to that reported by others [19,21,22], the percentage of mesangial cell showing angiotensin II-evoked contraction was 65% (69 of 106 cells) and 71% (72 of 101 cells), respectively, in the presence or absence of Ca^{++} in the incubation medium. The Ca^{++}-transients by angiotensin II was also present in mesangial cells incubated in Ca^{++}-free medium. It is of note that angiotensin II stimulated PGE_2 production, another well-recognized mesangial cell response to angiotensin II, both in the presence and absence of Ca^{++} in the incubation medium. These data are consistent with the view that an increase in $[Ca^{++}]^i$ due to Ca^{++} release from intracellular organellae, probably endoplasmic reticulum by inositol triphosphate, triggers cell contraction, activates Cl^- conductance of plasma membranes, and enhances PGE_2 production of the mesangial cell.

Effect of PGE_2 on mesangial cell function [8]

It is well recognized that mesangial cells are capable of producing a variety of prostaglandins [15,20,22]. Of these, PGE_2 is a major prostaglandin produced in rat mesangial cells. Since angiotensin II and arginine vasopressin stimulate PGE_2 production, it is possible that PGE_2 may modulate, as a feedback regulator, mesangial responses to these peptides as suggested for other cell systems. The percentage of mesangial cells showing unequivocal contraction in response to 100nM angiotensin II decreased significantly from 63% (136 of 217 cells) to 45% (137 of 303 cells) in the presence of 5μm PGE_2. Moreover, PGE_2 abolished a rise in $[Ca^{++}]^i$ by angiotensin II and arginine vasopressin as shown in Figure 2. These data indicate that PGE_2 suppresses angiotensin II-dependent mesangial cell contraction by inhibiting an increase in $[Ca^{++}]^i$ and suggest that angiotensin II-evoked PGE_2 production constitutes a feedback mechanism of mesangial cell function.

Effect of extracellular chloride ions on mesangial cell function [8,9]

The presence of Cl^--conductance which is activated by a rise in $[Ca^{++}]^i$ and $[Cl^-]^o$-dependent changes in the Vr in response to angiotensin II raise the possibility that a change in $[Cl^-]^o$ may modulate mesangial cell response to angiotensin II and arginine vasopressin. To test this possibility we have examined the effects of changes in $[Cl^-]^o$ on cell contraction, $[Ca^{++}]^i$, inositol triphosphate and PGE_2 production by mesangial cells. The percentage of contracting mesangial cells in response to angiotensin II decreased to 27±11% in the absence of $[Cl^-]^o$ ($Cl^-$was isoosmotically replaced by methanesulphonate) from the control value of 69±8% observed in the standard medium containing 140mM $[Cl^-]^o$. Similar changes were observed with arginine vasopressin. In addition, Ca^{++}-transients by angiotensin II and arginine vasopressin as well as inositol triphosphate levels were markedly attenuated in the absence of $[Cl^-]^o$ (Figure 2).

Since PGE_2 attenuates angiotensin II- and arginine vasopressin-evoked Ca^{++}-transients and cell contraction, the effects of ambient Cl^-depletion may be mediated by an enhanced PGE_2 production by mesangial cells. Indeed, it was the case; thus, PGE_2 production was 4.8±0.9, 6.3±1.2 and 10.7±0.7ng/mg protein/15 minutes at $[Cl^-]^o$ of 140, 70 and 0mM, respectively. Furthermore, addition of indomethacin to the Cl^--free incubation medium prevented the attenuation of cell contraction and the suppression of Ca^{++}-transients by angiotensin II.

These data clearly indicate that $[Cl^-]^o$ is an important determinant of mesangial function at least in part by modulating PGE_2 metabolism. The effects of decreased $[Cl^-]^o$ was specific to Cl^-in that replacement of $Cl^-$by propionate instead of methanesulphonate similarly attenuated cell contraction and increased PGE_2 production.

Causal relationship between cell contraction and membrane depolarization [5,6]
Results of our present study may suggest that the membrane potential change and cell contraction by changes in $[Ca^{++}]^i$ in response to angiotensin II (and also to arginine vasopressin) are causally related. The fact that the membrane depolarization with angiotensin II precedes cell contraction and that membrane repolarization to basal levels precedes cell relaxation strongly suggests the causal relationship between these two phenomena. Similar relationships were observed in response to A23187 and arginine vasopressin. However, membrane potentials depolarized without cell contraction in response to high $[K^+]^o$, indicate that membrane depolarization and cell contraction could be dissociated. The data also suggest that Ca^{++} influx through voltage-gated Ca^{++} channels activated by high $[K^+]^o$ is not involved in cell contraction and activation of Cl^-conductance in mesangial cells. Thus both phenomena are likely to represent two independent cellular responses following an increase in $[Ca^{++}]^i$. Nevertheless, since a change in $[Cl^-]^o$ affects cell contraction, these two events could modulate each other.

Physiological significance of the presence of calcium-activated chloride conductance in mesangial cells [5,6]
The presence of unique Ca^{++}-activated Cl^-conductance may suggest that mesangial cells may require to sense and respond to changes in Cl^-in their environment. In this regard, it is possible that this unique permeability to Cl^-may be important in the tubuloglomerular feedback system. The tubuloglomerular feedback mechanism is the regulation of glomerular filtration by distal tubular fluid [23,24]. Because of the anatomical proximity to the glomerulus, distal tubule, and efferent and afferent arterioles, it is likely that the macula densa cells of the juxtaglomerular apparatus are the sensing site of the tubuloglomerular feedback system [23,24]. Indeed, available data suggest that a change in the $[Cl^-]$ of the fluid perfusing the macula densa segment of the early distal nephron is the critical signal for the tubuloglomerular feedback.

The effector mechanisms involving the changes in glomerular filtration rate in response to alterations in distal fluid [Cl⁻] include changes in afferent and efferent vascular resistances and a change in Kf presumably caused by mesangial cell contraction [23–25]. An important structural relationship exists between the mesangium and juxtaglomerular apparatus. A group of interstitial cells called Goormaghtigh cells or lacis cells lie in the stalk region of the glomerulus. These cells are in direct contact with macula densa cells and with mesangial cells [23,24]. Indeed, the lacis cells are the cells in the juxtaglomerular apparatus that have the most intimate and regular contact with the cells of the macula densa. In addition, the lacis cells have myofilaments like mesangial cells and are extensively coupled with each other, intraglomerular mesangial cells and with afferent and efferent arterioles with gap junctions, thus forming a syncytium [23,24]. It is possible that the lacis cells are characterized by Cl^- conductance noted in the mesangial cells in the present study.

The structure and anatomical position of the lacis cells suggest a possibility that they may be the receptor cells which sense a change in the absorbate [Cl^-] of the macula densa cells and propagate the signal to the intraglomerular mesangial cells and to afferent and efferent arterioles through gap junctions. Since the interstitium surrounding lacis cells are characterized by the lack of capillaries and lymph vessels [23,24], it is possible that the $[Cl^-]^o$ of lacis cells may be directly altered by a change in [Cl^-] in the tubular fluid perfusing the macula densa. Such a change in $[Cl^-]^o$ may affect the lacis cell function which is then transmitted to intraglomerular mesangial cells via gap junctions, affecting glomerular haemodynamics and filtration. Thus, the presence of Cl^- channels in the mesangial cells may lend support for an important rôle of Cl^- as a mediator of the tubuloglomerular feedback system. The attenuation of mesangial cell contraction by low $[Cl^-]^o$ may be consistent with this view as a fall in tubular [Cl^-] is presumably attended by a rise in single nephron glomerular filtration rate, a condition thought to be associated with less mesangial cell contraction.

Effects of fetal calf serum on mesangial cell function [10]

It has been well established that the presence of fetal calf serum is necessary to promote and sustain mesangial cell growth in culture, presumably due to growth factors present in it. We have examined the effect of fetal calf serum on some properties of cultured mesangial cells. In addition to its growth promoting effect, we have found that application of fetal calf serum resulted in an immediate but sustained membrane potential depolarization with decreased input resistance (Figure 4). The Vr of the response in the standard medium with 140mM $[Cl^-]^o$ was about -20 to -30mV and it became less negative with decreasing $[Cl^-]^o$, identical to the Vr of the responses with angiotensin II. However, as can be seen in part by comparing Figures 1 and 4, there are several distinct differences in mesangial cell responses to fetal calf serum and angiotensin II. First, the membrane potential remained depolarized as long as fetal calf serum

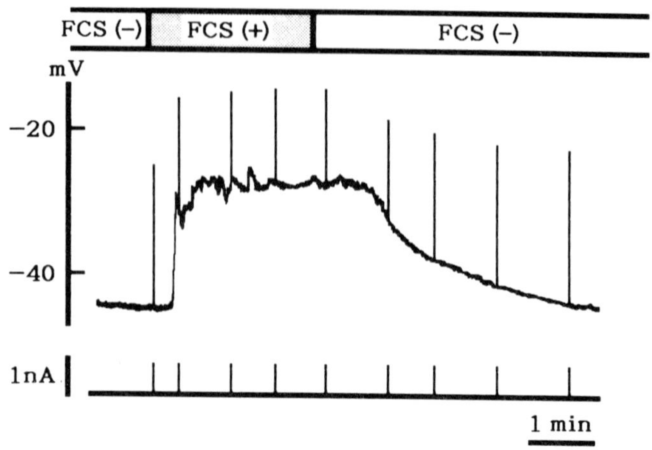

Figure 4. A representative tracing of membrane potential changes of a mesangial cell in response to fetal calf serum (FCS). The membrane potential depolarized and the input resistance decreased when the cell was superfused with a solution containing 5% fetal calf serum. Note that the depolarization was sustained as long as fetal calf serum was present and repolarized to the baseline upon removal of fetal calf serum, a response in contrast to that with angiotensin II as shown in Figure 1. The $[Cl^-]^o$ was 90mM in this experiment. See the legend for Figure 1

was present in the incubation medium and repolarized to the baseline upon removal of fetal calf serum while the depolarization in the presence of angiotensin II was transient. Second, tachyphylaxis was absent in the response to fetal calf serum but not to angiotensin II. Thus, repetitive application of fetal calf serum resulted in similar depolarization with decreased input resistance while repetitive application of angiotensin II failed to evoke membrane depolarization. Moreover, either fetal calf serum after angiotensin II application or angiotensin II after fetal calf serum could evoke membrane depolarization. These observations suggest that the depolarization stimulated by these two agonists are mediated through different mechanisms. Third, there was no visible cell contraction with fetal calf serum, a response quite different from that with angiotensin II.

It is not clear at present what is the significance of the mesangial cell membrane potential change in the regulation of cell growth by fetal calf serum. It is of interest that changes in ionic fluxes and membrane potentials may be the critical initial events of the action of growth promoting mitogens [26,27]. Thus, it is possible that these immediate responses of mesangial cells to fetal calf serum may be causally related to initiation of mesangial cell proliferation.

Effects of growth promoting peptides on mesangial cell proliferation [12]

It is not known what factors in fetal calf serum are responsible for mesangial cell proliferation. To further examine the factors which could promote mesangial cell proliferation, we tested several well characterized growth promoting peptides on mesangial cell growth in culture (4–8th passage). The cell proliferation was assessed by measuring a 48-hour radiolabelled thymidine incorporation to the TCA-precipitable fraction of growth arrested mesangial cells. We have found that insulin, insulin-like growth factor-I (IGF-I), and epidermal growth factor (EGF) stimulate the cell growth. Thus, insulin, IGF-I, and EGF at each maximum concentration stimulated mesangial cell thymidine incorporation, 1.22, 1.30 and 1.22-fold respectively. Fetal calf serum at 10% stimulated thymidine incorporation 4–6-fold. The maximum stimulation was achieved by about 200nM insulin and by 10nM IGF-I, suggesting that the effects of these two peptides are mediated through IGF-I receptors [28]. In addition, the effects of insulin and EGF are synergistic in that their combined effect was 1.72-fold, a value greater than the numerical sum of the stimulation expected by each of two agonists given separately.

Interestingly, we have found that transforming growth factor-β (TGF-β), a growth factor known to be present in normal, non-transformed cells [29], inhibited mesangial cell thymidine incorporation by approximately 50% at basal status as well as in the combined presence of insulin and EGF and also in the presence of fetal calf serum. These data indicate an important rôle and interactions of these peptides in the mesangial cell growth and suggest the possible involvement of these factors in the pathogenesis of certain glomerulonephritis.

Conclusion

There have been considerable advances in our understanding of physiological and biological properties of mesangial cells. Based on the results obtained in our

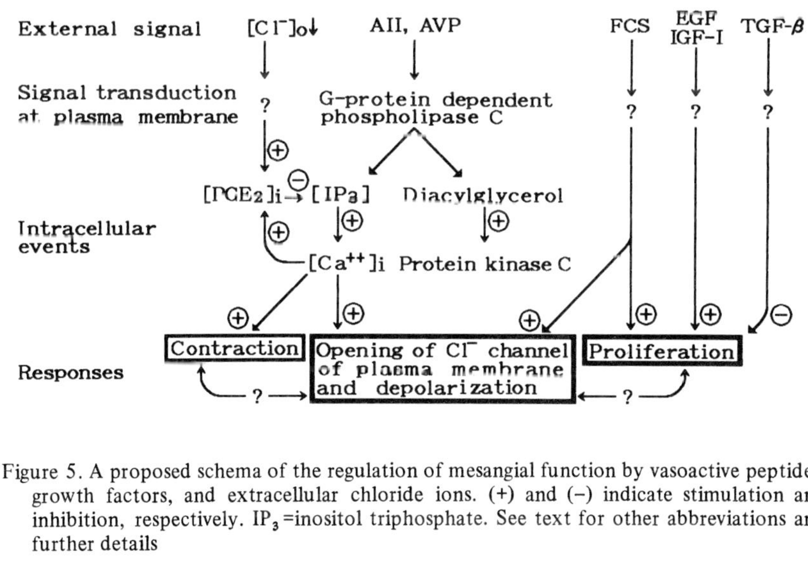

Figure 5. A proposed schema of the regulation of mesangial function by vasoactive peptides, growth factors, and extracellular chloride ions. (+) and (–) indicate stimulation and inhibition, respectively. IP_3 =inositol triphosphate. See text for other abbreviations and further details

and other laboratories, one can envisage the mesangial cell responses activated by several important external signals as depicted in Figure 5. We hope the schema outlined in the figure will be of value in directing research to further clarify the biological and physiological significance of mesangial cells and to better understand the pathogenesis and prevention of glomerulonephritis.

Acknowledgments

Portions of the studies described in this paper have been presented at the annual meetings of the American Society of Nephrology of 1985 (New Orleans, LO), 1986 (Washington DC), and 1987 (Washington DC), and of the American Society for Clinical Investigation, 1987 (San Diego, CA) and appeared as abstracts [7–12]. We thank Drs Etsuro Ogata and Itaru Kohima for their support, Ms Kazuko Sekizaki and Masako Yokokawa for technical, and Miss Ayko Nakamura for secretarial assistance. This work was supported in part by grants from the Ministry of Education of Japan (No59480197, No59440052, No61770436) and a grant for Cardiovascular Disease (59-C8) from the Ministry of Health and Welfare of Japan.

References

1 Dworkin LD, Ichikawa I, Brenner BM. Hormonal modulation of glomerular function. *Am J Physiol 1983; 244:* F95–104

2 Kreisberg JI, Karnovsky MJ. Glomerular cells in culture. *Kidney Int 1983; 23:* 439–447

3 Lovett DH, Ryan JL, Sterzel B. Stimulation of rat mesangial cell proliferation by macrophage interleukin I. *J Immunol 1983; 131:* 2830–2836

4 MacCarthy EP, Hsu A, Ooi YM, Ooi BS. Modulation of mouse mesangial cell proliferation by macrophage products. *Immunol 1985; 56:* 695–699

5 Okuda T, Yamashita N, Kurokawa K. Angiotensin II and vasopressin stimulate calcium activated chloride conductance in rat mesangial cells. *J Clin Invest 1986; 78:* 1443–1447

6 Kurokawa K, Okuda T, Yamshita N. Angiotensin II stimulates calcium activated chloride conductance in rat mesangial cells. In Shimizu F, Kihara I, Oite T, eds. *Cell Proliferation and Glomerulonephritis.* Niigata: Nishimura Co Ltd. 1986: 3–11

7 Okuda T, Yamashita N, Kohima I et al. Angiotensin II and vasopressin stimulate C^{++}-activated Cl^- conductance in cultured rat mesangial cells by releasing Ca^{++} from intracellular organellae. *Kidney Int 1987; 31 (Abstract):* 282

8 Kurokawa K, Kojima I, Okuda T. Extracellular chloride ion concentration is an important regulator of angiotensin II- and vasopressin-induced mesangial cell contraction: modulation of an increase in intracellular calcion ion levels via affecting PGE_2 production. *Clin Res 1987; 35 (Abstract):* 636A

9 Kurokawa K, Kojima I, Okuda T. Extracellular Cl ion concentration is an important determinant of mesangial cell function: modulation via inositol triphosphate (IP3), cell Ca^{++}, and PGE_2 metabolism. *Kidney Int 1988; Abstract:* in press

10 Okuda T, Yamashita N, Kurokawa K. Fetal calf serum stimulates Cl^- conductance and depolarizes membrane potential of cultured rat mesangial cells. *Kidney Int 1988; Abstract:* in press

11 Matsunaga H, Okuda T, Chang H, Kurokawa K. Analysis of single channel activities of mesangial cells: the presence of non-selective cation channels and Ca^{++}-activated K^+ channels. *Kidney Int 1988; Abstract:* in press

12 Chang H, Kurokawa K. Insulin, insulin-like growth factor-I and epidermal growth factor stimulate and transforming growth factor-β inhibits proliferation of cultured rat mesangial cells. *Kidney Int 1988; Abstract:* in press

13 Maruyama Y, Petersen OH. Voltage clamp study of stimulant-evoked currents in mouse pancreatic acinar cells. *Pfluegers Arch 1983; 399:* 54–62

14 Barish ME. A transient calcium dependent chloride current in the immature Xenopus oocyte. *J Physiol 1983; 342:* 309–325

15 Schlondorff D, Perez J, Satriano JA. Differential stimulation of PGE_2 synthesis in mesangial cells by angiotensin and A23187. *Am J Physiol 1985; 248:* C119–C126

16 Bonventre JV, Skorecki KL, Kreisberg JI, Cheung JY. Vasopressin increases cytosolic free calcium concentration in glomerular mesangial cells. *Am J Physiol 1986; 251:* F94–F102

17 Hassid A, Pidikiti N, Gamero D. Effects of vasoactive peptides on cytosolic calcium in cultured mesangial cells. *Am J Physiol 1986; 251:* F1018–F1028

18 Kojima I, Ogata E. Direct demonstration of adreno-corticotropin-induced changes in cytoplasmic free calcium with aequorin in adrenal glomerulosa cell. *J Biol Chem 1986; 261:* 9832–9838

19 Venkatachalam MA, Kreisberg JI. Agonist-induced isotonic contraction of cultured mesangial cells after multiple passage. *Am J Physiol 1985; 249:* C48–C55

20 Scharschmidt LA, Dunn MJ. Prostaglandin synthesis by rat glomerular mesangial cells in culture: effects of angiotensin II and arginine vasopressin. *J Clin Invest 1983; 71:* 1756–1764

21 Mahieu PR, Foidart JB, Dubois CH et al. Tissue culture of normal rat glomeruli: contractile activity of the cultured mesangial cells. *Invest Cell Pathol 1980; 3:* 121–128

22 Ardaillou N, Hagege J, Nivez MP et al. Vasoconstrictor-evoked prostaglandin synthesis in cultured human mesangial cells. *Am J Physiol 1985; 248:* F240–246

23 Schnermann J, Briggs JP. Function of the juxtaglomerular apparatus: local control of glomerular hemodynamics. In Seldin DW, Giebisch G, eds. *The Kidney: Physiology and Pathophysiology.* New York: Raven Press. 1985: 665–697

24 Briggs JP, Schnermann J. The tubuloglomerular feedback mechanism: functional and biochemical aspects. *Ann Rev Physiol 1987; 49:* 251–273

25 Ichikawa I. Direct analysis of the effector mechanism of the tubuloglomerular feedback system. *Am J Physiol 1982; 243:* F447–F455

26 Reuss L, Cassel D, Rothenberg P et al. Mitogens and ion fluxes. In Mandel LJ, Benos DJ, eds. *The Role of Membranes in Cell Growth and Differentiation, Current Topics in Membranes and Transport, Volume 27.* Orlando, FL: Academic Press. 1986: 3–54

27 Bell J, Nielsen L, Sariban-Sohraby S, Benos D. External triggers of ion transport systems: fertilization, growth, and hormone systems. In Mandel LJ, Benos DJ, eds. *The Role of Membranes in Cell Growth and Differentiation, Current Topics in Membranes and Transport, Volume 27.* Orlando, FL: Academic Press. 1986: 129–162

28 Rechler MM, Nissley SP. The nature and regulation of the receptors for insulin-like growth factors. *Ann Rev Physiol 1985; 47:* 425–442

29 Sporn MB, Roberts AB, Wakefield LM, Assoian RK. Transforming growth factor-β: biological function and chemical structure. *Science 1986; 233:* 532–534

MESANGIAL FUNCTION IN NORMAL AND DISEASED ANIMALS

M Kashgarian, R B Sterzel

Yale University School of Medicine, New Haven, Connecticut, USA

Introduction

The mesangium is involved in most pathological processes of the renal glomerulus. It is a highly specialized pericapillary tissue which is composed of mesangial cells [1–4], surrounded by an extracellular matrix which include types IV and V collagen, fibronectin, laminin, entactin and nidogen [5–8]. The pathological changes that involve the mesangium include swelling, extension and proliferation of mesangial cells, deposition of foreign material and ultimately, in chronic renal disease, hyalinization and sclerosis [3,8,9]. Arresting, ameliorating or preventing progressive glomerular lesions requires a precise understanding of the cell biology, physiology and pathology of the mesangium.

The mesangium as the centrilobular tissue of the glomeruli was first described by Zimmermann in 1929 [10] and has been the object of considerable interest. Functionally it is an integral part of the glomerular capillary ultrafilter and its function in the uptake and disposal of circulating substances and filtration residues is important to our understanding of its rôle in glomerular disease. The glomerular capillary serves as an ultrafilter of plasma and has a high hydraulic conductivity and a low permeability to proteins in the normal state. It consists of an endothelium with large fenestrae, a trilaminar basement membrane and a layer of epithelial cells. The capillaries are arranged radially around the mesangium. The interface between the mesangium and the glomerular capillary endothelium is devoid of the basement membrane and provides access of filtration residues to the mesangial space.

At least three cell types have been identified in the mesangium. They include intrinsic mesangial cells, resident Ia antigen bearing cells and transient monocyte macrophages [8,9]. Each of these cell types has properties which can contribute to the processing of macromolecules percolating into the mesangium.

Intrinsic mesangial cell

The predominant cell of the mesangium is the intrinsic mesangial cell. Both in vivo and in vitro studies have characterized this cell to be similar to a vascular smooth muscle-like cell or pericyte. The cells contain actin and myosin and bear receptors for angiotensin II and have been demonstrated to be contractile [11–15]. The cells have also been shown to be phagocytic and to contain a broad spectrum of acidic lysosomal hydrolases capable of degrading both filtration residues and glomerular structural components. These cells synthesize extracellular matrix components including glycosaminoglycans, types I, III and IV collagen, fibronectin, laminin and thrombospendin. In addition, they have been demonstrated to secrete eicosanoids (particularly vasodilatory prostaglandins), platelet activating factors, as well as various polypeptide cytokines, which may all act as inflammatory mediators [16,17]. As such, the intrinsic mesangial cell appears not only to provide structural support for the glomerular capillaries but also to participate in the clearing function and local regulation of inflammatory processes.

Ia cells

In addition to the intrinsic mesangial cell, a small subpopulation of Ia antigen bearing cells has been described to be present in the mesangium [18]. These cells appear to be bone marrow derived cells which bear Ia antigen and are similar to other tissue macrophage-like cells such as the Langerhans cell in the epidermis and dendritic cells in lymph nodes. It is thought that these resident Ia antigen bearing cells may be involved in recognizing and presenting foreign antigens to lymphocytes and to specifically stimulate lymphocyte proliferation. It is presently unclear whether they are also involved in endocytic processes in the clearance of the mesangium of macromolecules.

Monocyte macrophages

Finally, transient monocyte macrophages constitute another population of cells in the mesangium [19]. This population is extremely small under normal conditions, but monocyte macrophages are recruited in many instances of proliferative inflammatory processes involving the glomeruli such as acute glomerulonephritis or crescentic glomerulonephritis.

Mesangial matrix

The extracellular matrix is not a simple passive structural protein matrix in which the cells reside but rather it is involved in a dynamic interaction with the mesangial cells which can influence mesangial function. There is increasing evidence that growth and differentiation of cells is influenced directly by the extracellular matrix [20]. Endothelial cells that have been cultured on an extracellular matrix, secreted and deposited by other endothelial cells, have a different response to growth factors present in the serum than when grown on artificial substrates. Epithelial cell differentiation has also been demonstrated to be influenced by matrix. Indeed, in recent unpublished studies we have demonstrated that the morphology of mesangial cells is strikingly modified by the matrix on which they are grown. In addition, their attachment and proliferative response, as well as presumably their synthetic activities, may be modulated through these mechanisms.

Since the glomerulus has the unique function of a high pressure, high flow ultrafiltration apparatus, the mesangial space is predisposed to the deposition of macromolecular filtration residues. These residues may accumulate in the matrix or may be taken up by the mesangial cells by endocytosis. The process can be of particular importance if the filtration residues consist of phlogogenic immune complexes or other proteins which may activate the mesangial cells to proliferate, synthesize inflammatory mediators or produce new matrix components. The determinants of mesangial entry, uptake and removal of macromolecules are thus of importance not only in the regulation and maintenance of the function of the glomerular filter but also in the modulation of glomerular injury [8,9]. Multiple factors determine the rate of mesangial deposition and processing of macromolecules.

Mesangial function

Germuth et al [21] have observed a relationship between the size of immune complexes and their pattern of intraglomerular localization. Intermediate sized complexes with a molecular weight of approximately one million tend to localize predominantly in the mesangial region as opposed to smaller soluble complexes which are found mainly in the peripheral capillary wall. Molecular charge has also been demonstrated to be of importance in that increased mesangial entry and localization of cationized molecules such as ferritin or protamine sulphate has been observed [9,22,23]. Size and, in particular, biodegradibility of a molecule have been demonstrated to be important in the removal or clearing from the mesangium. The removal of ferritin is considerably delayed when it is conjugated to IgG as compared to when it is present as an unconjugated protein [24]. Clearly the phagocytic activity of the mesangial cells must also be of importance. Indeed, some studies suggest that it functions very much like other components of the reticuloendothelial system. Studies with colloidal carbon, radiolabelled aggregated IgG and antigen-antibody complexes have all revealed enhanced mesangial translocalization following saturation of the reticuloendothelial system associated with increased plasma levels.

A number of studies have examined how local microcirculatory alterations might affect mesangial function. Work in our own laboratory has confirmed that enhanced mesangial uptake of ferritin can be seen with acute angiotensin II infusion [3]. No significant correlations, however, were found between glomerular localization of ferritin and the mean systolic pressure or whole kidney filtration fraction. The strongest correlation was observed between mean urinary excretion of albumin and ferritin and the amount of glomerular ferritin. Similarly, work by Mauer et al [25] has demonstrated an increased mesangial deposition of filtered proteins in the mesangium of unclipped kidneys of rats with Goldblatt hypertension. Micropuncture studies in animals after 5/6th nephrectomy have revealed substantial increases in the transcapillary hydraulic pressure due to increases in glomerular capillary pressure with single nephron hyperfiltration leading to increased mesangial accumulation of plasma proteins followed by enhanced deposition of mesangial matrix and glomerular sclerosis [26]. These latter in vivo studies suggest that there is a dynamic interaction between the cells of the mesangium, the matrix and in their proliferative and synthetic responses.

Analysis of the structure and functional properties of the glomerular mesangial cells and matrix indicates that the interaction of mesangial matrix and mesangial cells play an important rôle in glomerular disease. Accumulation of macromolecules may modify the composition and configuration of the extracellular matrix, which in turn may modulate the proliferation and differentiation of mesangial cells and their synthetic activities. Indeed, studies by Grond et al [27] have compared the long-term effects of the nephrotic syndrome induced by adriamycin and that produced by aminonucleoside of puromycin. Using colloidal carbon as a tracer, they reported that mesangial uptake of carbon in adriamycin perfused animals did not differ significantly from that of contralateral, saline perfused kidneys. Glomerular sclerosis was more marked in aminonucleoside nephrosis where there was increased carbon accumulation, suggesting that increased accumulation and incorporation of macromolecular substances into the mesangium may lead to an overproduction of matrix substances and eventually to glomerular sclerosis.

Conclusion

Although we have much to learn about the rôle of the factors which modulate macromolecular deposition in the mesangium by altering access to and drainage from this space, we have come to realize that the mesangium is not merely an inert skeletal structure of the glomerulus but that it plays an active and important rôle in both health and disease. It participates in the regulation of glomerular filtration and serves in the disposal of macromolecular filtration residues as part of its normal physiological function. Perturbation of the mesangium by the accumulation of biologically active molecules or when its capacity to handle filtration residues is exceeded, may induce proliferation of both mesangial cells and matrix. A lack of control of this process can be self-destructive and may lead to glomerular sclerosis by a perpetuation of abnormal cell and matrix interaction. Continued investigation of the mesangial structure and function and the interrelationships between the matrix and cells is necessary to gain the information needed to better understand the pathogenesis of progressive glomerular sclerosis and renal insufficiency.

References

1 Farquhar MG, Palade GE. Functional evidence for the existence of a third cell type in the renal glomerulus. *J Cell Biol 1962; 13:* 55

2 Latta H, Maunsbach AB, Madden SC. The centralobular region of the renal glomerulus studied by electron microscopy. *J Ultrastruct Res 1960; 4:* 455

3 Stein HD, Federgreen W, Kashgarian M, Sterzel RB. The role of angiotensin II-induced renal functional charges for the mesangial deposition of exogenous ferritin in rats. *Lab Invest 1983; 49:* 270

4 von Mollendorff W. Der Exkretionsapparat. In von Mollendorff W, ed. *Handbuch der Mikroskopischen Anatomie des Menschen, Volume 7: Harn-und Geschlechtsapparat.* Berlin: Springer. 1930: 1–328

5 Kreisberg JI, Karnovsky MS. Glomerular cells in culture. *Kidney Int 1983; 23:* 439

6 Scheinman JI, Fish AJ, Matas AJ, Michael AF. The immunohistopathology of glomerular antigens. II. The glomerular basement membrane, actomyosin and fibroblast surface antigens in normal, diseased and transplanted human kidneys. *Am J Pathol 1978; 90:* 71

7 Scheinman JI, Foidart JM, Gehron-Robey P et al. The immunohistology of glomerular antigens. IV. Laminin, a defined non-collagen basement membrane glycoprotein. *Clin Immunol Immunopathol 1980; 15:* 175

8 Sterzel RB, Lovett DH, Stein HD, Kashgarian M. The mesangium and glomerulonephritis. *Klin Wochenschr 1982; 60:* 1077

9 Michael AF, Keane WF, Raij L et al. The glomerular mesangium. *Kidney Int 1980; 17:* 141

10 Zimmermann KW. Uber den Bau des Glomerulus der menschlichen Niere. *Z Mikroskanat Forsch 1929; 18:* 520–552

11 DeMartino C, Natali PG, Zamboni L, Accinni L. Ultrastructural study of mesangial cells and their relationship to smooth muscle cells of glomerular arterioles. *Contr Nephrol 1976; 2:* 17–24

12 Huhn D, Steiner JW, Movat HZ. Die Feinstruktur des Mesangiums in Nierenglomerulum von Hund und Maus. *Z Zellforsch 1962; 56:* 213–230

13 Latta H. The multipotential nature of mesangial cells. *Biol Cellulaire 1980; 39:* 245–248

14 Scheinman JI, Fish AJ, Matas AJ, Michael AF. The immunohistopathology of glomerular antigens. II. The glomerular basement membrane, actomyosin, and fibroblast surface antigens in normal diseased and transplanted human kidneys. *Am J Pathol 1978; 90:* 71–84

15 Osborne MJ, Droz B, Meyer P, Morel F. Angiotensin II: renal localization in glomerular mesangial cells by autoradiography. *Kidney Int 1975; 8:* 245–254

16 Lovett DH, Sterzel RB. Cell culture approaches to the analysis of glomerular inflammation. *Kidney Int 1986; 30:* 246

17 Lovett DH, Ryan JL, Sterzel RB. A thymocyte activating factor derived from glomerular mesangial cells. *J Immunol 1983; 131:* 2830

18 Schreiner GF, Kiely JM, Cotran RS, Unanue ER. Characterization of resident glomerular cells in the rat expressing Ia-determinants and manifesting genetically restricted interactions with lymphocytes. *Clin Invest 1981; 68:* 920

19 Cotran RS. Editorial. Monocytes, proliferation and glomerulonephritis. *J Lab Clin Med 1978; 922:* 837

20 Kashgarian M. Mesangium and glomerular disease. *Lab Invest 1985; 52:* 569–571

21 Germuth FG, Rodriguez E. *Immunopathology of the Renal Glomerulus.* Boston: Little Brown and Co. 1973: 15–161

22 Batsford SR, Takamiya H, Vogt A. A model of in situ immune complex glomerulonephritis in the rat employing cationized ferritin. *Clin Nephrol 1980; 14:* 211–216

23 Kanwar YS, Farquhar M. Anionic sites in the glomerular basement membrane. *J Cell Biol 1979; 81:* 137–153

24 Takamiya H, Batsford S, Kluthe R, Vogt A. Comparison of the handling of ferritin and ferritin-protein conjugates by the glomerular mesangium. *Lab Invest 1979; 40:* 18–24

25 Mauer SM, Steffes MW, Azar S et al. The effect of Goldblatt hypertension on development of the glomerular lesions of diabetes mellitus in the rat. *Diabetes 1978; 27:* 738

26 Hostetter TH, Olson JL, Rennke HG et al. Hyperfiltration in remnant nephrons: a potentially adverse response to renal ablation. *Am J Physiol 1981; 241:* F85

27 Grond J, Weening JJ, Elema JD. Glomerular sclerosis in nephrotic rats: comparison of long-term effects of adriamycin and aminonucleoside. *Lab Invest 1984; 51:* 277

MESANGIAL HANDLING OF IMMUNE DEPOSITS IN IgA NEPHROPATHY

R Sinniah
with the technical assistance of
C K Ow, L S Chia, T C Tan
National University of Singapore, Singapore

Introduction

In 1968 Jean Berger [1,2] described a lesion characterized by diffuse mesangial deposition of immunoglobulins, with IgA predominating. There were no systemic manifestations and secondary diseases being excluded, the lesion has come to be known as IgA nephropathy. Considerable evidence now exists to support the concept that mesangial deposits of IgA result from deposition of IgA-containing immune complexes [3–5]. The brunt of the immune complex deposition in IgA nephropathy is borne by the glomerular mesangium although glomerular capillary wall deposits of varying extent and severity do occur [6–9] and may contribute to, but seem unlikely to account for, the progressive decline in renal function. There is increased production of IgA antibodies and its polymers by both mucosal and peripheral blood lymphocytes directed against some as yet unidentified antigen [10]. Therefore a circulating factor is responsible, either IgA itself or a mediator leading to increased influx or to decreased mesangial clearance. To understand the fate of the deposits and the reaction of the mesangium, we need to have knowledge of the structure and functions of the mesangium; factors determining the accumulation and clearance of macromolecules, and the mesangial response to immunoprotein deposits leading to glomerular injury.

Possible mechanisms for mesangial uptake and disposal of IgA immune complexes

Mesangial localization of immune complexes is favoured by high blood levels, decreased efficiency of the systemic mononuclear phagocytic system, high avidity immune complexes, and the chemotactic and phlogogenic potential including complement fixing capacity [11–15]. Cationic circulating macromolecules can interact with anionic sites in the mesangial matrix and be an important factor in the enhanced uptake, localization and persistence of cationic antigens [16–18]. If either the antigen or antibody is cationic it can also initiate in situ immune complex formation in the mesangial matrix [19]. Experimental studies using dextran molecules with large latticed complexes, with cationic, neutral and anionic points as antigens for serum sickness resulted in production of IgA antibodies and IgA deposits in the glomerular mesangium [20]. Therefore the size, type, charge and biological properties of the IgA complex may determine its rate of accumulation and clearance [21,22].

In patients with Berger's disease there is increased production of IgA by peripheral B-cells [23] related to altered lymphocyte functions, an increase in T-helper cells [24] and a defect in IgA-specific suppressor T-cell activity [25]. It has also been proposed that there is an impairment in the removal of IgA immune complexes by receptors on phagocytic Kupffer cells in the liver [26,27], and by cells of the reticuloendothelial system including mononuclear phagocytes and polymorphonuclear neutrophils [28–31]. These and other factors summarized in Table I may lead to excessive deposition of IgA immunoproteins in the glomerular mesangium.

TABLE I Possible mechanisms of mesangial uptake and disposal of immune complexes*

Mesangial uptake	Mesangial disposal
1. Rate and quantity of immune deposits a) antigen exposure b) production c) clearance by systemic mononuclear phagocyte system	1. Phagocytosis by resident mesangial cells 2. Phagocytosis by infiltrating phagocytes 3. Transport via stalk to JG zone with exit via venules and lymphatics, digestion by lacis cells
2. Characteristics of macromolecules (size, charge, type etc)	4. Capillary regurgitation
3. Haemodynamic factors (especially hyperfiltration and hypertension)	5. Filtration into urinary space via para-mesangium-epithelium
4. Characteristics of glomerular capillary	6. Extracellular degradation by secreted enzymes 7. Complement-mediated solubilization 8. Haemodynamic factors – interruption of traffic by angiotensin II, prostaglandins

* Adapted from several sources including Michael, 1984 [32]

Most studies suggest limited phagocytosis and clearance of immune complexes by resident mesangial cells [32–34]. Phagocytic clearance of immune complexes by infiltrating mononuclear cells entering the mesangium have been suggested [35]. Monocytes/macrophages within the glomeruli have been observed in many types of immune-mediated experimental glomerulonephritis [36–39], and in some types of human proliferative glomerulonephritis, especially crescentic glomerulonephritis [40–45]. These cells might migrate as a non-specific inflammatory phagocytic response acting as scavangers of immune complexes, cellular debris or fibrin, or they play a specific rôle in the humoral response through their surface Fc and C3 receptors [46,47] or in cell-mediated immune mechanisms. Monocytes participate directly in glomerular injury through release of lytic enzymes that alter glomerular basement membrane [48], and factors stimulating the proliferation of fibroblasts and other glomerular cells [49,50].

The mesangium acts as a conduit for the passage of macromolecular particles by the matrix channels to the hilum and region of the lacis cells in the juxtaglomerular apparatus. Movement through these channels to the lymphatics, venules and renal interstitium have been proposed [51]. Regurgitation from the mesangium back into the glomerular capillary lumen has also been suggested [33], but not demonstrated [11,32]. The concentration of tracers and immune complexes beneath the basement membrane in the paramesangium, and the frequent finding of dense deposits in this region in human glomerulonephritis have suggested their possible removal to the urinary space through the overlying epithelium [52]. These and other possible mechanisms are also summarized in Table I. We have examined some of these possible mechanisms for the disposal of IgA associated proteins in IgA nephropathy.

Reaction of the mesangium in IgA nephropathy

Electron dense deposits are always in the mesangium, mostly between mesangial cells and basement membrane, and within the mesangial matrix. In the acute and active stages of the disease, the mesangial cells show abundant cytoplasm with numerous mitochondria and prominent endoplasmic reticulum. Despite this metabolic activity, no intracellular deposits are seen [6–9,53]. There is no clear correlation between the amount of mesangial IgA and the severity of glomerulonephritis [53,54], and one occasionally sees severe disease with only scant amounts of IgA. Some other factor may be necessary for the initiation and severity of injury. No evidence has been found for any significant intracellular phagocytosis and digestion by resident mesangial cells.

Disposal of IgA deposits by intrinsic glomerular structures

We could find no morphological evidence that mesangial cells have any significant phagocytic rôle in the removal of IgA immunoproteins in Berger's disease [53]. This is in accordance with the earlier observations that mesangial cells have no prominent phagocytic activity in the handling of larger molecules such as pre-formed antigen-antibody complexes.

The dense deposits are observed in the matrix of the mesangium with a preferential location in the paramesangium (Figure 1). We examined the hilus of each glomerulus for the possible presence of dense deposits in the lacis cells or other structures, but no deposits as ingested globules could be identified. Migration to the renal interstitium by the macula densa or to distal tubules, the lymphatics or venules could not be demonstrated. Regurgitation into the glomerular capillary lumen from the mesangial conduit could not be proven by

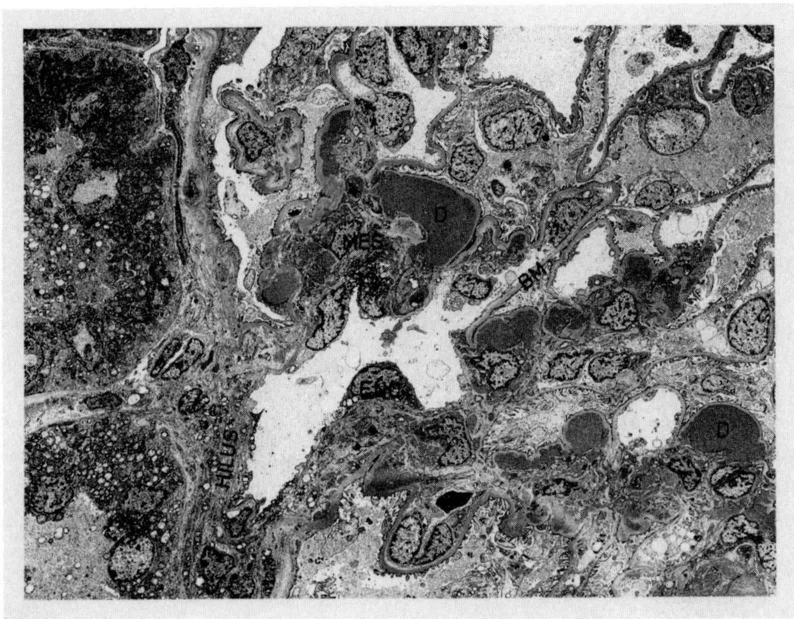

Figure 1. IgA nephropathy. Marked widening of the mesangium by electron dense deposits (D), with maximal concentration in the paramesangium. Structures of the hilus show no dense deposits. Mes=Mesangial cell; End=Endothelial cell; BM=Basement membrane. Electron micrograph ×2,250 – reduced for publication

ultrastructural or immunofluorescence microscopy. This possible exit route has not been proven to exist in experimental or human observations. Extraglomerular deposits have been found in afferent and small arterioles in a minority of cases but not in venules, lymphatics and intertubular capillaries, showing no evidence of removal by these routes.

The accumulation of deposits in the paramesangium may suggest exit through the overlying epithelial cells into the urinary space. Contraction of the mesangial cells, causing an accordion-like wrinkling of the juxta-mesangial epithelial basal lamina could aid in this movement of macromolecules [55]. IgA-containing casts and secretions within tubular lumen and epithelial cells are a common finding in IgA nephropathy, and their origin from the paramesangial deposits should be considered.

Rôle of infiltrating phagocytes in mesangial disposal of IgA deposits

Aggregated IgA, known to stimulate the alternate pathway of complement activation [56–58] has been considered responsible for local chemotaxis and inflammation. One often sees large amounts of mesangial C3 in IgA nephropathy with no inflammation or injury on light or electronmicroscopy. In acute immune-mediated glomerular injury infiltrating monocytes-macrophages have been shown to play an important rôle in glomerular damage [59], and these cells have an active rôle in a number of proliferative glomerulonephritis, including essential cryoglobulinaemia, systemic lupus erythematosus (SLE) and Henoch-Schönlein purpura [44,45].

We have studied the renal biopsies of 30 patients with IgA nephropathy, eight with SLE and 14 minimal change nephrotic syndrome. Sections cut from Bouin's fixed paraffin blocks were tested against commercially prepared monoclonal antibodies to leucocyte common antigen, and polyclonals of α_1-antitrypsin for monocytes/macrophages, both obtained from DAKO Labs. All sections were trypsinized before staining with the appropriate peroxidase anti-peroxidase complex using established techniques [60–63]. For each biopsy the total number of intraglomerular positive cells were counted, and then divided by the number of glomeruli, obtaining an index (M/G) which is the mean number of intraglomerular monocytes per glomerulus. The median and range of leucocytes positive with leucocyte common antigen, and monocytes positive with α_1-antitrypsin are shown in Table II. The number of positive cells per glomerular

TABLE II. Number of intraglomerular leucocytes and monocytes in IgA nephropathy, SLE and minimal change nephropathy

Disease	Number of cases	Leucocytes/glomerulus		Monocytes/glomerulus	
		Median	Range	Median	Range
Minimal change[1]	14	0	(0.00–0.30)	0	(0.0–0.30)
IgA nephropathy[2]	30	0	(0.00–2.33)	0	(0.0–1.00)
SLE nephritis[3]	8	6.45	(4.86–9.00)	4.65	(3.2–7.00)
Mann-Whitney U-test		p		p	
MC[1] versus IgA[2]		not significant		not significant	
MC[1] versus SLE[3]		< 0.001		< 0.001	
IgA[2] versus SLE[3]		< 0.01		< 0.01	

cross-section in the three groups are compared using a Mann-Whitney non-parametric-U-test, because the data are not normally distributed and are too small to allow critical assessment. Significant and large numbers of monocytes per glomerulus are found in proliferative SLE, and are negligible or absent in IgA nephropathy and minimal change nephropathy. These findings confirm the observations of Ferrario et al [44], Nolasco et al [45], and Stachura et al [64]. IgA nephropathy is clearly different from other forms of proliferative glomerulonephritis and the models of experimental immune-mediated glomerulonephritis with macrophages being involved. IgA nephropathy is also different from Henoch-Schönlein purpura. In IgA nephropathy, despite segmental or diffuse hypercellularity, no increase in the number of intraglomerular monocytes are seen, except in an occasional patient, unlike proliferative SLE nephritis where there is a substantial number of infiltrating monocytes contributing to the glomerular hypercellularity.

As in IgA nephropathy, monocytes are negligible in the glomeruli in renal amyloidosis, membranous nephropathy, mesangiocapillary glomerulonephritis, focal sclerosing nephritis and minimal change nephropathy [44,45]. In IgA nephropathy the mesangial hypertrophy and hypercellularity seem to result predominantly or exclusively from proliferation of resident mesangial cells which do not express leucocyte markers, confirming the earlier electronmicroscopy studies by Sinniah and Churg [53]. There does not appear to be a rôle for infiltrating phagocytes in mesangial disposal of IgA-associated immune complexes.

Extracellular degradation of IgA deposits by excretion of enzymes by mesangial cells

There is indolent progression of renal injury in many cases of IgA nephropathy. An IgA response appears to be much less phlogogenic than other classes of immunoglobulins such as IgG [65], and aggregated IgA in the mesangium is more inert than IgG aggregates [66]. With the absence of chemotactic factors and infiltrating phagocytes, the possible release of digestive enzymes and the activation of mesangial cells through specific cell membrane receptors may be responsible for degradation of mesangial deposits, and also glomerular damage.

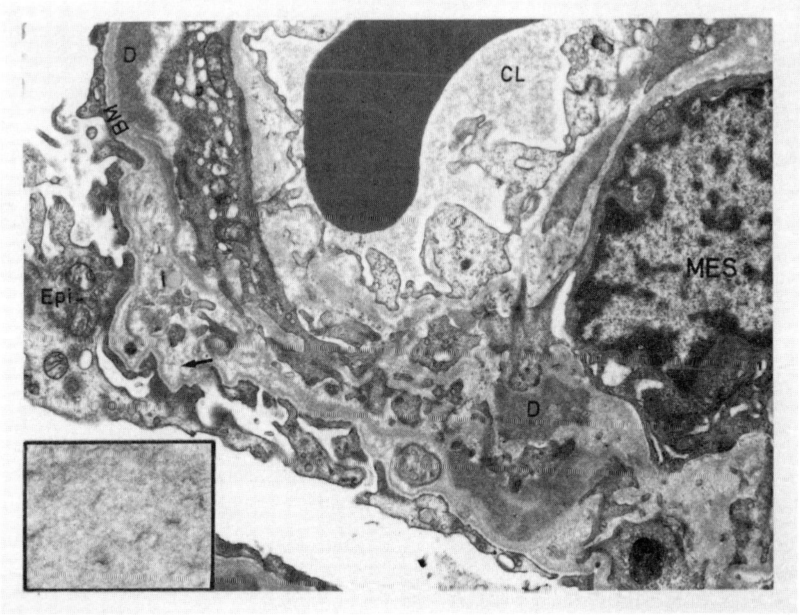

Figure 2. IgA nephropathy. Mesangial-paramesangial area and glomerular capillary basement membrane show lytic areas around and within the dense deposits. Microfibrils are admixed with the electron dense granular deposits (inset is higher magnification of area →). D=Dense deposits; Mes=Mesangial cell; CL=Capillary lumen; BM=basement membrane; Epi=Epithelial cell. Electron micrograph ×13,500; inset magnification ×81,000 – reduced for publication

Electronmicroscopic examinations show loosening of the matrix in the mesangium and paramesangial areas of the glomerulus. The lytic areas are around and within the dense deposits in the mesangial matrix, possibly by enzymes secreted by the mesangial cells. The matrix in and around the deposits is dissolved by a process of mesangiolysis, which also extends to the peripheral capillary loops containing dense deposits (Figure 2). Similar changes of lysis with loose fibrillar materials and dense deposits are seen to expand the mesangial channels at the glomerular hilus [53]. The mediators responsible for this lytic process are poorly understood, but the rôle of proteases, prostaglandins and other substances produced by the mesangial cells [67] have to be considered.

Chronic progressive glomerular disease in IgA nephropathy

The mesangial changes have been well documented in a number of studies [7,9,53,68–71], and the major changes are summarized in Table III. The mesangial deposits appear to stimulate increased production of matrix which may be preceded by mesangiolysis. In patients with more severe proliferation and sclerotic glomerular damage there is greater mesangial sclerosis and collagen fibres within the matrix. There is a good correlation between mesangial cell proliferation and sclerosis to collagen fibrils and amount of matrix formation. There is no definite correlation between the quantity of immune deposits and amount of mesangial matrix. The collagen fibres usually run together although some bend or curl in random directions. Further to our earlier observations of collagen fibres in the mesangial matrix [9,53] we can identify them also in the peripheral cytoplasmic processes of mesangial cells (Figure 3). The appearance of the fibres are similar to those of collagen fibres found in large quantities between the renal tubules. Within areas of mesangial lysis and dense deposits there are twisted collagen fibrils with accumulation of amorphous material, well away from the mesangial cell cytoplasm. A macromolecular precursor such as topocollagen could reach the centrilobular region by the bloodstream and polymerize there into collagen fibres.

Peripheral glomerular capillary abnormalities are seen in approximately 50% of patients [9,72,73]. Paramesangial subendothelial deposits are seen in nearly 80% of patients with diffuse mesangial cell proliferation with sclerotic glomeruli, and less frequently in non-sclerotic glomerulonephritis and minor changes. Mesangial interposition into subendothelial space and membranolysis with aneurysmal dilatation of some capillary loops are associated with the dense deposits. There is splitting, disruption of the lamina densa and irregular thickening of the glomerular basement membrane, and electron lucent substance admixed with granules (Figure 2). These seem to represent early lesions and later the glomerular basement membrane becomes irregularly thickened and in many of them entrapped mesangial and endothelial cell structures, and collagen fibrils can be identified. The peripheral capillary damage can lead to disruption of the basement membrane, and escape of intraluminal materials into Bowman's

TABLE III. Electronmicroscopic glomerular mesangial and capillary wall changes in IgA nephropathy*

Light microscopy	Number of cases	MESANGIAL CHANGES								CAPILLARY WALL CHANGES		
		Dense deposits 1+	2+	3+ (%)	Thickened Mesangial matrix 1+	2+	3+ (%)	Mesangio-lysis (%)	Collagen** fibrils (%)	Sub-endothelial deposits (%)	BM lysis/ aneurysms (%)	Thickening reduplication (%)
Minor change	28	3	5	20 (71)	16	12	–	2 (7)	5 (18)	12 (43)	3 (11)	13 (46)
Focal proliferation/ sclerosis	21	10	7	4 (19)	10	6	5 (24)	4 (19)	10 (48)	15 (71)	3 (14)	12 (57)
Diffuse mesangial proliferation	8	2	1	4 (50)	–	5	3 (37)	2 (25)	4 (50)	2 (25)	1 (12)	5 (62)
Diffuse mesangial proliferation and sclerosis	21	5	8	8 (38)	2	11	8 (38)	8 (38)	15 (71)	17 (81)	9 (43)	11 (52)

* Summary of data from Sinniah, 1987 [9]; Sinniah, Churg, 1983 [53].

** Inaccurately stated low incidence in reference [9].

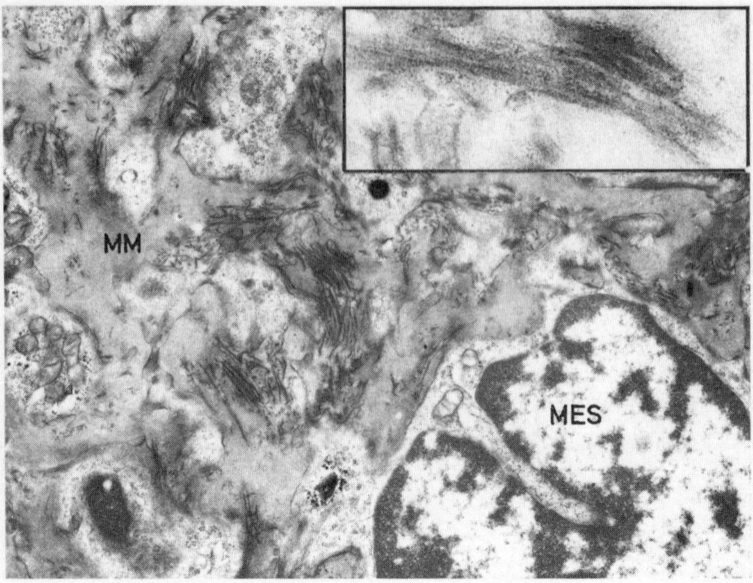

Figure 3. IgA nephropathy. Marked thickening of mesangial matrix (MM), with dense deposition of collagen fibrils within the matrix and in the cytoplasmic processes of mesangial cell (Mes). Inset shows the fibres to be similar in structure to collagen fibres between renal tubules. Electron micrograph ×22,500; inset magnification ×103,500 – reduced for publication

space with formation of adhesions and crescents. The combination of damage to mesangial and peripheral glomerular basement membrane leads to excessive production of matrix and collagen fibrils which encroach on mesangial and other intraglomerular structures with eventual glomerular sclerosis or obsolescence.

Immunohistochemical structure of extracellular matrix in IgA nephropathy

Monoclonal antibodies are useful in the study of extracellular components. Renal biopsies from 30 patients with IgA nephropathy, eight with proliferative SLE nephritis and eight with minimal change nephrotic syndrome were studied with the *'immunoperoxidase method'*, using established techniques [60–63].

Tissue preparation

Four micron sections were cut from Bouin's fixed paraffin blocks processed by the 24-hour cycle histokinette and placed on poly-L-lysin coated slides. The slides were dried overnight in a 37°C oven.

Antibodies

A panel of commercially prepared antibodies were used for the study. The monoclonals comprised leucocyte common antigen (DAKO), polyclonals of

α_1-antitrypsin (DAKO), fibronectin (DAKO), laminin (EY Lab), and collagen type IV (Pasteur Institute).

Immunoperoxidase staining

Briefly sections were incubated for one hour at room temperature with optimally diluted primary antibodies after prior treatment with 3% hydrogen peroxide and 10% ovalbumin. These were followed by a 30 minute incubation with appropriate secondary antibodies and then with appropriate peroxidase-anti-peroxidase complex. Three tris-buffer washings were used between incubations. Finally the peroxidase complex was revealed with DAB (0.5mg/ml in tris-buffer plus 0.01% H_2O_2). After washing, the slides were lightly stained with Gill's haematoxylin, dehydrated and mounted with Canada balsam. All sections were trypsinized with 0.1% trypsin type II (Sigma) for 20 minutes at 37°C.

Results

There is increased deposition of laminin, fibronectin and collagen type IV, in IgA nephropathy and SLE proliferative glomerulonephritis compared to minimal change nephrotic syndrome. The deposition of fibronectin and collagen type IV are markedly increased in IgA nephropathy with proliferative and sclerosing lesions, than in cases with minor changes only (Table IV). The deposits are

TABLE IV. Immunohistochemical structure of glomerular extracellular matrix in IgA nephropathy

Extracellular matrix	Grade	LIGHT MICROSCOPY Minor change (9 cases)	Proliferative and sclerosing glomerulonephritis (21 cases)
Lamin	1+	4	7
	2+	1	5
	3+	0	4 (19%)
Fibronectin	1+	4	4
	2+	2	7
	3+	2 (22%)	10 (48%)
Collagen type IV	1+	5	6
	2+	2	9
	3+	0	6 (29%)

present maximally in the mesangium, with peripheral subendothelial extensions in a segmental distribution (Figure 4). With sclerosis the extracellular glycoproteins and collagen are present as heavy deposits in both the mesangium and peripheral capillary loops (Figure 5), leading to total glomerular involvement. In diffuse proliferative SLE nephritis the distribution of fibronectin, laminin and

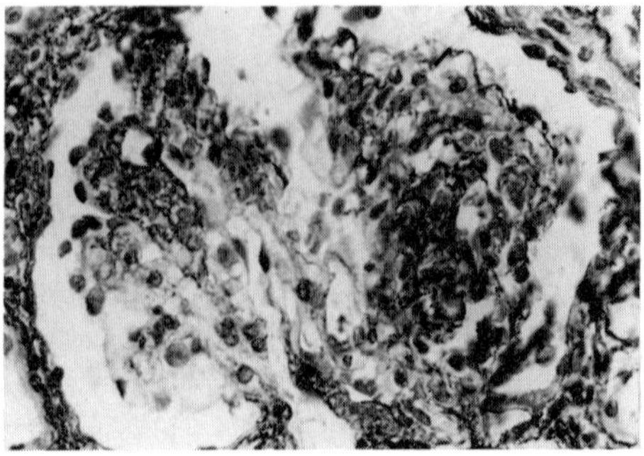

Figure 4. IgA nephropathy with diffuse proliferative glomerulonephritis on light microscopy, shows collagen type IV in the mesangium with peripheral subendothelial extensions. PAP technique ×640 – reduced for publication

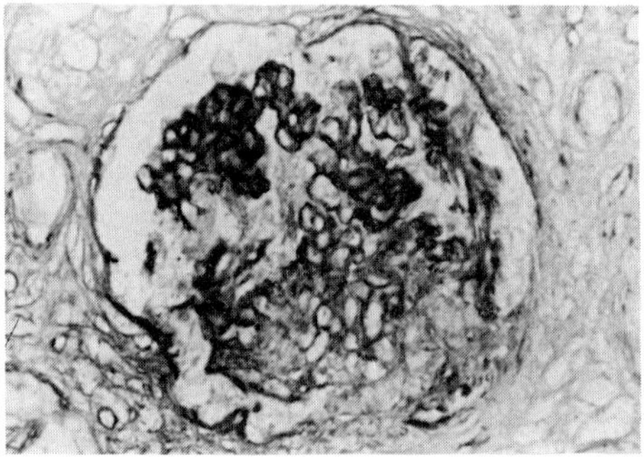

Figure 5. IgA nephropathy with diffuse proliferative and sclerosing glomerulonephritis with adhesion and crescents on light microscopy, shows heavy deposition of fibronectin in the mesangium and in the subendothelium of peripheral capillaries of a sclerosing glomerulus. PAP technique ×640 – reduced for publication

collagen type IV are maximal in the peripheral subendothelial location, with less intense granular mesangial deposits.

These preliminary studies in IgA nephropathy indicate progressive accumulation of fibronectin and collagen type IV in the mesangium, and later to peripheral glomerular capillaries, with incorporation of laminin as major components in the process of glomerular sclerosis. They reflect a marked increase in the secretion of endogenous mesangial matrix components by the endogenous mesangial cells. Contributing to this process may be the precipitation and polymerization of the circulating precursors of topocollagen into collagen fibres.

Haemodynamics and glomerular injury in IgA nephropathy

Glomerular hyperfiltration leading to focal glomerulosclerosis and hyalinosis may be an integral mechanism leading to progressive renal impairment in a variety of renal diseases [74]. Glomerular sclerosis and vascular abnormalities occur early and are interrelated in IgA nephropathy [75]. It has been postulated that glomerular damage in IgA nephropathy is related to altered intrarenal vasculature and increased hydraulic pressure and hyperfiltration due to decreased vascular resistance as an 'adaptive' haemodynamic change, rather than immunological glomerular injury. The vascular sclerosis and constriction lead to ischaemia with contraction and collapse glomerulosclerosis [6,76]. It has also been postulated that increased glomerular hydrostatic pressure may stimulate mesangial cells to increase deposition of excess mesangial matrix [77,78]. In our experience only one-third of IgA nephropathy patients with extensive mesangial matrix formation had hypertension, and sclerosis of glomeruli was related to hypertension in approximately 20% of cases [53]. Adhesions to Bowman's capsule and segmental crescents are frequent observations in IgA nephropathy [7,9], and not related to hypertension and ischaemic retraction of glomeruli. In a study by Feiner et al [76] 47% of kidneys with significant glomerular sclerosis were from subjects without hypertension, and 67% of these had vascular sclerosis associated with IgA nephropathy. Statistical association may not mean a cause and effect relation. In the pathogenesis of mesangial injury in IgA nephropathy it appears that mesangial entrapment of IgA-associated immune complexes initiate the glomerular injury, and alterations in glomerular haemodynamics and/or increased mesangial traffic may act independently or act synergistically in the development of glomerulosclerosis [11,79,80].

Summary

The resident mesangial cells show no significant phagocytic activity for macromolecules and have no major rôle in the removal of IgA deposits. In renal biopsies of IgA nephropathy patients there is no significant increase in the number of intraglomerular leucocytes, including monocytes/macrophages, and this could account for the reduction in the catabolic rate of polymeric IgA in these cases. There is little evidence for the removal of IgA immune complexes by regurgitation from the mesangium into capillary lumen or by the juxtaglomerular structures into the renal interstitium, venules or lymphatics. Escape to the urinary space by epithelial cells overlying the paramesangial deposits may possibly occur. The accumulated deposits probably lead to mechanical or functional disturbance of the mesangial draining system which stimulates hyperplasia and hypertrophy of cells, and the resident cells to produce excessive mesangial matrix. The deposits also stimulate the mesangial cells to secrete digestive enzymes which participate in mesangiolysis and membranolysis, whose frequent sequela is mesangial sclerosis. In chronic IgA nephropathy there is increased secretion of a number of different antigenic components, including

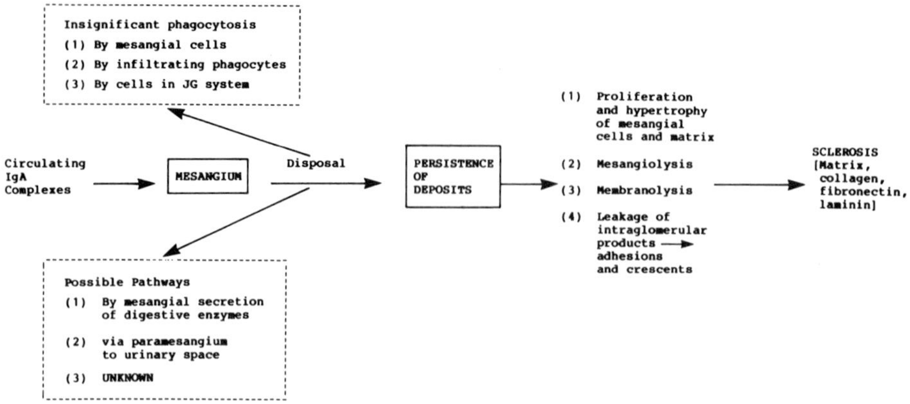

Figure 6. Pathways for mesangial handling of IgA immune complexes

fibronectin, collagen, including collagen type IV and laminin. These mesangial secretions extend through the subendothelium to peripheral capillary loops, and play an important rôle in mesangial interposition and eventual total glomerular sclerosis. These pathways for mesangial handling of IgA immune complexes are summarized in Figure 6.

More attention should be paid to the mechanisms involved in the removal of mesangial deposits in IgA nephropathy. Alterations in mesangial function and structure play an important rôle in progressive renal disease and unless this process is modulated it can lead to glomerular destruction and eventual glomerulosclerosis.

Acknowledgments

Our work has been supported by research grants from the National University of Singapore, PB Davar Memorial Fund, and Singapore Turf Club. Secretarial assistance was given by Ms Claire Lim.

References

1 Berger J, Hinglais N. Les depôts intercapillaires d'IgA. *J Urol (Paris) 1968; 74:* 694–695

2 Berger J. IgA glomerular deposits in renal disease. *Transplant Proc 1969; 1:* 934–944

3 Woodroffe AJ. Summary of the pathogenesis of IgA nephropathy. In Clarkson AR, ed. *IgA Nephropathy.* Boston: Martinus Nijhoff. 1987: 204–213

4 Berger J, Yaneva H, Naberra B, Barbanel C. Recurrence of mesangial deposition of IgA after renal transplantation. *Kidney Int 1975; 7:* 232–241

5 Berger J. Glomerulonephrites idiopathiques à dèpôts mesangiaux d'IgA. In Hamburger J, ed. *Nephrologie, 2nd Edition.* Paris: Flammarion. 1979: 541–549

6 Clarkson AR, Seymour AE, Thompson AJ et al. IgA nephropathy: a syndrome of uniform morphology, diverse clinical features, and uncertain prognosis. *Clin Nephrol 1977; 8:* 459–471

7 Sinniah R, Javier AR, Ku G. The pathology of mesangial IgA nephritis with clinical correlation. *Histopathology 1981; 5:* 469–490

8 Shigematsu H, Kobayashi Y, Tateno S, Tsukada M. Ultrastructure of acute glomerular injury in IgA nephritis. *Arch Pathol Lab Med 1980; 104:* 303–307
9 Sinniah R. The pathology of IgA nephropathy. In Clarkson AJ, ed. *IgA Nephropathy.* Boston: Martinus Nijhoff. 1987: 66–96
10 Tomino Y, Endoh M, Nomoto Y, Sakai H. Specificity of eluted antibody from renal tissues of patients with IgA nephropathy. *Am J Kidney Dis 1982; 1:* 276–280
11 Michael AF, Keane WF, Raij L et al. Editorial review. The glomerular mesangium. *Kidney Int 1980; 17:* 141–154
12 Germuth FG Jr, Rodriguez E, Lovelle CA et al. Passive immune complex glomerulonephritis in mice: models for various lesions found in human disease. I. High avidity complexes and mesangiopathic glomerulonephritis. *Lab Invest 1979; 41:* 360–365
13 Mannik M. Pathophysiology of circulating immune complexes. *Arthritis Rheum 1982; 25:* 783–787
14 Mannik M. Physiochemical and functional relationship of immune complexes. *J Invest Dermatol 1980; 74:* 333–338
15 Herbert LA, Waxman FJ, Birmingham DJ et al. Complement depletion accelerates the clearance of immune complexes from the circulation of primates. *Kidney Int 1983; 23 (Abstract):* 183
16 Brenner BM, Hostetter TH, Hunus HD. Molecular basis of proteinuria of glomerular origin. *N Engl J Med 1978; 298:* 826–833
17 Border WA. Role of antigen and antibody charge in immune complex disease. In Robinson RR, ed. *Nephrology. Proceedings of the IXth International Congress of Nephrology, Volume 1.* New York: Springer Verlag. 1984: 550–559
18 Venkatachalam MA, Rennke HG. The structural and molecular basis of glomerular filtration. *Circ Res 1978; 43:* 337–347
19 Cohen S, Vernier RL, Michael AF. The effect of charge on the renal distribution of ferritin. *Am J Pathol 1983; 110:* 170–181
20 Isaacs KL, Miller F. Role of antigen size and charge in immune complex glomerulonephritis. I. Active induction of disease with dextran and its derivatives. *Lab Invest 1982; 47:* 198–205
21 Mauer SM, Fish AJ, Blau EB, Michael AF. The glomerular mesangium. I. Kinetic studies of macromolecular uptake in normal and nephrotic rats. *J Clin Invest 1972; 51:* 1092–1101
22 Batsford SR, Weghaupt R, Takamiya H, Vogt A. Studies on the mesangial handling of protein antigens: influence of size, charge and biologic activity. *Nephron 1985; 41:* 146–151
23 Egido J, Blasco R, Sancho J, Lozano L. T-cell dysfunction in IgA nephropathy: specific abnormalities in the regulation of IgA synthesis. *Clin Immunol Immunopathol 1983; 26:* 201–212
24 Sakai H, Endoh M, Tomino Y, Nomoto Y. Increase of IgA specific helper T-cells in patients with IgA nephropathy. *Clin Exp Immunol 1982; 50:* 77–82
25 Sakai H, Nomoto Y, Arimori S. Decrease of IgA-specific suppressor T-cell activity in patients with IgA nephropathy. *Clin Exp Immunol 1979; 38:* 243–248
26 Rifai A, Mannik M. Clearance of circulating IgA immune complexes is mediated by a specific receptor on Kupffer cells in mice. *J Exp Med 1984; 160:* 125–137
27 Kater L, Jobsis AC, Baart de la Faille-Kuyper EH et al. Alcoholic hepatic disease: specificity of IgA deposits in liver disease. *Am J Clin Pathol 1979; 71:* 51–57
28 Roccatello D, Coppo R, Piccoli G. Monocyte-macrophage system function in primary IgA nephropathy. In D'Amico G, Minetti L, Ponticelli C, eds. *IgA Mesangial Nephropathy.* Basel: Karger. *Contr Nephrol 1984; 40:* 130–136
29 Egido J, Sancho J, Lorente F, Fontan G. Inhibition of neutrophil migration by serum IgA from patients with IgA nephropathy. *Clin Exp Immunol 1982; 49:* 709–716
30 Sato M, Kinugasa E, Ideura T, Koshikawa S. Phagocytic activity of polymorphonuclear leucocytes in patients with IgA nephropathy. *Clin Nephrol 1983; 19:* 166–171
31 Sato M, Morikawa S, Koshikawa S. Attachment of polymorphonuclear leukocytes to glomeruli in IgA nephropathy. *Clin Immunol Immunopathol 1983; 29:* 111–118

32 Michael AF. The glomerular mesangium. In D'Amico G, Minetti L, Ponticelli C, eds. *IgA Mesangial Nephropathy.* Basel: Karger. *Contr Nephrol 1984; 40:* 111–118
33 Sterzel RB, Lovett DH, Stein HD, Kashgarian M. The mesangium and glomerulonephritis. *Klin Wochenschr 1982; 60:* 1077–1094
34 Cattell V, Gaskin de Urdaneta A, Ailidge S et al. Uptake and clearance of ferritin by the glomerular mesangium. I. Phagocytosis by mesangial cells and blood monocytes. *Lab Invest 1982; 47:* 296–303
35 Striker GE, Mannik M, Tung MY. Role of marrow-derived monocytes and mesangial cells in removal of immune complexes from renal glomeruli. *J Exp Med 1979; 149:* 127–136
36 Holdsworth SR, Neale TJ, Wilson CB. The participation of macrophages and monocytes in experimental immune complexes glomerulonephritis. *Clin Immunol Immunopathol 1980; 15:* 510–524
37 Hunsickler LG, Shearer TP, Plattern SB, Weisenberger D. The role of monocytes in serum sickness nephritis. *J Exp Med 1979; 150:* 413–425
38 Schreiner GF, Cotran RS, Pardo V, Unanue ER. A mononuclear cell component in experimental immunological glomerulonephritis. *J Exp Med 1978; 147:* 369–384
39 Thompson NM, Holdsworth SR, Glasgow EF, Atkins RC. The macrophage in the development of crescentic glomerulonephritis. *Am J Pathol 1979; 94:* 223–240
40 Atkins RC, Glasgow EF, Holdsworth SR, Matthews FE. The macrophage in human rapidly progressive glomerulonephritis. *Lancet 1976; i:* 830–832
41 Magil AB, Wadsworth LD, Locwen M. Monocytes and human renal glomerular disease. A quantitative evaluation. *Lab Invest 1981; 44:* 27–31
42 Harry T, Bryant D, Coles GA et al. The detection of monocytes in human renal biopsies, a prospective study. *Clin Nephrol 1982; 18:* 29–33
43 Laohapand T, Cattell V, Gabriel JRT. Monocyte infiltration in human glomerulonephritis: alpha-1-antitrypsin as a marker for mononuclear phagocytes in renal biopsies. *Clin Nephrol 1983; 19:* 309–316
44 Ferrario F, Castiglione A, Colasanti G et al. The detection of monocytes in human glomerulonephritis. *Kidney Int 1985; 28:* 513–519
45 Nolasco FEB, Cameron JS, Hartley B et al. Intraglomerular T cells and monocytes in nephritis: study with monoclonal antibodies. *Kidney Int 1987; 31:* 1160–1166
46 Holdsworth SR. Fc dependence of macrophage accumulation and subsequent injury in experimental glomerulonephritis. *J Immunol 1983; 130:* 735–739
47 Bhan AK, Collins AB, Schneeberger EE, McCluskey RT. A cell-mediated reaction against glomerular-bound immune complexes. *J Exp Med 1979; 150:* 1410–1420
48 Kreisberg JI, Wayne DB, Karnowsky MJ. Rapid and focal loss of negative charge associated with mononuclear cell infiltration early in nephrotoxic serum nephritis. *Kidney Int 1979; 16:* 290–300
49 Foidart JB, Hautier MD, Dechenne CA et al. Proliferative glomerulonephritis in rats: evidence that mononuclear phagocytes infiltrating the glomeruli stimulate the proliferation of endothelial and mesangial cells. *Eur J Clin Invest 1981; 11:* 91–104
50 Leibovich SJ, Ross R. A macrophage-dependent factor that stimulates the proliferation of fibroblasts in vitro. *Am J Pathol 1976; 84:* 501–513
51 Raij L, Keane WF, Osswald H, Michael AF. Mesangial function in ureteral obstruction in the rat: blockade of the efferent limb. *J Clin Invest 1979; 64:* 1204–1212
52 Latta H, Fligiel S. Mesangial fenestrations, sieving, filtration and flow. *Lab Invest 1985; 52:* 591–598
53 Sinniah R, Churg J. Effect of IgA deposits on the glomerular mesangium in Berger's disease. *Ultrastructure Pathol 1983; 4:* 9–22
54 Sinniah R, Ku G. Clinicopathologic correlations in IgA nephropathy. In Robinson RR, ed. *Nephrology. Proceedings of the IXth International Congress of Nephrology.* New York: Springer Verlag. 1984: 665–686
55 Hung TW. Basal lamina heterogeneity in the glomerular capillary tufts of human kidneys. *J Exp Med 1979; 149:* 1450–1459
56 Pfaffenbach G, Lamm ME, Gigli I. Activation of the guinea pig alternative complement pathway by mouse IgA immune complexes. *J Exp Med 1982; 155:* 231–247

57 Götze O, Muller-Eberhard HJ. The C3-activation system: an alternative pathway of complement activation. *J Exp Med 1971; 134:* 905–1085

58 Evans DJ, Williams DG, Peters DK et al. Glomerular deposition of properdin in Henoch-Schönlein syndrome and idiopathic focal nephritis. *Br Med J 1973; 3:* 326–328

59 Cotran RS. Editorial. Monocytes, proliferation and glomerulonephritis. *J Lab Clin Med 1978; 92:* 837–840

60 Warnke RA, Gatter KC, Brunangelo Falini DP et al. Diagnosis of human lymphoma with monoclonal antileukocyte antibodies. *N Engl J Med 1983; 309:* 1275–1281

61 Kindblom LG, Jacobsen GK, Jacobsen M. Immunohistochemical investigations of tumours of supposed fibroblastic histiocytic origin. *Hum Pathol 1982; 13:* 834–840

62 Kurtin PJ, Pinkus S. Leucocyte common antigen-A diagnostic discriminant between hematopoietic and non-hematopoietic neoplasms in paraffin sections using monoclonal antibodies: correlations in the immunollgic studies and ultrastructural localization. *Hum Pathol 1985; 16:* 353–365

63 Roholl PJM, Kleyne J, Pijpers HW, Van Unnik JAM. Comparative immunohistochemical investigation of markers for malignant histiocytes. *Hum Pathol 1985; 16:* 763–771

64 Stachura I, Stachura A, Murphy WM. Mononuclear cell subsets in patients with IgA nephropathy. *Lab Invest 1985; 52:* 65A

65 Emancipator SN, Gallo GR, Lamm ME. Animal models of IgA nephropathy. In Clarkson AR, ed. *IgA Nephropathy.* Boston: Martinus Nijhoff. 1987: 188–203

66 Egido J. Handling of soluble IgA-aggregates by the mononuclear phagocyte system in mice. *Immunology 1982; 46:* 1–7

67 Scharschmidt LA, Dunn MJ. Prostaglandin synthesis by rat glomerular mesangial cells in culture: effect of angiotensin II and arginine vasopressin. *J Clin Invest 1983; 71:* 1756–1764

68 Levy M, Beaufils H, Gubler MC, Habib R. Idiopathic recurrent macroscopic haematuria and mesangial IgA-IgG deposits in children (Berger's disease). *Clin Nephrol 1973; 1:* 63–69

69 McCoy RC, Abramowsky CR, Tisher CC. IgA nephropathy. *Am J Pathol 1974; 76:* 123–144

70 D'Amico G. Idiopathic mesangial IgA nephropathy. In Bertani T, Remuzzi G, eds. *Glomerular Injury 300 Years after Morgagni.* Milan: Wichtig Editore. 1983: 205–228

71 Finlayson G, Alexander R, Juncos L et al. Immunoglobulin A glomerulonephritis: a clinicopathologic study. *Lab Invest 1975; 32:* 140–148

72 Shigematsu H, Kobayashi Y, Tateno S et al. Ultrastructural glomerular loop abnormalities in IgA nephropathy. *Nephron 1982; 30:* 1–7

73 Ng WL, Chan KW, Yeung CK, Kwan S. Peripheral glomerular capillary wall lesions in IgA nephropathy and their implications. *Pathology 1984; 16:* 324–330

74 Brenner BM, Meyer TW, Hostetter TH. Dietary protein intake and the progressive nature of kidney disease: the role of haemodynamically mediated glomerular injury in the pathogenesis of progressive glomerular sclerosis in ageing, renal ablation and intrinsic renal disease. *N Engl J Med 1982; 307:* 652–659

75 Feiner HD, Cabili S, Baldwin DS et al. Intrarenal vascular sclerosis in IgA nephropathy. *Clin Nephrol 1982; 18:* 183–192

76 Feiner HD, Galvin S, Neelakantappa K et al. Vessel sclerosis and progression in IgA nephropathy. In D'Amico G, Minetti L, Ponticelli C, eds. *IgA Mesangial Nephropathy,* Basel: Karger. *Contr Nephrol 1984; 40:* 222–227

77 Hostetter TH, Olson JL, Rennke HG et al. Hyperfiltration in remnant nephrons: a potentially adverse response to renal ablation. *Am J Physiol 1981, 241:* F85

78 Olson JL, Hostetter TH, Rennke HG et al. Altered glomerular permeability and progressive sclerosis following extensive ablation of renal mass. *Kidney Int 1982; 22:* 112–126

79 Raij L, Azar S, Keane WF. Role of hypertension in progressive glomerular immune injury. *Hypertension 1985; 7:* 398–404

80 Raij L, Azar S, Keane WF. Mesangial immune injury: hypertension and progressive glomerular damage in Dahl rats. *Kidney Int 1984; 26:* 137–143

MESANGIAL OVERLOADING AND GLOMERULAR SCLEROSIS IN SOME PROTEINURIC MODELS OF EXPERIMENTAL GLOMERULOPATHY

J D Elema, J Grond

University of Groningen, Groningen, The Netherlands

In the past several investigators have suggested either implicitly or explicitly, that overloading of the mesangium with macromolecular substances might lead to glomerulosclerosis [1–6]. These ideas were based on experiments that showed that under circumstances of increased flow, pressure and filtration there was an increased incidence of glomerulosclerosis [1,2,5] and on the observation that in certain experimental forms of glomerulopathy there was an increased deposition of macromolecular tracers in the mesangium [3,4,6–8]. The studies of Farquhar and Palade [9] and their hypothesis on the 'unclogging' functions of the mesangium played an important rôle in the conceptualization of overload as a possible mechanism of mesangial damage. As ideas on the character of the mesangium have further evolved and because suggestions on the possible rôle of mesangial overload were presented in an almost casual and general way without further elaborating on the matter or precisely defining what was meant by 'overload' and 'glomerulosclerosis', it seems appropriate to briefly review the modern concept of structure and function of the mesangium, and to define more precisely what will be meant by 'overload' and 'glomerulosclerosis'.

Structure and function of the mesangium

The mesangium constitutes the central core of the glomerulus around which the capillary loops are arranged. The mesangial areas of the glomerular lobules convene at the glomerular stalk which is in direct continuity with the so-called lacis area and renin-secreting juxtaglomerular apparatus. Mesangial cells have many properties in common with smooth muscle cells [10–14]. In fact the mesangium in a way can be viewed as an incomplete muscular wall of the glomerular capillaries, their peripheral stretch being 'naked' for filtering purposes, their centrally facing part bordering on the smooth muscle like mesangium. Mesangial cells are surrounded by a matrix containing anionic sites [15] and permeated by a labyrinth of an anastomosing channel system that is constantly perfused by plasma and its constituents, as can be demonstrated by immune-electron microscopy [16,17]. Circulating macromolecular substances have free access to this mesangial labyrinth from the capillary lumina as these are covered by fenestrated endothelium without an intervening basement membrane.

It is not clear how plasma leaves the mesangium and several possibilities have been suggested [18]. Plasma eventually could reach the extraglomerular interstitial space and be drained via the lymphatics; it could re-enter the glomerular capillaries in 'downstream' areas or it could be filtered in the mesangial waist still leaving residues in the mesangium. There are indications that differences exist between rats and mice. The transport of some tracers through the mesangium is much quicker in mice than in rats with their rapid appearance in the lacis area [19].

It has long been assumed that the mesangium basically functions as an 'unclogging system' or 'vacuum cleaner' of the capillary filter. This assumption was based on the studies of Farquhar and Palade [9] and seemed to gain further support from the studies showing increased mesangial accumulation of tracers in experimental proteinura [3,4]. This interpretation seems unlikely, however, because it is not expected that under circumstances of increased leakage there would be a demand for mesangial cells to remove filter residues. Moreover hydrostatic pressure being transmitted equally to all sides of the capillary circumference would prevent macromolecules from moving from the filter area in the direction of the mesangium but rather would drive them downstream in the direction of the efferent pole.

Studies on glomerular haemodynamics and the regulation of tubuloglomerular feedback [20–22] indicate that the main function of the mesangium is the regulation of glomerular filtration by modulating the surface area of the capillary system available for filtration. In this context it is unclear what, if any, is the significance of the existence of the mesangial channel system which allows plasma macromolecules to penetrate and do harm in the mesangium. It is possible that this channel system is an integral part of the tubuloglomerular feedback loop providing glomerular plasma samples to the juxtaglomerular apparatus and macula densa [23].

Mesangial overloading

When either implicitly or explicitly referring to mesangial overloading as a possible cause of glomerulosclerosis it appears that authors were considering an adverse effect on the mesangium of the presence of an increased bulk or mass of macromolecular substances circulating normally in the blood. It was implied on the basis of the studies by Farquhar and Palade [9] that these macromolecules represented filtration residues arriving in the mesangium from the peripheral filtering area. As argued above this seems unlikely. Considering the structural composition of the mesangium it can be assumed that plasma constituents have direct access from the capillary lumen. Because important amounts of macromolecular substances (proteins, lipids) cannot be demonstrated in normal glomeruli, it appears that there is a rapid clearance of these macromolecules from the mesangium. Deposition of circulating macromolecular substances (overloading) may therefore theoretically result from increased plasma concentration, increased flow or pressure in the glomerulus, increased uptake by mesangial cells, inadequate digestion and decreased clearance or any combination of these. Experimental studies have shown that each of these possibilities may be involved [7,16,24–26]. Moreover in view of the presence of anionic charges in the mesangium it is also conceivable that changes in the charge of mesangial cells or circulating macromolecules may lead to deposition [27]. The way in which these possible changes in mesangial behaviour are brought about is not yet completely clear. It appears from studies of Keane and Raij [18] and Stein et al [29] that angiotensin II causes increased uptake and decreased clearance of exogenous tracers from the mesangium and that the renin-angiotensin system may be involved in changes in mesangial behaviour in aminonucleoside nephrosis [28]. Immune complex deposition in the mesangium may interfere with clearance of tracers [30], possibly caused by inflammatory mediators, and the presence of non-immune macromolecules may also interfere with clearance of tracers [31]. Thus from these studies there is ample reason to speculate that mesangial overloading of circulating macromolecules such as proteins and lipids may occur under different circumstances.

Glomerular sclerosis

Sclerosis means hardening of tissue and, by inference, scarring through deposition of intercellular matrix consisting of collagens and proteoglycans. These substances take a pinkish red colour with conventional histological stains using eosin (hyalin material) or stain black with silver impregnations (methenamin silver). Glomerular scarring like any other scar can be caused in many different ways. Some types of scarring can be linked to specific causes. Chronic ischaemia typically gives rise to shrinking of the glomerular tuft and obliteration of Bowman's space by collagenous material produced by epithelial cells, membranoproliferative glomerulonephritis results in matrix deposition in the mesangial areas and on the inner side of the glomerular basement membrane. Focal and segmental glomerulonephritis as in vasculitic syndromes gives rise to focal and segmental scarring or sclerosis. Both 'diabetic intercapillary sclerosis', and focal and segmental glomerular hyalinosis and sclerosis [32] have been linked with overload because increased glomerular pressures exist in experimental diabetes [33] and because focal and segmental glomerular hyalinosis and sclerosis-like lesions develop in experimental models in which 50% or more of kidney tissue has been removed [2,5], increased mesangial deposition of tracers takes place or increased glomerular pressure has been measured [5,7,8].

Focal and segmental glomerular hyalinosis and sclerosis as a possible example of glomerular sclerosis caused by mesangial overload

There are several proteinuric models by which focal and segmental glomerular hyalinosis and sclerosis can be induced in rats. The two most frequently used are those employing chronic aminonucleoside treatment [34] and those using reduction of kidney mass [5,35]. In both models increased deposition of macromolecular tracers has been demonstrated before lesions develop [4,7] and increased glomerular pressure and flow have been measured in remaining glomeruli of rats developing focal and segmental glomerular hyalinosis and sclerosis after unilateral nephrectomy and 5/6 infarction of the remaining kidney. On the basis of these last experiments the development of focal and segmental glomerular hyalinosis and sclerosis is considered to be related to increased glomerular pressure and flow [5]. Experience in the aminonucleoside model suggests that this is not necessarily the only possibility leading to this type of glomerulopathy [36]. In passing it should be mentioned that the way in which increased pressure or flow would induce mesangial changes has not been further specified. More recently focal and segmental glomerular hyalinosis and sclerosis lesions have also been induced in rats made nephrotic by an intravenous injection of adriamycin [37,38].

Although mesangial pathology is an integral part of the focal and segmental glomerular hyalinosis and sclerosis lesions it is not certain that it is the basis of the completely developed hyalinosis and sclerosis that also entails obliteration of capillary lumina with hyaline material, endothelial and epithelial degeneration and adhesion with Bowman's capsule. Some authors consider the changes of the visceral epithelial cells as the primary lesions [34,39], others also put emphasis on the endothelial changes and clotting phenomena [40]. It is also quite possible that all these changes have their origin in different pathogenetic mechanisms all operating under conditions that eventually lead to focal and segmental glomerular hyalinosis and sclerosis.

Is there any indication of mesangial overload in models of focal and segmental glomerular hyalinosis and sclerosis?

In order to test the hypothesis that increased deposition of macromolecules could lead to focal and segmental glomerular hyalinosis and sclerosis we looked at the mesangial ability to process intravenously injected colloidal carbon in experimental circumstances that eventually would lead to focal and segmental glomerular hyalinosis and sclerosis. In both chronic aminonucleoside nephrosis and in the unilateral nephrectomy model we demonstrated increased uptake of colloidal carbon by the mesangium [7,8].

On the other hand induction of nephrosis of comparable severity by an intravenous injection of adriamycin did not lead to focal and segmental glomerular hyalinosis and sclerosis and under these circumstances there was no indication of increased uptake of tracer molecules [41]. Our experience with adriamycin treatment seems to be in contradiction with that of others [37,42]. It should be realized, however, that in these experiments higher doses of adriamycin were used resulting in a much more severe nephrosis and accompanying severe interstitial disease that may be indirectly responsible for the glomerular lesions [43,44]. It was also found that contrary to Wistar strain rats, PVG rats were resistant to the effect of unilateral nephrectomy [45] and less sensitive to the effect of chronic aminonucleoside treatment [46] as far as the development of focal and segmental glomerular hyalinosis and sclerosis is concerned. Studies of the mesangial handling of colloidal carbon showed that this was normal under these circumstances in PVG rats. Such observations at least are compatible with the suggestion that mesangial overloading as deduced from the functional studies mentioned above, precedes the development of focal and segmental glomerular hyalinosis and sclerosis.

However in order to further substantiate a possible relationship between mesangial overload and the development of focal and segmental glomerular hyalinosis and sclerosis (or any other type of glomerular damage) it is also necessary to show that such damage develops in the same area as where the presumed overloading takes place. To investigate this problem, Wistar rats were given a series of three intravenous injections of colloidal carbon shortly after they had been started on a regimen of chronic treatment with aminonucleoside or after they underwent unilateral nephrectomy. It could be expected from earlier experience that both experimental protocols eventually would lead to focal and segmental glomerular hyalinosis and sclerosis. As colloidal carbon is undigestible and disappears very slowly from the mesangium it could also be expected that the tracers would still be detectable at the end of the experiment and their relationship with focal and segmental glomerular hyalinosis and sclerosis lesions, that then would have developed, determined. In both experimental protocols a strong relationship was found between the localization of colloidal carbon and that of the focal and segmental glomerular hyalinosis and sclerosis lesions. As there was no difference in incidence of focal and segmental glomerular hyalinosis and sclerosis lesions in rats with the same experimental protocol but not treated with colloidal carbon it was concluded that colloidal carbon by itself did not induce focal and segmental glomerular hyalinosis and sclerosis and that therefore these lesions apparently developed in areas where already early in the course of the experiment increased deposition of the exogenous tracer (colloidal carbon) and presumably also of endogenous macromolecules took place [7,8]. These experiments provide a strong argument in favour of the hypothesis, that mesangial overloading (with macromolecules) may lead to focal and segmental glomerular hyalinosis and sclerosis or at least to the mesangial changes that are part of it.

What macromolecules could be involved?

Any suggestion on the nature of macromolecules involved in mesangial overloading can only be speculative. There are some restrictions, however. These macromolecules should be normally circulating substances and it should be possible to demonstrate their presence not only in the lesions, but also in the mesangium early in the experiment, before any appreciable amount of scarring has taken place.

The presence of immunoglobulins and complement in glomeruli of patients with a wide range of glomerular diseases has led to speculations on their immune nature. As considerable amounts of lipid are often present in focal and segmental glomerular hyalinosis and sclerosis lesions and because the mesangium has many properties in common with the medial wall of arterioles we have speculated on a possible rôle of lipids in the pathogenesis of focal and segmental glomerular hyalinosis and sclerosis [41,47]. Grond et al [41,46] have shown the presence of increased amounts of endogenous lipids in the mesangial areas of glomeruli in rats under experimental conditions that eventually lead to focal and segmental glomerular hyalinosis and sclerosis, but not in those models that do not lead to focal and segmental glomerular hyalinosis and sclerosis. Studies by Silva et al [48] and Kasiske et al [49] have demonstrated that the development of focal and segmental glomerular hyalinosis and sclerosis can be prevented by lipid lowering regimens in the remnant kidney model, without affecting intraglomerular pressure [50]. It is intriguing that cholesterol, the lipid preferentially found in focal and segmental glomerular hyalinosis and sclerosis lesions both in men and in rats [51], is mainly carried in high density lipoproteins in the rat. Further studies on the character and properties of the rat apoproteins are needed. Although the lipid hypothesis [52] seems attractive as a part of a possible pathogenesis of focal and segmental glomerular hyalinosis and sclerosis it is clear from our experience in the adriamycin model that hyperlipaemia by itself does not necessarily lead to focal and segmental glomerular hyalinosis and sclerosis [41]; apparently this only takes place when the mesangium itself is also changed in its behaviour regarding macromolecular traffic. It cannot be excluded that much higher levels of serum lipids than encountered in our experiments may lead to focal and segmental glomerular hyalinosis and sclerosis even in the face of a normal mesangial behaviour.

Interactions between lipids and the mesangium

To further substantiate any claim that mesangial lipid overloading may play an important rôle in the development of glomerulosclerosis and especially focal and segmental glomerular hyalinosis and sclerosis, it is necessary to demonstrate an adverse effect of lipids on the mesangial cell. For this in vitro studies on the interaction between lipoproteins and mesangial cells are needed. Although so far these are lacking, a parallel can be drawn with the numerous studies performed in the course of research on atherosclerosis. This parallelism is based on the similarities between mesangial cells and smooth muscle cells [10–14, 53,54] and on the importance of interaction between lipids and smooth muscle cells in the development of atherosclerosis [55–57]. It is obvious from these studies that lipoproteins are able to stimulate proliferation [58,59] of smooth muscle cells and their synthesis and secretion of collagens and proteoglycans [60,61]. Mesangial cells have also been shown to synthesize and secrete both collagens, glycoproteins and proteoglycans in a manner comparable to that of smooth muscle cells [62,63] and the formation of 'hillocks' in mesangial cell cultures [64] may even represent the glomerular pendant of the 'fibrous plaque' of atherosclerosis. Further research on the behaviour of mesangial cells under different in vitro conditions along the lines earlier used for atherosclerosis research should be fruitful.

Conclusion

Our tentative conclusions are depicted in Figure 1. Experimental studies support the concept of mesangial overload as a possible pathway for glomerulosclerosis. Lipids represent a likely candidate for the offending macromolecular substance involved in this mechanism. The smooth muscle cell-like character of the mesangial cells and the hyperlipaemia often encountered in chronic renal disease suggests some parallelism with the pathogenesis of atherosclerosis. It is likely that changes in the mesangial behaviour concerning the traffic of macromolecules are also important. Such changes might be induced by widely different mechanisms, such as increased local pressure (Pcap), activation of the renin-angiotensin system (RAS) and other humoral systems, toxic mechanisms, immunological mechanisms and so on. Basically, therefore, glomerulosclerosis caused by mesangial overload would be a multifactorial process with many risk factors working through hyperlipaemia and disturbed mesangial function.

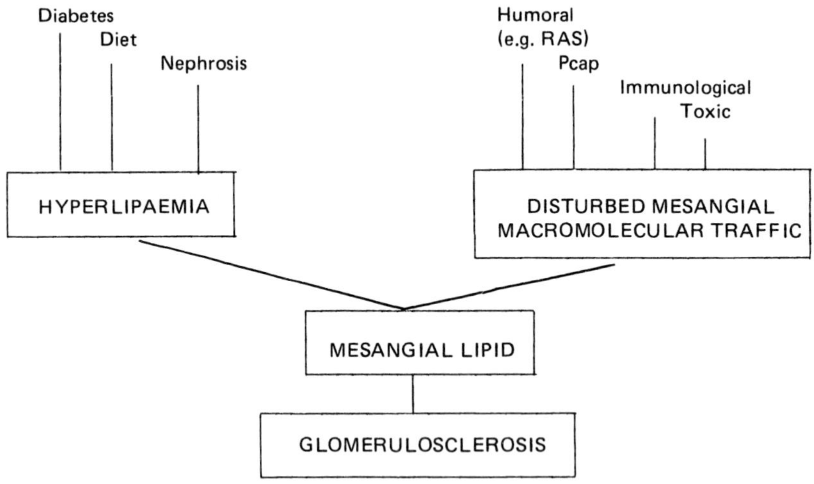

Figure 1

Acknowledgment

This work was supported by the Nier Stichting Nederland.

References

1 Elema JD, Arends A. Functional overload as a possible cause for non-immune glomerular damage. Effect of nephrectomy and irradiation of the contralateral kidney. *J Pathol 1971; 103 (Abstract):* 21

2 Elema JD, Koudstaal J, Lamberts HB, Arends A. Spontaneous glomerulosclerosis in the rat. Effect of nephrectomy and irradiation of the contralateral kidney. *Arch Pathol 1971; 91:* 418–425

3 Mauer SM, Fish AJ, Day NK, Michael AF. The glomerular mesangium. II. Studies of macromolecular uptake in nephrotoxic nephritis in rats. *J Clin Invest 1974; 53:* 431–439

4 Hoyer JR, Elema JD, Vernier RL. Unilateral renal disease in the rat. II. Glomerular mesangial uptake of colloidal carbon in unilateral amino-nucleoside nephrosis and nephrotoxic serum nephritis. *Lab Invest 1976; 34:* 250–255

5 Hostetter TH, Olson JL, Rennke HG et al. Hyperfiltration in remnant nephrons: a potentially adverse response to renal ablation. *Am J Physiol 1981; 241:* F85–F93

6 Foellmer HG, Sterzel RB, Kashgarian M. Progressive glomerular sclerosis in experimental antiglomerular basement membrane glomerulonephritis. *Am J Kidney Dis 1986; 7:* 5–11

7 Grond J, Schilthuis MS, Koudstaal J, Elema JD. Mesangial function and glomerulosclerosis in rats after unilateral nephrectomy. *Kidney Int 1982; 22:* 338–343

8 Grond J, Koudstaal J, Elema JD. Mesangial functions and glomerulosclerosis in rats with aminonucleoside nephrosis. *Kidney Int 1985; 27:* 405–410

9 Farquhar MG, Palade GE. Functional evidence of the existence of a third cell type in the renal glomerulus. Pathocytosis of filtration residues by a distinct 'third' cell. *J Cell Biol 1962; 13:* 55–87

10 Michielsen P, Creemers J. The structure and function of the glomerular mesangium. In Dalton AJ, Haguenau F, eds. *Ultrastructure of the Kidney.* New York: Academic Press. 1967: 57–72

11 Kazimierczak J. Histochemical observations on the developing glomerulus and juxtaglomerulus apparatus. *Acta Pathol Microbiol Scand 1970; 78A:* 401–413

12 Scheinman JI, Fish AJ, Brown DM, Michael AF. Human glomerular smooth muscle (mesangial) cells in culture. *Lab Invest 1976; 34:* 150–158

13 Osborne MJ, Droz B, Meyer M, Morel F. Angiotensin II: renal localization in glomerular mesangial cells by autoradiography. *Kidney Int 1975; 8:* 245–254

14 Hornych H, Beaufils M, Richet G. The effect of exogenous angiotensin on superficial and deep glomeruli in the rat. *Kidney Int 1972; 2:* 336–343

15 Grond J, Elema JD. Localization and distribution of anionic charges in the glomerular mesangium of normal and nephrotic rats. *Virchows Arch [Cell Pathol] 1985; 48:* 135–143

16 Grond J, Elema JD. Glomerular mesangium. Analysis of the increased activity observed in experimental acute aminonucleoside nephrosis in the rat. *Lab Invest 1981; 45:* 400–409

17 Lee S, Vernier RL. Immuno electron microscopy of the glomerular mesangial uptake and transport of aggregated human albumin in the mouse. *Lab Invest 1980; 42:* 44–58

18 Latta H, Fligiel S. Mesangial fenestrations, sieving, filtration, and flow. *Lab Invest 1985; 52:* 591–598

19 Suurmeyer AJH, Grond J, Elema JD. The glomerular mesangium: a comparative study of mesangial handling of iron dextran complex and endogenous IgG in mice and rats. *Virchows Arch [Cell Pathol] 1981; 37:* 357–368

20 Schor N, Ichikawa I, Brenner BM. Mechanisms of action of various hormones and vasoactive substances on glomerular ultrafiltration in the rat. *Kidney Int 1981; 20:* 442–451

21 Dworkin LD, Ichikawa I, Brenner BM. Hormonal modulation of glomerular function. *Am J Physiol 1983; 244:* F95–F104

22 Thurau K, Boylan JW. The unexpected logic of oligura in acute renal failure. *Am J Med 1976; 61:* 308–315

23 Rosivall L, Taugner R. The morphological basis of fluid balance in the interstitium of the juxtaglomerular apparatus. *Cell Tissue Res 1986; 243:* 525–533

24 Grond J, Daha MR, Elema JD. Glomerular mesangial uptake of intravenously injected colloidal carbon in the rat determined by an image analyzing method: lack of influence of platelet aggregation or complement activation. *Virchows Arch [Cell Pathol] 1980; 33:* 281–291

25 Sterzel RB, Krause PH, Kregeler M. Experimental changes in the mesangial capacity to handle glomerular immune deposits in rats. *Contrib Nephrol 1976; 2:* 66–75

26 Raij L, Keane WF, Osswald H, Michael AF. Mesangial function in ureteral obstruction in the rat. *J Clin Invest 1979; 64:* 1204–1212

27 Batsford SR, Weghaupt R, Takamiya H, Vogt A. Studies in the mesangial handling of protein antigens: influence of size, charge and biologic activity. *Nephron 1985; 41:* 146–151

28 Keane WF, Raij L. Relationship among altered glomerular barrier permselectivity, angiotensin II, and mesangial uptake of macromolecules. *Lab Invest 1985; 52:* 599–604

29 Stein HD, Feddergreen W, Kashgarian M, Sterzel RB. Role of angiotensin II induced renal function changes in mesangial deposition of exogenous ferritin in rats. *Lab Invest 1983; 49:* 270–280

30 Keane WF, Raij L. Impaired mesangial clearance of macromolecules in rats with chronic mesangial ferritin-antiferritin immune-complex deposition. *Lab Invest 1980; 43:* 500–508

31 Mauer SM, Numata M, Sutherland DER. The effects of polyvinyl alcohol on the uptake and processing of colloidal carbon by the glomerular mesangium in rats. *Lab Invest 1979; 41:* 475–482

32 Habib R. Focal glomerular sclerosis. *Kidney Int 1973; 4:* 355–361

33 Hostetter TH. Pathogenesis of diabetic nephropathy. In Mitch WE, Brenner BM, Stein JD, eds. *The Progressive Nature of Renal Disease.* New York: Churchill Livingstone. 1986: 149–166

34 Glaser RJ, Velosa JA, Michael AF. Experimental model of focal sclerosis. I. Relationship to protein excretion in aminonucleoside nephrosis. *Lab Invest 1977; 36:* 519–527

35 Elema JD, Arends A. Focal and segmental glomerular hyalinosis and sclerosis in the rat. *Lab Invest 1975; 33:* 554–561

36 Bohrer MP, Baylis C, Robertson CR, Brenner BM. Mechanism of the puromycin induced defects in the transglomerular passage of water and macromolecules. *J Clin Invest 1977; 60:* 152–161

37 Bertani T, Poggi A, Pozzoni R et al. Adriamycin induced nephrotic syndrome in rats: sequence of pathologic events. *Lab Invest 1982; 46:* 16–23

38 Bertani T, Rocchi G, Mecca G et al. Adriamycin-induced chronic proteinuria: a new model of glomerular focal sclerosis. *Kidney Int 1983; 23 (Abstract):* 192

39 Schwartz MM, Lewis EJ, Focal segmental glomerular sclerosis: the cellular lesion. *Kidney Int 1985; 28:* 968–974

40 Rennke HG. Structural alterations associated with glomerular hyperfiltration. In Mitch WF, Brenner BM, Stein JH, eds. *The Progressive Nature of Renal Disease.* New York: Churchill Livingstone. 1986: 111–131

41 Grond J, Weening JJ, Elema JD. Glomerular sclerosis in nephrotic rats. Comparison of the long term effects of adriamycin and aminonucleoside. *Lab Invest 1984; 51:* 227–285

42 Okuda S, Oh Y, Tsuruda H et al. Adriamycin induced nephropathy as a model of chronic progressive glomerular disease. *Kidney Int 1986; 29:* 502–510

43 Bertaini T, Cutillo F, Zoja C et al. Tubulo-interstitial lesions mediate renal damage in adriamycin glomerulopathy. *Kidney Int 1986; 30:* 488–496

44 Grond J, Weening JJ, van Goor H, Elema JD. The application of puromycin aminonucleoside and adriamycin to induce chronic renal failure in the rat. *Contrib Nephrol:* In press

45 Grond J, Beukers JJB, Schilthuis MS et al. Analysis of renal structural and functional features in two rat strains with a different susceptibility to glomerular sclerosis. *Lab Invest 1986; 54:* 77–83

46 Grond J, Muller EW, Van Goor H et al. Differences in puromycin aminonucleoside nephrosis in two rat strains. Submitted for publication

47 Elema JD, Schilthuis MS, Grond J, V d Hem GK. La pathogenie de la sclerose focale. *Nephrologie 1982; 3:* 59–64

48 Silva FG, David K, Edwards G, Pirani CL. Experimental focal glomerulosclerosis (GS): effects of hyperlipidemia and halofenate. *Kidney Int 1979; 16 (Abstract):* 789

49 Kasiske BL, O'Donnell MP, Daniels F, Keane WF. The lipid lowering agent clofibric acid ameliorates renal injury in the 5/6 nephrectomy model of chronic renal failure. *Clin Res 1985; 33 (Abstract):* 488A

50 O'Donnell MP, Kasiske BL, Daniels FX, Keane WF. Clofibric acid (CA) does not affect glomerular hemodynamics in rats with 5/6 nephrectomy (NX). *Kidney Int 1986; 29 (Abstract):* 324

51 Grond J, Van Goor H, Erkelens DW, Elema JD. Glomerular sclerotic lesions in the rat. Histochemical analysis of their macromolecular and cellular composition. *Virchows Arch [Cell Pathol] 1986; 51:* 521–534

52 Moorhead JF, El-Nahas M, Chan MK, Varghese Z. Lipid nephrotoxicity in chronic progressive glomerular and tubulo-interstitial disease. *Lancet 1982; ii:* 1309–1311

53 Michael AF, Keane WF, Raij L et al. The glomerular mesangium. *Kidney Int 1980; 17:* 141–154

54 Kashgarian M. Mesangium and glomerular disease. *Lab Invest 1985; 52:* 569–571

55 Ross R, Wight ThN, Strandness E, Thiele B. Human atherosclerosis. I. Cell constitution and characteristics of advanced lesions of the superficial femoral artery. *Am J Pathol 1984; 114:* 79–93

56 Ross R. The pathogenesis of atherosclerosis – an update. *N Engl J Med 1986; 314:* 488–500

57 Goldstein JL, Anderson RGW, Buja LM et al. Overloading human aortic smooth muscle cells with low density lipoprotein-cholesteryl esters reproduces features of atherosclerosis in vitro. *J Clin Invest 1977, 59:* 1196–1202

58 Fisher-Dzoga K, Fraser R, Wissler RW. Stimulation of proliferation in stationary primary cultures of monkey and rabbit aortic smooth muscle cells. I. Effects of lipoprotein fractions of hyperlipemic serum and lymph. *Exp Mol Pathol 1976; 24:* 346–359

59 Chamley-Campbell JH, Campbell GR, Ross R. Phenotype-dependent response of cultured aortic smooth muscle to serum mitogens. *J Cell Biol 1981; 89:* 379–383

60 Ronnemaa T, Doherty NS. Effect of serum and liver extracts from hypercholesterolemic rats on the synthesis of collagen by isolated aortas and cultured aortic smooth muscle cells. *Atherosclerosis 1977; 26:* 261–272

61 Burke JM, Ross R. Synthesis of connective tissue macromolecules by smooth muscle. *Int Rev Connect Tissue Res 1979; 8:* 119–157

62 Striker GE, Killen PD, Farin FM et al. Mesangial matrix and inflammatory cells. *Proc 8th Int Congr Nephrol.* Athens 1981: 879–887

63 Striker GE, Striker LJ. Biology of disease: glomerular cell culture. *Lab Invest 1985; 53:* 122–131

64 Sterzel RB, Lovett DH, Foellmer HG et al. Mesangial cell hillocks. Nodular foci of exaggerated growth of cells and matrix in prolonged culture. *Am J Pathol 1986; 125:* 130–140

MECHANISMS OF TUBULO-INTERSTITIAL NEPHRITIS

ANATOMY OF THE RENAL INTERSTITIUM

C Craig Tisher, Kirsten M Madsen

University of Florida College of Medicine, Gainesville, Florida, USA

Introduction

Investigations designed to elucidate the aetiology and pathogenesis of the many forms of tubulo-interstitial nephritis are legion. However, anatomical studies directed toward improving our understanding of the structural and functional relationships of the several components of the renal interstitium are relatively sparse.

General features

The renal interstitium is composed of insterstitial cells and a loose, flocculent extracellular matrix material consisting of sulphated and non-sulphated glucosaminoglycans [1]. There is very little interstitial tissue in the cortex and the tubules and capillaries are often directly opposed to each other. Morphometric studies have demonstrated that the interstitium constitutes 7% to 9% of the cortical volume in the rat [2,3]. It has been found that three of the 7% represents the interstitial cells and the remaining 4%, the extracellular space [1]. Estimates of the relative amount of renal cortical interstitial tissue have also been published for the human kidney. Dunnill and Halley [4] reported a value of 11.7± 5.5% of kidneys from patients less than 36 years of age and 15.7±3.0% in older patients. Bohle et al [5] found a mean value of 9% with a range of 5 to 11% in 20 kidneys. The age of the patients was not given. Hestbech et al [6] reported similar values with a mean of 13.6% and a range of 6.3 to 21.3% in 13 kidneys obtained from patients who ranged in age from 33 to 65 years. Kappel and Olsen [7] evaluated 54 donor kidneys that were unsuitable for transplantation and reported a range of 7.1 to 37.1% that was found to be age-dependent. In this latter series the age range was nine to 70 years.

In the medulla there is a gradual increase in the volume of the interstitium from 10 to 20% of the tissue in the outer medulla to approximately 30 to 40% at the papillary tip in both the rat and the rabbit [3,8]. The volume of the interstitium has also been estimated from the distribution volume of inulin and similar extracellular markers. The interstitial volume in the rat kidney constituted approximately 13% of the total kidney volume, whereas the value was 17.5% in the rabbit [9].

CORTICAL INTERSTITIUM

The interstitium in the cortex is compartmentalized. Several investigators have divided the cortical interstitium into a wide interstitial space located between two or more adjacent renal tubules and a narrow or slit-like interstitial space located between the basement membrane of a single tubule and the adjacent peritubular capillary [2,10,11] (Figure 1). Whether such a division has any functional significance is unknown; however, it is of interest that approximately two-thirds of the total peritubular capillary wall faces the narrow compartment and this portion of the vessel wall is fenestrated [2]. This relationship might facilitate the control of fluid reabsorption across the basolateral membrane of the proximal tubule by Starling forces.

Cortical interstitial cells

In the cortex two types of interstitial cells have been described, one that resembles a fibroblast (type 1 cortical interstitial cell) (Figure 2) and another less common mononuclear or lymphocyte-like cell (type 2 cortical interstitial cell) [1,10]. The type 1 cells are positioned between the basement membranes of adjacent tubules and peritubular capillaries. They have an irregular stellate appearance and contain a well-developed rough- and smooth-surfaced endoplasmic reticulum. The nucleus of these cells is often irregular in shape. Type 2 cells are generally round, the cytoplasm is sparse and cell organelles are few in number (Figure 3). The interstitial space contains a very loose flocculent material of low density and small bundles of collagen fibrils. Immunocytochemical staining of immature and mature human kidney has revealed the presence of types I and III collagen and fibronectin in the interstitium of the cortex [12]. The presence of type V collagen has been described in the cortical interstitium of rat kidney [13].

Function

The function of the two types of interstitial cells in the cortex is poorly understood. It is quite likely, however, that the type 1 cells are responsible for the secretion of collagen and reticular fibrils [14]. Phagocytic properties have also been described for these cells [14]. The origin and function of type 2 cells is unknown. They resemble lymphocytes and could be either blood-derived or represent an early cell of the monocyte series [1].

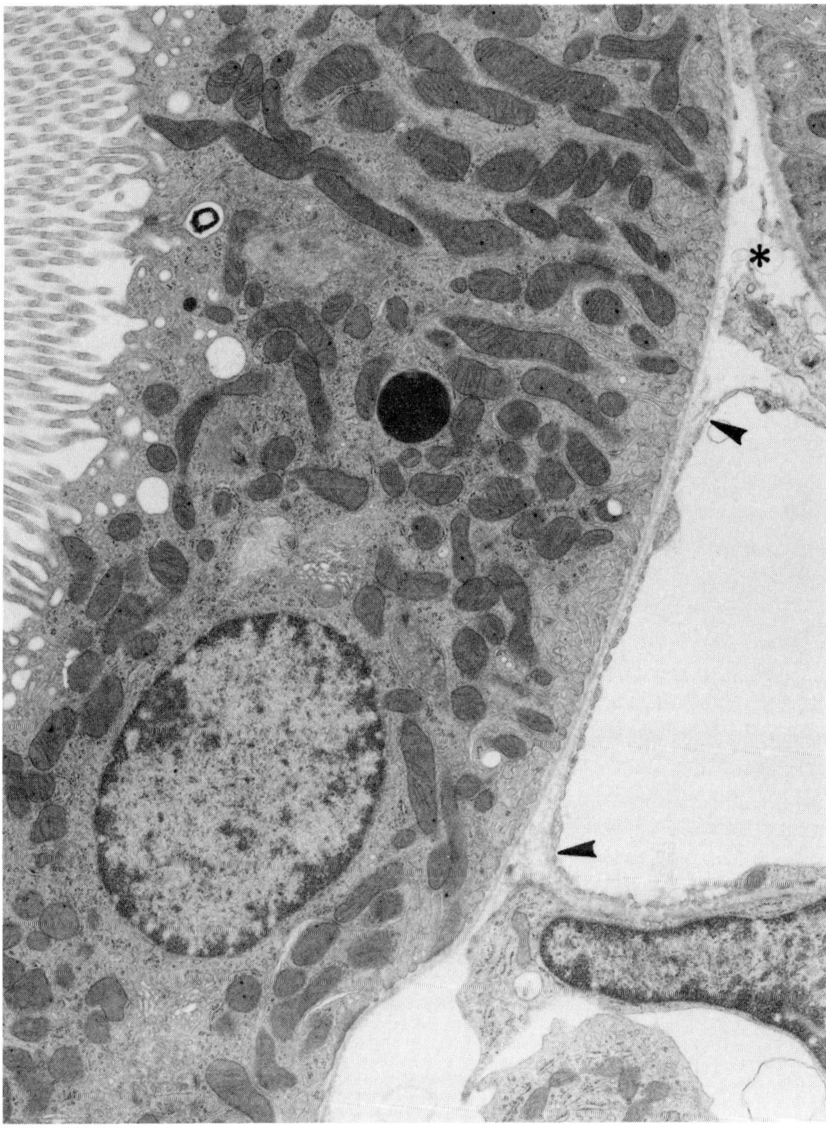

Figure 1. Low magnification electronmicrograph of rat renal cortex illustrating interstitial compartment. The wide interstitial compartment is depicted between two tubules (asterisk). The narrow interstitial compartment lies between the arrowheads and is in contact with the basement membrane of the proximal tubule on the left and the pertitubular capillary lined by fenestrated epithelium on the right. Portions of two type 1 interstitial cells are present at the lower right of the illustration. × 6,800

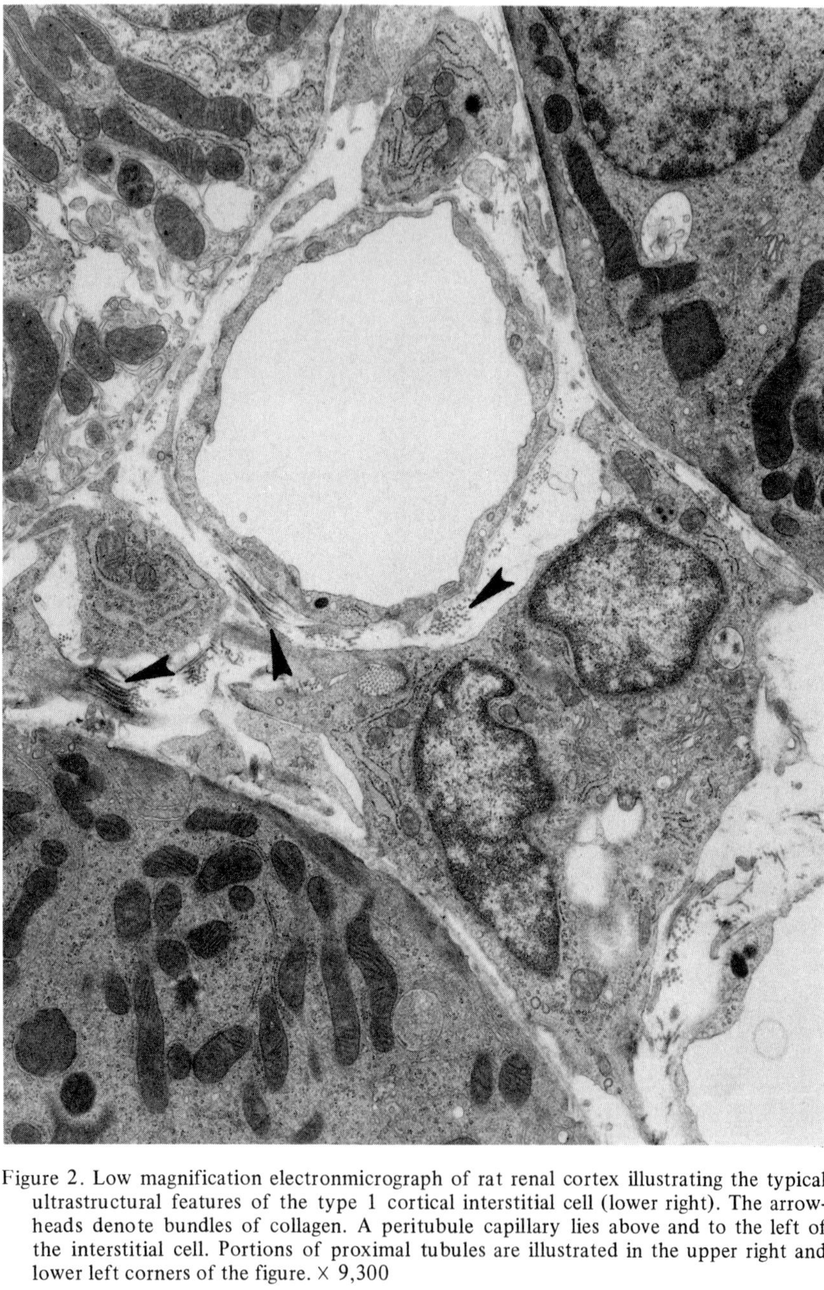

Figure 2. Low magnification electronmicrograph of rat renal cortex illustrating the typical ultrastructural features of the type 1 cortical interstitial cell (lower right). The arrowheads denote bundles of collagen. A peritubule capillary lies above and to the left of the interstitial cell. Portions of proximal tubules are illustrated in the upper right and lower left corners of the figure. × 9,300

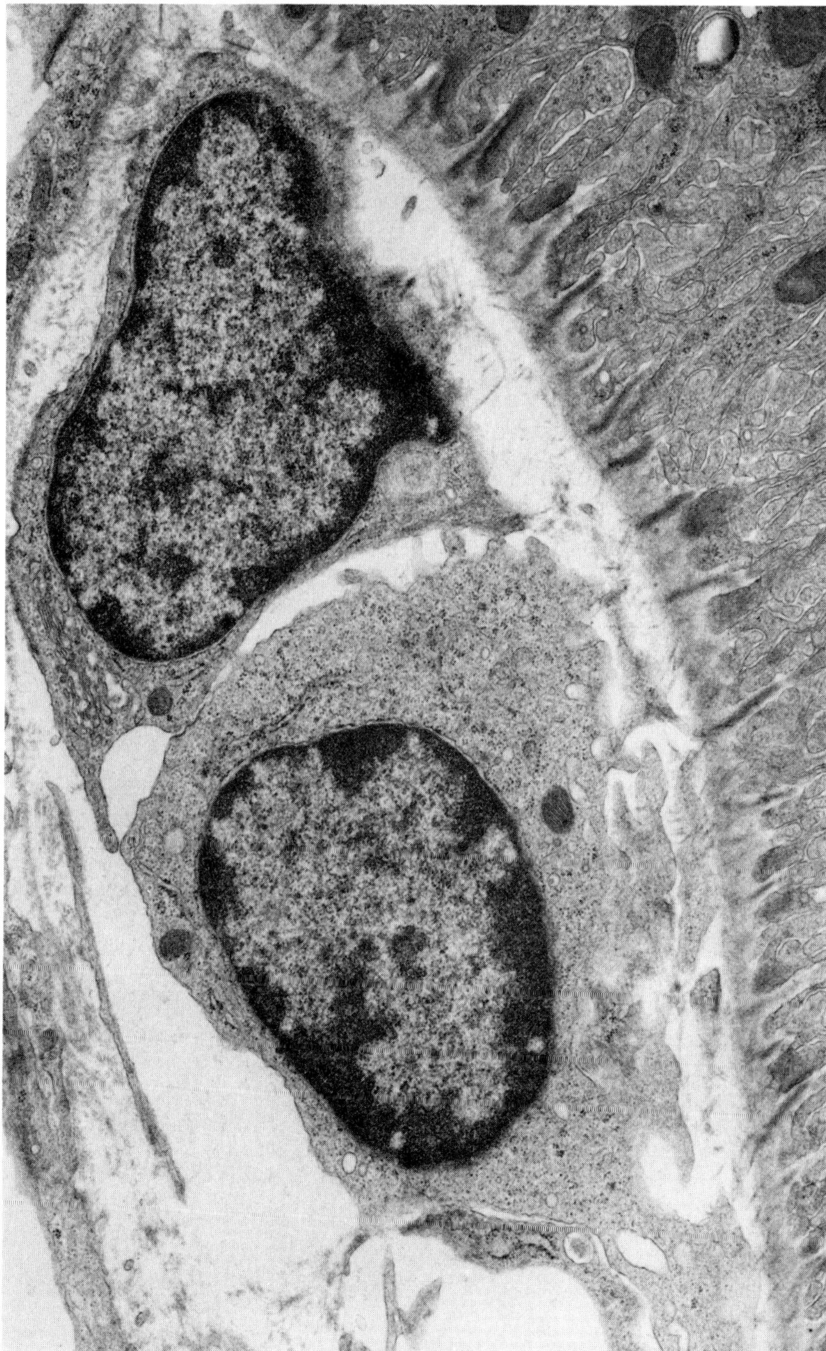

Figure 3. Electronmicrograph of type 2 cortical interstitial cell (lower centre). The nucleus is round, the cytoplasm is sparse and the cell organelles are few in number. × 14,600

Medullary interstitial cells

In a detailed study of the rat renal medulla, Bohman [11] described three different types of interstitial cells. Type 1 cells are the lipid-containing interstitial cells that are quite prominent in the renal medulla. Except for the presence of the lipid droplets, structurally these cells resemble the type 1 cells in the cortex. They are present throughout the inner medulla, and are also found in the inner

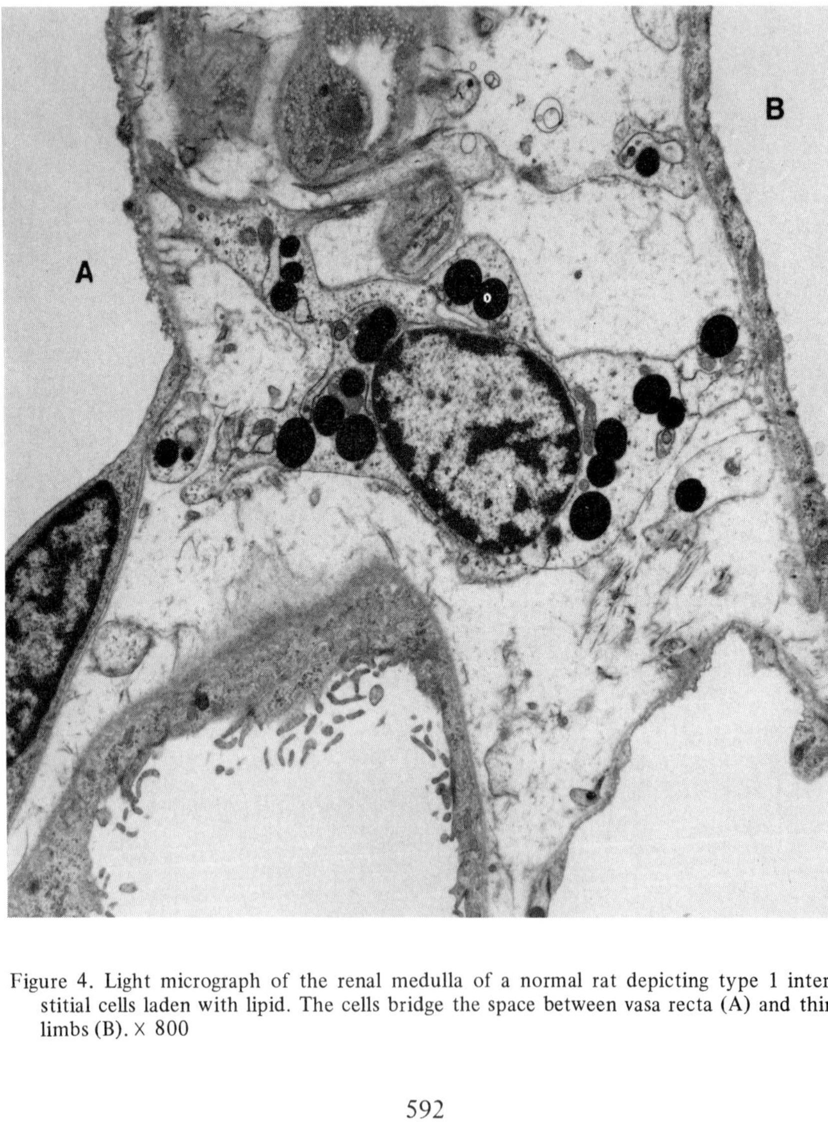

Figure 4. Light micrograph of the renal medulla of a normal rat depicting type 1 interstitial cells laden with lipid. The cells bridge the space between vasa recta (A) and thin limbs (B). × 800

stripe of the outer medulla. The type 2 medullary interstitial cell is a lymphocyte-like cell that is virtually identical to the mononuclear cell (type 2 interstitial cell) described in the cortex. It is present in the outer medulla and in the outer part of the inner medulla. The type 2 cell is free of lipid droplets, but lysosome-like bodies are often observed. Not infrequently type 2 cells are found together with type 1 cells. The type 3 cell is a pericyte that is located in the outer medulla and the outer portion of the inner medulla. It is closely related to the descending vasa recta where it is found between two leaflets of the basement membrane. These three types of interstitial cells have been described also in the rabbit [10].

In all species studied so far including the rat and the rabbit, most interstitial cells in the inner medulla are the lipid-containing type 1 renomedullary interstitial cells [15]. The cells have an irregular shape with long cytoplasmic projections which gives them a star-shaped appearance. The cells are often arranged between the loops of Henle and vasa recta in rows with their long axis perpendicular to that of adjacent tubules and vessels, thus resembling the rungs of a ladder [16] (Figure 4). The elongated cell processes are in close contact with thin limbs of Henle and the vasa recta, but direct contact with collecting ducts is observed only rarely. Often a single cell may be in contact with several vessels and thin limbs [11]. The long cytoplasmic processes from different cells are often connected by specialized cell junctions. Freeze fracture studies have demonstrated that these junctions vary in both size and shape, and they contain elements of both tight junctions and gap junctions [17]. Majack and Larsen [18] demonstrated the presence of gap junctions, tight junctions and intermediate junctions in the interstitial cells of the rat inner medulla using a combination of conventional transmission and freeze-fracture electronmicroscopy. Bicellular gap junctions occurred most frequently between elongated cell processes. So-called 'reflexive' gap junctions, formed by interactions between the plasma membrane of the same cell, were also present but varied greatly in their frequency.

Several investigators have described the ultrastructure of the type 1 medullary interstitial cells in both the rat [11,19,20] and rabbit [10,15] as well as the human kidney [21]. They are characterized by the presence of numerous lipid inclusions or droplets in the cytoplasm that vary considerably in both size and number (Figure 5). An average diameter of 0.4 to 0.5μm has been reported in the rat, but profiles with a diameter of up to 1μm were often observed [22]. In other species including the rabbit the lipid droplets are smaller [15]. They have a very homogeneous content and are without a limiting membrane, but are often surrounded by whorls of smooth cytomembranes with a thickness of 6 to 7nm. The cells contain large amounts of rough endoplasmic reticulum that often is continuous with elements of the smooth cytoplasmic membranes. Bohman [11] has stressed that the presence of a widely dilated perinuclear cisternae is indicative of poor fixation. Mitochondria are sparse and scattered randomly in the cytoplasm. A small number of lysosomes are present, but

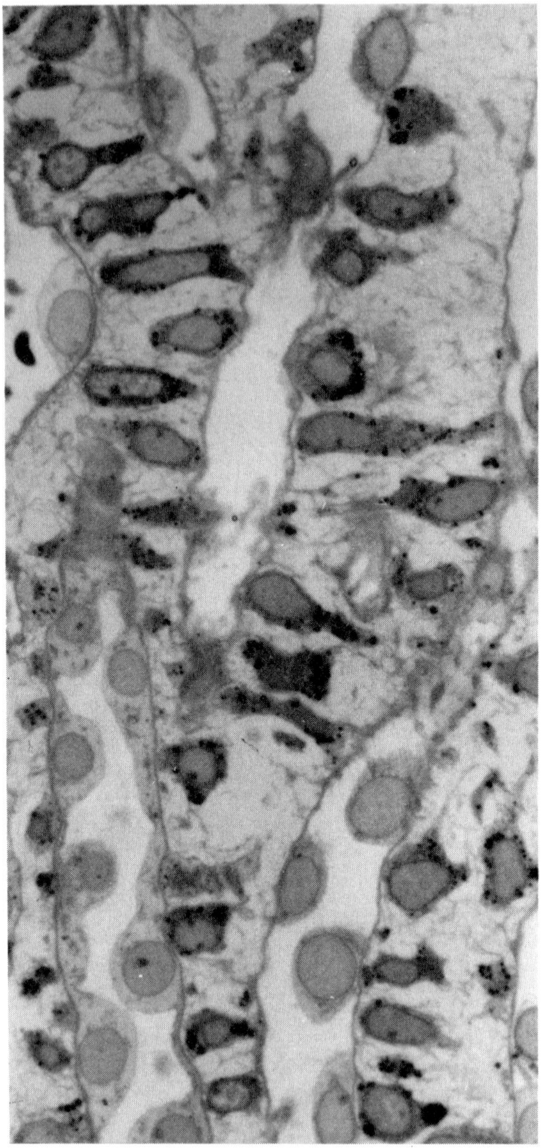

Figure 5. Electronmicrograph illustrating the ultrastructure of type 1 renal interstitial cell. Non-membrane-bound lipid droplets are present throughout the cytoplasm. Cell processes extend from the vasa recta on the left to the thin limb on the right. × 6,400

endocytic vacuoles are sparse. However, interstitial cells are capable of endocytosis of particulate material. Cavallo [23] has reported that in the rat the type 1 interstitial cells in the inner medulla contain endogenous peroxidase activity in the endoplasmic reticulum, the perinuclear cisterna and in small cytoplasmic vesicles. In contrast, no activity was observed in interstitial cells in the outer medulla or the cortex. Thus, type 1 interstitial cells in the cortex and medulla vary not only in their lipid content, but also in endogenous peroxidase activity. The functional significance of these observations remains unexplained.

An unusual type of cylindrical body measuring 0.1 to 0.2μm in diameter and up to 11μm in length has been described in the type 1 interstitial cells [1,24–26]. These structures were observed originally in dehydrated rats and were believed to represent a response to severe dehydration [24]. However, subsequent studies have demonstrated their presence under normal conditions [26]. They are believed to be derived from the endoplasmic reticulum. The wall of the cylinders consists of two triple-layered membranes, each measuring 6nm in thickness, and connections between the walls and the membranes of the endoplasmic reticulum have been observed [24]. The functional significance of these cylindrical structures remains unknown.

The structure of the type 2 medullary interstitial cells resembles that of type 2 cortical interstitial cells. It has been suggested they may be one and the same cell [1]. Type 3 medullary interstitial cells are typical pericytes and are located within the wall of the descending vasa recta. There they are surrounded by basement membrane material, and exhibit the usual complement of subcellular organelles.

The number and size of the lipid inclusions in the type 1 interstitial cells vary considerably depending on the physiological state of the animal [27,28] and the species of animal under investigation [15]. In the rat lipid droplets constitute 2 to 4% of the interstitial cell volume, and the volume depends largely on the physiological state of the animal [22]. It was reported originally that the lipid droplets were decreased in both size and number following 24 hours of dehydration [28]. However, Bohman and Jensen [22] could not confirm these findings in a more recent study. Those investigators examined the interstitial cells in both dehydrated and water-loaded rats and found no changes in the size or number of the lipid droplets following 24 hours of dehydration. However, there was an increase in both the size and the number of lipid droplets in water-loaded rats, whereas the interstitial cells were almost depleted of lipid inclusions in water-loaded rabbits [15]. Thus, although there appears to be a relationship between the lipid droplets and the diuretic state of an animal, the exact nature of this relationship remains to be established.

Function

The function of type 1 interstitial cells is not known with certainty. It is quite likely they have a supporting function in the medulla because of their special arrangement perpendicular to the tubules and vessels. The close relationship between these cells and the thin limbs and capillaries also suggests some kind of interaction between these structures. Because of the presence of a well developed endoplasmic reticulum and prominent lipid droplets, it has been suggested that the type 1 interstitial cells may have a secretory function [29]. However, the lipid droplets are not secretory granules in the usual sense, since they have no limiting membrane, and there is no evidence that they are secreted by the cell. The droplets have been isolated from homogenates of both rat [30,31] and rabbit [32] renal medulla. Biochemical studies have established that they consist mainly of triglycerides and small amounts of cholesterol esters and phospholipids [31]. The triglycerides are rich in unsaturated fatty acids including arachidonic acid, a prostaglandin precursor [30,32]. Since the renal medulla is a major site of prostaglandin synthesis [32], several investigators have suggested that the type 1 interstitial cells are specialized prostaglandin producing cells. Studies using tissue cultures of renal medullary interstitial cells have demonstrated synthesis of prostaglandins by these cells [33,34] with the major product being PGE_2 [35,36]. However, direct measurements of prostaglandin synthetase activity in rabbit renal papillary slices have revealed that 39% of the activity was located in the collecting duct cells suggesting that prostaglandin synthesis is not limited to the interstitial cells [37].

The results of recent studies suggest that angiotensin may regulate prostaglandin production in the renal medulla. Investigators [38] have demonstrated that angiotensin receptors are present in cultured rabbit renomedullary interstitial cells, and prostaglandin E_2 biosynthesis is stimulated by angiotensin. Kugler [39], using histochemical techniques has demonstrated the presence of aminopeptidase A (E.C. 3.4.11.7), an angiotensinase that is capable of degrading angiotensin, in the type 1 renomedullary interstitial cells of the rat, rabbit, golden hamster and guinea pig. Thus, another possible mechanism to control angiotensin stimulation of prostaglandin production appears to be present in the medulla.

The type 1 renomedullary interstitial cells may have an endocrine antihypertensive function [33]. In various types of experimental hypertension, a decrease in the number of lipid droplets in the interstitial cells has been reported. Muirhead and co-workers have demonstrated that transplantation of renal papillary tissue [40,41] and cultured renomedullary interstitial cells [33] into hypertensive animals was followed by a decrease in blood pressure. It is believed that the lipid droplets are in some way related to the antihypertensive function of the interstitial cells, but the precise mechanism is yet to be established. In addition to a possible endocrine function, the interstitial cells are believed to be responsible for the synthesis of glucosaminoglycans that are present in the matrix material of the interstitium.

Even less is known about the function of the type 2 and type 3 medullary interstitial cells. Bohman [1] has suggested that the type 2 cells are probably phagocytic, but the function of the type 3 cells remains unknown.

Acknowledgments

A portion of this work was supported by US Public Health Service Grant AM-28330 (Dr Tisher). The authors acknowledge the technical assistance of James Cannon, Isabelle Williams and Fred Kopp. Linda Michael provided secretarial support. The authors thank Dr W Fischlschweiger, Director of the Electron Microscope Facility of the College of Dentistry at the University of Florida where the electron microscope studies were performed.

References

1 Bohman S-O. The ultrastructure of the renal medulla and the interstitial cells. In Mandal AK, Bohman S-O, eds. *The Renal Papilla and Hypertension.* New York: Plenum Medical Book Co. 1980: 7–33

2 Pedersen JC, Persson AE, Maunsbach AB. Ultrastructure and quantitative characterization of the cortical interstitium in the rat kidney. In Maunsbach AB, Olsen TS, Christensen EI, eds. *Functional Ultrastructure of the Kidney.* London: Academic Press. 1980: 443–456

3 Pfaller W. Structure function correlation in rat kidney. *Adv Anat Embryol Cell Biol 1982: 70:* 1–106

4 Dunnill MS, Halley W. Some observations on the quantitative anatomy of the kidney. *J Pathol 1973; 110:* 113–121

5 Bohle A, Grund KE, Mackensen S, Tolon M. Correlations between renal interstitium and level of serum creatinine. *Virchows Arch [Path Anat] 1977; 373:* 15–22

6 Hestbech J, Hansen HE, Amdisen A, Olsen S. Chronic renal lesions following long-term treatment with lithium. *Kidney Int 1977; 12:* 205–213

7 Kappel B, Olsen S. Cortical interstitial tissue and sclerosed glomeruli in the normal human kidney, related to age and sex. A quantitative study. *Virchows Arch [Path Anat] 1980; 387:* 271–277

8 Knepper MA, Danielson RA, Saidel GM, Post RS. Quantitative analysis of renal medullary anatomy in rats and rabbits. *Kidney Int 1977; 12:* 313–323

9 Wolgast M, Larson M, Nygren K. Functional characteristics of the renal interstitium. *Am J Physiol 1981; 241:* F105–F111

10 Bulger RE, Nagle RB. Ultrastructure of the interstitium in the rabbit kidney. *Am J Anat 1973; 136:* 183–204

11 Bohman S-O. The ultrastructure of the rat renal medulla as observed after improved fixation methods. *J Ultrastruct Res 1974; 47:* 329–360

12 Mounier F, Foidart J-M, Gubler M-C. Distribution of extracellular matrix glycoproteins during normal development of human kidney. An immunohistochemical study. *Lab Invest 1986; 54:* 394–401

13 Martinez-Hernandez A, Gay S, Miller EJ. Ultrastructural localization of type V collagen in rat kidney. *J Cell Biol 1982; 92:* 343–349

14 Romen W, Thoenes W. Histiocytaro und fibrocytare Eigenschaften der interstitiellen Zellen der Nierenrinde. *Virchows Arch [Cell Pathol] 1970; 5:* 365–375

15 Bohman S-O, Jensen PKA. The interstitial cells in the renal medulla of rat, rabbit and gerbil in different states of diuresis. *Cell Tiss Res 1978; 189:* 1–18

16 Lapp H, Nolte A. Vergleichende elektronenmikroskopische Untersuchungen am Mark der Rattenniere bci Harnkonzentrierung und Harnverdunnung. *Frankfurter Zeitschrift fur Pathologie 1962; 71:* 617–633

17 Schiller A, Taugner R. Junctions between interstitial cells of the renal medulla: a freeze-fracture study. *Cell Tissue Res 1979; 203:* 231–240

18 Majack RA, Larsen WJ. The bicellular and reflexive membrane junctions of renomedullary interstitial cells: functional implications of reflexive gap junctions. *Am J Anat 1980; 157:* 181–189

19 Osvaldo L, Latta H. Interstitial cells of the renal medulla. *J Ultrastruct Res 1966; 15:* 589–613

20 Bulger RE, Trump BF. Fine structure of the rat renal papilla. *Am J Anat 1966; 118:* 685–721

21 Bulger RE, Tisher CC, Myers CH, Trump BF. Human renal ultrastructure. II. The thin limb of Henle's loop and the interstitium in healthy individuals. *Lab Invest 1967; 16:* 124–141

22 Bohman S-O, Jensen PKA. Morphometric studies on the lipid droplets of the interstitial cells of the renal medulla in different states of diuresis. *J Ultrastruct Res 1976; 55:* 182–192

23 Cavallo T. Fine structural localization of endogenous peroxidase activity in inner medullary interstitial cells of the rat kidney. *Lab Invest 1974; 31:* 458–464

24 Bulger RE, Griffith LD, Trump BF. Endoplasmic reticulum in rat renal interstitial cells: molecular rearrangement after water deprivation. *Science 1966; 151:* 83–86

25 Moffat DB. A new type of cell inclusion in the interstitial cells of the medulla of the rat kidney. *J Microsc 1967; 6:* 1073–1076

26 Ledingham JM, Simpson FO. Bundles of intracellular tubules in renal medullary interstitial cells. *J Cell Biol 1973; 57:* 594–598

27 Nissen HM. On lipid droplets in renal interstitial cells. II. A histological study on the number of droplets in salt depletion and acute salt repletion. *Z Zellforsch Mikrosk Anat 1968; 85:* 483–491

28 Nissen HM. On lipid droplets in renal interstitial cells. III. A histological study on the number of droplets during hydration and dehydration. *Z Zellforsch Mikrosk Anat 1968; 92:* 52–61

29 Mandal AK, Frohlich ED, Chrysant K et al. A morphologic study of the renal papillary granule: analysis in the interstitial cell and in the interstitium. *J Lab Clin Med 1975; 85:* 120–131

30 Nissen HM, Bojesen I. On lipid droplets in renal interstitial cells. IV. Isolation and identification. *Z Zellforsch Mikrosk Anat 1969; 97:* 274–284

31 Bohman S-O, Maunsbach AB. Ultrastructure and biochemical properties of subcellular fractions from rat renal medulla. *J Ultrastruct Res 1972; 38:* 225–245

32 Anggard E, Bohman S-O, Griffin JE III et al. Subcellular localization of the prostaglandin system in the rabbit renal papilla. *Acta Physiol Scand 1972; 84:* 231–246

33 Muirhead EE, German GS, Armstrong FB et al. Endocrine-type antihypertensive function of renomedullary interstitial cells. *Kidney Int 1975; 8:* S271–S282

34 Dunn MJ, Staley RS, Harrison M. Characterization of prostaglandin production in tissue culture of rat renal medullary cells. *Prostaglandins 1976; 12:* 37–49

35 Zusman RM, Keiser HR. Prostaglandin biosynthesis by rabbit renomedullary interstitial cells in tissue culture: stimulation by angiotensin II, bradykinin and arginine vasopressin. *J Clin Invest 1977; 60:* 215–223

36 Zusman RM. Prostaglandin E_2 biosynthesis by renomedullary interstitial cells. In Mandal AK, Bohman S-O, eds. *The Renal Papilla and Hypertension.* New York: Plenum Medical Book Co. 1980; 187–207

37 Bohman S-O. Demonstration of prostaglandin synthesis in collecting duct cells and other cell types of the rabbit renal medulla. *Prostaglandins 1977; 14:* 729–744

38 Brown CA, Zusman RM, Haber E. Identification of an angiotensin receptor in rabbit renomedullary interstitial cells in tissue culture. Correlation with prostaglandin biosynthesis. *Circ Res 1980; 46:* 802–807

39 Kugler P. Angiotensinase A in the renomedullary interstitial cells. *Histochemistry 1983; 77:* 105–115

40 Muirhead EE, Brooks B, Pitcock JA, Stephenson P. Renomedullary antihypertensive function in accelerated (malignant) hypertension. Observations on renomedullary interstitial cells. *J Clin Invest 1972; 51:* 181–189

41 Muirhead EE, Brooks B, Pitcock JA et al. Role of the renal medulla in the sodium-sensitive component of renoprival hypertension. *Lab Invest 1972; 27:* 192–198

AMMONIA, THE KIDNEY, AND COMPLEMENT COMPONENT C3

Margaret K Hostetter, K A Nath, J P Tolins, T H Hostetter

University of Minnesota, Minneapolis, USA

More than 60 years have passed since Gordon and colleagues reported that ammonia abolished the function of complement proteins [1]. In these early experiments, the incubation of ammonium chloride (NH_4Cl) or ammonium hydroxide (NH_4OH) with guinea pig serum halted the complement-mediated haemolysis of sensitized erythrocytes. Although the inhibition of haemolysis was greatest at pH values between 8 and 10, alkalinization alone, in the absence of ammonia, caused no inhibition. These investigators rightly implicated free base ammonia as the cause of complement dysfunction.

Fifteen years later, Pillemer and colleagues established the rôle of nucleophile amines in the inhibition of complement-mediated haemolysis [2]. These investigators were the first to correlate nucleophilic structure with inhibitory effect: small compounds such as hydrazine were the most active in their inhibition, followed by methylamine, ethylamine, and ammonia in close order, while the presence of a phenyl ring reduced the inhibitory effect of phenylhydrazine by two-thirds. Polar amino compounds, such as urea, glycine, or acetamide were wholly inactive. These investigators then proposed that the active amino compounds exerted their inhibitory effect by converting a carbonyl group on the complement component to a 'less active' form.

Beeson and Rowley [3] proposed that the intrarenal production of ammonia inhibited complement-mediated bactericidal activity against coliform bacteria in a rat model of pyelonephritis.

These early papers, some of them more than half-a-century old, have proved to be uncanny predictors of biochemical truths. The functional inactivation of the human complement proteins C3 and C4 by nucleophilic amines was definitively proven in the early sixties with the first purification of these complement proteins [4]. The characterization of the reactive thiolester bond, first in C3 and later in other members of what we now know as the extended thiolester family –C4, α_2-macroglobulin, and pregnancy zone protein – has enabled us to understand both the biochemistry of this reaction and the functional implications which derive from it [5–8]. In this paper, we shall review (a) the structure of the reactive thiolester bond; (b) the mechanism by which ammonia, as a physiological nucleophile, attaches to the reactive carbonyl of the C3 thiolester to form amidated C3; and (c) the functional ramifications of the formation of amidated C3 at sites of increased ammoniagenesis, such as the kidney in chronic renal failure.

Structure of the reactive thiolester bond

Human C3 is a two-chain protein in which the alpha chain of 115,000 daltons is connected to the beta chain of 75,000 daltons by a single disulfide bond [9]. Activation of C3 by the convertases of the classical or the alternative pathway is a proteolytic event in which the C3a fragment is cleaved from the amino terminal end of the alpha chain by the scission of an arginine-serine bond at residue 77; the remainder of the α-chain and the uncleaved β-chain constitute C3b (Figure 1). Only with substantial refinements in the purification procedure

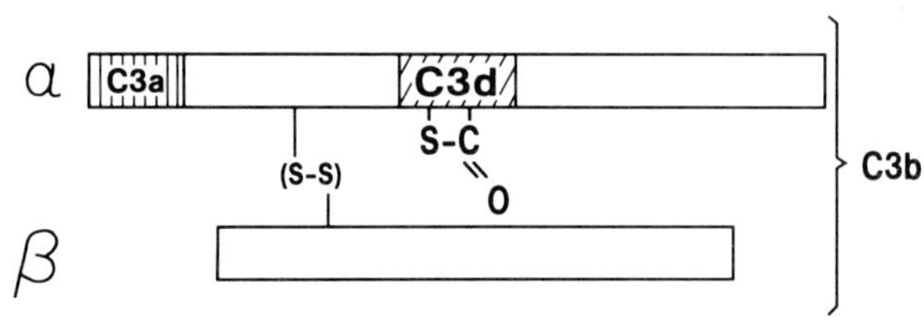

Figure 1. Schematic diagram of the C3 molecule, showing C3a, C3b, and the C3d subdomain. Reprinted from *Reviews of Infectious Diseases 1987; 9:* 97–109

[10] was it possible to show that inactivation of isolated human C3 nucleophiles (or by chaotropes such as KSCN or KBr) was accompanied by the expression of a single -SH group on a cysteinyl residue located on the alpha chain of the C3 molecule within the C3d subdomain [5,11]. For each mole of C3 inactivated, one mole of sulfhydryl was measured: a stoichiometry of 1:1. Such chemically inactivated C3 was incapable of supporting a haemolytic activity; thus, the appearance of the sulfhydryl group was both a marker for the inactivation of C3 and an indicator of a change in the chemical nature of the protein.

Studies with α_2-macroglobulin, another protein inactivated by nucleophiles, had shown that reaction with methylamine resulted in the incorporation of the nucleophile into a particular glutamyl residue on the α_2-macroglobulin molecule [12]. Although methylamine-reactive glutamyl residues were also found in C3 and C4 [13,14], it remained for Tack and colleagues to establish, by sequence analysis, that the site of sulfhydryl expression was located only three amino-acid residues distant from the methylamine-reactive glutamyl residue on C3 [5]. After inactivating C3 with [^{14}C] methylamine, these investigators excised a 33-residue peptide from the alpha chain and carboxymethylated it with [^{3}H] iodoacetic acid. Upon Edman degradation, this peptide contained the tritium label at the cysteinyl sulfhydryl, while the [^{14}C] methylamine was found at the glutamyl carbonyl. Tack and colleagues then proposed an internal thiolester bond linking a cysteinyl and a glutamyl residue within native C3. Subsequent papers placed the C3 thiolester within the C3d subdomain [15] and provided biochemical confirmation for the sequence analysis [16]. Characterization of homologous sites in C4, α_2-macroglobulin, and pregnancy zone protein quickly followed (Figure 2).

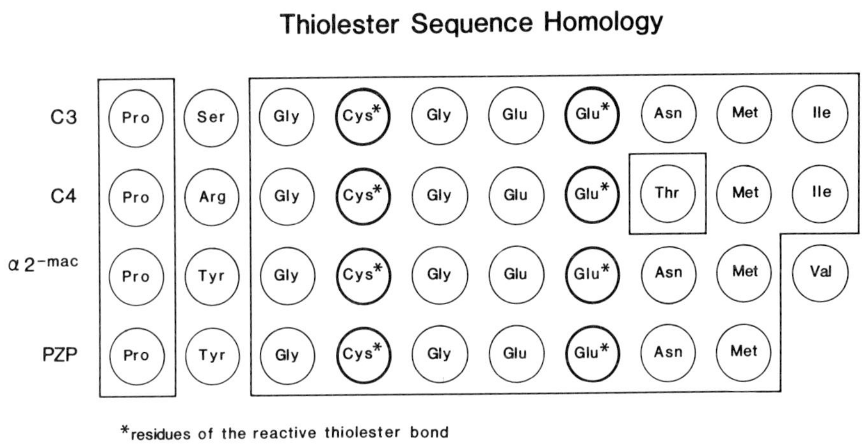

Figure 2. Sequence homology surrounding the thiolester bond in C3, C4, α_2-macroglobulin, and pregnancy zone protein. Reprinted from *Reviews of Infectious Diseases 1987; 9: 97–109*

The covalent binding reaction

The characterization of the C3 thiolester provided biochemical foundation for many important observations regarding its function. For several years, it had been known that the binding of C3 to surfaces such as zymosan, bacteria, or cell membranes occurred only upon activation of the protein, that is, as C3 was cleaved to C3b by the action of the classical or the alternative pathway convertases. When C3b bound to acceptor surfaces such as zymosan or sheep erythrocytes, the bond formed was a covalent oxy-ester, in which the carbonyl group derived from the α chain of the C3 molecule, rather than from some component of the cell surface [17]. Surface constituents which served as acceptors for C3b included a wide variety of carbohydrates – mannose, glucose, galactose, 5-thiol-D-glucose, and even bacterial polysaccharides – as well as compounds with free amino groups, such as threonine, lysine, or putrescine [18–20]. However, although C3b bound covalently to the acceptor molecule in each of these experimental systems, the site of attachment on C3b was not known.

Hostetter and colleagues then chose a representative carbohydrate ([^{14}C] glycerol) and amino compound ([^{14}C] threonine) and, after cleaving purified human C3 to C3b with trypsin, demonstrated specific and covalent binding of the labelled compound to C3b [21]. These investigators then isolated the thiolester peptide from the C3d subdomain, removed noncovalently bound ligand by dialysis in SDS, and radioalkylated the sulfhydryl group exposed during trypsin cleavage with [^{3}H] iodoacetic acid. On Edman degradation of the threonine peptide, for example, the tritium counts were found at the cysteinyl residue of the thiolester peptide, and the [^{14}C] label, representing threonine covalently bound to the labile binding site, was recovered at the thiolester glutamyl residue.

These experiments revealed how C3b binds covalently to small molecules which are themselves incapable of disrupting the C3 thiolester (Figure 3).

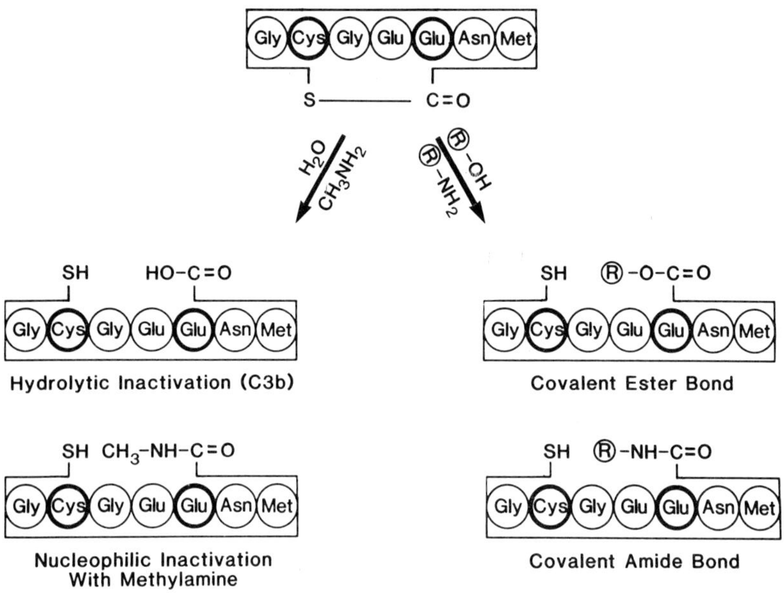

Figure 3. Diagram of the aminoacid sequence of the thiolester site in native human C3 (top). Inactivation of the thiolester site is represented by the reactions on the lower left. The transacylation reaction leading to covalent bond formation with carbohydrates or amino groups is represented at the lower right. Reprinted from *The Journal of Infectious Diseases 1984; 150:* 653–661

Upon cleavage of C3 to C3b by the convertases of the classical or alternative pathway, or by trypsin in vitro, the thiolester bond is disrupted; the reactive glutamyl residue, now freed from the thiolester bridge with the cysteinyl sulfhydryl group, denotes its carbonyl group in a transacylation reaction which results in the formation of either an oxy-ester bond with carbohydrate acceptors, or an amide bond with amino acceptors. These reactions can, of course, occur in the fluid phase as an interesting biochemical phenomenon, but they have physiological relevance in the process of bacterial opsonization, whereby carbohydrate or amino groups expressed on the bacterial surface serve as acceptor sites for the covalent attachment of C3b [22].

Nucleophilic disruption of the C3 thiolester

The covalent binding reaction between C3b and carbohydrates or amino compounds requires the cleavage of C3 to C3b and the concomitant exposure of the reactive thiolester. In contrast, nucleophilic amines are inheritantly reactive with the C3 thiolester; these compounds, which disrupt the thiolester solely by virtue of nucleophilic attack, bind directly to the glutamyl carbonyl in amide linkage but do not cleave the C3a fragment.

The biological consequences of this reaction were first made apparent by the independent studies of Isenman and von Zabern and their co-workers, who established that nucleophilic modification of the C3 thiolester endowed the protein with the ability to bind factor B and form the alternative pathway convertase [23,24]. In von Zabern's work, for example, treatment of isolated human C3 and C4 with hydrazine, ammonium hydroxide, or neutral ammonium salts resulted in total loss of haemolytic activity but preserved the ability of the molecule to function as the alternative pathway convertase [23]. Isenman's

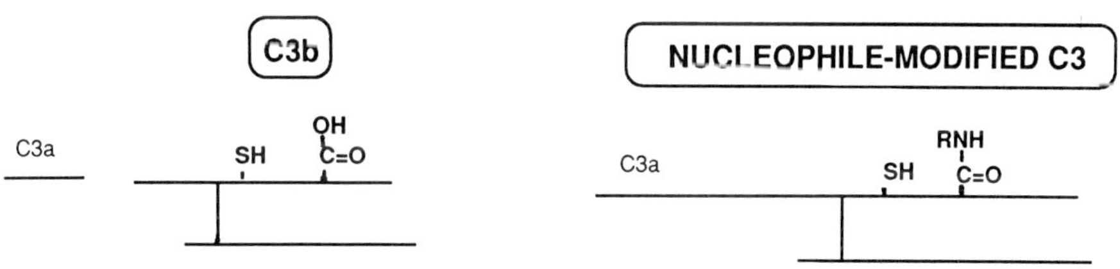

- FORMS THE C3/C5 CONVERTASE FOR THE ALTERNATIVE PATHWAY
- FOSTERS C3 CLEAVAGE AND DEPOSITION
- PROMOTES THE ASSEMBLY OF THE MEMBRANE ATTACK COMPLEX, C5b-9
- BINDS TO COMPLEMENT RECEPTORS ON PHAGOCYTES AND TRIGGERS OXIDATIVE METABOLISM

Figure 4. A comparison of the structures and functions of C3b and its amidated analogues work demonstrated that methylamine-treated C3, although still retaining the C3a fragment, nevertheless assumed the conformation of C3b, bound factor B, and served as an alternative pathway convertase [24]. A comparison of the structures of C3b and its analogue, nucleophile-modified C3, is shown in Figure 4. Clearly, the functional similarities in the binding of factor B and in the formation of the alternative pathway convertase derive from this structural correspondence.

Amidated C3: formation, structure and function

Nucleophilic disruption of the C3 thiolester by nucleophiles such as methylamine or hydrazine carries little physiological relevance, since these compounds are rarely, if ever, present in normal body fluids. Assuredly, the nucleophile of physiological importance is ammonia, just as Gordon suggested more than 60 years ago. Confirmation of the incorporation of ammonia into the C3 thiolester was first obtained by Hostetter and colleagues [21]; when the C3d peptide of previous studies was incubated with 1.0M ammonium acetate at pH for two hours at 37°C, sequence analysis yielded a cysteinyl residue at step 9 and a glutamine, rather than a glutamyl, residue at step 12. Under these circumstances then, the ester linkage at the glutamyl carbonyl had been replaced with a covalent amide linkage, and ammonia had been directly incorporated into the C3 thiolester. A diagram of this reaction is shown in Figure 5. However, as Gordon and

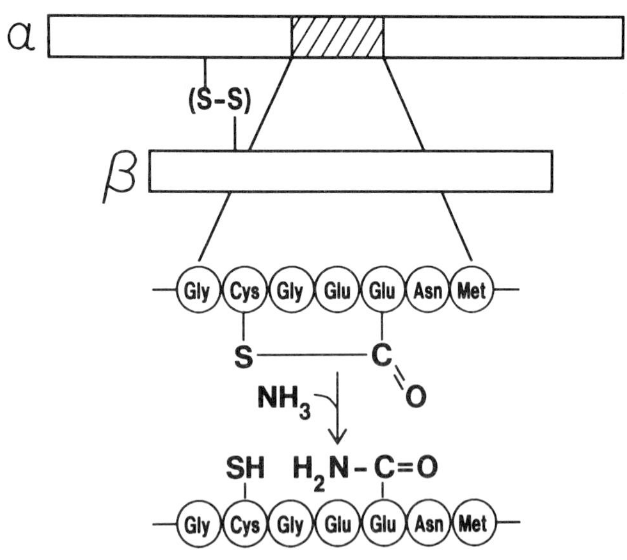

Figure 5. The reaction of ammonia with human C3. Nucleophilic attack by ammonia disrupts the thiolester site and permits the incorporation of ammonia at the thiolester glutamyl. Reprinted from *Reviews of Infectious Diseases 1987; 9:* 97–109

later investigators have suggested, the reaction of ammonia with complement proteins can and indeed does occur at lesser pH values in the range of 7.5 to 8, even though the concentration of free base ammonia is reduced some 100-fold at these more physiological values.

Data from our laboratory readily support the contention that thiolester disruption by ammonia can occur at physiologic pH and at concentrations of ammonia which are achievable within the human body. For example, disruption of the C3 thiolester can be quantitated by the use of [^{3}H] iodoacetic acid to alkylate the sulfhydryl group which is expressed after nucleophilic attack [11]. When preparations of purified human C3, which typically express a titrable sulfhydryl group on 3–5% of molecules as a result of the purification procedure, are incubated at pH 7.45 with NH_4Cl in concentrations ranging from 0 to 4mM, expression of the sulfhydryl group doubles after incubation with ammonia in concentrations as low as 0.1mM. More importantly, if normal human plasma at physiological pH is incubated with NH_4Cl in concentrations ranging from

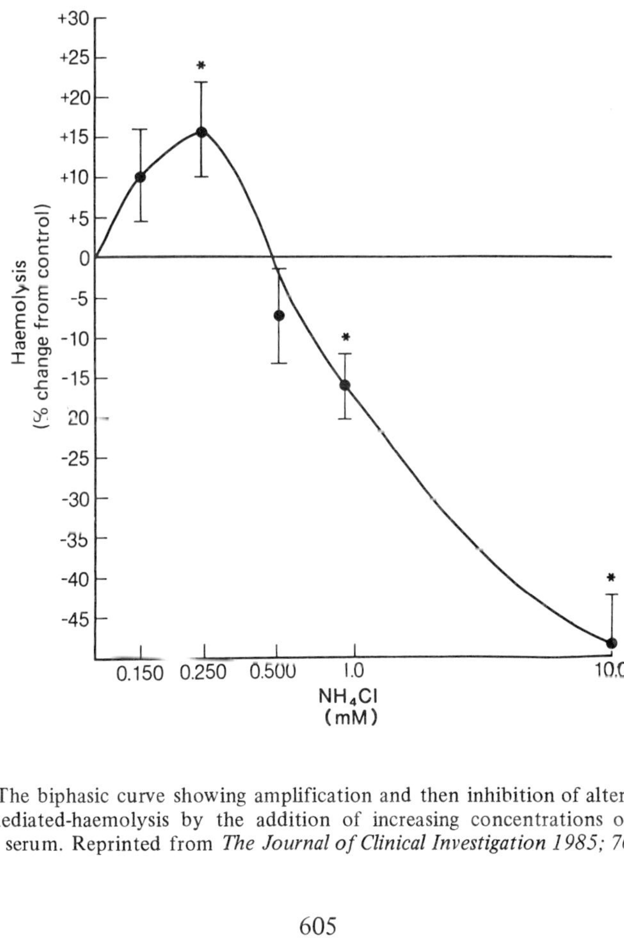

Figure 6. The biphasic curve showing amplification and then inhibition of alternative pathway mediated-haemolysis by the addition of increasing concentrations of NH_4Cl to human serum. Reprinted from *The Journal of Clinical Investigation 1985; 76:* 667–675

0.15 to 10mM, removal of C3 by affinity chromatography and titration of the C3 sulfhydryl by [^{3}H] iodoacetic acid again document an increase in thiolester disruption in response to increasing concentrations of ammonium chloride.

The physiological consequences of the disruption of the C3 thiolester by free base ammonia are shown in Figure 6, which compares the haemolytic activity of the alternative pathway in normal human serum in the absence and presence of ammonium chloride.

As can be seen from the figure, concentrations of NH_4Cl >1mM depressed the haemolytic activity of normal serum. Similar observations were reported by Tack, who noted that incubation of purified human C3 with 10mM methylamine reduced the haemolytic activity of the protein by 50% [11], and these experiments were subsequently confirmed with other nucleophiles [23,24]. Concentrations of NH_4Cl in excess of 1mM readily amidate all available C3 molecules, thereby exhausting the supply of thiolester-reactive C3 (native C3), which alone is haemolytically active.

Of greater interest, however, is the stimulation of alternative pathway activity observed by us [25] at concentrations ranging from 0.15 to 0.5mM ammonium chloride, a range not studied in earlier papers. At these lesser concentrations, which can readily be attained at sites of increased ammoniagenesis such as the renal vein, the activity of the alternative pathway is amplified beyond that observed in the absence of ammonia. At these lower concentrations, ammonia disrupts the thiolester site in only a small (but significant) percentage of all available C3 molecules to form the C3/C5 convertase of the alternative pathway. This increment in convertase activity amplifies the enzymatic cleavage of native C3, which in turn binds directly to the erythrocyte cell membrane, fosters the formation of the membrane attack complex, C5b–9, and results in haemolysis.

Formation of amidated C3 at sites of ammoniagenesis

Based on these in vitro studies, we predicted that concentrations of ammonia in the range of 0.15 to 0.5mM could lead to increased activity of the alternative complement pathway in vivo, through the formation of amidated C3 and its activity as a C3/C5 convertase. Such convertase activity would serve to cleave not only thiolester-reactive C3, which could then bind directly to tissue surfaces, but also C5, thereby generating the chemoattractant C5a and triggering the assembly of the membrane attack complex, C5b-9. As a prelude to our experiments, Falk and colleagues had noted that peritubular deposition of complement proteins was present in a wide variety of chronic human renal disease, both nephritic and non-nephritic [26]. For non-nephritic diseases such as diabetic nephropathy, antigen/antibody complexes that activate the classical pathway are not present, and the mechanism by which complement proteins including C3 and C5b-9 are deposited about the tubules was unknown.

The remnant kidney in the rat is the experimental analogue of non-nephritic disease in humans, with a histological picture dominated by chronic tubulo-interstitial disease and associated abnormalities of haemodynamic and tubular transport function. In the remnant model, reductions in renal mass produce compensatory changes in renal function. For example, despite reductions in total ammonia production, ammonia excretion factored for glomerular filtration rate is increased several fold, as is ammonia production per surviving nephron [27].

In the published studies of Nath and colleagues [25], adult rats with one and three-quarter nephrectomy were paired for serum creatinine, in order to assure similar degrees of renal injury after ablation. The diet of the experimental group consisted of 20% protein supplemented with sodium chloride (NaCl), while the control group received 20% protein supplemented with equimolar sodium bicarbonate ($NaHCO_3$), in order to suppress ammonia production. At the appropriate time points, animals in both groups were studied for tubular and glomerular functions, and remnant kidney tissue was obtained for histology and immunofluorescence.

Mean renal vein total ammonia concentration in the rats with high dietary acid load was 0.24±0.02mM, statistically greater than the renal vein total ammonia concentration in the $NaHCO_3$-supplemented rats, 0.145±0.020mM ($p<0.05$). Rats with the higher renal vein ammonia concentration demonstrated a near two-fold increase in total urinary protein excretion and in the urinary excretion of low molecular weight protein (molecular weight <10.000). In addition, although there was no difference in glomerular filtration rate between the rats with high renal vein ammonia and their $NaHCO_3$-supplemented controls, rats with elevated renal vein ammonia had a significantly reduced ability to secrete para-amino-hippuric acid per unit glomerular filtration rate ($p<0.05$). Thus, those animals with higher renal vein ammonia concentrations had evidence of significantly greater impairment in urinary protein excretion and para-aminohippuric acid secretion than did their bicarbonate-supplemented controls. Bicarbonate supplementation and reduction of ammonia production were thus correlated with improvement of renal function.

Similarly, rats with increased renal vein ammonia concentrations had significantly greater evidence of histological injury, as assessed by cast formation, interstitial infiltration, and tubular dilation and atrophy. More importantly, however, immunofluorescence studies demonstrated markedly different patterns in the remnant kidney of NaCl-supplemented versus $NaHCO_3$-supplemented rats. In rats with a higher renal vein ammonia concentration, there was widespread peritubular immunofluorescence for C3 and for C5b-9, the membrane attack complex. In those rats in which renal vein ammonia concentration was reduced by systemic alkalinization with bicarbonate supplementation, peritubular fluorescence for C3 and for C5b-9 was much reduced. In addition, there was no peritubular immunofluorescence for IgG and albumin in either group, a result which negates the possibility that deposition of complement proteins was simply the result of non-specific entrapment of macromolecules within the kidney.

Based on these experiments, we proposed that ammonia reacted biochemically with the third component of complement to provoke tubulo-interstitial injury. At concentrations of ammonia attained in the renal vein of animals fed a high dietary acid load (0.25mM), there was a significant increase in functional injury, in indices of histological damage, and in the peritubular deposition of complement proteins C3 and C5b-9. Control animals with reduced renal vein ammonia (0.15mM) exhibited significant improvements, both in tubular function and in histology. Most importantly, immunofluorescence of remnant kidneys in the $NaHCO_3$-supplemented rats also showed a marked decrease in peritubular deposition of C3 and C5b-9.

Thus, the in vivo model correlates well with the in vitro experiments presented in Figure 6. Alternative pathway activity, whether manifest by haemolysis or by peritubular deposition of C3 and C5b-9, is significantly increased at levels of ammonia readily attained in the renal veins of animals with chronic tubulo-interstitial disease. Although peritubular deposition of complement proteins has been observed in a wide variety of chronic human renal disease, both nephritic and non-nephritic [26], our results provide a mechanism for the antibody-independent activation of the alternative complement pathway through the formation of amidated C3.

Experimental models of hypokalaemic nephropathy also link increased ammoniagenesis and progressive tubulo-interstitial injury. In studies of chronic potassium deficiency, Tolins and colleagues induced hypokalaemia by dietary deficiency; experimental animals received 150mM sodium chloride in drinking water, while controls received equimolar $NaHCO_3$ to suppress renal ammoniagenesis. Once again, increases in renal hypertrophy, histological evidence of injury, and proteinuria were found in the hypokalaemic animals given NaCl. Mean renal vein ammonia concentration in these animals was 0.392±0.110mM, while the hypokalaemic cohorts supplemented with bicarbonate had a markedly reduced mean renal vein ammonia concentration, 0.214±0.028mM ($p<0.05$), a result which did not differ significantly from values in control animals (0.179± 0.057mM). Once again, immunofluorescence studies revealed circumferential peritubular deposition of C3 in potassium-deficient, NaCl-supplemented rats, with the additional observation that C3 deposition was most prominent in tubules immediately adjacent to renal venules. Such peritubular immunofluorescence was reduced in $NaHCO_3$-supplemented rats when comparable perivascular areas were observed.

Because the focality of C3 deposition precluded definitive comparisons between the two groups of potassium-deficient rats, direct deposition of C3 and its fragments was quantitated by a radiolabelled antibody binding assay using affinity purified [^{3}H] goat anti-rat C3. Corticotubular fragments from normal rats were incubated in normal rat serum supplemented with increasing concentrations of NH_4Cl (1–0.5mM); in normal rat serum without NH_4Cl, or in buffer (pH 7.45) with identical concentrations of NH_4Cl. Analysis of C3 deposition on renal tubules by antibody binding assay showed a 58% increase in the tubular deposition of C3 on corticotubular fragments incubated with normal rat serum and NH_4Cl, as compared to tubules incubated with normal rat serum alone. Thus, concentrations of ammonia comparable to those in hypokalaemic rats significantly enhanced deposition of C3 on rat tubules.

These results provided quantitative support for our contention that concentrations of ammonia in the range of 0.25 to 0.5mM are sufficient for the generation of amidated C3 and for the subsequent triggering of the alternative complement pathway by this amidated mediator. Ammonia, generated in the proximal tubule, diffuses into the peritubular capillaries and reacts directly with fluid-phase C3 [21]. Formation of amidated C3 triggers the alternative complement pathway, cleaves unreacted C3, mediates the peritubular deposition of C3 and C5b-9, and generates multiple molecular mediators of tissue injury.

Functional effects of high ammonia concentrations

Our discussion to this point has focused on those effects engendered by ammonia concentrations ranging from 0.25 to 0.5mM. As shown by the biphasic curve in Figure 6, higher concentrations of ammonia (1mM and above) effectively inhibit pathway activation. At these high ammonia concentrations, the thiolester site in every available C3 molecule is amidated, leaving no unreacted C3 to serve as substrate for the convertase. Amidated C3 cannot itself bind covalently to cell surface macromolecules, because the glutamyl carbonyl – the site of covalent attachment – is occupied by ammonia. However, amidated C3 can indeed interact with membrane receptors for complement proteins, again by virtue of its structural correspondence with C3b [28,29]. Using monomeric amidated C3 prepared by the incubation of purified human C3 and 1.0M NH_4Cl at pH 8.0, Gordon and colleagues demonstrated that the incubation of amidated C3 with polymorphonuclear leucocytes and monocytes evoked a significantly greater chemiluminescent response than did equimolar amounts of the physiological mediator C3b [28]. Amidated C3 proved to be a more potent stimulator of the oxidative response of polymorphonuclear leucocytes and monocytes whether presented on the surface of inert microspheres, or more physiologically, in the fluid phase.

Since antibodies to complement receptor type 3 (CR3) did not inhibit the binding of amidated C3 to the neutrophil, this reaction most likely takes place at CR1, the C3b receptor. Although the affinity of CR1 for amidated C3 is equal to that for C3b with a Ka of 5.7×10^7 L/M, the number of binding sites for amidated C3 on the neutrophil is increased approximately four-fold. In addition, amidated C3 greatly outstrips C3b in the elicitation of such inflammatory mediators as superoxide, myeloperoxidase, and lactoferrin from neutrophils [29]. Thus, although high concentrations of ammonia will lead to the amidation of virtually all C3 molecules, amidated C3 formed under these conditions has potent effects upon the white cell and, by virtue of its structural similarity with C3b, can bind to membrane receptors for complement proteins and stimulate the release of inflammatory mediators such as superoxide, myeloperoxidase, and lactoferrin. The binding of amidated C3 to complement receptors on the glomerulus [30], as well as the physiological consequences which may ensue, deserve vigorous investigation.

Summary

In this paper, we have traced the historical evolution of our understanding of the biochemical reaction between ammonia and complement component C3. By aminoacid sequencing, we have confirmed both the disruption of the C3 thiolester and the binding of ammonia to the reactive carbonyl group at the thiolester glutamyl residue. We have further shown the importance of the biphasic nature of this reaction. At low concentrations of ammonia, akin to those attainable in the renal veins of animals with chronic renal disease, the reaction of ammonia with complement component C3 leads to a significant increase in the activity of the alternative pathway, with the resultant deposition of C3b and C5b-9 on tubular membranes. Correlated with this deposition are significant increases in functional damage and in histological injury. The reduction of ammoniagenesis by systemic alkalinization ablates these changes, which can be qualitatively assessed by immunofluorescence and quantitated by radiolabelled antibody binding.

In contrast, at ammonia concentrations >1mM, all available C3 thiolesters are readily amidated, and there is no unreacted C3 to serve as substrate for the enzymatic convertase. Even under these conditions, however, the formation of amidated C3 engenders inflammatory consequences, in that the binding of amidated C3 to leucocyte receptors for C3 fragments stimulates the release of potent oxidants and destructive enzymes.

The system is thus purely physiological. A given concentration of ammonia determines the extent to which C3 molecules are amidated; the degree of amidation determines whether the effects are predominantly those of alternative pathway activation, with covalent deposition of C3b, formation of the membrane attack complex, and the consequences attendant on its binding, or whether the effects are ascribable to the binding of amidated C3 to membrane receptors for C3 fragments. In either case, the concentration of ammonia incites a series of self-perpetuating, injurious effects. For the kidney, the physiology of ammonia production and excretion engenders immunological mediators which have profound consequences for renal function.

References

1 Gordon J, Whitehead HR, Wormall A. The action of ammonia on complement. The fourth component. *Biochem J 1926; 20:* 1028–1035

2 Pillemer L, Seifter J, Eicker EE. The effect of amino compounds on the fourth component of complement. *J Immunol 1941; 40:* 89–95

3 Beeson PB, Rowley D. The anticomplementary effect of kidney tissue. Its association with ammonia production. *J Exp Med 1959; 110:* 201–215

4 Muller-Eberhard HJ, Nilsson UR, Aronsson T. Isolation and characterization of two β_1-glycoproteins of human serum. *J Exp Med 1960; 111:* 201–215

5 Tack BF, Harrison RA, Janatova J et al. Evidence for presence of an internal thiolester bond in third component of human complement. *Proc Natl Acad Sci USA 1980; 77:* 5764–5768

6 Harrison RA, Thomas ML, Tack BF. Sequence determination of the thiolester site of the fourth component of human complement. *Proc Natl Acad Sci USA 1981; 78:* 7388–7392

7 Sottrup-Jensen L, Peterson TE, Magnusson S. A thiol-ester in α_2-macroglobulin cleaved during proteinase complex formation. *FEBS Lett 1980; 121:* 275–279

8 Sand O, Folkersen J, Westergaard JG, Sottrup-Jensen L. Characterization of human pregnancy zone protein: comparison with human α_2-macroglobulin. *J Biol Chem 1985; 260:* 15723–15735

9 Tack BF, Morris SC, Prahl JW. Third component of human complement: structural analysis of the polypeptide chains of C3 and C3b. *Biochemistry 1979; 18:* 1497–1503

10 Tack BF, Prahl JW. Third component of human complement: purification from plasma and physiochemical characterization. *Biochemistry 1976; 15:* 4513–4521

11 Janatova J, Lorenz PE, Schechter AN et al. Third component of human complement: appearance of a sulfhydryl group following chemical or enzymatic inactivation. *Biochemistry 1980; 19:* 4471–4478

12 Swenson RP, Howard JB. Characterization of alkylamine-sensitive site in α_2-macroglobulin. *Proc Natl Acad Sci USA 1979; 76:* 4313–4316

13 Howard JB. Methylamine reaction and denaturation-dependent fragmentation of complement component 3: comparison with α_2-macroglobulin. *J Biol Chem 1980; 255:* 7082–7084

14 Gorski JP, Howard JB. Effect of methylamine on the structure and function of the fourth component of human complement, C4. *J Biol Chem 1980; 255:* 10025–10028

15 Thomas ML, Janatova J, Gray WR, Tack BF. Third component of human complement: localization of the internal thiolester bond. *Proc Natl Acad Sci USA 1982; 79:* 1054–1058

16 Thomas ML, Davidson FF, Tack BF. Reduction of the α-cys-γ-glu thiol ester bond of human C3 with sodium borohydride. *J Biol Chem 1983; 258:* 13580–13586

17 Law SK, Levine RP. Interaction between the third complement protein and cell surface macromolecules. *Proc Natl Acad Sci USA 1977; 74:* 2701–2705

18 Capel PJA, Groeneboer O, Grosveld G, Pondman KW. The binding of activated C3 to polysaccharides and immunoglobulins. *J Immunol 1978; 121:* 2566–2572

19 Mann J, O'Brien R, Hostetter MK et al. The third component of complement: covalent attachment of a radioactive sugar to the labile binding site of C3 via the alternative pathway. *J Immunol 1981; 126:* 2370–2372

20 Sim RB, Twose TM, Paterson DS, Sim E. The covalent-binding reaction of complement component C3. *Biochem J 1981; 193:* 115–127

21 Hostetter MK, Thomas ML, Rosen FS, Tack BF. Binding of C3b proceeds by a transesterification reaction at the thiolester site. *Nature 1982; 298:* 72–75

22 Hostetter MK, Krueger RA, Schmeling DJ. The biochemistry of opsonization: central role of the reactive thiolester bond of the third component of complement. *J Inf Dis 1984; 150:* 653–661

23 Isenman DE, Kells DI, Cooper NR et al. Nucleophilic modification of human complement protein C3: correlation of conformational changes with acquisition of C3b-like functional properties. *Biochemistry 1981; 20:* 4458–4467

24 Von Zabern I, Nolte R, Vogt W. Treatment of human complement components C4 and C3 with amines or chaotropic ions. *Scand J Immunol 1981; 13:* 413–431

25 Nath KA, Hostetter MK, Hostetter TH. Pathophysiology of chronic tubulo-interstitial disease in rats: interactions of dietary acid load, ammonia, and complement component C3. *J Clin Invest 1985; 76:* 667–675

26 Falk RJ, Dalmasso AP, Kim Y et al. Neoantigen of the polymerized ninth component of complement: characterization of a monoclonal antibody and immuno-histochemical localization in renal disease. *J Clin Invest 1983; 72:* 650–573

27 Tolins JP, Hostetter MK, Hostetter TH. Hypokalemic nephropathy in the rat: the role of ammonia in chronic tubular injury. *J Clin Invest 1987; 79:* 1447–1458
28 Gordon DL, Krueger RA, Quie PG, Hostetter MK. Amidation of C3 at the thiolester site: stimulation of chemiluminescence and phagocytosis by a new inflammatory mediator. *J Immunol 1985; 134:* 3339–3345
29 Hostetter MK, Johnson GM, Retsinas EM. The erythrocyte as instigator of inflammation. *Clin Res 1986; 34:* 460A
30 Gelfand MC, Frank MM, Green I. A receptor for the third component of complement in the human renal glomerulus. *J Exp Med 1975; 142:* 1029–1034

INTERSTITIAL NEPHRITIS: A UNIVERSAL FEATURE OF ALLOIMMUNITY POST-KIDNEY TRANSPLANTATION

T B Strom

Beth Israel Hospital, Harvard Medical School, Boston, Massachusetts, USA

Before end-stage renal failure patients and their physicians take 'the plunge' and opt for a renal transplant, the hosts' immune system is relatively unperturbed (Figure 1). Obligatory recognition of mismatched histocompatibility antigens by host T-cells follows every allogeneic kidney transplant (Figure 2). Consequently, all renal allografts show evidence of an interstitial nephritis. Hence, the nature and severity of the interstitial nephritis in any given case must be viewed in the context of a continuum of biological responses in which subclinical 'rejection' and irreversible rejection are the polar extremes of this process. Although a significant proportion of renal allografts are never the subject of severely destructive recipient anti-donor immune mechanisms, a lymphocytic infiltrate is present in such well-functioning allografts. This should not be surprising since cyclosporin, azathioprine and corticosteroids – the medications used to prevent allograft rejection – do not block antigen recognition [1,2]. Each of these medications blocks certain distinctive aspects of T-cell activation

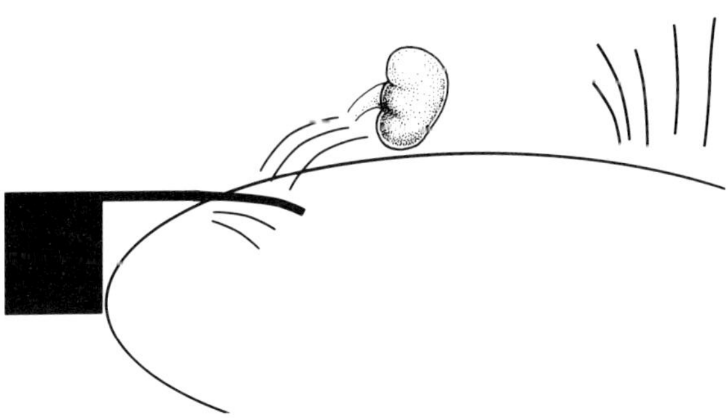

Figure 1. The plunge

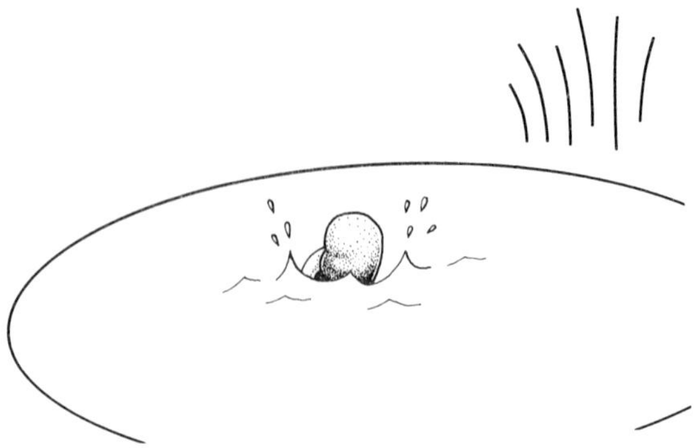

Figure 2. Alloactivation occurs at the time of transplantation

through drug effects that are exerted in the T-cell activation cascade distal to the point of antigen recognition. What is the nature of the interstitial nephritis noted in 'trivial' alloimmune-induced interstitial nephritis, i.e. subclinical rejection? In the absence of clinical rejection, a patchy infiltration of T-lymphocytes is noted; this infiltrate is primarily confined to the interstitium. Interestingly, the majority of the invading lymphocytes bear the $CD4^+$ phenotype. This pattern of infiltration can also be seen in patients plagued with cyclosporin activity in the absence of rejection [3]. These pieces of clinical evidence indicate that the first wave of graft invading lymphocytes consist of $CD4^+$ T-cells (Figure 3). In the absence of $CD8^+$ cell infiltration, interstitial oedema and haemorrhage, pathological hallmarks of rejection, do not occur.

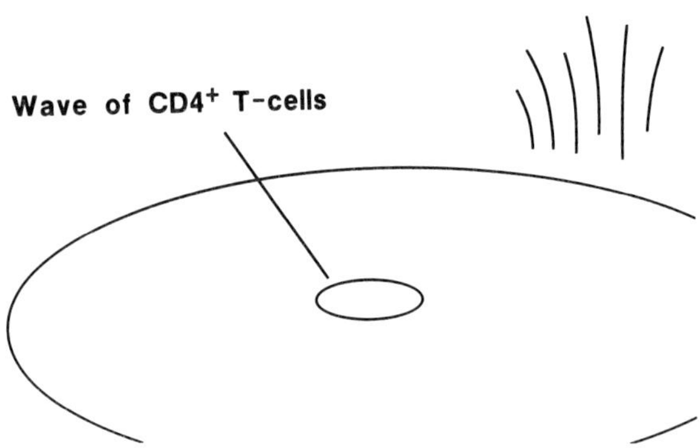

Figure 3. The wave of patchy infiltration by $CD4^+$ T-cells into the interstitium

Mild corticosteroid-sensitive rejection episodes are characterized by a more diffuse infiltration of T-cells primarily noted in the medullary regions [4,5]. Extensive interstitial and tubular infiltration and modest endothelial invasion are noted. While $CD8^+$ T-cells are not abundant in the infiltrate associated with

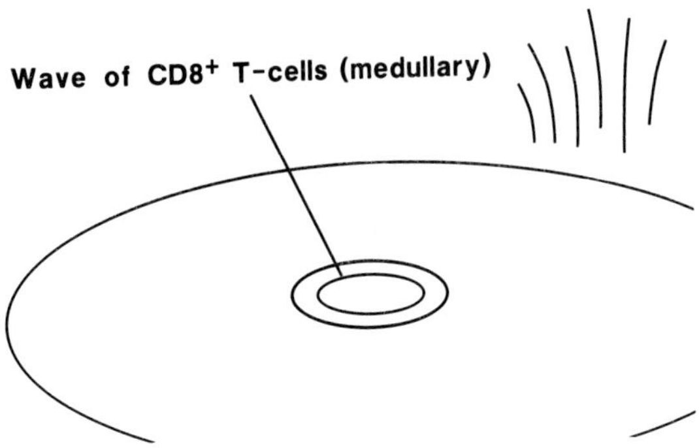

Figure 4. The wave infiltration by $CD8^+$ T-cells into the interstitium

'subclinical rejection' (see Figure 3), the infiltrate in corticosteroid-sensitive rejection episodes contains a relatively balanced population of $CD4^+$ and $CD8^+$ T-cells (Figure 4). Thus, while the first wave of graft infiltrating cells consists of $CD4^+$ T-cells, the second wave of infiltration by medullary homing, $CD8^+$ T-cells results in graft rejection (Figure 4).

More vexing corticosteroid-sensitive cellular rejection episodes are characterized by cortical as well as interstitial infiltration by host T-cells. Diffuse infiltration of $CD4^+$ and $CD8^+$ T-cells, noted in corticosteroid-sensitive rejection episodes, is also observed in corticosteroid-insensitive rejection episodes. What characteristic distinguishes these more severe rejection episodes from corticosteroid-sensitive rejection? In corticosteroid-insensitive cellular rejection, a diffuse cortical and glomerular invasion, by $CD8^+$ T-cells is also present [4,5]. Hence, the third wave of invading leucocytes consists of cortex homing $CD8^+$ T-cells (Figure 5). Since OKT3/anti-thymocyte globulin (ATG) can reverse some steroid-insensitive rejection episodes, it appears likely that this form of rejection is corticosteroid-insensitive but frequently OKT3/ATG-sensitive (Figure 5).

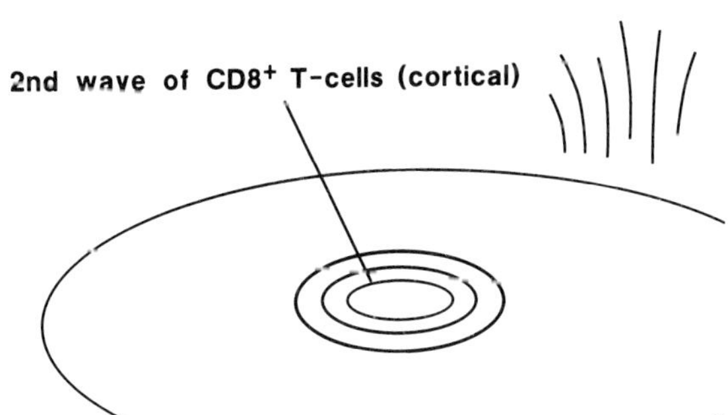

Figure 5. The wave of infiltration by $CD8^+$ cells into the cortex and glomeruli

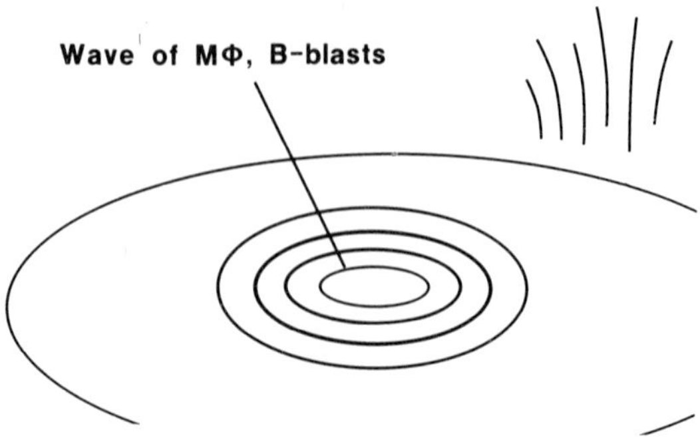

Figure 6. The wave of infiltration by macrophages and beta blasts

Other forms of cellular rejection are even more resistant to therapy. While the infiltrate noted in subclinical rejection and in treatment-sensitive forms of rejection is dominated by T-cells, more severe rejection episodes are characterized by concomitant infiltration with abundant numbers of macrophages and B-cells (Figure 6). Endothelial cell injury often accompanies this pattern of cellular infiltration. It is likely that the appearance of antibody producing B-blasts in the interstitium and the presence of endothelial injury are two morphologically distinct manifestations of humoral alloimmunity. These corticosteroid-insensitive rejection episodes are not uniformly sensitive to OKT3/ATG. As these rejection episodes are often resistant to OKT3 treatment, the appearance of this more varied cellular pattern of an infiltration, including abundant macrophages and B-cells, denotes that the rejection process has now progressed to the point that T-cell dependent mechanisms are not necessarily required to sustain the cytodestructive activities of the invading host cells.

In the most virulent pattern of interstitial nephritis, immunological mechanisms of graft injury are accompanied by, or even given way to, frank inflammation (Figure 7). Infiltration by T-cells and B-cells is now joined by more abundant

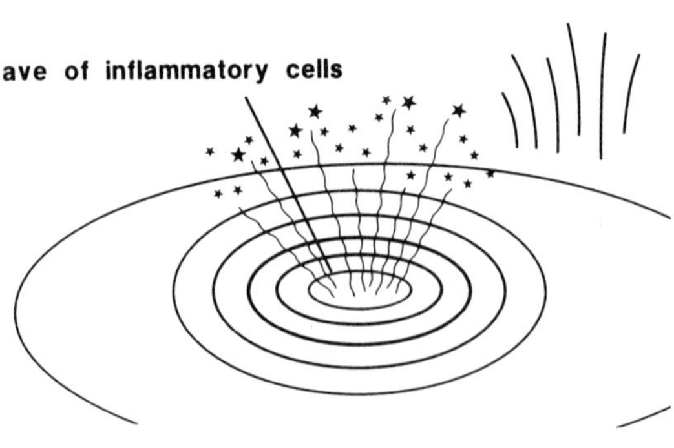

Figure 7. A wave of infiltration by inflammatory cells destroys the graft

numbers of invading macrophages. Polymorphonuclear neutrophils, eosinophils and basophils are also noted. Evidence of vasculitic injury and thrombosis accompanies this sinister pattern of graft inflammation. Anti-rejection therapy is counter-productive. Graft nephrectomy is frequently required to relieve the unremitting sequelae of gross inflammation.

It seems evident that transplant physicians must learn to characterize each invading wave of leucocytes into the graft in order to navigate the graft toward safe engraftment.

References

1 Bach SF, Strom TB. *The Mode of Action of Immunosuppressive Agents, 2nd Edition.* Amsterdam: Elsevier. 1986

2 Strom TB. Basic transplant immunobiology on the mode of action of immunosuppressive agents utilized in clinical renal transplantation. *Kidney Int 1984; 26:* 353–365

3 Platt JL, Ferguson RM, Sibley RK et al. Renal interstitial cell populations in cyclosporine nephrotoxicity: identification using monoclonal antibodies. *Transplantation 1983; 36:* 343–346

4 Bishop GA, Hall BM, Duggin GG et al. Immunopathology of renal allograft rejection analyzed with monoclonal antibodies to mononuclear cell markers. *Kidney Int 1986; 29:* 708–717

5 Sanfilippo F, Kolbeck PC, Vaughan WK, Bollinger RR. Renal allograft cell infiltrates associated with irreversible rejection. *Transplantation 1985; 40:* 679–685

IMMUNOLOGICAL MECHANISMS IN EXPERIMENTAL MODELS OF TUBULO-INTERSTITIAL NEPHRITIS

K M Bannister, *T R Ulich, †C B Wilson

Royal Adelaide Hospital, Adelaide, South Australia,
**University of California, Irvine Medical Center, South Orange,*
†Research Institute of Scripps Clinic, La Jolla, California, USA

As in glomerulonephritis, much of our understanding of the immunological mechanisms of tubulo-interstitial nephritis has come from studies of animal models which resemble the human disease. In glomerulonephritis, this has been very productive since both the human disease and its models are largely humorally mediated, thereby allowing meaningful extrapolations. In contrast, although anti-tubular basement membrane (TBM) antibody is associated with most of the animal models of tubulo-interstitial nephritis studied, these antibodies are unusual in human disease [1–3]. The animal models of anti-TBM antibody-associated tubulo-interstitial nephritis have been useful to attempt to determine the individual contributions of the humoral and cellular immune mechanisms and to begin to understand the cellular events suspected in the human situation; however, these models may incompletely address the major cellular rôle suspected to be present in most forms of human tubulo-interstitial nephritis. It has therefore been more difficult than in glomerulonephritis to extrapolate from the animal studies to the human situation, and models in which cellular immunity is the prominent or sole mechanism have been sought.

In the anti-TBM antibody-associated models, the contributions of humoral and cellular immunity appear to vary with the species. For example, transfer of disease using immune serum is easily and rapidly accomplished in the guinea pig [4]. In the rat, such transfer is feasible only with certain high titre sera [5]. In the mouse, the rôle of the accompanying anti-TBM antibody in the slowly developing (weeks) lesion is much less clear, and transfer of the lesions with immune lymph node cells or cloned T-cells provides evidence for a prominent rôle for cellular immune processes [6–9]. The response can be inhibited by adoptive transfer of suppressor T-cells from donor mice primed with tubular antigen-derived syngeneic lymphocytes [10]. Transfer with cells in rats was accomplished only with some difficulty [11,12] and has not as yet been possible in the guinea pig [13]. Models of cell-mediated tubulo-interstitial nephritis have been difficult to produce until recently. An interstitial delayed type hypersensitivity using aggregates of protein [14], and a model in the Lewis rat produced by immunization with syngeneic kidney [15] represent two examples of mild interstitial disease transferable with immune cells. The spontaneous tubulo-interstitial nephritis of kd/kd mice also has a strong cellular immune pathogenesis [16].

The present discussion will focus on experimentally induced tubulo-interstitial nephritis in certain rat strains and the relationship of the lesions to the variable expression of nephritogenic tubular basement membrane antigens. It will attempt to analyse the relative rôles of antibody and cell-mediated mechanisms in the production of tubulo-interstitial nephritis in the rat. The development and study of an interesting new model of cell-mediated tubulo-interstitial nephritis in the Lewis rat will be presented in detail [17,18]. This new model appears to be independent of anti-TBM antibody and fulfils the criteria of a purely cell-mediated process; as such it may provide a closer parallel to human disease.

RAT MODELS OF ANTI-TBM ANTIBODY-ASSOCIATED TUBULO-INTERSTITIAL NEPHRITIS

Shortly after the description of anti-TBM antibody-associated tubulo-interstitial nephritis in the guinea pig [19], Sugisaki et al described an autoimmune tubulo-interstitial nephritis associated with anti-TBM antibody in rats [20]. Brown Norway rats immunized with homologous (Sprague-Dawley) kidney suspension in complete Freund's adjuvant (CFA) and an injection of *Bordetella pertussis* vaccine developed anti-TBM antibodies and an interstitial disease characterized by the deposition of IgG and C3 in a linear fashion along the tubular basement membrane. This was associated with a cellular infiltrate comprising polymorphonuclear leucocytes initially and lymphocytes, macrophages and giant cells later. The rats also developed a delayed glomerular lesion resembling Heymann's nephritis.

Lehman et al reported a similar tubulo-interstitial nephritis in Brown Norway rats following immunization with heterologous (bovine) tubular basement membrane in CFA plus pertussis [21]. In this instance the glomerular lesion was avoided. The development of tubulo-interstitial nephritis was shown to relate to the quantity of antibody deposited and highlighted the strain-specific presence of immunofluorescence detectable tubular basement membrane antigen which was a requirement for the disease to develop. Thus the Lewis rat, known to lack this tubular basement membrane antigen, produced large quantities of circulating anti-TBM antibody after immunization with bovine tubular basement membrane but failed to bind the antibody to the kidney and lesions of tubulo-interstitial nephritis were not detected. Robertson et al [22] later used bovine glomerular basement membrane to immunize Brown Norway rats, first producing tubulo-interstitial nephritis, followed by glomerular disease associated with the linear deposition of IgG along the glomerular basement membrane.

A number of heterologous TBM-rich renal basement membranes have been used for induction of similar lesions in the Brown Norway rat. Ulich et al reported that the lesion could be induced in the Brown Norway rats using very small amounts of a soluble chaotropic extract of bovine tubular basement membrane together with adjuvants [11]. The tubulo-interstitial nephritis so produced was shown, in terms of the cellular and humoral responses, to be the same as that described using particulate tubular basement membrane [23,24]. This soluble immunogen allowed cell culture and propagation experiments to be more easily performed (see later sections).

Immunogenetics of anti-TBM antibody-associated tubulo-interstitial nephritis

The development of anti-TBM antibody-associated tubulo-interstitial nephritis in the rat appears to be most critically dependent on the genetically determined presence of the relevant antigen [21,25]. The expression of this antigen is independent of the MHC (RT1) and is controlled by one dominant gene [25,26] which is linked to the gene for albinism on the first linkage group [27].

Although in guinea pig models of tubulo-interstitial nephritis genetic control of an effective humoral immune response has been shown to be important [28], the situation is less clear in the rat. As noted above, early studies demonstrated a correlation between severity and the amount of anti-TBM antibody eluted from the kidneys of Brown Norway and AC1 rats after immunization with bovine tubular basement membrane [21]. More recent extensions of this work have shown a further relationship between the amount of antibody directed against antigens present in collagenase solubilized (CS) tubular basement membrane and the extent of disease [23]. This anti-CS-Brown Norway-TBM antibody was shown to be over 500 times more concentrated in the kidneys than in the serum of immunized Brown Norway rats, thereby indicating its selective binding. Neilsen et al, although agreeing with strain differences in the amount of anti-TBM antibody produced, found little or no effect of genes controlling such a response on disease susceptibility based on measurement of circulating rather than eluted anti-TBM antibody [27]. Using F1 hybrid rats, these authors concluded that the important genetically controlled response to heterologous tubular basement membrane is cell-mediated and determined by an RT1-linked gene.

Finally, although Brown Norway rats develop severe tubulo-interstitial nephritis after immunization with heterologous tubular basement membrane, the disease does not develop if autologous membrane is used. Kelly et al investigated this tolerance to autologous basement membrane using the delayed type hypersensitivity response to Brown Norway-TBM as a marker of cell-mediated immunity [29]. Their data suggest the immunization of tubular basement membrane antigen-positive rat strains with Brown Norway-TBM results in the development of antigen specific, cyclophosphamide sensitive, RT1 restricted suppressor T-cells. This suppression could be overcome with cyclophosphamide, with the subsequent development of significant tubulo-interstitial nephritis. It would therefore appear that maintenance of tolerance to autologous tubular basement membrane in the Brown Norway rat is the result of a potent suppressor cell mechanism.

Characterization of anti-TBM antibodies

Anti-TBM antibodies produced in the rat show a broad cross species (including human) reactivity. However, as described previously, certain strains of rat including the Lewis, Maxx, Wistar Furth and Wistar Munich do not express the reactive antigen in a detectable form (without alteration) and do not bind the anti-TBM antibody to their kidneys.

Immunization of Brown Norway rats with bovine tubular basement membrane results in the production of circulating antibody against tubular basement membrane antigens of both heterologous and autologous origin. However, the relevant nephritogenic antibody, i.e. that bound in the kidney, reacts primarily with Brown Norway-TBM in radioimmunoassay (RIA) or by immunofluorescence, and most of this reactivity is directed at a CS-TBM fraction [23]. Heterologous or autologous anti-idiotypic antibodies modify the anti-TBM antibody response in guinea pigs or rats [30,31]. Using passive administration of heterologous anti-idiotypic antibody, Zanetti et al found a correlation between reduced intensity of tubulo-interstitial nephritis in Brown Norway rats and a selective decrease in circulating antibody directed towards CS-Brown Norway-TBM [32], supporting the nephritogenic potential of this antibody.

Characterization of nephritogenic tubular basement membrane antigens

Early studies on CS human tubular basement membrane isolated a 70 kD moiety which was used to establish a RIA for tubular basement membrane antibodies [33]. This antigen appeared to be tubular basement membrane-specific and was a glycoprotein. Using trypsin digestion of human tubular basement membrane, Wakashin et al [34] isolated a 30 kD protein which did not cross-react with glomerular basement membrane antigens but did cross-react with tubular basement membrane antigens from goats, guinea pigs and mice using immunodiffusion. This antigen preparation was able to induce tubulo-interstitial nephritis in a limited number of goats and mice studied.

More recently, Zanetti et al showed that eluted antibody from the kidneys of Brown Norway rats immunized with bovine tubular basement membrane precipitated a major CS-Brown Norway-TBM antigen of about 42 kD using polyacrylamide gel electrophoresis (PAGE) of immunoprecipitates [23]. Of interest in this study, a small amount of a similar sized reactive material was recovered from CS-Lewis-TBM, suggesting that the Lewis rat does not actually lack the reactive antigen but that its reactive epitope(s) is normally inaccessible to antibody. Subsequent studies demonstrated that anti-TBM antibody from Lewis rats immunized with Brown Norway renal basement membrane reacted with a 45 kD moiety in CS-Brown Norway-TBM using SDS-PAGE and immunoblotting [5].

Using a monoclonal anti-TBM antibody and affinity chromatography, Clayman et al [35] isolated a 48 kD glycoprotein from CS rabbit tubular basement membrane. This non-collagenous glycoprotein was capable of inducing tubulo-interstitial nephritis in strain 13 guinea pigs, while selective removal of this antigen from rabbit tubular basement membrane resulted in the inability of the latter to produce disease. Although the nephritogenic potential of the antigen was not tested in rats, electron immunohistochemical localization demonstrated the presence of the antigen on the most lateral aspects of Brown Norway tubular but not glomerular basement membrane. As expected, the antigen was not found in Lewis tubular basement membrane. This antigen is probably similar to that described above [5,23].

Recently, Fliger et al [36] characterized a 58 kD antigen from human tubular basement membrane which reacted with anti-TBM antibodies from two patients with primary anti-TBM antibody mediated tubulo-interstitial nephritis. An antigen from human tubular basement membrane of 54 kD was reported by Yoshioka et al [37]. In contrast, Clayman et al, using affinity chromatography, recovered a reactive antigen of 48 kD from human CS tubular basement membrane [38]. The apparent cross-reactivity of the rat and human tubular basement membrane antigen, as well as the genetic absence of the antigen in certain humans [39] analogous to that in the Lewis rat, suggests a similar structure which is not accounted for by the variation in size of reactive antigens detected to date. The explanation may relate to either the presence of multiple reactive antigens or to partial degradation of a common tubular basement membrane antigen depending on the methods employed.

Transfer of tubulo-interstitial nephritis by antibody

Although there is good indirect evidence of the pathogenetic importance of anti-TBM antibodies in the initiation of tubulo-interstitial nephritis in the rat, in contrast to guinea pigs [4] and mice [6], it has been difficult [11], until recently, to passively transfer the disease by serum to naive recipients. The difficulty may relate to the presence of only small quantities of nephritogenic antibody in the circulation of immunized rats from which the serum was collected. Lewis rats immunized with Brown Norway renal basement membrane and adjuvants produce significantly higher titres of anti-CS-Brown Norway-TBM antibody than Brown Norway rats immunized with heterologous tubular basement membrane, presumably in part because the Lewis rat cannot bind this antibody to its kidneys. The pooled immune Lewis sera had 10 times the reactivity of bovine tubular basement membrane immunised Brown Norway rat serum when tested by RIA against CS-Brown Norway-TBM [5] (Figure 1).

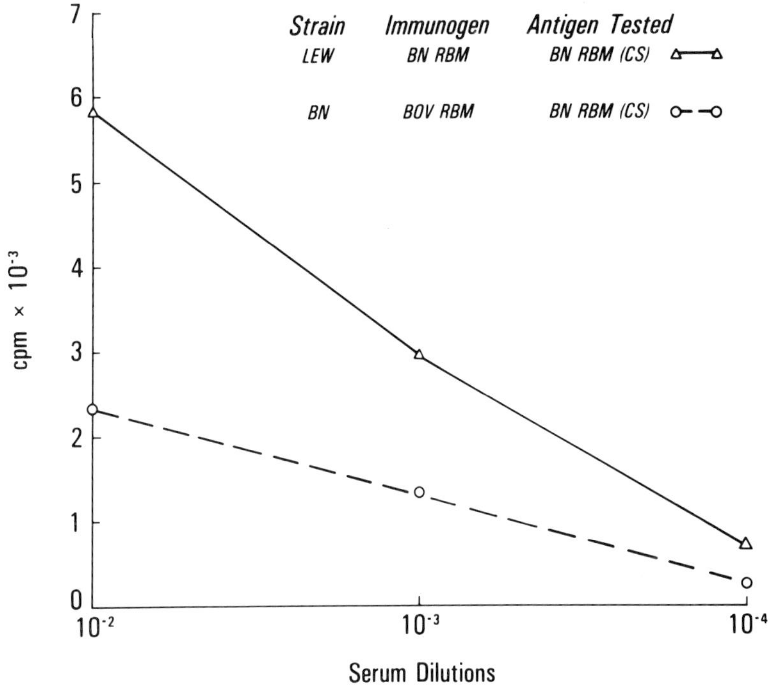

Figure 1. Comparison of reactivity of Lewis (LEW) anti-CS-Brown Norway (BN) renal basement membrane (RBM) and Brown Norway anti-CS-bovine (BOV) renal basement membrane serum pools on RIA. (Background reactivity of normal Lewis and Brown Norway sera subtracted)

This pooled Lewis sera was used for passive transfer experiments. Transfer of as little as 3ml of the Lewis serum to recipient Brown Norway rats resulted in focal lesions of tubulo-interstitial nephritis within 24 hours, histologically similar to that seen after active immunization of Brown Norway rats [5]. The only discernible difference appeared to be that the earliest lesions contained only up to 20% polymorphonuclear leucocyte influx compared to over 90% in the active model. In contrast, a total of 45ml of pooled sera (in divided doses) from actively immunized Brown Norway rats (having a lower reactive antibody titre) produced only one small debatable lesion of tubulo-interstitial nephritis in a recipient Brown Norway rat [5].

Using paired isotope quantitative binding studies of a passively transferred Lewis anti-Brown Norway-RBM IgG fraction, a slow accumulation of renal-bound antibody was demonstrated over six days [5]. This data correlated with immunofluorescence and elution studies after transfer of nephritogenic quantities of immune Lewis sera to normal Brown Norway rats. This slow binding of anti-TBM antibody is in contrast to the extremely rapid binding of anti-GBM antibodies in the rat [40], and may be similar to the binding of anti-TBM antibodies in the guinea pig [13]. From the quantitative binding experiments, approximately 167μg of kidney-fixing antibody per gram of kidney was required for the development of the earliest cellular infiltrate in the Brown Norway rat. These experiments quantitate the initiating rôle for anti-TBM antibody in tubulo-interstitial nephritis in the Brown Norway rat, but do not exclude an additional rôle for cell-mediated mechanisms in the progression of disease.

The rôle of complement

Circumferential linear deposition of C3 along the tubular basement membrane in areas of tubulo-interstitial nephritis is one of the hallmarks of anti-TBM-associated diseases in the rat. Although suggested in the guinea pig [41], it is only recently that evidence of a functional rôle for complement has been forthcoming in the rat model.

The very rapid induction of disease by antibody transfer is presumably largely independent of cell-mediated mechanisms and provides a setting to study the effects of complement. Complement depletion with purified cobra venom factor before intravenous transfer of Lewis anti-Brown Norway-RBM serum antibody resulted in a major reduction in the number and area of destructive tubular lesions seen in Brown Norway rat kidneys over the next five days [5]. However, complement depletion did not completely prevent minor cellular infiltrates, suggesting a possible rôle for non-complement-dependent immune processes.

The effects of decomplementation were studied in the active model of tubulo-interstitial nephritis in the Brown Norway rat produced by immunization with bovine tubular basement membrane [42]. Decomplementation with cobra venom factor was instituted just before the predicted onset of antibody deposition, i.e. day six or seven, in order that serum C3 levels could be maintained at less than 5% of control sera during the initial phase of injury. Decomplementation significantly reduced the neutrophilic inflammatory infiltrate seen on days 8–10 but did not affect the mild mononuclear inflammatory cell influx also seen on those days. By day 12, however, a significant reduction in the mononuclear cell infiltrate compared to controls was evident. However, non-complement-dependent immune processes may play some rôle in the full development of the mononuclear cell infiltrate.

Anti-idiotypic antibodies

Anti-idiotypic immunity has provided another means of demonstrating the importance of antibody in the induction of anti-TBM antibody-associated tubulo-interstitial nephritis in the rat. After reports of the efficacy of anti-idiotypic antibodies in the suppression of tubulo-interstitial nephritis in the guinea pig [23], our laboratory utilized heterologous anti-idiotypic antibody directed against eluted anti-TBM antibodies from the kidneys of Brown Norway rats immunized with bovine tubular basement membrane [32]. This anti-idiotypic antibody selectively blunted only the anti-Brown Norway-TBM response to CS-Brown Norway-TBM antigen when given 48 hours prior to active immunization, and this effect correlated with impairment of induction of tubulo-interstitial nephritis in the Brown Norway rats.

In a slightly different approach using tubular basement membrane reactive T-lymphoblasts to stimulate auto-anti-idiotypic immunity, Neilsen et al [31] reached similar conclusions about the protective effects of anti-idiotypic antibodies in tubulo-interstitial nephritis in the Brown Norway rat. However, the actual rôle of such antibodies in the control of the anti-TBM antibody response in this model is uncertain. Auto-anti-idiotypic antibodies have not been demonstrated in the Brown Norway rat model of tubulo-interstitial nephritis, and it has been suggested that the failure of development of such a regulatory response may be the result of a suppressor T-cell effect which develops shortly after immunization [43]. Further work in this area is needed to clarify the rôle, if any, of anti-idiotypic immunity in the tubulo-interstitial nephritis in the rat.

Cell mediated immunity in anti-TBM antibody associated tubulo-interstitial nephritis

Immunization of Brown Norway rats with bovine tubular basement membrane and adjuvants results in the development of a progressive tubulo-interstitial nephritis characterized by antibody deposition along the tubular basement membrane and the sequential infiltration of the renal interstitium by distinct cell types and subsets. Anti-TBM antibody and C3 deposits can be initially found at days 8–10 after immunization along with a prominent polymorphonuclear leucocyte influx. This initial phase is followed by a mononuclear cell infiltrate with giant cells and eventual interstitial fibrosis. Quantitative analysis of the infiltrating cells, utilizing both tissue sections and cell suspensions from the affected kidneys and monoclonal antibodies, showed that the majority of cells were T-cells between days 13–21 [24]. Most of these were T helper cells and expressed the Ia antigen [11,24]. B cells and macrophages were present in much smaller numbers, but by four weeks esterase positive cells became predominant. These results support a rôle for cell-mediated mechanisms in the progression of tubulo-interstitial nephritis in the Brown Norway rat.

Using isolated and purified renal infiltrate cells from diseased Brown Norway kidneys, we attempted to demonstrate the presence of specifically sensitized cells in blast transformation assays. Although reactivity against the immunogen was found, a variety of autologous renal antigen preparations failed to cause a response [11]. Inappropriate antigen presentation or a suppressor mechanism may have explained these results as well as an absolute lack of sensitized cells.

Adoptive transfer of anti-TBM antibody associated tubulo-interstitial nephritis

The most conclusive evidence for a rôle for cell-mediated immunity is, of course, transfer of disease by cells. Lehman et al demonstrated that subcapsular renal transfer of lymph node cells and peritoneal exudate cells obtained from Brown Norway rats immunized with bovine tubular basement membrane could transfer a very mild form of tubulo-interstitial nephritis [12]. Recently, Ulich et al transferred tubulo-interstitial nephritis using lymph node cells from Brown Norway rats (immunized with a soluble chaotropic extract of bovine tubular basement membrane) which were propagated for five days with immunogen and interleukin-2 [11]. Both circulating and bound anti-TBM antibody was present in recipients, therefore making the quantitative contributions of either antibody or cells indeterminate. However, since large volumes of serum from similarly immunized Brown Norway rats failed to passively transfer tubulo-interstitial nephritis, the activated cells may well be of pathogenic importance.

Immunomodulation of anti-TBM antibody-associated tubulo-interstitial nephritis
Attempts to modulate the immune mechanisms involved in anti-TBM antibody-associated tubulo-interstitial nephritis in the Brown Norway rat have generally resulted in an apparent dissociation of cell-mediated and humoral responses [9]. Thus pre-immunization of the rats with antigen in incomplete Freund's adjuvant [44], dietary protein restriction [45], and the use of high dose cyclophosphamide from day 12 [46] in Brown Norway rats immunized with rabbit tubular basement membrane reduced the intensity of histological tubulo-interstitial nephritis, but serum titres of anti-TBM antibody showed little change. The disease has also been modulated with (15S)-15-methyl prostaglandin E_1 [47].

In general, these experiments seem to add weight to the evidence that cell-mediated mechanisms are important in the development and progression of anti-TBM antibody-associated tubulo-interstitial nephritis in the rat, although the quantitative contribution of antibody remains to be determined.

CELL-MEDIATED MODELS OF TUBULO-INTERSTITIAL NEPHRITIS IN THE RAT

The development of models of tubulo-interstitial nephritis mediated purely by T-cells has proved difficult. This has been especially frustrating as the majority of cases of human tubulo-interstitial nephritis appear to be mediated by just this mechanism, as evidenced by mononuclear cell infiltrates with many T-cells and the lack of antibody [48–51].

Extrarenal antigens can be used to induce delayed type hypersensitivity reactions in the kidney interstitium. The intra-cortical injection of aggregated, but not of soluble, bovine gamma globulin in guinea pigs or rats previously sensitized with the same antigen resulted in mononuclear cell infiltrates with focal tubular destruction [14]. This reactivity was transferable with cells but not with serum. The physical nature of the antigen, presumably related to its retention in the interstitium, was apparently important in determining whether a delayed type hypersensitivity reaction would occur.

Tubulo-interstitial nephritis in Lewis rats following immunization with autologous renal antigens

In relation to the above concept, Sugisaki et al [15] described a model of tubulo-interstitial nephritis in the Lewis rat that appears to be the result of cell-mediated reactivity against unknown autologous renal antigens. Immunization with syngeneic kidney homogenate and adjuvants resulted in irregular mononuclear cell interstitial infiltrates without immunofluorescence detectable antibody deposition. Mild lesions could be transferred by cells, but not serum, within 24 hours. In our experience syngeneic renal basement membrane preparations produce extremely mild or no cellular infiltrates at all when used to immunize Lewis rats [17,18]. However, the Lewis rat seemed the logical choice in which to study cellular mechanisms in the initiation of tubulo-interstitial nephritis as the inability of the Lewis tubular basement membrane to bind antibody would hopefully allow the contribution of humoral mechanisms to be ruled out.

Tubulo-interstitial nephritis in Lewis rats following immunization with homologous renal basement membranes

A wide range of homologous and heterologous renal basement membrane preparations were tested for their ability when combined with adjuvants to produce a reliable model of tubulo-interstitial nephritis in the Lewis rat. Immunization with homologous renal basement membrane from strains expressing the immunofluorescent detectable tubular basement membrane antigen emulsified in CFA and, together with *Bordetella pertussis* vaccine, resulted in the consistent appearance of a severe nodular form of tubulo-interstitial nephritis useful for characterization in terms of the contribution of humoral and cellular immunity.

Temporal characterization of Lewis tubulo-interstitial nephritis

Following immunization with 4mg Brown Norway renal basement membrane and adjuvants, mild focal mononuclear cell infiltration between tubules was first evident at day 9, increasing until day 21. A polymorphonuclear leucocyte influx did not occur. By days 12–14, over 35% of the surface of the kidneys was involved with very characteristic focal, nodular lesions which could be seen on gross examination, and which histologically appeared granulomatous with a central area containing epithelioid cells, occasional giant cells and a surrounding infiltrate of mononuclear cells (Figure 2). These focal inflammatory lesions occurred throughout the cortex (and outer medulla), where they always surrounded collapsed and severely damaged tubules and often had a

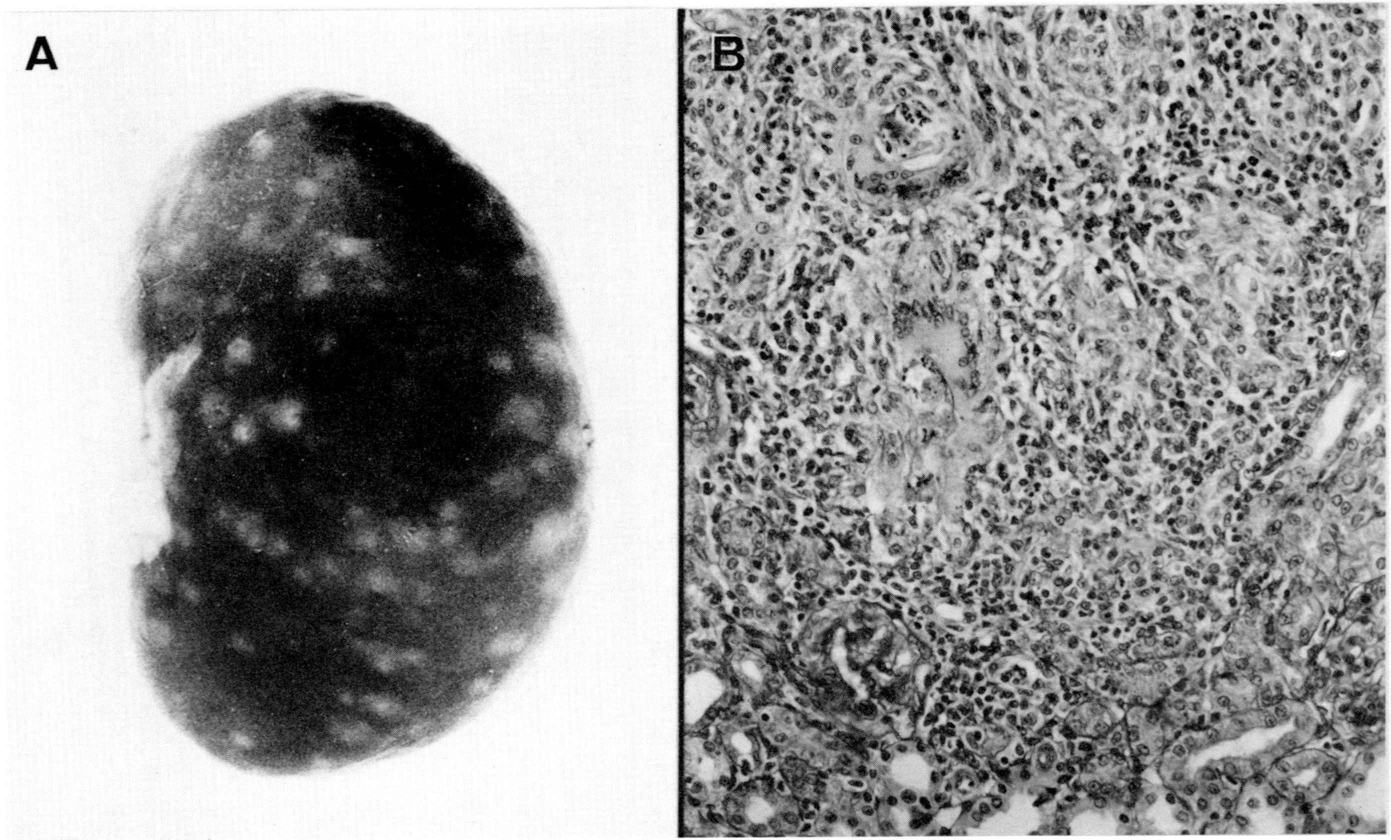

Figure 2. A) Macroscopic appearance of kidney at day 14 from a Lewis rat immunized with Brown Norway renal basement membrane and adjuvants. B) Day 14 histology showing granuloma-like infiltrate with giant cell. × 250

periglomerular localization. By days 21–28, the mononuclear cell infiltrate decreased, leaving dilated tubules with peritubular fibrosis and increased numbers of giant cells.

Serum creatinine was significantly elevated in immunized Lewis rats (1.3± 0.11mg/dl) at day 14 compared to controls (0.60±0.03mg/dl), but by day 28 the values were no longer significantly different. Significant proteinuria or glycosuria was not present in the rats at either days 14 or 28.

Characterization of the humoral response in the Brown Norway renal basement membrane immunized Lewis rat

Tubular or glomerular basement membrane IgG fixation was not found on days 5–14 except in occasional areas of inflammation, where portions of tubular basement membrane showed linear IgG staining at day 14. As noted above, CS-Lewis-TBM does contain small amounts of the tubular basement membrane antigen reacting with Brown Norway anti-TBM antibody in inhibition RIA studies [23], suggesting that exposure of these antigens may occur in Lewis tubular basement membrane in the presence of enzymes related to the inflammatory process. At later time points some rats were found to have weak linear glomerular basement membrane staining, indicating the occasional emergence of an auto-anti-basement membrane antibody different from the allo-reactive anti-Brown Norway-TBM response seen in all Brown Norway renal basement membrane immunized Lewis rats. This antibody may be similar to that noted earlier in the studies of Robertson et al [22] or reported recently by Sado et al [52]. Further studies suggested that the anti-GBM antibody from our rats also reacted with human glomerular basement membrane antigens by RIA separating it from the typical anti-TBM antibody response seen in humans.

In view of the findings of occasional fixation of anti-basement membrane antibodies on direct immunofluorescence, elution studies were undertaken. The eluate of day 14 kidneys failed to bind to normal Lewis kidney targets, but day 28 eluates did react to some extent with linear glomerular and tubular basement membrane staining and showed a selective concentration of anti-Lewis-RBM antibody over serum on RIA. However, the relatively late fixation of these auto-antibodies compared to the development of histological disease suggests their pathogenetic rôle to be minimal.

As previously mentioned, the Lewis rats immunized with Brown Norway renal basement membrane produced a high titre (1:12, 800 at day 14) circulating allo-antibody reactive with Brown Norway tubular basement membrane on immunofluorescence and RIA. In addition, low titres of an auto-antibody reactive with Lewis particulate and CS-RBM could be detected by RIA, presumably corresponding to the day 28 eluted auto-antibody.

Characterization of the cellular immune response in immunized Lewis rats

All cells within inflammatory foci expressed the Ia antigen (OX 6^+). The central epithelioid cells in granulomatous foci did not react with a pan T-cell antibody (OX 19), but 50–60% of the surrounding mononuclear cells were OX 19 positive and W3/25 (T-helper) positive, with minimal numbers of OX 8 positive (T-suppressor) cells and B-cells. Many cells therefore expressed both T-cell markers and Ia, suggesting T-cell activation within inflammatory foci.

Although lymph node cells from immunized Lewis rats incorporated thymidine in response to the immunizing antigen and also to other renal basement membranes expressing the immunofluorescence detectable tubular basement membrane antigen, minimal proliferation occurred after stimulation with autologous renal basement membrane. These data correlate with the relevance of the tubular basement membrane antigen in producing tubulo-interstitial nephritis in the Lewis rat, but the lack of stimulation by autologous renal basement membrane was surprising, especially since the lymph node cells were able to transfer the disease to Lewis recipients, implying sensitization to Lewis tubular basement membrane. It is unclear whether this was a technical problem, in that the proper antigen was not used, or perhaps was due to the presence of suppressor mechanism.

Adoptive transfer of tubulo-interstitial nephritis by lymph node cells

Intravenous transfer of day 14 immune cells (spleen and/or lymph node, including some B-cell depleted transfers) from immunized Lewis rats resulted in renal interstitial cell infiltration in 21 of 22 recipient rats. No histological lesions were seen after transfer of any control cells, including irradiated immune cells from Brown Norway renal basement membrane immunized Lewis rats and cells from ovalbumin immunized rats incubated with Brown Norway renal basement membrane prior to transfer. The latter findings strongly suggest that passive antigen transfer was not responsible for these lesions. At the earliest time point examined (day seven after transfer), severe focal tubular destruction was often present along with frequent giant cells and mononuclear cell infiltrates (Figure 3). Histologically, the lesions were the same as days 14–21 lesions in the active model. Immunofluorescence studies showed an absence of fixation of antibody to tubular or glomerular basement membranes in recipient kidneys. Characterization of the inflammatory infiltrates in the recipient kidneys, using monoclonal antibodies, again showed that nearly all cells were OX 6 positive (Ia) with the same proportions of T-cells and T-cell subsets as in the active model.

The lack of in vivo fixation of antibody to Lewis tubular basement membrane at the time of the developing disease and the successful transfer of the full-blown histological lesions with immune cells strongly suggests that cell-mediated immunity plays a central rôle in this model of tubulo-interstitial nephritis in the Lewis rat. Similar granulomatous-like lesions have been reported in the interstitial lesions of drug-induced tubulo-interstitial nephritis in humans [53].

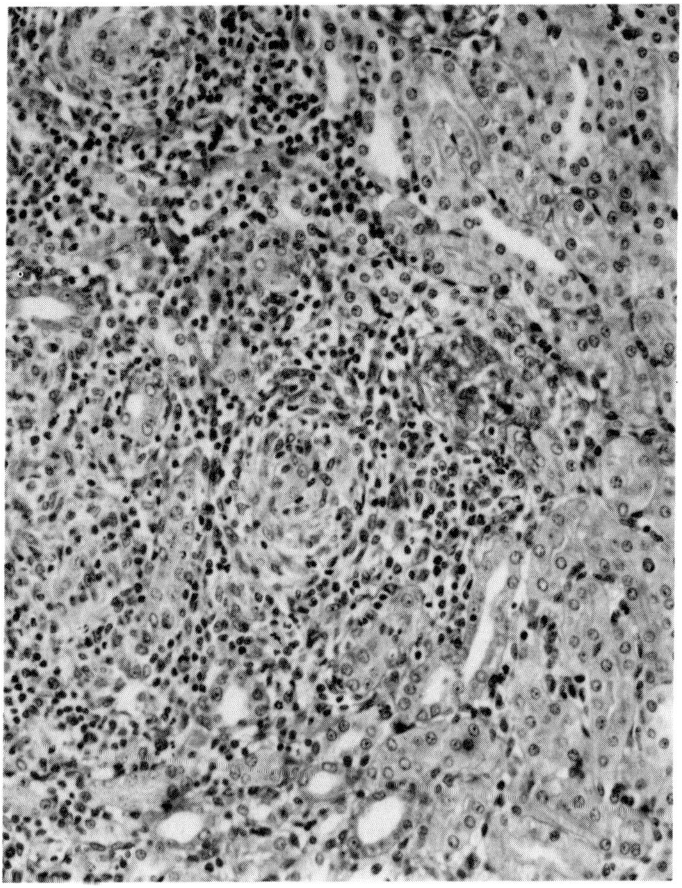

Figure 3. Histology of a portion of Lewis interstitial infiltrate seen at day seven following adoptive transfer of lymph node cells from Lewis rats immunized with Brown Norway renal basement membrane and adjuvants. × 250

Summary

We present an overview of the participation of humoral and cellular immune mechanisms involved in tubulo-interstitial nephritis in the rat. Antibody transfer demonstrates that anti-TBM antibody is responsible for the initiation of tubulo-interstitial nephritis in the Brown Norway rat, the strain most commonly used for such studies. The quantitative kinetics of antibody binding are slow and about 167μg are needed for disease induction. The complement dependence of both the active and passively transferred lesions has been demonstrated. There is also strong indirect evidence that cell-mediated immune mechanisms play a rôle in the progressive nature of the anti-TBM antibody-associated interstitial lesions. Several different molecular weight tubular basement membrane target antigens with some unexplained variation in reported molecular weight have been identified in the rat and in humans, who share this antigen system and its genetically variable appearance.

We present evidence of a purely cell-mediated mechanism which can cause tubulo-interstitial nephritis in the Lewis rat. The Lewis rat, when immunized with homologous tubular basement membrane antigen positive renal basement membrane, has provided evidence of the considerable importance of both anti-TBM antibody, by virtue of the successful serum transfer of tubulo-interstitial nephritis to Brown Norway rats, and of cellular mechanisms by the adoptive transfer of a different form of tubulo-interstitial nephritis to Lewis recipients. This new model of cell-mediated tubulo-interstitial nephritis provides a useful link to advance the understanding of cellular immune mechanisms as they may apply to human tubulo-interstitial nephritis.

Acknowledgments

This is publication No 4961-IMM from the Department of Immunology, Research Institute of Scripps Clinic, La Jolla, California, USA. This work was supported in part by United States Public Health Service Grants DK-20043, DK-32353, and Biomedical Research Support Grant RRO-5514. Dr Bannister was the recipient of a National Kidney Foundation of America Fellowship and a Royal Australasian College of Physicians Travelling Fellowship.

References

1 McCluskey RT. Immunologically mediated tubulointerstitial nephritis. In Cotran RS, Brenner BM, Stein JH, eds. *Contemporary Issues in Nephrology, Volume 10.* New York: Churchill Livingstone. 1983: 121–149

2 Andres GA, McCluskey RT. Tubular and interstitial renal disease due to immunologic mechanisms. *Kidney Int 1975; 7:* 271–289

3 Wilson CB, Dixon FJ. The renal response to immunological injury. In Brenner BM, Rector FC Jr, eds. *The Kidney, 3rd Edition.* Philadelphia: Saunders. 1986; 800–889

4 Steblay RW, Rudofsky U. Transfer of experimental autoimmune renal cortical tubular and interstitial disease in guinea pigs by serum. *Science 1973; 180:* 966–968

5 Bannister KM, Wilson CB. Transfer of tubulointerstitial nephritis in the Brown-Norway rat with anti-tubular basement membrane antibody: quantiation and kinetics of binding and effect of decomplementation. *J Immunol 1985; 135:* 3911–3917

6 Zakheim B, McCafferty E, Michael-Phillips S et al. Murine interstitial nephritis. II. The adoptive transfer of disease with immune T lymphocytes produces phenotypically complex interstitial lesion. *J Immunol 1984; 133:* 234–239

7 Neilson EG, McCafferty E, Mann R et al. III. The selection of phenotypic (Lyt and L3t4) and idiotypic (RE-Id) T cell preferences by genes in Igh-1 and H-2k characterizes the cell mediated potential for disease expression: susceptible mice provide a unique effector T cell repertoire in response to tubular antigen. *J Immunol 1985; 134:* 2375–2382

8 Mann R, Zakheim B, Clayman M et al. IV. Long term cultures L3T4$^+$ T cell lines transfer delayed expression of disease as I-A-restricted inducers of the effector T cell repertoire. *J Immunol 1985; 135:* 286–293

9 Neilson EG, Clayman MD, Haverty T et al. Experimental strategies for the study of cellular immunity in renal disease. *Kidney Int 1986; 30:* 264–279

10 Neilson EG, McCafferty E, Mann R et al. Tubular antigen-derivatized cells induce a disease-protective, antigen-specific, and idiotype-specific suppressor T cell network restricted by I-J and Igh-V in mice with experimental interstitial nephritis. *J Exp Med 1985; 162:* 215–230

11 Ulich TR, Bannister KM, Wilson CB. Tubulointerstitial nephritis induced in the Brown-Norway rat with chaotropically solubilized bovine tubular basement membrane: the model and the humoral and cellular responses. *Clin Immunol Immunopathol 1985; 36:* 187–200

12 Lehman DH, Wilson CB. Role of sensitized cells in antitubular basement membrane interstitial nephritis. *Int Arch Allergy Appl Immunol 1976; 51:* 168–174

13 Van Zweiten MJ, Bhan AK, McCluskey RT, Collins AB. Studies on the pathogenesis of experimental anti-tubular basement membrane nephritis in the guinea pig. *Am J Pathol 1976; 83:* 531–546

14 Van Zweiten MJ, Leber PD, Bhan AK, McCluskey RT. Experimental cell-mediated interstitial nephritis induced with exogenous antigens. *J Immunol 1977; 118:* 589–593

15 Sugisaki T, Yoshida T, McCluskey RT et al. Autoimmune cell-mediated tubulointerstitial nephritis induced in Lewis rats by renal antigens. *Clin Immunol Immunopathol 1980; 15:* 33–43

16 Kelly CJ, Korngold R, Mann R et al. II. Characterization of a tubular antigen-specific, H-2K-restricted Lyt-2$^+$ effector T cell that mediates destructive tubulointerstitial injury. *J Immunol 1986; 136:* 526–531

17 Bannister KM, Ulich TR, Wilson CB. Cell-mediated autoimmune tubulo-interstitial nephritis (TIN) in the Lewis (LEW) rat. *Kidney Int 1985; 27 (Abstract):* 205

18 Bannister KM, Ulich TR, Wilson CB. Induction, characterization, and cell transfer of autoimmune tubulointerstitial nephritis in the Lewis rat. *Kidney Int 1987:* in press

19 Steblay RW, Rudofsky U. Renal tubular disease and autoantibodies against tubular basement membrane induced in guinea pigs. *J Immunol 1971; 107:* 589–594

20 Sugisaki T, Klassen J, Milgrom F et al. Immunopathologic study of an autoimmune tubular and interstitial renal disease in Brown-Norway rats. *Lab Invest 1973; 28:* 658–671

21 Lehman DH, Wilson CB, Dixon FJ. Interstitial nephritis in rats immunized with heterologous tubular basement membrane. *Kidney Int 1974; 5:* 187–195

22 Robertson JL, Hill GS, Rowlands DT. Tubulointerstitial nephritis and glomerulonephritis in Brown-Norway rats immunized with heterologous glomerular basement membrane. *Am J Pathol 1977; 88:* 53–68

23 Zanetti M, Wilson CB. Characterization of anti-tubular basement membrane antibodies in rats. *J Immunol 1983; 130:* 2173–2179

24 Mampaso F, Wilson CB. Characterization of inflammatory cells in autoimmune tubulointerstitial nephritis in rats. *Kidney Int 1983; 23:* 448–457

25 Krieger A, Thoenes GH, Gunther E. Genetic control of autoimmunetubulointerstitial nephritis in rats. *Clin Immunol Immunopathol 1981; 21:* 301–308

26 Sugisaki T, Kano K, Andres GA, Milogrom F. Antibodies to tubular basement membrane elicited by stimulation with allogeneic kidney. *Kidney Int 1982; 21:* 557–564

27 Neilson EG, Gasser DI, McCafferty E et al. Polymorphism of genes involved in antitubular basement membrane disease in rats. *Immunogenetics 1983; 17:* 55–65

28 Hyman LR, Steinberg AD, Colvin RB, Bernard EF. Immunopathogenesis of autoimmune tubulointerstitial nephritis. II. Role of an immune response gene linked to the major histocompatibility locus. *J Immunol 1976; 117:* 1894–1897

29 Kelly CJ, Silvers WK, Neilson EG. Tolerance to parenchymal self. Regulatory role of major histocompatibility complex-restricted OX8$^+$ suppressor T cells specific for autologous renal tubular antigen in experimental interstitial nephritis. *J Exp Med 1985; 162:* 1892–1903

30 Brown CA, Carey K, Colvin RB. Inhibition of autoimmune tubulointerstitial nephritis in guinea pigs by heterologous antisera containing antiidiotype antibodies. *J Immunol 1979; 123:* 2102–2107

31 Neilson EG, Phillips SM. Suppression of interstitial nephritis by auto-anti-idiotypic immunity. *J Exp Med 1982; 155:* 179–189

32 Zanetti M, Mampaso F, Wilson CB. Anti-idiotype as a probe in the analysis of autoimmune tubulointerstitial nephritis in the Brown Norway rat. *J Immunol 1983; 131:* 1268–1273

33 Graindorge PP, Majieu PR. Radioimmunologic method for detection of antitubular basement membrane antibodies. *Kidney Int 1978; 14:* 594–606

34 Wakashin Y, Takei I, Ueda S et al. Autoimmune interstitial disease of the kidney and associated antigen purification and characterization of a soluble tubular basement membrane antigen. *Clin Immunol Immunopathol 1981; 19:* 360–371

35 Clayman MD, Martinez-Hernandez A, Michaud L et al. Isolation and characterization of the nephritogenic antigen producing anti-tubular basement membrane disease. *J Exp Med 1985; 161:* 290–305

36 Fliger FD, Wieslander J, Brentjens JR et al. Identification of a target antigen in human anti-tubular basement membrane nephritis. *Kidney Int 1987; 31:* 800–807

37 Yoshioka K, Morimoto Y, Iseki T et al. Characterization of tubular basement membrane antigens in human kidney. *J Immunol 1986; 136:* 1654–1660

38 Clayman MD, Michaud L, Brentjens J et al. Isolation of the target antigen of human anti-tubular basement membrane antibody-associated interstitial nephritis. *J Clin Invest 1986; 77:* 1143–1147

39 Wilson CB, Lehman DH, McCoy RC et al. Antitubular basement membrane antibody after renal transplantation. *Transplantation 1974; 18:* 447–431

40 Unanue ER, Dixon FJ. Experimental glomerulonephritis. V. Studies on the interaction of nephrotoxic antibodies with tissue of the rat. *J Exp Med 1965; 121:* 697–714

41 Rudofsky UH, Steblay RW, Pollara B. Inhibition of experimental autoimmune renal tubulointerstitial disease in guinea pigs by depletion of complement with cobra venom factor. *Clin Immunol Immunopathol 1975; 3:* 396–407

42 Ulich TR, Bannister KM, Wilson CB. Inhibition of the neutrophilic infiltrate of experimental tubulointerstitial nephritis in the Brown-Norway rat by decomplementation. *Clin Immunol Immunopathol 1987; 42:* 288–297

43 Neilson EG, McGafferty E, Phillips SM et al. Antiidiotypic immunity in interstitial nephritis. II. Rats developing anti-tubular basement membrane disease fail to make an antiidiotypic regulatory response: the modulatory role of an $RT7.1^+$, $OX8^-$ suppressor T cell mechanism. *J Exp Med 1984; 159:* 1009–1026

44 Kelly CJ, Clayman MD, Neilson EG. Immunoregulation in experimental interstitial nephritis: immunization with renal tubular antigen in incomplete Freund's adjuvant induces major histocompatibility complex-restricted, $OX8^+$ suppressor T cells which are antigen-specific and inhibit the expression of disease. *J Immunol 1986; 136:* 903–907

45 Agus D, Mann R, Cohn D et al. Inhibitory role of dietary protein restriction on the development and expression of immune-mediated antitubular basement membrane-induced tubulointerstitial nephritis in rats. *J Clin Invest 1985; 76:* 930–936

46 Agus D, Mann R, Clayman M et al. The effects of daily cyclophosphamide administration on the development and extent of primary experimental interstitial nephritis in rats. *Kidney Int 1986; 29:* 635–640

47 Ulich TR, Ni R-X. Inhibition of experimental autoimmune tubulointerstitial nephritis in Brown-Norway rats by (15S)-15-methyl prostaglandin E_1. *Am J Path 1986; 124:* 286–293

48 Gimenez A, Mampaso F. Characterization of inflammatory cells in drug-induced tubulointerstitial nephritis. *Nephron 1986; 43:* 239–240

49 Brunati C, Brando B, Confalonieri R et al. Immunophenotyping of mononuclear cell infiltrates associated with renal disease. *Clin Nephrol 1986; 26:* 15–20

50 Boucher A, Droz D, Adafer E et al. Characterization of mononuclear cell subsets in renal cellular interstitial infiltrates. *Kidney Int 1986; 29:* 1043–1049

51 Husby G, Tung KSK, Williams RC Jr. Characterization of renal tissue lymphocytes in patients with interstitial nephritis. *Am J Med 1981; 70:* 31–38

52 Sado Y, Okigaki T, Takamiya H et al. Experimental autoimmune glomerulonephritis with pulmonary hemorrhage in rats. The dose-effect relationship of the nephritogenic antigen from bovine glomerular basement membrane. *J Clin Lab Immunol 1984; 15:* 199–204

53 Magil AB. Drug-induced acute interstitial nephritis with granulomas. *Hum Pathol 1983; 13:* 36–41

INHERITED RENAL DISEASES

ADVANCES IN THE UNDERSTANDING OF INHERITED RENAL DISEASES

J P Grünfeld, L H Noël, G Bobrie, C Ferran, G Albouze, R Charbonneau, *C M Lockwood, *C O S Savage, †L Bachner, †J C Kaplan, **M C Hors-Cayla, **S Szpiro-Tapia

*Hôpital Necker, Paris, France, *Royal Postgraduate Medical School, Hammersmith Hospital, London, United Kingdom, †INSERM U129, Institut de Pathologie moléculaire, CHU Cochin, Paris, **INSERM U12, Hôpital des Enfants Malades, Paris, France*

Inherited diseases have long been considered a consequence of immutable fate and characterized by an inexorable course, unresponsive to therapy. Recent progress in various fields of medicine and biology has dramatically changed our mind and has allowed us to achieve (or to expect) better understanding, prevention and, in some cases, specific therapy. This is the case for hereditary renal diseases and further progress may be expected in the coming decades.

A prerequisite to advances in understanding is adequate evaluation of prevalence of these diseases and description of their specific clinical and pathological features. In adult patients, hereditary kidney diseases represent approximately 15 to 20% of all renal diseases (excluding diabetic nephropathy) and their prevalence is readily underestimated if genetic investigation is not routinely performed. Rambausek et al [1] have indicated that among 860 patients with glomerular diseases, 10% had a positive family history of kidney involvement. Among the 45 index families, 21 had unclassified, progressive or non-progressive, glomerular diseases. Efforts have been made to better categorize these so far unclassified hereditary diseases. Various forms of hereditary glomerulonephritis associated [2,3] or not with complement defects, have been identified and described as familial idiopathic membranous glomerulonephritis [4]. X-linked mesangiocapillary glomerulonephritis [5] or characterized by mesangial deposits of C3 [6] or of IgA (Berger's disease) [7]. With regard to the latter disease, M Lévy [personal communication] collected data in France in 26 unrelated families with idiopathic IgA nephropathy, each having at least two affected members. In 16 additional families, Berger's disease and Henoch-Schönlein purpura coexisted.

A new familial syndrome has been recently identified and characterized by small vessel hyalinosis involving kidneys and the digestive tract [8]. Diarrhoea, intestinal bleeding, malabsorption and protein-losing enteropathy are the most prominent features. Retinal ischaemic changes, poikiloderma, early hair greying, cerebral calcification and subarachnoid haemorrhage due to ruptured cerebral aneurysm are also associated abnormalities. In two patients [8,9], kidney involvement led to renal failure.

TABLE I. Heredofamilial diseases with renal involvement in adults. Adapted from [17]

1. Cystic kidney diseases
   - Adult-type (autosomal dominant)
   - Medullary cystic disease (or nephronophthisis)
   - Other cystic diseases

2. Hereditary nephritis
   - Progressive hereditary nephritis
     - with nerve deafness (Alport's syndrome)
     - without hearing impairment
     - variants
   - Familial benign haematuria

3. Hereditary metabolic disorders
   - Diabetes mellitus
   - Fabry's disease
   - Lecithin cholesterol acyltransferase deficiency
   - Primary hyperoxaluria
   - Familial urate nephropathy
   - Wilson's disease
   - Refsum's disease
   - Adult-type cystinosis
   - Other identified or unidentified storage diseases
   - Various complement defects
   - Genetic amyloidosis (including familial Mediterranean fever, Muckle-Wells syndrome, other nephropathic systemic amyloidosis and type 1 familial amyloid polyneuropathy)
   - Sickle cell disease

4. Diseases with extrarenal defects (in the absence of detected metabolic abnormalities)
   - Nail-patella syndrome
   - Tuberous sclerosis
   - Hereditary osteolysis
   - Juvenile megalolastic anaemia
   - Familial dysautonomia
   - Alström's syndrome
   - Laurence-Moon-Bardet-Biedl syndrome

5. Hereditary tubular disorders
   - Cystinuria
   - Other tubular defects

6. Renal diseases, usually sporadic, occasionally heredofamilial, such as:
   - Berger's disease
   - Vesicoureteric reflux with renal scars
   - Haemolytic-uraemic syndrome
   - Bartter's syndrome

7. Unclassified

In this review, we will mainly focus on inherited renal diseases observed in adults (Table I). We will, however, mention some hereditary diseases which occur exclusively or predominately in children, such as cystinosis or nephronophthisis.

Progress in the understanding of pathogenesis: the various inherited defects of renal basement membranes

Various defects involving renal basement membranes have been found by electronmicroscopy or other techniques in various renal diseases.

Nail-patella syndrome

This syndrome (or hereditary osteo-onychodysplasia) is inherited as an autosomal dominant trait. The incidence of kidney involvement ranges from 30 to 55% of the cases [10]. The rate of progression of the renal disease is often slow. A characteristic lesion of the glomerular basement membrane has been identified by electronmicroscopy [11–13]: it consists of areas of glomerular basement membrane rarefaction, containing bundles of cross-striated collagen fibrils. The tubular basement membrane is not affected. Immunochemical composition of the glomerular basement membrane has not been so far studied in the syndrome. Of note, Goodpasture's syndrome developed in one patient with the nail-patella syndrome [14]. It was postulated that the glomerular basement membrane alteration found in the latter disease might predispose to the development of anti-glomerular basement membrane antibody. To our knowledge, no case of anti-glomerular basement membrane nephritis has been described after kidney transplantation in patients with the nail-patella syndrome.

Glomerular basement membrane abnormalities similar to those seen in the nail-patella syndrome have been observed in two kindreds, in the absence of osteo-onychodysplasia [15,16]. In one of them, autosomal recessive inheritance was suggested [16]. Does the ultrastructural glomerular basement membrane lesion correspond to a specific pathogenetic mechanism, whatever the mode of inheritance or the extrarenal features?

Alport's syndrome

This syndrome is characterized by the association of hereditary renal disease and sensorineural hearing loss. Ocular defects are also observed, involving the lens and retina [17]. Among the variants of Alport's syndrome, the cases with leiomyomatosis and those with platelet abnormalities deserve mention. The association of oesophageal, tracheobronchial and genital leiomyomatosis with Alport's syndrome was first underlined by Garcia-Torres and Guarner and the syndrome of hereditary macrothrombocytopenia, nephritis and deafness by Epstein et al. Twenty-one cases have so far been reported. Granulocyte inclusions were detected in three kindreds [see review in 18]. In addition to Alport's syndrome, X-linked hereditary thrombocytopenia may be associated with elevated serum IgA and renal disease. This disorder may be a variant of the Wiskott-Aldrich syndrome [19].

Several lines of evidence have pointed out that a molecular defect in the structure of the glomerular basement membrane is involved in the pathogenesis of Alport's syndrome [20]: 1) characteristic changes of the glomerular basement membrane are found by electronmicroscopy in most but not all patients with Alport's syndrome [see review in 21]; 2) human anti-glomerular basement membrane antibodies do not bind to the glomerular basement membrane of some patients with Alport's syndrome; 3) some patients with Alport's syndrome develop anti-glomerular basement membrane mediated glomerulonephritis after kidney transplantation; most, though have satisfactorily functioning grafts [22]. It is of interest, however, that a significant percentage of transplanted kidneys in patients with Alport's syndrome have transient IgG linear fixation along the glomerular basement membrane in the absence of detectable circulating anti-glomerular basement membrane antibodies [22].

The preceding renal histopathological features are characteristic of hereditary nephritis and may therefore be used for diagnosis. Similar glomerular basement membrane defects have been found by electronmicroscopy and by immunofluorescence study [23,24] in patients who had neither positive family history of renal disease nor deafness, and have diseases probably related to Alport's syndrome. Jansen et al have described hereditary renal disease in a line of Samoyed dogs. The renal involvement bears some similarities with human hereditary nephritis: it progresses to renal failure in affected male dogs whereas female carriers show less severe disease; the pattern is consistent with X-linked dominant inheritance; the glomerular basement membrane appears normal at birth but thickening and splitting of the glomerular basement membrane develop subsequently in affected males [25,26]. Of great interest, a single human anti-glomerular basement membrane antibody was reactive with the glomerular basement membrane of normal dogs (except in the neonatal period) but did not bind to the glomerular basement membrane of affected male dogs, even after acid-urea treatment [27].

Analysis of altered glomerular basement membrane antigenicity in hereditary nephritis has been made possible by recent progress in the structure and composition of glomerular basement membrane [28–31]. The 'Goodpasture antigen' has been located, at least in part [30], in the globular non-collagenous 1 (NC1) domain of type IV collagen, a component of the basement membrane. Type IV collagen consists of three chains, generally considered to be two α-1(IV) and one α-2(IV). The central region is occupied by the triple helical domain; the globular NC1 domain is at the carboxyl terminus, whereas at the amino terminus of the molecule there is a collagenase-resistant region, referred to as the '7 S domain'. In addition to NC1 domain, there is a second non-collagenous region, the NC2 domain, which is found near the amino terminus. The NC1 domain receives contributions from both the α-a(IV) and α-2(IV) chains. It is felt to function as the site of initiation of assembly of the triple helix and to connect adjacent molecules of type IV collagen. The Samoyed dog provides an interesting model to study the rôle of the Goodpasture antigen and its ability to maintain integrity of the normal trilaminar glomerular basement membrane [27].

We will focus on the globular NCl domain of type IV collagen which contains Goodpasture antigen: sera from patients with Goodpasture's syndrome react with components of this domain and in contrast, do not react with the glomerular basement membrane of some patients with hereditary nephritis, pointing to a glomerular basement membrane defect in these subjects. This hypothesis has been further elaborated by the use of a mouse monoclonal antibody (MCA-P_1) to the Goodpasture antigen [28–31], an antigen which can be released in soluble form from human glomerular basement membrane by collagenase digestion (CS-GBM) and of sera from patients with Alport-type familial nephritis (FNS) who developed circulating anti-glomerular basement membrane antibodies and nephritis following renal transplantation [32]. The studies by Savage, Lockwood and their co-workers have clearly shown reduced or absent binding of MCA-P_1 to glomerular basement membrane of some patients with hereditary nephritis, using indirect immunofluorescence or immunoperoxidase techniques [33,34]. This subgroup of patients is also characterized by typical ultrastructural changes of the glomerular basement membrane. In contrast, these lesions were absent in most cases of hereditary nephritis with normal glomerular binding of MCA-P_1 [18]. Similar conclusions bearing on heterogeneity of Alport's syndrome were reached by Mounier et al by the use of anti-M_2 antibodies (the subunit M_2, a monomer of 26kD, contains the Goodpasture antigen) [35]. Defects in other constituents of normal glomerular basement membrane might be identified by using other monoclonal antibodies Melvin et al showed that in the glomerular basement membrane of patients lacking the Goodpasture antigen, amyloid P component was also selectively absent whereas it is detected in normal glomerular basement membrane. The amyloid P component, however, was found in the same patients in the mesangial region and in the internal elastic lamina of blood vessels [36]. It should be pointed out that absence of binding by immunofluorescence and typical ultrastructural glomerular basement membrane changes may be found in patients with hereditary nephritis without hearing loss, as well as in those with classical Alport's syndrome [18]. This suggests that the pathogenesis of these nephropathies is closely related and that the clinical separation between them may not be warranted.

The immunogenicity of the glomerular basement membrane was more directly studied by immunoblotting by using on the one hand CS-HGBM and collagenase solubilized glomerular basement membrane from kidneys of patients with hereditary nephritis (CS-HNK), and on the other hand, MCA-P_1, Goodpasture sera and familial nephritis sera. The immunoblotting studies on CS-HNK showed a discrete loss of certain antigenic bands of 54, 30 and 26kD, but the other bands (50, 42 and 22kD) retained their antigenicity. This suggests that the gene coding for the Goodpasture antigen is probably normal and that the abnormality may reside in carrier molecules to which the antigen is attached. In addition, preparations of CS-HNK failed to inhibit binding of anti-glomerular basement membrane antibodies to CS-HGBM in solid-phase radioimmunoassay. The latter result suggests that the remaining sites, carried on bands of 50, 42 and 22kD are hidden and not available for binding, whereas they are well exposed in the immunoblotting procedures [37]. Similarly Kleppel et al have recently indicated that a 28kD NC1 subunit was not detected in X-linked dominant Alport-type familial nephritis by protein staining or immunoblotting of digests of glomerular basement membrane, whereas 26 and 24kD subunits were present. They suggest a defect in the synthesis, secretion or membrane integration of the 28kD parent molecule [38].

Heterogeneity in Alport's syndrome is further demonstrated by the data of Kashtan et al dealing with the epidermal basement membrane of acid-urea denatured skin [32]. The binding of familial nephritis sera to control epidermal basement membrane was enhanced by acid-urea denaturation which uncovers antigenic determinants in basement membranes. In contrast, familial nephritis sera did not react with epidermal basement membrane of eight affected males, even after acid-urea denaturation, but the reactivity was normal in two additional male patients. Goodpasture sera and familial nephritis sera did not stain glomerular basement membrane in non-urea treated kidneys from affected males. After urea preincubation familial nephritis sera did not stain renal basement membranes but Goodpasture sera bound to epidermal basement membrane, tubular basement membrane and Bowman's capsules of affected males while the glomerular basement membrane remained unreactive. It was concluded that the familial nephritis antigen was distinct from the Goodpasture antigen [32]. In the study by Savage et al, the three familial nephritis sera used did not bind to normal epidermal basement membrane, either before or after acid-urea treatment [37]. This emphasizes again how the antibodies developing after transplantation in patients with Alport's syndrome are heterogeneous, and that various glomerular basement membrane defect(s) are probably involved in this syndrome.

Thinning of the glomerular basement membrane can be seen in children, at the early stages of Alport's syndrome, associated with segments of normal or thickened glomerular basement membrane [39], in cases of benign familial or non-familial haematuria [40,41], or in rare adult patients with progressive hereditary nephritis [1,21]. Thus the lesion is not specific for any hereditary renal disease. Immunogenicity of the thin glomerular basement membrane has not yet been studied, especially in patients with familial benign haematuria.

Nephronophthisis (or nephronophthisis-medullary cystic disease complex)
This autosomal recessive disease is a frequent cause of end-stage renal failure in children. Tapetoretinal degeneration is associated in some families. Skeletal

changes and liver fibrosis are less frequently found [42]. In the rare cases of adult-onset nephronophthisis, both autosomal recessive and autosomal dominant modes of inheritance have been observed [43].

Renal histopathological features are characterized by severe tubular atrophy, interstitial fibrosis and, in most cases, cysts at the corticomedullary junction and in the medulla. It has long been noted that thickening of the tubular basement membrane is an early and prominent morphological finding in nephronophthisis [42].

Two studies have recently been devoted to ultrastructural and immunohistochemical analysis of the tubular basement membrane in this disease [44,45]. Various types of tubular basement membrane changes have been observed. They include thickening, layering, duplication, wrinkling and splitting, with areas of extreme thinning and attenuation [44]. The extent of the changes and the abrupt transitions are remarkable. Indirect immunofluorescence staining demonstrated the presence of laminin and type IV collagen in the tubular basement membrane. Some thickened segments were heavily stained, but in most segments, Gubler et al found diffuse reduction of binding. The results of immunostaining with anti-tubular basement membrane antibodies are heterogeneous. With the use of anti-tubular basement membrane serum, Cohen and Hoyer found fixation in only 25% of tubular basement membrane whereas the great majority of cortical tubular basement membrane in controls stained. With the monoclonal anti-tubular basement membrane antibodies, staining was identical in control and patient kidneys [44]. Gubler et al observed decreased binding with one anti-tubular basement membrane antibody, and no staining in renal specimens from eight of nine patients with the use of the other antibody tested. The latter antibody, however, did not stain fetal kidneys and three of nine mature kidneys [45]. Grateau et al noted normal staining with anti-tubular basement membrane serum in the renal specimens of three adult patients. Atrophic tubules did not stain, in nephronophthisis as in other renal diseases [43].

Cohen and Hoyer have suggested that the fundamental defect in nephronophthisis may be the production of abnormal tubular basement membrane, analogous to the glomerular basement membrane abnormality found in Alport's syndrome. Further studies, however, are required to test this hypothesis: the ultrastructural tubular basement membrane changes are non-specific and no decisive conclusion can be drawn from immunochemical studies. The tubular defect might predispose to the development of anti-tubular basement membrane antibodies in some patients with nephronophthisis who receive a normal kidney transplant. This occurred in a single patient with nephronophthisis who developed massive linear deposition of IgG and C3 along both the tubular basement membrane and glomerular basement membrane. The nephrotic syndrome responded to plasmapheresis [46]. Such a complication has not been observed, however, in large series of transplanted patients with nephronophthisis [42].

Cystic kidney diseases

Autosomal dominant (or adult-type) polycystic kidney disease is the most frequent hereditary renal disease and one of the most frequent inherited diseases (approximately 1:1,000). Besides its inheritance and its inexorable course, adult-type polycystic kidney disease was penalized by its 'uninteresting' primary lesion, a cyst, i.e. water and solutes surrounded by an unspecific wall. Despite the pioneer work of Lambert in 1947, Dalgaard in 1953 and by Potter et al in the sixties, few studies have been devoted to the pathophysiology of cysts in adult-type polycystic kidney disease until recent years [see review in 47].

The question of how cysts function in situ has recently been raised. Cysts are not impermeable bags that store urine originating from more proximal nephron segments. Analysis of cyst content has shown that cyst epithelium was capable of carrying on active transport and that cysts retain some functional features of the tubule segments from which they arise. For example, 'distal' cystic fluid has low sodium ion and high hydrogen ion concentrations whereas fluid from a 'proximal' cyst has sodium ion concentration and pH similar to those of plasma [47,48]. Perrone has studied cyst epithelium from a human adult-type polycystic kidney disease, in vitro, using Ussing chamber techniques. He provided direct evidence for active transport mechanisms of cyst epithelium. Cysts with low sodium ions demonstrate characteristics consistent with distal nephron origin [49]. Ultrastructure of the cyst epithelium is correlated with function of the cyst wall. Distal cysts are lined by epithelial cells with tight apical junctions that appear permeable to lanthanum, whereas cells from proximal cysts have open or short closed junctions permeable to lanthanum [50]. In contrast, Grantham et al found by scanning electronmicroscopy that most cysts (84%) could not be correlated with any typical renal tubule segment [51].

Three pathophysiological mechanisms for cyst formation and progression have been proposed (they are not mutually exclusive).

Intratubular obstruction. This view has been developed by Evan, Gardner, Bernstein and co-workers [52]. In experimental cystic kidney diseases induced by various antioxidants, such as diphenylamine or nordihydroguaiaretic acid, cellular proliferation and micropolyp formation along outer medullary collecting ducts have been found. While the relevance to adult-type polycystic kidney disease might be questioned the authors point out that similar histopathological findings have been demonstrated in adult-type polycystic kidney disease. In contrast, in a more recent study, Grantham et al indicated that micropolyps, adenomas or linear cell hyperplasia were seen in only 4.9% of the cysts in adult-type polycystic kidney disease [51]. In addition, Welling and Welling [quoted in 47] have calculated that increased luminal pressure alone cannot explain the enlargement of renal cysts. The fluid-absorptive rate of the cyst epithelium should also decrease as the lesions progress.

Alteration of the tubular basement membrane, thereby increasing tubular compliance. Cuppage et al have indicated that cyst basement membranes appeared abnormal in adult-type polycystic kidney disease by electronmicroscopy but there was no consistent pattern [50]. Increased renal excretion of 3-hydroxy-proline may reflect abnormal synthesis or catabolism of renal type IV collagen [53]. Of great interest are the results of cell culture experiments. Wilson et al have grown proximal straight tubules and cortical collecting tubules of adult-type polycystic kidney disease. These epithelia grew more rapidly than normal tubular cells, and showed cyst-like areas. Ultrastructural study showed striking abnormalities of the tubular basement membrane consisting of some banded collagen and numerous blebs or spheroids stained with ruthenium red, suggesting a proteoglycan composition. The authors hypothesized that adult-type polycystic kidney disease cells synthesize an abnormal basement membrane [54]. These data have been obtained from end-stage cystic kidneys; they need to be extended by studying polycystic kidneys at an earlier stage.

Administration of various steroids, mainly to newborn animals, has been shown to induce renal cysts, arising from collecting ducts. Avner et al have found that addition of hydrocortisone induced cystic maldevelopment in serum-free murine metanephric organ culture. The most striking changes consisted of basolateral intercellular spreading and irregular thickening and lamellation of tubular basal laminae [55].

A more generalized defect in basement membranes might also be found in adult-type polycystic kidney disease, accounting for the systemic manifestations of the disease, such as aneurysms of the cerebral arteries, possibly diverticuli of the colon and cardiovascular abnormalities [47,56]. In this regard, the high incidence (approximately 30%) of asymptomatic mitral valve prolapse and/or incompetence found by echo/doppler studies in patients with adult-type polycystic kidney disease is striking [57]. Scarce information is available on the mechanisms involved in formation of liver cysts. It is generally accepted that liver cysts derive from segmentation and progressive dilatation of the von Meyenburg complexes. Liver cysts develop more slowly than kidney cysts, and are detected in 70 to 80% of dialysis patients [58]. Complications of liver cysts, which are rare before end-stage renal failure, may be severe in dialysis patients, including infection of cyst fluid or cholangiocarcinoma originating from cyst epithelium [58].

Increased transepithelial secretion of solutes and water, possibly related to epithelial cell hyperplasia. Grantham et al have long put forward this hypothesis [47]. They have recently provided evidence that the number of epithelial cells increases strikingly as tubule segments enlarge to form cysts, and that transepithelial secretion is the only way to fill cysts which are not connected with proximal segments [51]. Indeed by scanning microscopy, they found clear evidence of at least one tubule opening in only 27.3% of selected spherical cysts and in 10.2% of the randomly examined cysts [51]. Kidneys from azotaemic patients (9 of 10 cases) were studied and morphological exmination at earlier stages of adult-type polycystic kidney disease is required.

It had been assumed from inulin measurements in cyst fluid after bolus parenteral injections that glomerular filtration was the primary mechanism by which solutes enter the cysts of adult-type polycystic kidney disease. This assumption has been questioned [59,60]. Cyst fluid may derive not only from glomerular filtrate, but also from transepithelial secretion, non-ionic diffusion and ion trapping. These findings are of clinical interest when penetration of antibiotics into cysts is considered. It was found that highly lipid-soluble and non-polar antibiotics equilibrate into cysts by diffusion across cyst walls [61]. Trimethoprim, chloramphenicol, metronidazole, and ciprofloxacin (and probably related compounds) were shown to be effective agents in the treatment of renal cyst infections in adult-type polycystic kidney disease [61,62].

Animal models of autosomal recessive polycystic kidney disease have been developed in inbred strains of Springboks [63] and of C57 BL/6 J (cpk/cpk) mice. These models are appropriate for studying expression of the genes involved in the control of tubular cell proliferation and of basement membrane synthesis [64]. Crocker et al have suggested that renal cyst formation in homozygous cpk/cpk mice might be related in part to a transient abnormal increase of corticosterone (the major glucocorticoid in rats) in the post-natal period [65]. Of interest, the cystic tubular changes completely regressed when the kidneys from this mutant strain were cultured in serum-free organ culture, demonstrating that environmental factors (possibly glucocorticoids) regulate the expression of the defective gene(s) [66]. Corticosteroids are known to stimulate various transport systems, including Na^+, K^+-ATPase and Na^+/H^+ exchange, in kidney tubules and other tissues; the activity of these transport systems needs to be evaluated in the polycystic kidney diseases [54]. Crocker et al also found cystic dilatations of liver biliary ducts in heterozygous (cpk/+), but not in homozygous mice. It is not clear whether the liver changes are reminiscent of the cysts observed in adult-type polycystic kidney disease or of the intrahepatic biliary dilatations found in recessive (infantile) polycystic kidney disease [65].

Some key questions concerning renal cyst formation and progression are unsolved. Solitary cysts readily develop in the ageing kidney. Are the mechanisms involved in the genesis of solitary cysts similar to those implicated in adult-type polycystic kidney disease? Why is the formation of solitary cysts limited whereas cysts progress in adult-type polycystic kidney disease? Is there some analogy between the development of acquired multiple renal cysts in end-stage renal failure and that of adult-type polycystic kidney disease? How many nephrons are involved in cyst formation in adult-type polycystic kidney disease? Grantham and his co-workers suggested from β_2-microglobulin measurements in cystic fluid and from morphological data that cysts develop in relatively few nephrons and collecting ducts, and that the renal disease progresses, not because more tubules are recruited to form cysts, but because the established cysts enlarge, compress and atrophy the adjacent parenchyma [51,67]. This view may justify surgical or pharmacological attempts at reducing early cyst size. This hypothesis has stimulated renewed interest in the surgical procedures proposed in the past for reducing cyst volume [68]. If the hypothesis of Grantham et al is valid and if there is a renal defect in cell metabolism (whatever it is) in adult-type polycystic kidney disease, why are only some nephrons affected? In vitro studies on cystic and non-cystic areas from affected kidneys may clarify this issue.

In addition to adult-type polycystic kidney disease, other rare cystic kidney diseases may be found in adults. In medullary cystic disease (or nephronophthisis), cysts may be detected by ultrasonography [43]. Glomerulocystic kidney disease has been reported either as the only major anomaly, progressing to renal failure, or as part of a well-defined syndrome (such as Zellweger – a peroxisomal disorder, trisomy 13, or short-rib polydactyl syndrome [69] or associated with various congenital abnormalities of the cardiac, gastrointestinal and genito-urinary systems, mainly in children [7]). Familial glomerulocystic kidney disease without extrarenal defects has been identified in rare adult patients. The transmission is compatible with autosomal dominant inheritance [70,71]. Ultrasonographic findings are not homogeneous: renal cysts may be detected [70] but in other cases, the cortical microcysts had a mean diameter of 328μm and were not seen by ultrasonography [71]. In the oro-facial-digital syndrome (an X-linked dominant condition), a cystic kidney disease is found which is probably of the 'glomerulocystic' type; no liver cysts were detected, except in one case [72].

Advances in some inherited metabolic disorders with kidney involvement

For several decades, the inherited metabolic diseases with renal involvement (Table I) have been identified on clinical and biochemical grounds. Therapeutic progress, however, has long been minimal, limited to symptomatic management. In some cases, decisive advances have been made in recent years and effective therapy may be expected in the next decade.

Cystinosis is a rare autosomal recessive disorder, resulting from cystine accumulation within the lysosomes of various cell types. Normal lysosomal transport of cystine requires a carrier system which is impaired in cystinosis. Kidney involvement leads to end-stage renal failure in children, generally by 10 years of age. The diagnosis is based on the early-onset Fanconi syndrome, failure to thrive and rickets, on the pathognomonic finding of cystine crystals in the cornea by slit-lamp examination, and on a large increase in the level of free cystine in polymorphonuclear leucocytes and cultured fibroblasts [73,74]. Besides the most common form, nephropathic cystinosis, two other variants have been recognized, benign cystinosis (with only eye involvement) and late-onset or juvenile or adolescent cystinosis [75,76]. In the latter form, the Fanconi syndrome is slight or incomplete, and heavy proteinuria is associated with focal and segmental glomerular hyalinosis and with multinucleated glomerular epithelial cells (polykaryocytosis). The renal disease progresses to end-stage, usually by 20 years of age or less [75,76].

Recently it has been demonstrated that cysteamine constitutes the current treatment of choice of nephropathic cystinosis in children [74]. Cysteamine freely traverses the lysosomal membranes, and reacts with lysosomal cystine to form cysteine and cysteine-cysteamine which leave cystinotic lysosomes. Thus oral cysteamine by depleting cells of cystine, helps maintain glomerular filtration rate and improves growth. Pre-existing renal injury, as indicated by the Fanconi syndrome and/or renal failure is, however, not reversible by cystine depletion. Oral cysteamine induces significant side effects, accounting for 14% non-compliance rate. More palatable and effective cystine-depleting agents, such as phosphocysteamine, may be expected to be clinically available in the near future [74].

Topical cysteamine, in eyedrops, has been shown to decrease the number of corneal crystals in two children in whom therapy had been initiated before two years of age [77]. It should, however, be kept in mind that visual disturbances, leading to blindness, are mainly related to specific retinal changes which develop late during regular dialysis and/or kidney transplantation [73].

Fabry's disease is characterized by the deficiency in the lysosomal α-galactosidase A, resulting in the accumulation of globotriaosylceramide and related α-galactosyl terminating glycosphingolipids. It is inherited as a recessive X-linked trait. Hemizygous males progress to renal failure due to glycolipid accumulation in the kidneys [78].

Attempts at enzyme replacement therapy have been so far disappointing. Normal plasma or purified placental or splenic human α-galactosidase infusion restores transiently some circulating enzyme activity; plasma exchange removes glycosphingolipid; intraperitoneal injection of human fetal liver cells induces slight clinical and biochemical effects [79] but none of these procedures modify cell enzyme deficiency or affect the long-term clinical course. Similarly, after earlier enthusiastic reports, the results of kidney transplantation have been disappointing in restoring general tissue α-galactosidase A activity and removing accumulated glycolipid [see discussion in 78]. Glycolipid deposition does not recur in glomeruli or tubules of the transplant (except in the case described by Faraggiana et al [80]), demonstrating that the local tissue level of galactosidase A is of crucial importance [78,81].

Recent biochemical data provide important information on the synthesis and processing of the human α-galactosidase A in normal and Fabry fibroblasts [82]. In normal cells, this enzyme is synthesized as a precursor which is processed in several days, via ill-defined intermediates to a mature form and then secreted in a final form. In fibroblasts from five unrelated Fabry patients, a marked heterogeneity with respect to the synthesis and processing was noted: synthesis of a normal enzyme, no synthesis of immunologically cross-reacting polypeptides, retarded maturation of the enzyme (probably due to resistance to processing proteinases), or rapid degradation of α-galactosidase A polypeptides [82]. These findings are not surprising since the lysosomal storage disorders are due not only to failure to synthetize an active form of the relevant enzyme, but also to various defects affecting processing, stability, packaging and transport to the lysosome [83]. In this regard, the diagnosis of two lysosomal storage diseases, cystinosis and Fabry's disease, has been made in a single sibship [84]. It is possible that different lysosomal disorders occur together because of a defect in a shared processing or stabilizing step (but the reported family does not provide an example of such a phenomenon).

Primary hyperoxaluria is a rare autosomal recessive disorder of oxalate metabolism. Type I primary hyperoxaluria is the most frequent form, characterized by increased urinary excretion of both glycolate and oxalate (whereas type II hyperoxaluria is accompanied by augmented L-glycerate excretion). Increased synthesis of oxalate induces urolithiasis, nephrocalcinosis and extrarenal calcium oxalate deposition (systemic oxalosis). The disease mainly affects children. The prognosis is poor despite end-stage renal failure supportive therapy. Conventional dialysis does not prevent the disabling and fatal consequences of systemic (bone and cardiovascular) oxalosis and to date the results of kidney transplantation have been poor [85].

Urological surgery may trigger irreversible renal failure. A non-surgical approach, such as extracorporeal shock-wave lithotripsy, may facilitate the treatment of renal stones [88]. Some progress has been made in the management of primary hyperoxaluria. In approximately one-third of the patients, oxalate production is reduced by administration of pyridoxine [86,87]. Strategies have been developed to improve prognosis of kidney transplantation. These measures include good donor match, vigorous perioperative dialysis, and administration of thiazide, phosphate and magnesium to minimize oxalate deposition in the graft [85].

The major advance in primary hyperoxaluria resides in the revision of the biochemical defect involved. It had been stated that the defective enzyme was 2-oxoglutarate:glyoxylate cystosolic carboligase but it was subsequently shown that carboligase does not normally exist in the cytosol of human liver. Danpure et al have found that activity of the peroxisomal alanine:gloxylate aminotransferase (AGT) was substantially reduced or absent in the liver of patients with type I pyridoxine-resistant primary hyperoxaluria whereas glutamate-gloxylate aminotransferase (GGT) activity was preserved [89]. Primary hyperoxaluria is phenotypically heterogeneous, ranging from the severe neonatal forms to the milder variants which may not be symptomatic until early adulthood. Liver residual AGT activity is inversely correlated to the severity of the disease. In addition high levels of GGT may compensate for the decrease of AGT and blunt severity of the disease [90].

Since the deficient enzyme in primary hyperoxaluria is normally expressed in hepatic tissue, it was logical to attempt liver transplantation (combined with kidney transplantation) to restore normal enzyme activity. This was performed in the case reported by Watts et al [91]. The plasma oxalate concentration, oxalate production rate and oxalate metabolic pool size decreased dramatically after liver transplantation despite very poor renal function. Unfortunately the patient died from sepsis [91]. Further attempts are warranted to assess the value of combined liver and kidney transplantation in primary hyperoxaluria.

Progress afforded by modern molecular biology

DNA technology has provided a breakthrough in many fields of medicine. Obviously, it has already contributed to our understanding of the basic mechanisms involved in genetic disorders. The clinical consequences include not only early diagnosis, but also new insights into the pathogenesis of these diseases.

In recent years various strategies have been devised to characterize the molecular defects in genetic diseases. In some cases, the abnormal gene products causing the clinical disorders are known. When the aminoacid sequence of the gene product is known or an antibody to it is available, the gene associated with the disease can be isolated. The mutation or the point mutation, producing the defective gene, can then be identified by analysing DNA from affected persons.

In other cases, the strategy is based on DNA-sequence polymorphisms. These polymorphic sequences are detectable by digesting DNA with enzymes called restriction endonucleases, which cleave DNA wherever a specific sequence occurs. Fragments of discrete well-defined length are obtained when DNAs from normal subjects are studied. In the human genome, single base-pair change may abolish an existing restriction-enzyme recognition site and therefore alter the length of these fragments. The term 'restriction-fragment-length polymorphism' (RFLP) has been coined to describe the variation in fragment length generated. Since 1978, more than a thousand DNA polymorphisms have been identified and some have been successfully linked to disease loci. The RFLPs have become useful as genetic markers.

The progress afforded by DNA analysis allows early diagnosis and better clinical classification. The data available on gene location in heredofamilial diseases with kidney involvement are summarized in Table II. Additional information on more precise gene mapping may be found in the original publications. It should be kept in mind that in the coming decades, the genes will be isolated and cloned; the gene products causing the expression of the diseases will be identified. This will help to clarify the pathogenesis of the genetic diseases. Advances in cell and molecular biology will be complementary in this regard. Concomitantly, in diseases with dominant inheritance, gene transfer to transgenic animals will reproduce an experimental disease similar to the human

TABLE II. Heredofamilial diseases with kidney involvement: data on gene location

Disease	Chromosome
Adult-type (autosomal dominant) polycystic kidney disease	16
X-linked dominant Alport's syndrome	X (provisional)
Fabry's disease	X
LCAT deficiency	16
Wilson's disease	13
Type I familial amyloidotic polyneuropathy (with amyloid deposition in the kidney)	18
C2 and C4 deficiency	6
C1q and H deficiency	1
Sickle-cell anaemia	11
Hypoxantine-guanine phosphoribosyl transferase deficiency (Lesch-Nyhan syndrome)	X
Adenine-phosphoribosyl transferase deficiency (2,3 dihydroadenine urolithiasis)	16
Nail-patella syndrome	9
Tuberous sclerosis of Bourneville	9
Torticollis, keloids, cryptorchidism and renal dysplasia	X
Carbonic anhydrase II deficiency (osteopetrosis, renal tubular acidosis and cerebral calcifications)	8
Lowe oculocerebral syndrome	X

disease. Finally it will be possible to test whether abnormalities caused by the defective genes are amenable to treatment.

We will briefly review information provided by DNA analysis in some inherited diseases with kidney involvement.

Adult-type polycystic kidney disease

Reeders et al located the adult-type polycystic kidney disease locus on the short arm of chromosome 16 by using a RFLP located at a probe site called 3′hyperviarable region (3′HVR) because it was immediately adjacent to the α-globin gene cluster on its 3′site. Adult type polycystic kidney disease has been mapped to within 11 centimorgans of the α-globin cluster [92]. Another marker, at the phenotypic level, the phosphoglycolate phosphatase locus was subsequently linked to both the locus for adult-type polycystic kidney disease and the α-globin gene cluster [93]. This gene, however, has not yet been cloned. Both markers are located downstream from the α-globin locus but the exact location of the adult-type polycystic kidney disease locus is unknown. The availability of a flanking marker will improve reliability of detection.

We have investigated the 3′HVR RFLPs in 127 individuals belonging to four large families, including 26 patients with adult-type polycystic kidney disease. The reliability was nearly 100% using two restriction enzymes (Pvu II and Bgl I; see Figure 1). We confirmed the tight linkage with the adult-type polycystic kidney disease locus since no recombinant was found [L Bachner, JC Kaplan et al, unpublished results].

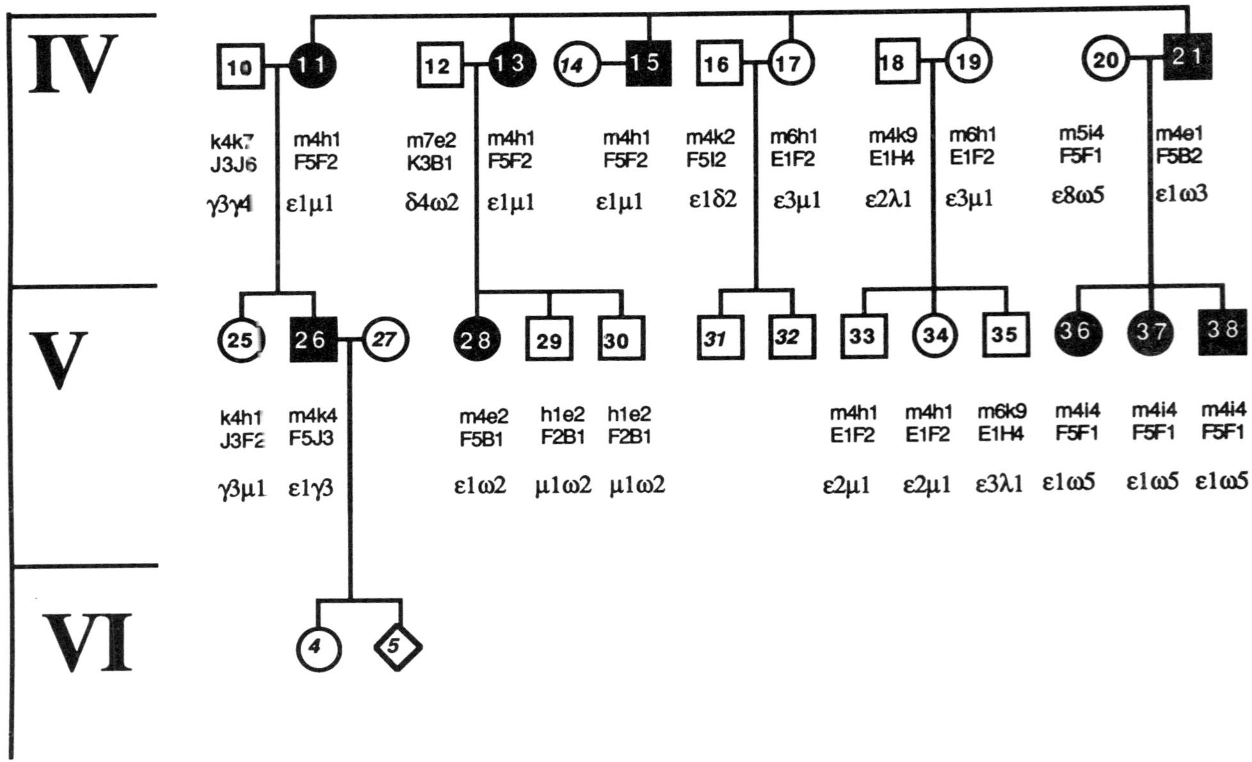

Figure 1. Part of a pedigree of a family with adult-type polycystic kidney disease. Cosegregation of the alleles m4 F5 (haplotype ε1) with the disease. Probe: 3′HVR. RFLPs: Pvu II (lower cases); Bgl I (capitals). Haplotypes are given in greek letters [L Bachner et al, unpublished results]

The question is open whether there is a single locus for all phenotypic variants of adult-type polycystic kidney disease. The data by Reeders et al suggest a single locus [92]. Further studies are required in families with unusual clinical manifestations to assess the possible genetic heterogeneity of adult-type polycystic kidney disease: for example, is the occurrence of cerebral artery aneurysms genetically determined or not? One of the most important issues concerns the progression of adult-type polycystic kidney disease: is the rate of progression dependent on genetic factors, environmental factors or both? Several studies have shown that a relatively large percentage of patients with adult-type polycystic kidney disease do not progress to end-stage renal failure or reach this stage after 70–80 years of age. Churchill et al have stated that persons with ultrasonographically detectable adult-type polycystic kidney disease may be advised that, conservatively, their chances of developing end-stage renal failure are 48% by the age of 73 years [94]. In the Olmsted County, the initial diagnosis of adult-type polycystic kidney disease was made at autopsy, over 80 years of age, in a significant number of cases [95]. Adult-type polycystic kidney disease has been identified as late as 96 years of age by autopsy [96]. In contrast, some children with adult-type polycystic kidney disease have early progression to renal failure, especially when clinical manifestations appear and the disease is diagnosed under one year of age [96]. Can these different rates of progression be predicted from DNA analysis?

The 3′HVR probe was used by Reeders et al in linkage studies for prenatal diagnosis in a nine-week fetus at risk for adult-type polycystic kidney disease. The fetus was judged to have inherited the adult-type polycystic kidney disease mutation. Pregnancy was terminated during the 12th week of gestation. Microscopical examination revealed multiple glomerular (with diameter up to 300μm) and tubular cysts in the renal cortex [97]. In very rare cases, the diagnosis of adult-type polycystic kidney disease has been made in the fetus by ultrasonography [98,99].

The availability of prenatal diagnosis of adult-type polycystic kidney disease raises ethical questions, similar to those in other disorders with onset in middle or late life. As indicated above, the rate of progression of adult-type polycystic kidney disease is heterogeneous and some affected patients may have a normal life span. In addition, regular dialysis and/or kidney transplantation are currently available to patients who progress to end-stage renal failure. The reliability of the 3′HVR marker is roughly 95% and the diagnosis is possible in approximately 92% of cases. Phophoglycolate phosphatase typing may be contributory in a few additional cases [93]. Genetic investigation implies DNA analysis and ultrasonography in many members of an affected family, including asymptomatic patients. This may have social and professional consequences, as well as negative psychological impact, especially if the medical information is not clearly delivered. All these drawbacks should be kept in mind and should be balanced with the hope of eradicating a debilitating disease and with the need to cope with the wishes of some heavily affected families. At present, nephrologists should avoid the wide and indiscriminate use of prenatal diagnosis of adult-type polycystic kidney disease. The position may change if the rate of progression of the disease could be predicted on a genetic basis.

It should be recalled that no data are available on the location of the defective gene responsible for autosomal recessive (infantile-type polycystic kidney disease.

Alport's syndrome and related hereditary nephritis

Genetic heterogeneity has been recognized in Alport's syndrome [100,101], which does not facilitate DNA studies. In many families, the mode of transmission is compatible with X-linked dominant inheritance, but in others, autosomal dominant and recessive inheritances have been identified [100].

Attention was first focused on X-linked forms. Indeed many genetic markers have been identified on the X chromosome. Menlove et al [102] and Brunner et al [103] have located the defective gene on the long arm of the X chromosome. The data by Brunner et al indicate close linkage between the gene and a DNA marker DXS 17 defined by probe S9, locating the gene near band Xq22 in the middle of the long arm [103]. Our preliminary results, obtained in three different families, in which the mode of transmission is compatible with an X-linked dominant inheritance, show one recombinant out of 11 meiosis with the marker DXS 17 and one recombinant out of 7 meiosis with the marker DXS 3. Those results are in keeping with the above data.

The question remains open as to how to relate the gene defect (possibly located on chromosome X in some kindreds) with the abnormality in type IV collagen found by immunochemical studies (see above). Indeed, human collagen genes encoding α_1 and α_2 chains of type IV collagen have been mapped to the distal long arm of chromosome 13 [104]. The genes encoding type IV collagen have a structure different from that of types I–III genes. Many questions cannot yet be answered. What is encoded for on the X chromosome which could influence type IV collagen synthesis? Effort should be made to better characterize the molecular defect(s) involved in hereditary nephritis. Attempts should also be made to classify affected families according to immunochemical findings. Are the various glomerular basement membrane defects related to discrete mutations in a given gene, as has been shown for other genetic diseases? Altered regulation may also reside in the collagen gene expression, e.g. resulting in increased transcriptional activity of the genes or in increased stability of type IV collagen mRNA transcripts.

Inherited metabolic disorders with kidney involvement

The human enzyme α-galactosidase A is encoded by a structural gene on the long arm of the X-chromosome, Xq21→q22. The gene has been cloned [see reference in 105]. Various mutations have been identified in unrelated families:

partial gene deletions, partial duplication or point mutation. This again shows how heterogeneous are the gene defects in a given lysosomal disease, as are the various metabolic defects (see above). In addition RFLPs have been defined for precise heterozygote detection [106]. Efforts have been undertaken to express full-length cDNA and to achieve production of large amounts of active enzyme for evaluation of enzyme replacement therapy [RJ Desnick, personal communication]. Similar progress may be expected in the following years with regard to lecithin-cholesterol acyltransferase (LCAT) deficiency. The defective gene has been located on the long arm of chromosome 16. The aminoacid sequence of human LCAT has been recently determined [107].

Recent advances in type I familial amyloidotic polyneuropathy (an autosomal dominant disease with lower limb neuropathy, gastrointestinal disorders, ocular abnormalities and renal involvement) are also exemplary. Prealbumin (or transthyretin) is the major component of the amyloid substance. In type I familial amyloidotic polyneuropathy, a variant of prealbumin is found, characterized by a single aminoacid substitution (a methionine in place of a valine at position 30). Investigations at the DNA level have resulted in the cloning of human prealbumin cDNA, the prealbumin gene and the location of this gene to chromosome 18. A single base change in the first position of the valine codon of the gene was found and this resulted in a new recognition site for a restriction enzyme, leading to a detectable RFLP [108,109].

Concomitantly, transgenic mice producing the variant prealbumin have been generated. Significant concentrations of the variant were found in the serum but it is not known so far whether these mice will develop amyloid deposition and polyneuropathy [110].

Inherited diseases with renal and extrarenal abnormalities, but without known metabolic disturbance

Two such diseases, nail-patella syndrome and tuberous sclerosis of Bourneville [111] are listed in Table II.

Inherited tubular disorders

Two such examples are quoted in Table II. Carbonic anhydrase II (CA II) deficiency is an autosomal recessive syndrome. Using a cloned mouse CA II cDNA probe and a panel of mouse-human somatic cell hybrids, the structural gene for human CA II was located on chromosome 8 [112]. More recently, the Lowe oculocerebrorenal syndrome (an X-linked hereditary disorder characterized by congenital cataract, mental retardation and Fanconi syndrome) has been mapped to Xq24–q26 by use of two RFLPs [113].

References

1 Rambausek G, Hartz G, Waldherr R et al. Familial glomerulonephritis. *Pediatr Nephrol:* in press

2 Coleman TH, Forristal J, Kosaka T, West CD. Inherited complement component deficiencies in membranoproliferative glomerulonephritis. *Kidney Int 1983; 24:* 681–690

3 Lévy M, Halbwachs-Mecarelli L, Gubler MC et al. H deficiency in two brothers with atypical dense intramembranous deposit disease. *Kidney Int 1986; 30:* 949–956

4 Vasmant D, Murnaghan K, Bensman A et al. Familial idiopathic membranous glomerulonephritis. *Int J Pediatr Nephrol 1984; 5:* 193–196

5 Stutchfield PR, White RHR, Cameron AH et al. X-linked mesangiocapillary glomerulonephritis. *Clin Nephrol 1986; 26:* 150–156

6 Kourilsky O, Gubler MC, Morel-Maroger L et al. A new form of familial glomerulonephritis. *Nephron 1982; 30:* 97–105

7 Julian BA, Quiggins PA, Thompson JS et al. Familial IgA nephropathy. Evidence of an inherited mechanism of disease. *N Engl J Med 1985; 312:* 202

8 Rambaud JC, Galian A, Touchard G et al. Digestive tract and renal small vessel hyalinosis, idiopathic nonarteriosclerotic intracerebral calcifications, retinal ischemic syndrome and phenotypic abnormalities. *Gastroenterology 1986; 90:* 930–938

9 Touchard G, Rambaud JC, Galian A et al. Hyalinose systémique familiale avec mésangiolyse: un nouveau syndrome (Abstract). *Néphrologie 1983; 4:* 94

10 Bennett WM, Musgrave JE, Campbell RA et al. The nephropathy of the nail-patella syndrome. Clinicopathologic analysis of 11 kindreds. *Am J Med 1973; 54:* 304–319

11 Silverman ME, Goodman RM, Cuppage FE. The nail-patella syndrome. *Arch Intern Med 1967; 120:* 68–74

12 Del Pozo E, Lapp H. Ultrastructure of the kidney in the nephropathy of the nail-patella syndrome. *Am J Clin Pathol 1970; 54:* 845–851

13 Ben-Bassat M, Cohen L, Rosenfeld J. The glomerular basement membrane in the nail-patella syndrome. *Arch Pathol 1971; 92:* 350–355

14 Curtis JH, Bhathena D, Leach RP et al. Goodpasture's syndrome in a patient with the nail-patella syndrome. *Am J Med 1976; 61:* 401–406

15 Dombros N, Katz A. Nail patella-like renal lesions in the absence of skeletal abnormalities. *Am J Kidney Dis 1982; 1:* 237–240

16 Salcedo JR. An autosomal recessive disorder with glomerular basement membrane abnormalities similar to those seen in the nail patella syndrome: report of a kindred. *Am J Med Gen 1984; 19:* 579–584

17 Grünfeld JP. The clinical spectrum of hereditary nephritis. *Kidney Int 1985; 27:* 83–91

18 Grünfeld JP, Grateau G, Noël LH et al. Variants of Alport's syndrome. *Pediatr Nephrol:* in press

19 Standen GR, Lillicrap DP, Matthews N, Bloom AL. Inherited thrombocytopenia, elevated serum IgA renal disease: identification as a variant of the Wiskott-Aldrich syndrome. *Q J Med 1986; 59:* 401–408

20 Spear GS. Hereditary nephritis (Alport's syndrome) – 1983. *Clin Nephrol 1984; 21:* 3–6

21 Habib R, Gubler MC, Hinglais N et al. Alport's syndrome: experience at Hôpital Necker. *Kidney Int 1982; 21:* S20–S28

22 Quérin S, Noël LH, Grünfeld JP et al. Linear glomerular IgG fixation in renal allografts: incidence and significance in Alport's syndrome. *Clin Nephrol 1986; 25:* 134–140

23 Resnik VM, Griswold WR, Vazquez MD et al. Glomerulonephritis with absent glomerular basement membrane antigens. *Am J Nephrol 1985; 5:* 296–298

24 Hara M, Asada R, Miura IK et al. Glomerulonephritis with absent glomerular basement membrane antigens and no family history of renal diseases. *Am J Nephrol 1987; 7:* 69–70

25 Jansen B, Tryphonas L, Wong J et al. Mode of inheritance of samoyed hereditary glomerulopathy: an animal model for hereditary nephritis in humans. *J Lab Clin Med 1986; 107:* 551–555

26 Jansen B, Thorner P, Baumal R et al. Samoyed hereditary glomerulopathy (SHG). Evolution of splitting of glomerular capillary basement membranes. *Am J Pathol 1986; 125:* 536–545

27 Thorner P, Jansen B, Baumal R et al. Samoyed hereditary glomerulopathy. *Lab Invest 1987; 56:* 435–443

28 Weber S, Engel J, Widemann H et al. Subunit structure and assembly of the glomerular domain of basement-membrane collagen type IV. *Eur J Biochem 1984; 139:* 401–410

29 Butkowski RJ, Wieslander J, Wisdom BJ et al. Properties of the globular domain of type IV collagen and its relationship to the Goodpasture antigen. *J Biol Chem 1985; 260:* 3739–3747

30 Kefalides NA. The Goodpasture antigen and basement membranes: the search must go on. *Lab Invest 1987; 56:* 1–3

31 Pusey CD, Dash A, Kershaw MJ et al. A single autoantigen in Goodpasture's syndrome identified by a monoclonal antibody to human glomerular basement membrane. *Lab Invest 1987; 56:* 23–31

32 Kashtan C, Fish AJ, Kleppel M et al. Nephritogenic antigen determinants in epidermal and renal basement membranes of kindreds with Alport-type familial nephritis. *J Clin Invest 1986; 78:* 1035–1044

33 Savage COS, Kershaw M, Pusey CD et al. Use of a monoclonal antibody in differential diagnosis of children with haematuria and hereditary nephritis. *Lancet 1986; i:* 1459–1461

34 Savage COS, Pusey CD, Kershaw MJ et al. The Goodpasture antigen in Alport's syndrome: studies with monoclonal antibody. *Kidney Int 1986; 30:* 107–112

35 Móunier F, Gros F, Wieslander J et al. Alport's syndrome. Immunohistochemical study of glomerular basement membrane. *Kidney Int (Abstract):* in press

36 Melvin T, Kim Y, Michael AF. Amyloid P component is not present in the glomerular basement membrane in Alport-type hereditary nephritis. *Am J Pathol 1986; 125:* 460–464

37 Savage COS, Noël LH, Cashman S et al. Hereditary nephritis: immunoblotting studies of the glomerular basement membrane. Submitted for publication

38 Kleppel MM, Kashtan C, Butkowski RJ et al. Absence of 28 kDa type IV collagen NC1 domains in glomerular basement membrane (GBM) in Alport-type familial nephritis (FN). *Kidney Int 1987; 31 (Abstract):* 206

39 Gubler M, Lévy M, Broyer M et al. Alport's syndrome. A report of 58 cases and a review of the literature. *Am J Med 1981; 70:* 493–505

40 Rogers PW, Kurtzman NA, Bunn SM Jr, White MG. Familial benign essential hematuria. *Arch Intern Med 1973; 131:* 257–262

41 Abe S, Amagasaki Y, Iyori S et al. Thin basement membrane syndrome in adults. *J Clin Pathol 1987; 40:* 318–322

42 Kleinknecht C. Néphronophtise. In Royer P, Habib R, Mathieu H, Broyer M, eds. *Néphrologie Pédiatrique.* Paris: Flammarion Médecine-Sciences. 1983: 48–53

43 Grateau G, Grünfeld JP, Droz D, Noël LH. La néphronophtise de l'adulte: une seule ou deux maladies? *Néphrologie 1986; 7:* 104–108

44 Cohen AH, Hoyer JR. Nephronophthisis. A primary tubular basement membrane defect. *Lab Invest 1986; 55:* 564–572

45 Gubler MC, Mounier F, Foidart JM et al. Ultrastructural and immunohistochemical study of RBM in familial juvenile nephronophthisis. In Price RG, Hudson BG, eds. *Renal Basement Membranes in Health and Disease.* London: Academic Press. 1987: 389–398

46 Zevin D, Ben-Bassat M, Weinstein T et al. Rejection-related nephrotic syndrome associated with massive antiglomerular and antitubular basement membrane deposits. *Israel J Med Sci 1985; 21:* 915–918

47 Grantham JJ. Polycystic kidney disease: a predominance of giant nephrons. *Am J Physiol 1983; 244:* F3–F10

48 Huseman R, Grady A, Welling D, Grantham JJ. Macropuncture study of polycystic disease in adult human kidneys. *Kidney Int 1980; 18:* 375–385

49 Perrone RD. In vitro function of cyst epithelium from human polycystic kidney. *J Clin Invest 1985; 76:* 1688–1691

50 Cuppage FE, Huseman RA, Chapman A, Grantham JJ. Ultrastructural and function of cysts from human adult polycystic kidneys. *Kidney Int 1980; 17:* 372–381
51 Grantham JJ, Geiser JL, Evan AP. Cyst formation and growth in autosomal dominant polycystic kidney disease. *Kidney Int 1987; 31:* 1145–1152
52 Evan AP, Gardner KD Jr, Bernstein J. Polypoid and papillary epithelial hyperplasia: a potential cause of ductal obstruction in adult polycystic disease. *Kidney Int 1979; 16:* 743–750
53 Chanard J, Szymanowicz A, Brunois JP et al. Increased renal excretion of 3-hydroxy-proline in patients with active glomerular nephropathies and with polycystic renal disease. *Clin Nephrol 1982; 17:* 64–69
54 Wilson PD, Schrier RW, Breckon RD, Gabow PA. A new method for studying human polycystic kidney disease epithelia in culture. *Kidney Int 1986; 30:* 371–378
55 Avner ED, Piesco NP, Sweeney WE Jr et al. Hydrocorticone-induced cystic metanephric maldevelopment in serum-free organ culture. *Lab Invest 1984; 50:* 208–218
56 Leier CV, Baker PB, Kilman JW, Wooley CF. Cardiovascular abnormalities associated with adult polycystic kidney disease. *Ann Intern Med 1984; 100:* 683–688
57 Hossack KF, Leddy CL, Schrier RW, Gabow PA. Incidence of cardiac abnormalities associated with autosomal dominant polycystic kidney disease (ADPKD). *Kidney Int 1987; 31 (Abstract):* 203
58 Grünfeld JP, Albouze G, Jungers P et al. Liver changes and complications in adult polycystic kidney disease. In Bach JF, Crosnier J, Funck-Brentano JL et al, eds. *Advances in Nephrology, Volume 14.* Chicago: Year Book Medical Publishers. 1985: 1–20
59 Muther RS, Bennett WM. Cyst fluid antibiotic concentrations in polycystic kidney disease: differences between proximal and distal cyst. *Kidney Int 1981; 20:* 519–522
60 Wickre CG, Bennett WM. Renal cyst epithelial transport in non-uremic polycystic kidney disease. *Kidney Int 1983; 23:* 514–518
61 Schwab SJ, Bander SJ, Klahr S. Renal infection in autosomal dominant polycystic kidney disease. *Am J Med 1987; 82:* 714–718
62 Carr M, Elzinga L, Rashad A et al. Ciprofloxacin for the treatment of cyst infection in cystic kidney disease (CKD). *Kidney Int 1987; 31 (Abstract):* 193
63 Iverson WO, Fetterman GH, Jacobson ER et al. Polycystic kidney and liver disease in Springbok: I. Morphology of the lesions. *Kidney Int 1982; 22:* 146–155
64 Ebihara I, Killen PD, Yamada Y et al. Sustained expression of basement membrane genes in murine congenital polycystic kidney disease (ckp/ckp). *Kidney Int 1987; 31 (Abstract):* 165
65 Crocker JFS, Blecher SR, Givner ML, McCarthy SC. Polycystic kidney and liver disease and corticosterone change in the cpk mouse. *Kidney Int 1987; 31:* 1088–1091
66 Avner ED, Sweeney WE Jr, Piesco NP, Ellis D. Regression of genetically determined polycystic kidney disease in murine organ culture. *Experientia 1986; 42:* 77–78
67 Birenboim N, Donoso VS, Huseman RA, Grantham JJ. Renal excretion and cyst accumulation of β_2 microglobulin in polycystic kidney disease. *Kidney Int 1987; 31:* 85–92
68 Bennett WM, Elzinga L, Golper TA, Barry JM. Reduction of cyst volume for symptomatic management of autosomal dominant polycystic kidney disease. *J Urol 1987; 137:* 620–622
69 Joshi VV, Kasznica J. Clinicopathologic spectrum of glomerulocystic kidneys: report of two cases and a brief review of literature. *Pediatr Pathol 1984; 2:* 171–186
70 Carson RW, Bedi D, Cavallo T, DuBose TD Jr. Familial adult glomerulocystic kidney disease. *Am J Kidney Dis 1987; 9:* 154–165
71 Melnick SC, Brewer DB, Oldham JS. Cortical microcystic disease of the kidney with dominant inheritance: a previously undescribed syndrome. *J Clin Pathol 1984; 37:* 494–499
72 Stapleton FB, Bernstein J, Koh G et al. Cystic kidneys in a patient with oral-facial-digital syndrome type I. *Am J Kidney Dis 1982; 1:* 288–293

73 Broyer M, Guillot M, Gubler MC, Habib R. Infantile cystinosis: a reappraisal of early and late symptoms. In Hamburger J, Crosnier J, Grünfeld JP, Maxwell MH, eds. *Advances in Nephrology, Volume 10.* Chicago: Year Book Medical Publishers. 1981: 137–166
74 Gahl WA, Reed GF, Thoene JG et al. Cysteamine therapy for children with nephropathic cystinosis. *N Engl J Med 1987; 316:* 865–877
75 Hauglustaine D, Corbeel L, Van Damme B et al. Glomerulonephritis in late-onset cystinosis. Report of two cases and review of the literature. *Clin Nephrol 1976; 6:* 529–535
76 Pabico RC, Panner BJ, McKenna BA, Bryson MF. Glomerular lesions in patients with late-onset cystinosis with massive proteinuria. *Renal Physiol 1980; 3:* 347–354
77 Kaiser-Kupfer MI, Fujikawa L, Kuwabara J et al. Removal of corneal crystals by topical cysteamine in nephropathic cystinosis. *N Engl J Med 1987; 316:* 775–779
78 Gubler MC, Lenoir G, Grünfeld JP et al. Early renal changes in hemizygous and heterozygous patients with Fabry's disease. *Kidney Int 1978; 13:* 223–235
79 Touraine JL, Malik MC, Maire I et al. Fetal liver transplantation in congenital enzyme deficiencies in man. *Exp Hematol 1982; 10:* 46–47
80 Faraggiana T, Churg J, Grishman E et al. Light- and electron-microscopic histochemistry of Fabry's disease. *Am J Pathol 1981; 103:* 247–262
81 Friedlaender MM, Kopolovic J, Rubinger D et al. Renal biopsy in Fabry's disease eight years after successful renal transplantation. *Clin Nephrol 1987; 27:* 206–211
82 Lemansky P, Bishop DF, Desnick RJ et al. Synthesis and processing of α-galactosidase A in human fibroblasts. Evidence for different mutations in Fabry disease. *J Biol Chem 1987; 262:* 2061–2065
83 Kornfeld S. Trafficking of lysosomal enzymes in normal and disease states. *J Clin Invest 1986; 77:* 1–6
84 Gahl WA, Adamson M. Biochemical phenotyping of a single sibship with both cystinosis and Fabry disease. *J Inherited Metab Dis 1985; 8:* 127–131
85 Scheinman JI, Najarian JS, Mauer SM. Successful strategies of renal transplantation in primary oxalosis. *Kidney Int 1984; 25:* 804–811
86 Gibbs DA, Watts RWE. The action of pyridoxine in primary hyperoxaluria. *Clin Sci 1970; 38:* 277–286
87 Yendt ER, Cohani MM. Response to a physiologic dose of pyridoxine in type I primary hyperoxaluria. *N Engl J Med 1985; 312:* 953–957
88 Grateau G, Grünfeld JP, Beurton D et al. Post-surgical deterioration of renal function in primary hyperoxaluria. *Nephrol Dial Transplant 1987; 1:* 261–264
89 Danpure CJ, Jennings PR. Peroxisomal alanine: glyoxylate aminotransferase deficiency in primary hyperoxaluria type I. *FEBS Letters 1986; 201:* 20–24
90 Danpure CJ, Jennings PR, Watts RWE. Enzymological diagnosis of primary hyperoxaluria type 1 by measurement of hepatic alanine: glyoxylate aminotransferase activity. *Lancet 1987; i:* 289–291
91 Watts RWE, Calne RY, Williams R et al. Primary hyperoxaluria (type I): attempted treatment by combined hepatic and renal transplantation. *Q J Med 1985; 57:* 697–703
92 Reeders ST, Breuning MH, Davies KE et al. A highly polymorphic DNA marker linked to adult polycystic kidney disease on chromosome 16. *Nature 1985; 317:* 542–544
93 Reeders ST, Breuning MH, Corneyt G et al. Two genetic markers closely linked to adult polycystic kidney disease on chromosome 16. *Br Med J 1986; 292:* 851–853
94 Churchill DN, Bear JC, Morgan J et al. Prognosis of adult onset polycystic kidney disease re-evaluated. *Kidney Int 1984; 26:* 190–193
95 Iglesias GC, Torres VE, Offord KP et al. Epidemiology of adult polycystic kidney disease, Olmsted County, Minnesota: 1935–1980. *Am J Kidney Dis 1983; 2:* 630–639
96 Sedman A, Bell P, Manco-Johnson M et al. Autosomal dominant polycystic kidney disease in childhood: a longitudinal study. *Kidney Int 1987; 31:* 100–105
97 Reeders ST, Gal A, Propping P et al. Prenatal diagnosis of autosomal dominant polycystic kidney disease with a DNA probe. *Lancet 1986; ii:* 6–8

98 Zerres K, Weiss H, Bulla M, Ropth B. Prenatal diagnosis of an early manifestation of autosomal dominant adult-type polycystic kidney disease. *Lancet 1982; ii:* 988

99 Fryns JP, Vandenberghe K, Moerman F. Mid-trimester ultrasonographic diagnosis of early manifesting 'adult' form of polycystic kidney disease. *Hum Genet 1986; 74:* 461

100 Feingold J, Bois E, Chompret A et al. Genetic heterogeneity of Alport syndrome. *Kidney Int 1985; 27:* 672–677

101 Hasstedt SJ, Atkin CI, San Juan AC Jr. Genetic heterogeneity among kindreds with Alport syndrome. *Am J Hum Genet 1986; 38:* 940–953

102 Menlove L, Kirschner N, Nguyen K et al. In De la Chapelle A, ed. *Human Gene Mapping 8.* Basel: Karger. 1985: 697–698

103 Brunner H, Van Bennekon C, Schröder C et al. X-linked Alport syndrome: localization of the gene in three families. *Kidney Int 1987; 31:* 1044

104 Griffin CA, Emanuel BS, Hansen JR et al. Human collagen genes encoding basement membrane α1(IV) and α2(IV) chains map to the distal long arm of chromosome 13. *Proc Natl Acad Sci USA 1987; 84:* 512–516

105 Bishop DF, Calhoun DH, Bernstein HS et al. Human α-galactosidase A: nucleotide sequence of a cDNA clone encoding the mature enzyme. *Proc Natl Acad Sci USA 1986; 83:* 4859–4863

106 Morgan SH, MacDermot K, Cheshire J et al. Restriction fragment length polymorphisms (RFLP) in Anderson-Fabry disease. *Eur J Clin Invest 1987; 17 (Abstract):* A12

107 Yang CY, Manoogian D, Pao Q et al. Lecithin:cholesterol acyltransferase. *J Biol Chem 1987; 262:* 3086–3091

108 Wallace MR, Conneally RM, Long GL, Benson MD. Molecular detection of carriers of hereditary amyloidosis in a Swedish-American family. *Am J Med Genet 1986; 25:* 335–341

109 Yoshioka K, Sasaki H, Yoshioka N et al. Structure of the mutant prealbumin gene responsible for familial amyloidotic polyneuropathy. *Mol Biol Med 1986; 3:* 319–328

110 Sasaki H, Toné S, Nakazato M et al. Generation of transgenic mice producing a human transthyretin variant: a possible mouse model for familial amyloidotic polyneuropathy. *Biochem Biophys Res Commun 1986; 139:* 794–799

111 Fryer AE, Chalmers A, Connor JM et al. Evidence that the gene for tuberous sclerosis is on chromosome 9. *Lancet 1987; i:* 659–661

112 Venta PJ, Shows TB, Curtis PJ, Tashian RE. Polymorphic gene for human carbonic anhydrase II: a molecular disease marker located on chromosome 8. *Proc Natl Acad Sci USA 1983; 80:* 4437–4440

113 Silver DN, Lewis RA, Nussbaum RL. Mapping the lower oculocerebrorenal syndrome Xq24–q26 by use of restriction fragment length polymorphisms. *J Clin Invest 1987; 79:* 282–285

DISORDERS OF SODIUM AND WATER EXCRETION

EFFECTIVE BLOOD VOLUME REVISITED: PATHOGENESIS OF OEDEMATOUS DISORDERS

R W Schrier

University of Colorado School of Medicine, Denver, Colorado, USA

There are several circumstances in which renal sodium and water retention occur when measured total blood volume is normal or increased. These include high and low output cardiac failure, nephrotic syndrome, cirrhosis and pregnancy. Since the kidney is the primary organ responsible for the regulation of sodium and water excretion and thus extracellular fluid volume, these clinical circumstances of continued sodium and water retention despite normal or increased blood volume are perplexing. In 1948 John Peters suggested that some component of total blood volume must be diminished in these oedematous disorders thus providing a signal to the kidney to retain sodium and water in an effort to replenish this 'effective blood volume" [1]. Although the term 'effective blood volume' has been provocative in stimulating efforts to understand the pathogenesis of oedematous disorders, the specific definition of the component of total blood volume which best deserves the name 'effective blood volume' has remained illusive and ill-defined.

In this paper a hypothesis will be presented with supporting data whereby the variety of oedematous disorders can be understood by a specific definition of effective blood volume. This hypothesis is not intended to exclude other mechanisms but rather to provide a framework to explain the renal regulation of sodium and water excretion as a physiological response to extrarenal circumstances created by disease. In this context we will examine a specific notion of effective blood volume as the 'fullness of the arterial vascular tree as defined by the interrelationship between cardiac output and peripheral vascular resistance'. A diminution of this effective arterial blood volume (EABV) during various oedematous disorders then triggers neurohumoral reflexes which attempt to restore the integrity of this compartment. Thus, a fall in cardiac output may signal a diminution in EABV which results in compensatory responses in an effort to restore the fullness of the arterial vascular tree by diminishing its size. Thus, an increase in arterial peripheral vascular resistance, as well as renal sodium

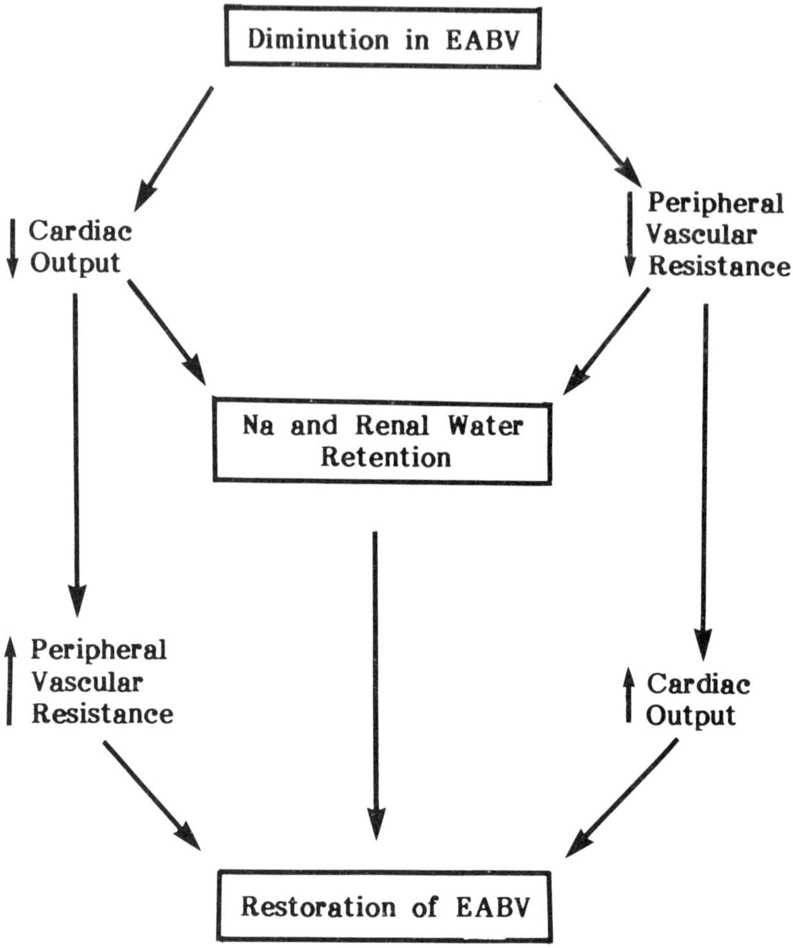

Figure 1. Schema to show the responses to a diminution in effective arterial blood volume (EABV)

and water retention in the presence of a diminution in cardiac output will tend to restore the fullness of the arterial vascular tree. On the other hand, a decrease in arterial vascular resistance may signal a decrease in EABV and result in compensatory responses including a rise in cardiac output and renal and sodium water retention. This schema is summarized in Figure 1 and will now be used as the basis to analyse several of the oedematous states.

Congestive heart failure

Renal sodium and water retention is an important hallmark of both high and low output cardiac failure. The trigger event to decrease EABV in high output cardiac failure is a fall in peripheral vascular resistance with a compensatory increase in cardiac output. In low output cardiac failure the trigger event to decrease EABV is a fall in cardiac output with a secondary rise in peripheral vascular resistance. Considerable evidence has been obtained that a decrease in EABV, due either to a fall in cardiac output or a decrease in peripheral vascular resistance, is associated with the complementary activation of three pressor systems, namely the non-osmotic release of vasopressin, the renin-angiotensin-aldosterone system and the sympathetic nervous system [2]. The arterial baroreceptors in the aortic arch and carotid sinus appear to be the critical modulator of this three-compartment response to circulatory stress as defined by EABV [3]. A decrease in stretch, stroke volume, or arterial pressure at these baroreceptors is associated with a diminution in the afferent inhibitory pathways to the central nervous system via the glossopharyngeal nerve. This results in an increase in noradrenergic discharge which affects several end-organ responses. In the peripheral circulation an increase in adrenergic discharge causes vasoconstriction of arterioles and activation of renal beta and baroreceptors which activate the renin-angiotensin-aldosterone system. Angiotensin II then further increases peripheral vascular resistance and both norepinephrine and angiotensin II exert inotropic effects on myocardial contractility. Recent results demonstrate that the baroreceptor-mediated, non-osmotic release of vasopressin involves stimulation by the adrenergic nervous system. Pathways have been tracked from the entry of the glossopharyngeal fibres at the nucleus tractus solitarii to the supraoptic and paraventricular nuclei where catecholamine nerve endings have been shown to abut neurons which synthesize vasopressin [4]. Moreover, electrophysiological studies by Renaud et al [5] have demonstrated that the phasic discharge of vasopressin neurons in the supraoptic nucleus is altered by changes in systemic arterial blood pressure. Miller et al [6] have also shown that catecholamine depletion of the central nervous system with intraventricular 6-hydroxy dopamine in the rat diminishes the release of vasopressin to non-osmotic stimuli. Recent studies in the dog have also shown vasopressin release in response to central adrenergic stimulation [7].

On this background, the response of these three vasoconstrictor hormones to high and low cardiac output has been shown to occur in a number of studies in humans and animal models of cardiac failure. Activation of the renin-angiotensin and sympathetic systems has been demonstrated to occur in both low [8] and high output heart failure [9]. In this regard, plasma norepinephrine concentrations appear to be a reasonable index of enhanced sympathetic activity. Blockade of these two hormone systems have also been shown to reduce cardiac overload and thereby enhance cardiac output. Specifically, both angiotensin converting enzyme inhibitors and the alpha-1 adrenergic blocker, prazosin, have been used to treat congestive heart failure.

In 1981 Szatalowicz et al [10], using a sensitive radioimmunoassay, initially demonstrated elevations in plasma vasopressin in a large number of hyponatraemic patients with congestive heart failure independent of diuretic use. This observation has recently been confirmed by several other groups of investigators [11,12]. In several animal models of low-output cardiac failure a rôle of vasopressin has been incriminated, including inferior vena caval constriction in the dog [13] and rat [14], myocardial infarction secondary to coronary artery ligation [15], adriamycin-induced cardiomyopathy [16], and high-output failure due to a large aortocaval shunt [17]. It is also interesting that a vascular V_1 antagonist of vasopressin has been shown to decrease peripheral vascular resistance in two of these models: myocardial infarction and adriaymycin-induced cardiomyopathy. In fact, in the adriamycin model this effect was observed despite no detectable increase in plasma vasopressin; however, an increase in the vascular sensitivity to an exogenous vasopressin infusion was demonstrable in rabbits with cardiac failure as compared to normal controls. It is interesting to note that subpressor doses of either angiotensin II or norepinephrine have been shown to convert subpressor doses of vasopressin into a pressor response [18]. Thus, the interaction between these three pressor systems not only occurs at the afferent reflex limb which modulates hormone release but also at the efferent cellular level. In this regard, evidence both in vivo [19] and in vitro [20] supports an interaction in the post-receptor signal transduction events, particularly relating to cellular calcium kinetics.

It should be noted that in the aortocaval model of high-output failure a V_1 antagonist of vasopressin failed to decrease peripheral vascular resistance [17]. This parameter is difficult to measure in this setting, however, because of the presence of shunting. In a study of patients with stable cardiac failure and no increase of plasma vasopressin, a V_1 antagonist exerted no effect except in a single patient with severe unstable heart failure [21]. In this regard, it is important to emphasize that patients with cardiac failure with the most significant hyponatraemia and the highest plasma renin activity have the worst prognosis. It thus seems that the lower the cardiac output the more striking will be the decrease in EABV and thus the baroreceptor activation of the non-osmotic vasopressin, renin-angiotensin and sympathetic nervous systems. Indeed, Bichet et al [22] have demonstrated that treatment of patients with Class III and IV heart failure with either the converting enzyme inhibitor, captopril, or the alpha-1-adrenergic antagonist, prazosin, not only increases cardiac output but also suppresses plasma concentrations of vasopressin and improves renal water excretion. In this study it is important to note that mean arterial pressure diminished slightly (approximately 5mmHg), thus suggesting that ventricular receptors [23] or arterial receptors, sensing stroke volume [24] rather than mean arterial pressure, led to reflex suppression of the three-component vasoconstrictor response as cardiac output and thus EABV increased.

Nephrotic syndrome

On the background of the aforementioned definition of EABV the interpretation of the mechanism of renal sodium and water retention in nephrotic syndrome might seem to be straightforward. Increased glomerular permeability to albumin would cause albuminuria (>3.5 grams/day) and thus hypoalbuminuria and diminished plasma oncotic pressure. Such a diminution in plasma oncotic pressure would decrease the net intravascular Starling force and thus lead to increased transudation of fluid into the interstitium. In this setting there would be no divergence between a decrease in total blood volume and a decrease in EABV. Indeed it is clear that consistent diminutions in total plasma and blood volumes have been measured in patients with nephrotic syndrome [25]. This decrease in total and EABV with nephrotic syndrome has been shown to be associated with increases in plasma vasopressin, activation of the renin-angiotensin-aldosterone system and the sympathetic nervous system [26]. Indeed, head-out-water immersion (HWI) has been demonstrated to increase central blood volume and enhance sodium and water excretion in patients with nephrotic syndrome [26–28]. Shapiro et al [28] showed, however, that the best correlation between the renal excretory response to HWI in patients with nephrotic syndrome was the rate of glomerular filtration. This observation may explain the findings of Meltzer et al [29] that nephrotic patients with minimal change disease demonstrated the hormonal indices of a decrease in EABV, namely stimulation of the renin-angiotensin-aldosterone and sympathetic nervous system as assessed by plasma norepinephrine. In contrast, another group of nephrotic patients exhibited low plasma renin and aldosterone values, hypertension, mild renal insufficiency and chronic glomerulonephritis on histological examination. Thus, nephrotic syndrome can be categorized into a classical 'underfilling' state which predominates in children with minimal change disease and the 'overfilling' syndrome in those patients, predominantly adults, who have chronic glomerular disease, diminished glomerular filtration rate and expanded blood volumes [30], and which have suppression of the renin-angiotensin-aldosterone system. The glomerular disease per se may also be associated with primary involvement of the juxtaglomerular apparatus, thereby also accounting for the hyporeninaemic hypoaldosteronism. It is interesting to note that, although the impaired water excretion in adults with nephrotic syndrome which occurred secondary to a variety of glomerular diseases correlated best with the level of glomerular filtration rate [28], micropuncture studies in rats [31] suggest a primary intrarenal enhancement of distal tubular reabsorption of sodium and water. In this latter study unilateral, intrarenal aminonucleoside was associated with a lower glomerular filtration rate in the aminonucleoside-treated kidney which demonstrated heavy proteinuria and enhanced reabsorption of sodium and water. The nephron site of this enhanced reabsorption was distal to the micropuncture site in the superficial proximal convoluted tubules or in deeper nephron sites which were not accessible to the micropuncture pipette. Perhaps it is this intrarenal mechanism of sodium and water retention which accounts for the finding of the Dorhout-Mees group that increased total plasma volume may be observed in adult patients with not only chronic glomerular but also minimal change disease. There are no data which examine the intrarenal mechanism of such sodium and water retention in nephrotic syndrome. Thus a primary tubular effect cannot be distinguished from an effect secondary to enhanced sensitivity to aldosterone and vasopressin.

Cirrhosis

The classical 'underfilling' theory of sodium and water retention in cirrhosis indicated that portal hypertension and hypoalbuminaemia causes ascites formation. This ascites formation was purported to decrease intravascular blood volume which then caused a secondary increase in tubular reabsorption of sodium and water in an effort to return intravascular volume to normal. Lieberman and associates [32] challenged this underfilling theory because measured blood volume was normal or increased in patients who had cirrhosis with ascites and this did not change during spontaneous diuresis. Since hepatic wedge pressure as an index of portal hypertension also did not change during spontaneous diuresis, these authors felt that splanchnic venous sequestration seemed to be an unlikely cause of underfilling and secondary renal sodium and water retention. These authors therefore proposed that in cirrhosis primary renal sodium retention occurs which then leads secondarily to ascites formation – the so-called overflow hypothesis. Using a nitrosamine-induced model of cirrhosis in the dog, Levy and associates [33] performed a careful series of studies which supported this 'overflow' hypothesis. These studies in dogs demonstrated renal sodium retention prior to ascites formation and at a time when total splanchnic and non-splanchnic blood volume was increased. This renal sodium retention was suggested to occur secondary to a hepatorenal reflex which is initiated by an increased intrahepatic pressure. This possibility was supported by an observation in dogs with chronic bile duct obstruction that a side-to-side, but not end-to-side, portal-caval shunt lowered intrahepatic pressure and diminished the renal retention of sodium [34].

On the background of these classical underfilling and overflow hypotheses a recent series of studies has been performed in cirrhotic patients to examine the pathogenesis of sodium and water retention. Studies by Bichet et al [35,36] in cirrhotic patients who exhibited impaired water excretion (non-excretors), showed that plasma concentrations of vasopressin as measured by radioimmunoassay were not suppressed despite a degree of plasma hypo-osmolality which would suppress plasma vasopressin to undetectable concentrations ($<$0.5pg/ml) in normal subjects. These non-excretor patients were also found to have the hormonal indices of intravascular underfilling, namely significantly increased plasma concentrations of renin, aldosterone and norepinephrine compared to cirrhotic patients who excreted a water load normally (excretors). The non-excretor patients, as defined by their response to a standard water load, could also be differentiated from the excretor patients by the presence of significantly lower plasma concentration of sodium and albumin, more avid sodium retention, a higher incidence of ascites (non-excretors: 19 out of 19 versus excretors: 2 out of 7) and increased pulse rates (90 versus 76 beats/min, $p<0.001$).

Previous efforts to reverse sodium and water retention with HWI have been undertaken in heterogenous groups of cirrhotic patients and the results have been variable with normal, decreased and increased diuretic and natriuretic responses [37]. Bichet et al [38] examined the response of non-excretor patients to HWI and monitored the haemodynamic changes during this manoeuvre. Consistent evidence of central blood volume expansion was observed during HWI including a significant increase in cardiac output, right atrial pressure and pulmonary wedge pressure. Blood pressure did not change because a fall occurred in peripheral vascular resistance which counterbalanced the rise in cardiac output. These sytemic haemodynamic effects were associated with a significant diminution in plasma concentrations of vasopressin, renin, aldosterone and norepinephrine. The resultant increase in sodium and water excretion during HWI were not attributable to detectable differences in renal haemodynamics. Whereas these results with HWI clearly supported the underfill hypothesis of sodium and water retention in cirrhosis, it is important to emphasize that the sodium and water excretion was improved but not normalized by HWI in these patients. This finding either provided indirect evidence for the overflow hypothesis or indicated that HWI alone is insufficient to normalize EABV. The latter possibility was examined by studying in a random manner the effect of HWI when the fall in peripheral vascular resistance was avoided by an exogenous infusion of norepinephrine [39]. This combined manoeuvre led to the normal ization of both water and sodium excretion in the non-excretor cirrhotic patients. Since the improved excretion of water occurred in the absence of further suppression of plasma vasopressin than that observed by HWI alone, this suggested an increase in fluid delivery to the more distal nephron. Such an increase in distal delivery would also tend to enhance the 'escape' from the sodium retaining effect of aldosterone and the natriuretic response to atrial natriuretic factor, events which occur in the cortical, medullary, and papillary collecting ducts. In this regard, the rise in right atrial pressure was the variable which correlated most significantly with the natriuretic response to HWI [38], a manoeuvre which is associated with a rise in atrial natriuretic factor [40]. The systemic and renal haemodynamic responses to HWI versus HWI with exogenous norepinephrine were no different except for the peripheral vascular resistance which was higher during the infusion of norepinephrine. Since the increase in cardiac output was no different, mean systemic, and thus renal perfusion, pressure was much higher with the combined manoeuvre than with HWI alone (136/76 versus 105/64mmHg). This increase in renal perfusion pressure most likely caused a diminution in proximal tubular reabsorption, as demonstrated in micropuncture studies [41], and thus accounted for the increase in distal fluid delivery.

Thus, when extrarenal systemic haemodynamics were normalized in cirrhotic patients with HWI and norepinephrine infusion combined, renal excretory capacity also could be normalized. Whereas these dramatic results in hyponatraemic cirrhotic patients with ascites who were diuretic-resistant do not exclude the presence of a hepatorenal reflex as proposed in the overflow hypothesis, they do not necessitate the existence of such a theory. In this regard, the results of the studies of Levy and associates [42] in the nitrosamine-induced cirrhotic dog indicated that a very small positive sodium balance (+20mEq/day) occurred prior to a detectable decrease in peripheral vascular resistance (although mean blood pressure had decreased by approximately 10mmHg); more profound renal sodium retention occurred, however, at a time when the peripheral vascular resistance had fallen significantly.

The cause(s) of the peripheral vasodilatation which decreases EABV with cirrhosis is not clear. Certainly, the known arteriovenous shunting in the splanchnic, pulmonary, dermal and muscular beds contribute to this arterial vascular underfilling, but other hormonal factors may also be involved. Since arterial blood volume constitutes only 15% of total blood volume, it is clearly apparent that an increased venous blood volume, as might occur with portal hypertension and splanchnic venous pooling, can increase total blood volume even though EABV is decreased. The measurement of cardiac output and mean arterial pressure allows the calculation of peripheral vascular resistance as a primary determinant of EABV. It must be rememembered, however, that when peripheral vascular resistance is the initial cause of a decrease in EABV, the patient is generally studied after varying degrees of neurohumoral and haemodynamic compensation have occurred. Thus, mean arterial pressure alone is not a sensitive index of a decrease in EABV caused by a fall in peripheral vascular resistance, since a compensatory rise in cardiac output secondary to this afterload reduction and the activation of three pressor systems has occurred. In this regard, it is interesting that Rascher and colleagues [personal communication] have recently demonstrated that decompensated cirrhotic patients may have a varied natriuretic response to volume expansion with hyperoncotic colloid (25%). Those patients with the most profound evidence of underfilling, including greater diminutions in plasma atrial natriuretic factor and increases in plasma vasopressin, renin and aldosterone, demonstrated a diuretic and natriuretic response to the colloid infusion. Those cirrhotic patients with less evidence of underfilling responded, as do normal subjects, to hyperoncotic albumin with very little diuresis or natriuresis. Since cirrhotic patients may be seen at any stage in the primary peripheral vasodilation and secondary compensatory response, a functional classification of cirrhosis would be helpful.

Although sequential studies of cirrhotic patients are inadequate to provide sufficient information to establish such a functional classification, the results of some recent studies have been useful in addressing this question. Nicholls et al [43] analysed the non-excretor patients with respect to the degree of their impaired water excretion. Those with the most profound impairment in response to a 20ml/kg water load (<20%) over five hours demonstrated, both under control and HWI conditions, that plasma concentrations of vasopressin, renin, aldosterone and norepinephrine concentrations were higher and that glomerular filtration rates and effective renal plasma flows were lower when compared to non-excretor cirrhotic patients who excreted between 20 to 80% of the water load over five hours. A follow-up study over 24 months [44] demonstrated that in the group with evidence for the most severe underfilling, the only patient who survived longer than five months received a LeVeen shunt and survived longer than 24 months. This patient's water excretion increased from 12 to 90% after the LeVeen shunt. The poor prognosis in this group occurred even though only one of seven patients continued to consume alcohol. In those non-excretor patients who excreted between 20 to 80% of the water load, 24-month survival was considerably better, even though the majority continued to consume alcohol (4 of 8 patients).

These results therefore suggest that, even though the LeVeen shunt has recently been shown not to prolong life in cirrhotic patients with hepatorenal syndrome [45], early prophylactic placement of the LeVeen shunt may be of value in patients whose diminution in EABV is most severe as assessed by an acute water load test (<20% excretion). A prospective randomized study will be necessary, however, to test this hypothesis.

Pregnancy

Pregnancy has been considered to be a volume expanded state by many observers because of the 30 to 50% increase in plasma volume, extracellular fluid volume, cardiac output, glomerular filtration rate and renal plasma flow. There are, however, several findings in humans and experimental animals which suggest that pregnancy may indeed be another example where sodium and water retention occur secondary to a decrease in EABV. In humans, blood pressure is known to be decreased in the first trimester of pregnancy [46], a finding most compatible with the notion that the increase in cardiac output occurred secondary to after-load reduction rather than to primary volume expansion. Moreover, it is also known that the early rise in glomerular filtration rate and renal plasma flow in pregnancy occur prior to, and thus cannot be attributed to, plasma volume expansion. These renal haemodynamic changes seem most likely to occur secondary to some of the hormonal changes of pregnancy including the increases in plasma oestrogen, progesterone, prolactin, placental lactogen and chorionic gonadotrophin [47]. Moreover, recently an increase in plasma cyclic GMP, a known secondary messenger of vasodilation, has been shown to occur in the conscious, trained pregnant rat [47].

The humoral profile of pregnancy is most compatible with a state of under-filling secondary to peripheral vasodilation. The osmotic stimulation of vasopressin in rat [48] and human pregnancy [49] has been shown to occur at a lower plasma osmolality than the virgin state, a circumstance which is known to occur secondary to volume depletion [3]. In contrast, volume expansion should increase the osmotic threshold for vasopressin release [3]. Similar to vasopressin release, the threshold for thirst has also been shown to occur at a lower plasma osmolality in pregnancy compared to the non-pregnant state [49]. The pregnant rat is also known to ingest significantly greater volumes of water (42 versus 35ml/kg, $p<0.001$) as compared to the virgin rat [48]. If such an increase in water intake were secondary to a primary polydipsia of pregnancy, then restricting water intake to the level of the virgin rat should not alter the hormonal indices of a decrease in EABV. However, in a study in which both the virgin and pregnant rats ingested 35–37ml/day of water, the pregnant rat's plasma vasopressin increased 9-fold (2.7 to 19.0pg/ml, $p<0.001$), and the plasma aldosterone increased 5-fold (235 to 1143pg/ml, $p<0.001$) – findings more compatible with underfilling than volume expansion. It is also interesting to note that sodium restriction worsens the hyponatraemia of pregnancy in the pregnant, whereas no effect on plasma sodium concentration is observed during sodium restriction in the virgin rat [50]. Another finding which supports pregnancy as being an underfilling state is the observation that the decreased vascular sensitivity and increased adrenal sensitivity to angiotensin II in the pregnant state [Broughton Pipkin and Brown, personal communication] can be mimicked by sodium restriction [51].

Analysis of the tubulo-glomerular feedback mechanism in the pregnant rat was also not compatible with a volume expanded state [52]. Increased rather than decreased sensitivity of the tubulo-glomerular feedback response was observed in the pregnant rat, another finding most compatible with a decrease in EABV. It is also interesting to note that the administration of the converting enzyme inhibitor, captopril, lowered blood pressure in the anaesthetized pregnant but not in the non-pregnant rat [53]. This finding suggests that activation of the renin-angiotensin-aldosterone system is a secondary event elicited in an effort to return EABV to normal. The non-osmotic stimulation of vasopressin during volume depletion secondary to intraperitoneal polyethylene glycol in the pregnant rat is also compatible with a state of diminished EABV [54]. The volume depleted pregnant rat stimulates vasopressin release at a mean blood volume of 8.5ml/kg whilst the virgin rat does not exhibit non-osmotic vasopressin release until a blood volume of 6.0ml/kg is reached.

The exact cause(s) of the peripheral vasodilation ('plethora') of pregnancy is not known but several factors may be involved. The placental circulation constitutes an anteriovenous shunt and increased synthesis of vasodilating prostaglandins, such as prostacyclin, also is known to occur with pregnancy [55]. Whilst the rôle of prostacyclin in the vascular resistance to angiotensin II, norepinephrine and vasopressin in pregnancy [56] remains to be proven, this vascular resistance to the normal response to a decrease in EABV may contribute to the maintenance of the peripheral vasodilation and enhanced renal haemodynamic response to pregnancy. Lastly, it should be emphasized that the major difference between pregnancy and other vasodilated states, such as high-output failure, large arteriovenous fistulae, and cirrhosis, is that the latter states are characterized by diminished renal haemodynamics. The increased filtered load of sodium and water in pregnancy may allow sufficient sodium and water delivery to the distal nephron to allow escape from aldosterone as well as a normal response to an acute sodium or water load. In contrast, the decreased filtered load of sodium and water in the other oedematous diseases, causing a diminished EABV, are associated with diminished distal fluid and sodium delivery, failure to escape from aldosterone and more avid sodium and water retention than during pregnancy.

Thus, in high- and low-output failure, nephrotic syndrome, cirrhosis and pregnancy the kidney may be responding in a totally normal manner to a decrease in EABV, whether initiated by a decrease in cardiac output or a decrease in peripheral vascular resistance. In these settings EABV is the conductor of a hormonal symphony in which the kidney is the master organ responding predictably in an elegant manner to orchestrate the ensemble of the living body.

References

1 Peters JP. The role of sodium in the production of edema. *N Engl J Med 1948; 239:* 353–362

2 Bichet DG, Schrier RW. Cardiac failure, liver disease and nephrotic syndrome. In Schrier RW, Gottschalk C, eds. *Diseases of the Kidney.* Boston: Little Brown. 1987

3 Schrier RW, Berl T, Anderson RJ. Osmotic and nonosmotic control of vasopressin release. *Am J Physiol 1979; 236:* F321–F332

4 Sladek JR Jr. Central catecholamine pathways to vasopressin neurons. In Schrier RW, ed. *Vasopressin.* New York: Raven Press. 1985: 343–352

5 Renaud LP, Day TA, Randle JCR et al. In vivo and in vitro electrophysiological evidence that central noradrenergic pathways enhance the activity of hypothalamic vasopressinergic neurosecretory cells. In Schrier RW, ed. *Vasopressin.* New York: Raven Press. 1985

6 Miller TR, Handelman WA, Arnold PE et al. Effect of central catecholamine depletion on the osmotic and nonosmotic stimulation of vasopressin (antidiuretic hormone) in the rat. *J Clin Invest 1979; 64:* 1599–1607

7 Brooks DP, Share L, Crofton JT. Central adrenergic control of vasopressin release. *Neuroendocrinol 1986; 42:* 416–420

8 Cohn JN, Levine TB, Francis GS, Goldsmith S. Neurohumoral control mechanisms in congestive heart failure. *Am Heart J 1981; 102:* 509–514

9 Riegger AJG, Liebau G. The renin-angiotensin-aldosterone system, antidiuretic hormone and sympathetic nerve activity in an experimental model of congestive heart failure in the dog. *Clin Sci 1982; 62:* 465–469

10 Szatalowicz VL, Arnold PE, Chaimovitz C et al. Radioimmunoassay of plasma arginine vasopressin in hyponatremic patients with congestive heart failure. *N Engl J Med 1981; 305:* 263–266

11 Pruszezynski W, Vahaniau A, Ardaillou R, Acar J. Role of antidiuretic hormone in impaired water excretion of patients with congestive heart failure. *J Clin Endocrinol Metab 1984; 58:* 599–605

12 Riegger GAJ, Lieban G, Kochsiek K. Antidiuretic hormone in congestive heart failure. *Am J Med 1982; 72:* 49–53

13 Anderson RJ, Cadnapaphornchai P, Harbottle JA et al. Mechanism of effect of thoracic inferior vena cava constriction on renal water excretion. *J Clin Invest 1974; 54:* 1473–1479

14 Ishikawa S, Saito T, Okada K et al. Effect of vasopressin antagonist on water excretion in inferior vena cava constriction. *Kidney Int 1986; 30:* 49–55
15 Yared A, Kon V, Brenner BM, Ichikawa I. Role for vasopressin (AVP) in rats with congestive heart failure (CHF). *Kidney Int 1985; 27 (Abstract):* 337
16 Arnolda L, McGrath BP, Cocks M, Johnston CI. Vasoconstrictor role for vasopressin in experimental heart failure in the rabbit. *J Clin Invest 1986; 78:* 674–679
17 Riegger GAJ, Liebau G, Bauer E, Kochsiek K. Vasopressin and renin in high output heart failure of rats: hemodynamic effects of elevated plasma hormone levels. *J Cardiovasc Pharmacol 1985; 7:* 1–5
18 Ishikawa S, Goldberg JP, Schrier D et al. Interrelationship between subpressor effects of vasopressin and other vasoactive hormones in the rat. *Mineral Electrolyte Metab 1984; 10:* 184–189
19 Goldberg JP, Schrier RW. Effect of calcium membrane blockers on in vivo vasoconstrictor properties of norepinephrine, angiotensin II and vasopressin. *Mineral Electrolyte Metab 1984; 10:* 178–183
20 Caramelo C, Tsai P, Kim J et al. Interaction of angiotensin II and arginine vasopressin on calcium mobilization and contraction in rat cultured vascular vascular smooth muscle cells. *Abstracts Xth International Congress of Nephrology.* London. 1987: 248
21 Nicod P, Waeber B, Bussien J et al. Acute hemodynamic effect of a vascular antagonist of vasopressin in patients with congestive heart failure. *Am J Cardiol 1985; 55:* 1043–1047
22 Bichet DG, Kortas C, Mettauer B et al. Modulation of plasma and platelet vasopressin by cardiac function in patients with heart failure. *Kidney Int 1986; 29:* 1188–1196
23 Thames MD, Peterson MG, Schmid PG. Stimulation of cardiac receptors with veratrum alkaloids inhibit ADH secretion. *Am J Physiol 1980; 239 (Heart Circ Physiol 8):* H784–H788
24 Hakumaki MOK, Wang BC, Sundet WD, Goetz KL. Aortic baroreceptor discharge during nonhypotensive hemorrhage in anesthetized dogs. *Am J Physiol 1985; 249:* H393–H403
25 Brown E, Hopper J Jr, Wennesland R. Blood volume and its regulation. *Ann Rev Physiol 1957; 19:* 231–254
26 Rascher W, Tulassay T. Hormonal regulation of water metabolism in children with nephrotic syndrome. *Kidney Int:* in press
27 Krishna GG, Danovitch GM. Effects of water immersion on renal function in the nephrotic syndrome. *Kidney Int 1982; 21:* 395–401
28 Shapiro MD, Nicholls KM, Groves BM, Schrier RW. Role of glomerular filtration rate in the impaired sodium and water excretion of patients with the nephrotic syndrome. *Am J Kidney Dis 1986; 8:2 (Aug):* 81–87
29 Meltzer JI, Keim HJ, Laragh JH. Nephrotic syndrome: vasoconstriction and hypervolemic types indicated by renin-sodium profiling. *Ann Int Med 1979; 91:* 688–696
30 Dorhout-Mees EJ, Geers AB, Koomans HA. Blood volume and sodium retention in the nephrotic syndrome: a controversial pathophysiology concept. *Nephron 1984; 36:* 201–211
31 Ichikawa I, Rennke HG, Hoyer JR et al. Role of intrarenal mechanisms in the impaired salt excretion of experimental nephrotic syndrome. *J Clin Invest 1983; 71:*91–103
32 Lieberman FL, Denison EK, Reynolds TB. The relationship of plasma volume, portal hypertension, ascites, and renal sodium retention in cirrhosis: the overflow theory of ascites formation. *Ann NY Acad Sci 1970; 170:* 202–212
33 Levy M. Observations on renal function and ascites formation in dogs with experimental portal cirrhosis. In Epstein M, ed. *The Kidney in Liver Disease.* New York: Elsevier/North Holland. 1978: 131–142
34 Unikowsky B, Wexler MJ, Levy M. Dogs in experimental cirrhosis of the liver but without intrahepatic hypertension do not retain sodium or form ascites. *J Clin Invest 1983; 72:* 1594–1604
35 Bichet O, Szatalowicz V, Chaimovitz C, Schrier RW. Role of vasopressin in abnormal water excretion in cirrhotic patients. *Ann Int Med 1982; 96:* 413–417

36 Bichet DG, Van Putten VJ, Schrier RW. Potential role of the increased sympathetic activity in impaired sodium and water excretion in cirrhosis. *N Engl J Med 1982; 307:* 1552–1557

37 Epstein M. Renal effects of head-out water immersion in man: implications for an understanding of volume homeostasis. *Physiol Rev 1978; 58:* 529–581

38 Bichet DG, Groves BM, Schrier RW. Mechanisms of improvement of water and sodium excretion by enhancement of central hemodynamics in decompensated cirrhotic patients. *Kidney Int 1983; 24:* 788–794

39 Shapiro MD, Nicholls KM, Groves BM et al. Interrelationship between cardiac output and vascular resistance as determinants of "effective arterial blood volume" in cirrhotic patients. *Kidney Int 1985; 28:* 206–211

40 Yee B, Durr J, Cosby R et al. Effect of head-out water immersion (HWI) on atrial natriuretic factor (ANF), proximal and distal sodium reabsorption in cirrhotic patients. *Abstracts Xth International Congress of Nephrology.* London. 1987: 224

41 Schrier RW, de Wardener HE. Factors other than aldosterone which influence the tubular reabsorption of sodium. (Medical Progress). *N Engl J Med 1971; 285:* 1231–1243; 1292–1301

42 Levy M, Wexler MJ. Renal sodium retention and ascites formation in dogs with experimental cirrhosis but without portal hypertension or increased splanchnic vascular capacity. *J Lab Clin Med 1978; 91:* 520–536

43 Nicholls KM, Shapiro MD, Groves BS, Schrier RW. Factors determining renal response to water immersion in non-excretor cirrhotic patients. *Kidney Int 1986; 30:* 417–421

44 Cosby RL, Yee B, Shapiro M et al. Prognostic factors in cirrhosis. *Kidney Int 1986; 29 (Abstract):* 184

45 Linas SL, Schaefer JW, Moore EE et al. Peritoneal venous shunt in the management of the hepatorenal syndrome. *Kidney Int 1986; 30:* 736–740

46 MacGillivray I, Rose GA, Rowe B. Blood pressure survey in pregnancy. *Clin Sci 1969; 37:* 395–407

47 Conrad KP. Possible mechanisms for changes in renal hemodynamics during pregnancy: studies from animal models. *Am J Kidney Dis 1987; 9:* 253–259

48 Durr JA, Stamoutsos B, Lindheimer MD. Osmoregulation during pregnancy in the rat. Evidence for resetting of the threshold for vasopressin secretion during gestation. *J Clin Invest 1981; 68:* 337–346

49 Davison JM, Gilmore EA, Durr JA et al. Altered osmotic thresholds for vasopressin and thirst in human pregnancy. *Am J Physiol 1984; 246:* F105–F109

50 Barron WM. Volume homeostasis during pregnancy in the rat. *Am J Kidney Dis 1987; 9:* 296–302

51 Oelkers W. Schoneshofer M, Schultze G. Prolonged infusions of Ile^5-angiotensin-II in sodium replete and deplete man: effects on aldosterone, ACTH, cortisol, blood pressure and electrolyte balance. *J Clin Endocrinol Metab 1978; 46:* 402–413

52 Baylis C, Blantz RC. Tubuloglomerular feedback activity in virgin and 12-day pregnant rats. *Am J Physiol 1985; 249:* F169–F173

53 Baylis C, Collins RC. Angiotensin II inhibition on blood pressure and renal hemodynamics in pregnant rats. *Am J Physiol 1986; 250:* F308–F314

54 Barron WM, Stamoutsos BA, Lindheimer MD. Role of volume in regulation of vasopressin secretion during pregnancy in the rat. *J Clin Invest 1984; 73:* 923–932

55 Whalen JB, Clancey CJ, Farley DB, Van Orden DE. Plasma prostaglandins in pregnancy. *Obstet Gynecol 1978; 51:* 52–55

56 Paller MS. Mechanism of decreased pressor responsiveness to Ang II, NE and vasopressin in pregnant rats. *Am J Physiol 1984; 247:* H100–H108

CENTRAL NERVOUS SYSTEM EFFECTS OF ACUTE AND CHRONIC DISTURBANCES OF PLASMA SODIUM – CONSEQUENCES OF RAPID VERSUS SLOW CORRECTION

A I Arieff

Veterans Administration Medical Center and University of California School of Medicine, San Francisco, California, USA

Introduction

Hyponatraemia (serum sodium less than 130mM/litre) is probably the most common electrolyte abnormality to be found in a hospital population, with an incidence of about 1% [1]. Among post-operative patients, the incidence of hyponatraemia is greater than 4% [2]. Although the incidence of hyponatraemia is high, permanent brain damage appears to occur less frequently than might be expected [1–8]. In addition to hyponatraemia itself, there are many other circumstances associated with hyponatraemia which might lead to permanent brain damage. These include pressure necrosis of the brain due to oedema, herniation of the brain stem into the foramen magnum, seizures and hypoxia or anoxia. The possible rôle of hypoxia or anoxia in the genesis of hyponatraemic brain damage has not been well explored. In many instances, patients who have developed permanent neurological damage in association with hyponatraemia or its subsequent therapy have also suffered an assocated episode of hypoxia or anoxia [9].

The ideal mode of correction of hyponatraemia has been the subject of much controversy in recent years. In particular, the ideal rate of its correction has been hotly debated in the literature [10–12]. The arguments for rapid versus slow correction of severe symptomatic hyponatraemia will be reviewed.

Classification

Hyponatraemia may be found in association with many different systemic diseases and in many different clinical situations, including the post-operative state [2,3,5–8,13]. Hyponatraemia is almost always the result of dilution of extracellular fluid sodium. The condition may be either acute or chronic, and total body water may be either high, low or normal. The causes of hyponatraemia can be divided into nine major groups, on the basis of the patient's volume status and the underlying mechanisms. If there is extracellular fluid volume depletion, due to losses of fluid by either (a) renal, or (b) extrarenal routes, hyponatraemia may occur when the patient ingests hypotonic fluid. If the extracellular fluid volume is normal or only modestly decreased, hyponatraemia is probably related to either (c) hormone deficiency (hypothyroidism, Addison's disease), (d) hormone excess (antidiuretic hormone), (e) drugs which inhibit the ability of the kidney to excrete water, or (f) post-surgical non-osmotic stimuli to retain water. If the extracellular fluid volume is expanded, hyponatraemia is usually associated with (g) hepatic cirrhosis, nephrotic syndrome, or congestive heart failure or (h) acute or chronic renal failure. In a more simplistic sense, hyponatraemia is almost always associated with dilution, as it is nearly impossible to lose body fluid (such as urine, diarrhoea or emesis) which has a higher sodium concentration than does plasma. Acute water intoxication (i) is an example of dilution where there is administration of water (usually as intravenous 280mmol/litre glucose in water) at a time when there is impairment in the ability of the kidney to excrete water. Renal sodium wasting (j) is a rare potential cause of hyponatraemia. In most instances, one thinks of hyponatraemia as being a primary condition, and any associated disturbance in the central nervous system as secondary. However, there are at least two clinical conditions where the central nervous system disturbance is primary and the hyponatraemia is secondary. These are 'reset osmostat' and 'cerebral salt wasting'.

Symptoms of hyponatraemia

The symptoms of acute hypontraemia depend on the aetiology, magnitude and acuteness of the condition, as well as the age and sex of the individual involved. In general, symptoms of sustained hyponatraemia, which can be due to various combinations of sodium depletion and water ingestion, differ substantially from those which accompany acute water intoxication. The symptoms of water intoxication are related to both the extent of the fall in serum sodium and rapidity with which serum sodium is lowered. Neurological manifestations of acute water intoxication are not usually observed until the plasma sodium has fallen below about 125mmol/litre and may include nausea, emesis, muscular twitching, grand mal seizures and coma [5,10,13].

Acute (less than 24 hours) water intoxication (plasma sodium less than 125mmol/litre) has a mortality greater than 50% with a substantial morbidity (usually brain damage) [5,10]. However, when plasma sodium is slowly lowered (several days to several weeks) to 125mmol/litre or less by salt depletion and water ingestion, patients usually are less symptomatic [5]. In both patients and experimental animals, the severity of the neurological manifestations seems to be related to both the degree and the rapidity of onset of the hyponatraemia and the sex of the individual. Chronic hyponatraemia, compared with acute hyponatraemia, usually causes less fulminant symptoms and a lower morbidity and mortality. Several studies have shown that in individuals with depression of serum sodium below 120mmol/litre, symptoms of nausea, emesis and abdominal cramps may occur [14]. With even more severe hyponatraemia (below 115mmol/litre),

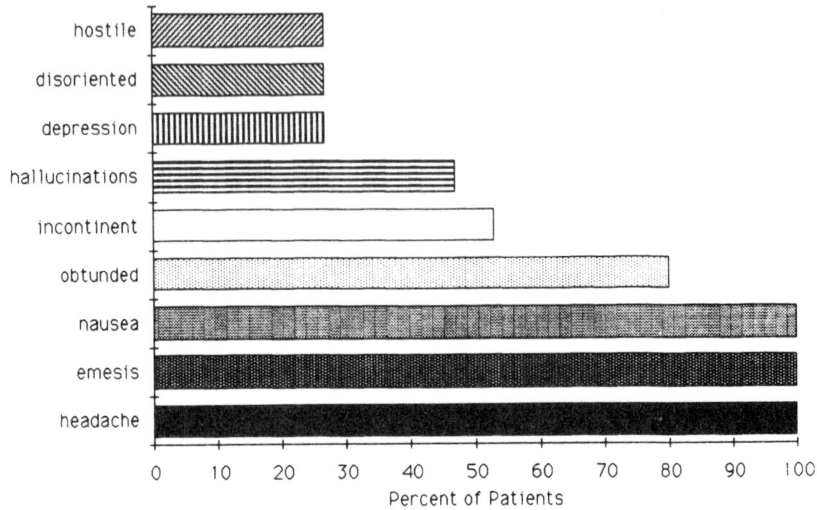

Figure 1. The post-operative signs and symptoms in 15 patients who developed symptomatic hyponatraemia. These findings occurred prior to the onset of grand mal seizures. Data from [7]

subjects may manifest weakness, lethargy, restlessness, confusion, delirium, and impaired mentation (Figure 1). In addition, muscle twitching is often present, and convulsions may occur. Many other neurological abnormalities have been reported in patients with chronic hyponatraemia, including focal weakness,

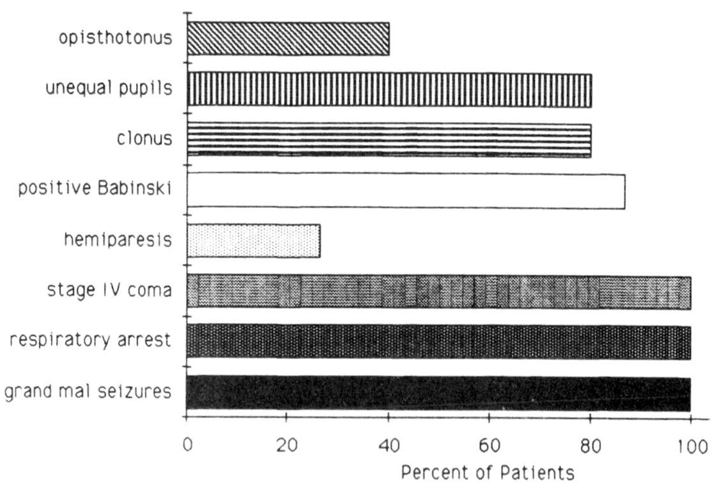

Figure 2. The neurological manifestations that developed in 15 patients with post-operative hyponatraemia. The grand mal seizures predated all other neurological findings. Data from [7]

hemiparesis, ataxia, unequal pupils and Babinski sign [5] (Figure 2). Patients with chronic hyponatraemia may also have organic brain syndrome and cognitive impairment, whereas depression, overt psychosis and anxiety may occur but are rare. In patients with severe symptomatic hyponatraemia and plasma sodium less than 120mM/litre, overall mortality exceeds 40% (Figure 3) while with a plasma sodium less than 106mM/litre, mortality is greater than 60% (Figure 4).

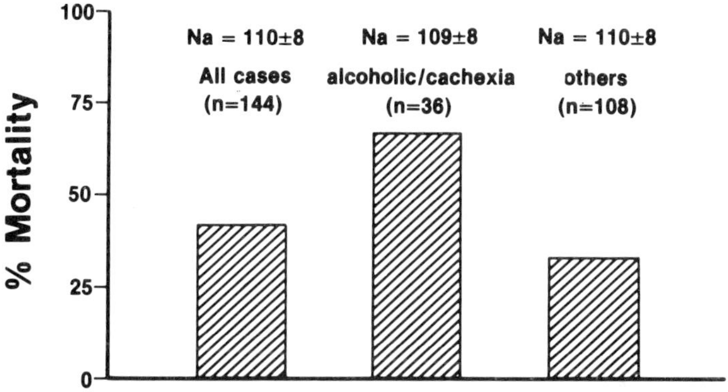

Figure 3. Overall mortality of patients with symptomatic hyponatraemia whose serum sodium (Na) was ≤120mM. In 114 cases from 29 articles, mean serum Na was 109mM. Of these patients, 36 had either alcoholism or other debilitating medical illness, and their mean serum Na was 109mM. The mortality was 67% in alcoholic/cachetic subjects, versus only 33% in other patients. Data from [5]

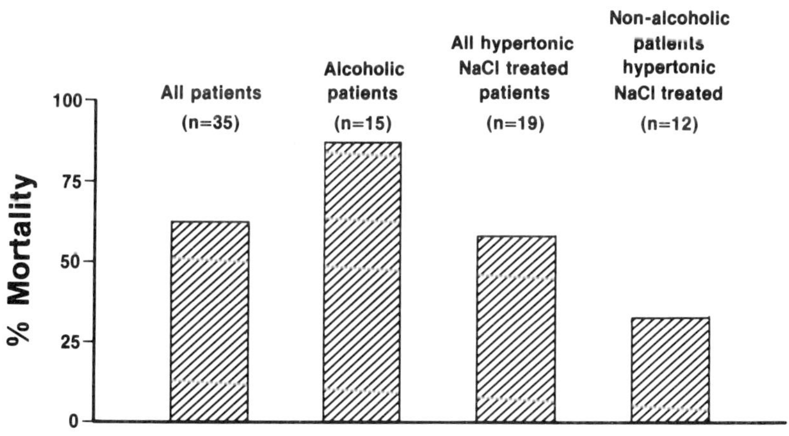

Figure 4. Mortality for patients whose serum sodium (Na) was ≤105mM. Overall mortality was 63%, but among alcoholic/cachetic subjects the mortality was 87%. Among relatively healthy subjects who were not alcoholic/cachetic, who did not have debilitating medical illness, and who were treated with hypertonic saline, the mortality was 33%. Data from [5]

Chronic hyponatraemia is common in patients with any of several oedematous states such as congestive heart failure, nephrotic syndrome, renal insufficiency, or liver failure, in all of which both total body water and sodium are increased. Chronic hyponatraemia is also frequently seen in patients with the syndrome of inappropriate secretion of ADH (SIADH), which may be caused by various tumours, many central nervous system diseases or lung disease. Among hospitalized patients, an inappropriate ADH-like syndrome is commonly seen with the administration of various drugs, including oral hypoglycaemics (particularly chlorpropamide), tricyclic antidepressant agents, anticancer agents, diuretics, clofibrate, and morphine-like analgesics [14]. Chronic hyponatraemia may also be seen in patients with salt-losing states, such as salt losing renal disease, excessive sweating, Addison's disease, and gastrointestinal electrolyte loss, and has also been reported in patients ingesting massive quantities of beer [14].

In unselected individual hyponatraemic patients, the severity of symptoms does not always correlate with the degree of hyponatraemia [5]. Some patients with a plasma sodium of 115mmol/litre are asymptomatic, whereas others with a plasma sodium of 120mmol/litre are in stupor or coma. In general, however, when plasma sodium is less than 120mmol/litre, most patients have some depression of sensorium and many have seizures [11].

Central pontine myelinolysis

Central pontine myelinolysis (CPM) is a rare neurological disorder of uncertain aetiology which was initially described in alcoholic and/or malnourished individuals [15]. Subsequently, it has been described in over 170 patients, virtually all of whom had either some chronic debilitating medical illness, malnourishment, or chronic alcoholism. Only a small minority of these patients (less than 20%) have ever had a history of hyponatraemia. In fact several have had hypernatraemia [14].

The anatomic lesion in CPM usually involves the centre of the basis pontis and often extends from midbrain to nerves in the lower pons. Most medullary sheaths are destroyed within the area of the lesion. There is destruction of myelin involving all tracts, regardless of site of origin, termination, or function. In contrast, however, to the complete destruction of myelin which usually occurs in the axis cylinders, the nerve cells and blood vessels are relatively well-preserved [15]. There are a number of reported cases where extrapontine cerebral demyelinating lesions are present. These lesions are most likely anoxic in nature, and are probably different lesions than CPM [11]. The clinical characteristics of CPM may be quite variable among patients with documented lesions. In the original description, patients had flaccid quadriplegia, facial weakness, inability to speak and swallow, and impaired response to painful stimuli [11]. The symptoms appear to vary according to the extent of the lesion. A majority of cases have a history of alcoholism and most of the remainder have had a variety of severe debilitating medical illness, including cancer, lymphoma, leukaemia, sepsis and severe malnutrition.

It has been suggested that 'rapid correction' of hyponatraemia may lead to CPM [6]. However, the data in human studies which might suggest such a relationship are scanty. Further insight into the possible relationship between hyponatraemia, its correction and the development of CPM or other demyelinating brain lesions is provided in several recent reports. In most previous reports, CPM actually is equated with the presence of diffuse demyelinating lesions of the brain which are largely extrapontine and resemble lesions found in hypoxia or anoxia. In a recent study [16], the severe post-operative symptomatic hyponatraemia in 15 women was corrected from 106 to 130mmol/litre at a mean rate of less than 0.7mmol/litre/hour, which has been defined as 'slow' correction of hyponatraemia [14]. All of the women died or suffered permanent brain damage. However, none had CPM, either on the basis of CAT scan, autopsy or brain biopsy. In a recent study, Ayus, Krothapalli and Arieff have demonstrated the development of CPM in humans when normonatraemic subjects with hepatic encephalopathy who had their serum sodium elevated to hypernatraemic (above 145mmol/litre) levels [12]. However, when patients with symptomatic hyponatraemia had their serum sodium elevated from 113 to 130mmol/litre in 24 hours, there was no evidence of either CPM or other neurological disability by CAT scan or neurological examination [12]. In these studies

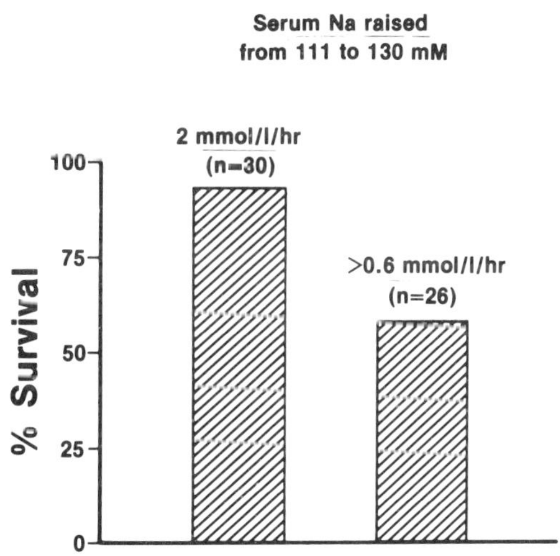

Figure 5. The survival of symptomatic hyponatraemia (serum sodium concentration of 120mM or less) among patients who were treated with hypertonic saline in two different eras (1973–1982 and 1951–1965) with two different regimens (rapid and slow treatment). In patients treated with the rapid regime, the mean rate of increase in serum sodium concentration was 2mmol/litre/hour. Patients with a history of alcoholism and/or cachexia are not included. The overall survival for these patients exceeds 90% and no patient developed central pontine myelinolysis. Data from [5]

then, when symptomatic hyponatraemia is treated 'slowly', there is often a high morbidity (permanent brain damage) and mortality when compared to the reported survival of greater than 90% with 'rapid' treatment (Figure 5) [14]. Thus, there is little evidence in clinical studies to support the contention that rapid correction of symptomatic hyponatraemia to mildly hyponatraemic levels can in itself cause CPM.

Delayed neurological deterioration following hypoxia or anoxia

The causes of permanent brain damage in hyponatraemic subjects are not well defined. Although not yet reported in association with hyponatraemia, hypoxic brain damage may be an important factor in the neurological disability observed in some hyponatraemic subjects. The syndrome of delayed post-anoxic encephalopathy (DPAE) has been known at least since 1925. The disorder can follow anoxia or hypoxia from any cause but most cases are related to either carbon monoxide intoxication or cardiopulmonary arrest with resuscitation. The clinical characteristics of this disorder have been described by Ginsberg [17]. Whatever the cause, patients are initially deeply comatose, often requiring artificial ventilation. Characteristically, they begin to regain consciousness within one to three days. Initial improvement may be rapid enough that patients are discharged from the hospital within a week of the initial intoxication. As early as two days, or as late as several weeks, patients begin to relapse. The onset may be abrupt and heralded by disorientation, confusion, restlessness, apathy or inappropriate behaviour. There may be cortical dysfunction which may be multifocal in character, with dysphasias, agnosias and apraxias. Motor control is impaired, with resultant rigidity or spasticity.

Seizures may occur in patients with delayed post-anoxic encephalopathy. Seven patients with symptomatic hyponatraemia who had been comatose were treated and awoke during the time that the serum sodium was increased from a mean of 105 to 131mmol/litre. Then, two-and-a-half days after awakening from coma to the point of communicating, eating and ambulating, all seven patients again manifested grand mal seizures and became comatose. None recovered from this recurrent episode of coma, which occurred when serum sodium was at least 128mmol/litre. Although the cause of recurrent coma is uncertain, the syndrome appears similar to that previously described in patients who have suffered hypoxic or anoxic episodes from other causes [17,18]. In common with previously reported subjects with delayed post-anoxic encephalopathy, the hyponatraemic patients have also generally been quickly resuscitated, and appeared to recover, usually within a few days. These patients seemed relatively normal for two to 10 days, but then developed apathy, irritability and confusion, often with agitation or manic behaviour. There are no obvious features during the initial anoxic insult which serve to distinguish those patients destined to relapse from those who have uncomplicated recoveries. Many such patients are initially misdiagnosed and are felt to have primary cerebral pathology, such as subdural haematoma [17,18]. In the hyponatraemic patients the diagnosis must be made on clinical grounds, but appears to be the most likely cause of the recurrent seizures and coma, with either death or a persistent vegetative state as the outcome.

Female preponderance of brain damage with symptomatic hyponatraemia

Post-operative hyponatraemia is quite common, and can develop in two days or less. The causes of the abrupt fall of serum sodium are probably multiple, but the most important one appears to be excessive post-operative administration of hypotonic fluid. However, excessive administration of free water alone does not generally result in hyponatraemia. Normal male subjects can ingest up to 15 litres a day of water with little or no change in serum sodium. In hyponatraemic subjects, both total body water and sodium can be high, low or normal [12]. In most clinical situations, hyponatraemia is associated with water retention and elevated plasma levels of vasopressin (ADH). Chung and associates [12] found that among 48 post-operative patients with hyponatraemia, most had elevated plasma levels of ADH. Several investigators have shown that almost all post-operative patients have elevated plasma ADH levels [15,20]. Post-operative hyponatraemia is actually quite common and may include over 4% of all patients who undergo surgery [2]. It is, however, rarely symptomatic, plasma sodium does not usually fall below 130mmol/litre, and neurological morbidity appears to be uncommon [2].

There are several reports of post-operative hyponatraemia accompanied by coma and seizures. Most of these reports appear in the older surgical literature [14]. Despite the fact that serum sodium below 115mmol/litre with symptomatology was present, neurological morbidity and mortality were very infrequent Since many of the aforementioned patients were in generally good health, and were usually undergoing elective surgical procedures, the lack of serious associated medical illness was thought to be a major factor in the low morbidity and mortality. Several reported cases of hyponatraemia with associated brain damage have occurred in patients with other co-morbid conditions [14]. However, one very vital bit of information appears to have escaped analysis.

With very few exceptions, most patients who had symptomatic hyponatraemia with sodium less than 120mmol/litre but did not suffer permanent neurological damage were men. In contrast, most patients who died or suffered permanent brain damage have been women [11]. The reasons for such a female predeliction to brain damage from hyponatraemia are not clear. However, when the serum sodium is lowered to as low as 102mM within five hours in men, respiratory arrest may not occur [21], whereas lowering serum sodium to 115mM in 1.5 days will generally result in respiratory arrest and permanent brain damage in menstruating women [11,21,22].

It may be that the adaptive mechanisms whereby the brain is able to decrease its volume in response to hyponatraemia is less efficient in females than in males.

This may be related to the fact that these mechanisms can be inhibited by certain female sex hormones. It has recently been shown that progesterone and certain of its derivatives can in several tissues inhibit certain enzymes (Na-K ATPase) which may act to prevent increases in brain cell volume [11]. In addition, both sexual and racial differences in the amount and the activity of Na-K ATPase in other cells have been demonstrated [14]. Such differences may be present in the brain as well.

Rapid versus slow correction of severe symptomatic hyponatraemia

There is not a consensus of opinion as to the optimal rate of correction of symptomatic hyponatraemia. Despite the incomplete and retrospective nature of currently available data, substantial clinical evidence is provided that rapid correction of severe symptomatic hyponatraemia to mildly hyponatraemic levels (in non-alcoholic patients) does not usually result in CPM or an increase in mortality. Retrospective data demonstrate that the survival of patients treated 'rapidly' is significantly greater than in those treated 'slowly' (Figure 5). It now appears that rate of correction of hyponatraemia is not a major factor in survival [11,12,16,24]. Recent studies suggest that a major determinant of survival may in fact be the occurrence of a hypoxic episode, usually respiratory arrest. In six recent prospective studies containing over 60 patients with severe symptomatic hyponatraemia where serum sodium was increased at a rate of about 2mmol/litre/hour to a new level of about 130mmol/litre, all survived with no evidence of permanent brain damage [11,12,23,24]. Thus, rapid correction of severe symptomatic hyponatraemia per se is not the cause of brain damage in such patients. Rather, recent evidence suggests that the presence of a hypoxic episode may be a major factor in determining the presence of neurological dysfunction.

It still appears, however, that rapid therapy of severe symptomatic hyponatraemia is desirable. In three recent studies [10,16,22], 18 patients with symptomatic hyponatraemia were alert and responsive with serum sodiums of 102 to 124mmol/litre. All such patients were women between the ages of 18 and 46 years. These patients had an abrupt onset (within 30 minutes) of seizures and respiratory arrest, and all suffered permanent brain damage. There is no obvious way to determine which symptomatic hyponatraemic patients are going to suffer an acute hypoxic episode. This appears to provide a major rationale for rapid institution of therapy. Additionally, both hyponatraemia and hypoxia would tend to reduce the brain oedema quickly. Such an effect may improve survival in some patients.

In summary, the major factors which are associated with permanent brain damage in patients with severe symptomatic hyponatraemia appear to be the following [12]: (a) the presence of an episode of hypoxia or anoxia, such as respiratory arrest with seizures; (b) a change in serum sodium of more than 20–25mmol/litre in the initial 24 hours of therapy; (c) the presence of associated medical conditions known to result in abnormalities of the blood-brain barrier, such as hepatic cirrhosis or metastatic cancer; (d) correction of serum sodium to normonatraemic (in excess of 134mmol/litre) or hypernatraemic levels. In particular, it is especially dangerous to acutely (within the initial two days) elevate plasma sodium to hypernatraemic levels (serum sodium greater than 145mmol/litre); (e) delay in institution of therapy for symptomatic hyponatraemia. The untreated mortality in patients with serum sodium less than 120mmol/litre accompanied by central nervous symptoms is greater than 50% [14].

Acknowledgments

Supported by the Research Service of the Veterans Administration Medical Center, San Francisco, California.

References

1 Anderson RJ. Hospital associated hyponatremia. *Kidney Int 1986; 29:* 1237–1247

2 Chung HM, Kluge R, Schrier RW, Anderson RJ. Postoperative hyponatremia: a prospective study. *Arch Intern Med 1986; 146:* 333–336

3 Kennedy PGE, Mitchell DM, Hoffbrand BI. Severe hyponatraemia in hospital patients. *Br Med J 1978; 2:* 1251–1253

4 Baran D, Hutchinson TA. The outcome of hyponatremia in a general hospital population. *Clin Nephrol 1984; 22:* 72–76

5 Arieff AI, Llach F, Massry SG. Neurological manifestations and morbidity of hyponatremia: correlation with brain water and electrolytes. *Medicine (Baltimore) 1976; 55:* 121–129

6 Tomlinson BE, Pierides AM, Bradley WG. Central pontine myelinolysis. *Q J Med 1976; 65:* 373–386

7 Zimmermann B, Wangensteen OH. Observations on water intoxication in surgical patients. *Surgery 1952; 31:* 654–659

8 Ashraf N, Locksley R, Arieff AI. Thiazide-induced hyponatremia associated with death or neurologic damage in outpatients. *Am J Med 1981; 70:* 1163–1168

9 Posner JB, Ertel NH, Kossmann RJ, Scheinberg LC. Hyponatremia in acute polyneuropathy. *Arch Neurol 1967; 17:* 530–541

10 Arieff AI, Fraser CL. Detrimental consequences of untreated hyponatremia in children. *Kidney Int 1987; 31:* 190

11 Arieff AI. Hyponatremia associated with permanent brain damage. *Adv Intern Med 1987, 32:* 325 344

12 Ayus JC, Krothapalli R, Arieff AI. Treatment of symptomatic hyponatremia and relationship to brain damage: a prospective study. *Abstracts Xth Int Cong Nephrol 1987:* 105

13 Plum F, Posner JB. Metabolic brain diseases causing coma. Hypo-osmolar states. In *Diagnosis of Stupor and Coma.* Philadelphia: F A Davis Co. 1966: 151–153

14 Arieff AI. Effects of water electrolyte and acid-base disorders on the central nervous system: hyponatremia. In Arieff AI, DeFronzo RA, eds. *Fluid, Electrolyte and Acid-base Disorders.* New York: Churchill Livingstone. 1985: 992–1007

15 Adams RD, Victor M, Mancall EL. Central pontine myelinolysis. *Arch Neurol Psychiat 1959, 81:* 154–172

16 Arieff AI. Hyponatremia, convulsions, respiratory arrest, and permanent brain damage after elective surgery in healthy women. *N Engl J Med 1987; 314:* 1529–1535

17 Ginsberg MD. Delayed neurological deterioration following hypoxia. *Adv Neurol 1979; 26:* 21–44

18 Plum F, Posner JB, Hain RF. Delayed neurological deterioration after anoxia. *Arch Intern Med 1962; 110:* 18–25

19 Ayus JC, Krothapalli R, Arieff AI. Treatment of symptomatic hyponatremia and relationship to brain damage: a prospective study. *Abstracts Xth Int Cong Nephrol 1987:* 105
20 Robertson GL. Abnormalities of thirst regulation. *Kidney Int 1984; 25:* 460–469
21 Ayus JC, Krothapalli R, Arieff AI. Sexual difference in survival with severe symptomatic hyponatremia. *Kidney Int 1988; 33 (Jan)*
22 Arieff AI, Fraser CL. Severe symptomatic hyponatremia complicated by hypernatremia, central diabetes mellitus and central diabetes insipidus: a new syndrome. *Abstracts Xth Int Cong Nephrol 1987:* 105
23 Ashouri OS. Severe diuretic induced hyponatremia: a series of eight patients. *Arch Intern Med 1986; 146:* 1295–1296
24 Decaux G, Unger J, Brimioulle S, Mockel J. Hyponatremia in the syndrome of inappropriate secretion of antidiuretic hormone. *JAMA 1982; 247:* 471–474

SUBJECT AND AUTHOR INDEXES

SUBJECT INDEX

AUTHOR INDEX

Badalamenti J 481
Renal Section
The University Hospital
75 East Newton Street
Boston
Massachusetts
USA

Badr KF 57
Vanderbilt University School of Medicine
Nashville
Tennessee
USA

Bailey RR 835
Department of Nephrology
Christchurch Hospital
Christchurch
New Zealand

Bannister KM 618
Renal Unit
Royal Adelaide Hospital
North Terrace
Adelaide
South Australia

Baud L
INSERM 64
Hôpital Tenon
Paris
France

Bergerson B 1255
Hennepin County Medical Center
Division of Nephrology
Minnesota
USA

Bergström J 1192
Department of Renal Medicine
Karolinska Institute
Huddinge University Hospital
Stockholm
Sweden

Bernstein K 402
Metabolic Diseases Branch
National Institute of Diabetes and Digestive and Kidney Diseases
National Institutes of Health
Bethesda, Maryland 20892, USA

Berry CA 196
Cardiovascular Research Institute
University of California, San Francisco
San Francisco
California 94143-0532, USA

Beurton D 1333
Department of Urology
Hôpital Necker
Paris, France

Bichara M 275
Hôpital Louis Mourier
92701 Colombes, France

Bing RF 917
Department of Medicine
Clinical Sciences Building
Leicester Royal Infirmary
PO Box 65
Leicester
LE2 7LX
United Kingdom

Blantz RC 453,509
University of California, San Diego School of Medicine and Veterans Administration Medical Center
3350 La Jolla Village Drive
San Diego
California 92161
USA

Bobrie G 637
Département de Néphrologie
Hôpital Necker
Paris
France

Bommer J 1126
University of Heidelberg
Im Neuenheimer Feld 220/221
D-6900 Heiderlberg
FRG

Bonjour J-P 1059
Division of Clinical Pathophysiology
Department of Medicine
University Hospital of Geneva
1211 Geneva 4
Switzerland

Bonomini V 1042
Institute of Nephrology and Dialysis
St Orsola University Hospital
via Massarenti 9
40138 Bologna
Italy

Border WA 689
University of Utah Health Sciences Center
Salt Lake City
Utah 84132
USA

Boron WF 213
Department of Cellular and Molecular Physiology
Yale University School of Medicine
New Haven
Connecticut 06510
USA

Boyce NW 523
Monash University
Department of Medicine
Prince Henry's Hospital
Melbourne
Australia

Brady HR 1319
Division of Nephrology
Toronto Western Hospital
ECW 7-042
399 Bathurst Street
Toronto
Ontario M5T 2S8
Canada

Brentjens JR 392
Renal Research Laboratory
Buffalo General Hospital
Buffalo
NY 14214
USA

Brezis M 937,945
Department of Medicine
Hadassah University Hospital
Mount Scopus
PO Box 24035
Jerusalem
Israel 91240

Briggs JD 1353
Renal Unit
Western Infirmary
Glasgow
G11 6NT
United Kingdom

Brown A 1067
The Renal Division
Department of Medicine
Washington University School of Medicine
St Louis
Missouri 63110
USA

Brown D 332
Harvard Medical School
The Renal Unit
Massachusetts General Hospital
Boston
Massachusetts 02114
USA

Broyer M 1333
Department of Pediatrics
Hôpital des Enfant Malades
149 rue de Sèvres
75743 Paris Cedex 15
France

Brunner FF 1276
EDTA Registry
St Thomas' Hospital
London
SE1 7EH
United Kingdom

Brunner HR 896
Division of Hypertension
University Hospital
CH-1011 Lausanne
Switzerland

Bucht H 1192
Department of Renal Medicine
Karolinska Institute
Huddinge University Hospital
Stockholm
Sweden

Druet E 462
Hôpital Broussais
INSERM U28
96 rue Didot
Paris
France

Druet Ph 462
Hôpital Broussais
INSERM U28
96 rue Didot
Paris
France

Druml WJ 1003
University of Vienna
Lazarettgasse 14
A-1090 Wien
Austria

Dubyak GR 98
Department of Physiology
Case Western Reserve University
Cleveland
Ohio
USA

Dunn MJ 98
Department of Medicine
Division of Nephrology
University Hospitals of Cleveland
2074 Abington Road
Cleveland
Ohio 44106
USA

Dusso A 1067
The Renal Division
Department of Medicine
Washington University School of Medicine
St Louis
Missouri 63100
USA

Elalouf JM 255
Département de Biologie
Service de Biologie Cellulaire
CEN Saclay
91191 Gif-sur-Yvette Cedex
France

Edmunds ME 917
Department of Medicine
Clinical Sciences Building
Leicester Royal Infirmary
PO Box 65
Leicester
LE2 7LX
United Kingdom

Elema JD 574
Department of Pathology
University of Groningen
Oostersingel 63
9713 EZ Groningen
The Netherlands

Elliot SJ 402
Metabolic Diseases Branch
National Institute of Diabetes and Digestive and Kidney Diseases
National Institutes of Health
Bethesda
Maryland 20892
USA

El Nahas AM 1206
Department of Renal Medicine
Northern General Hospital
Herries Road
Sheffield
S5 7AU
United Kingdom

Elseviers MM 1086
University of Antwerp
Department of Nephrology-Hypertension
B-2610 Wilrijk (Antwerp)
Belgium

Eschbach JW 1050
University of Washington
Seattle
Washington 98195
USA

Fabre JW 1312
Blond McIndoe Centre for Medical Research
Queen Victoria Hospital
East Grinstead
Sussex RH19 3D2
United Kingdom

Faugere MC 1082
Division of Nephrology, Bone and Mineral Metabolism
University of Kentucky
Lexington
Kentucky, USA

Ferran C 637
Département de Néphrologie
Hôpital Necker
Paris
France

Friedrich T 217
Max-Planck Institut für Biophysik
Kennedyallee 70
D-6000 Frankfurt/Main 70
FRG

Fukatsu A 441
State University of New York at Buffalo
and Renal Research Laboratory of the Buffalo General Hospital
Buffalo
NY 14214, USA

Gabbai FB 453
University of California
San Diego School of Medicine
and Veterans Administration Medical Center
San Diego
California, USA

Gagnadoux MF 1333
Hopital des Enfants Malades
149 rue de Sèvres
75743 Paris Cedex 15
France

Garibotto G 1011
Istituto Scientifico di Medicina Interna
Section of Nephrology
Viale Benedetto XV, 6
16132 Genova
Italy

Geerlings W 1276
EDTA Registry
St Thomas' Hospital
London SE1 7EH
United Kingdom

Giebisch G 179
Department of Physiology
Yale University School of Medicine
333 Cedar Street
New Haven
Connecticut 06510, USA

Gögelein H 159
Max-Planck-Institut für Biophysik
Kennedyallee 70
D-6000 Frankfurt/Main 70, FRG

Gokal R 1268
Department of Renal Medicine
Manchester Royal Infirmary
Manchester
M13 9WL
United Kingdom

Goodship THJ 1003
Department of Medicine
University of Newcastle upon Tyne
Newcastle upon Tyne
NE2 4HH
United Kingdom

Grantham JJ 1119
Nephrology Division
University of Kansas School of Medicine
Kansas City
Kansas 66103, USA

Green R 179
Department of Physiological Sciences
University of Manchester
Stopford Building
Oxford Road
Manchester, M13 9PT
United Kingdom

Greenfeld Z 937
Department of Medicine
Hadassah University Hospital
Mount Scopus
Jerusalem, Israel

Greger R 159
Lehrstuhl II Physiologisches Institut der Universität Freiburg
Hermann-Herder-Strasse 7
D-7800 Freiburg, FRG

Gresser I 790
Institute de Recherches Scientifiques sur le Cancer
Villejuif
France

Grond J 574
Department of Pathology
University of Groningen
Oostersingel 63
9713 EZ Groningen
The Netherlands

Grünfeld JP 637
Département de Néphrologie
Hôpital Necker
Paris
France

Guest G 1333
Hôpital des Enfants Malades
149 rue de Sèvres
75743 Paris Cedex 15
France

Gutierrez A 1192
Department of Renal Medicine
Karolinska Institute
Huddinge University Hospital
Stockholm
Sweden

Hakim RM 1245
Harvard Medical School
Brigham and Women's Hospital
75 Francis Street
Boston
Massachusetts 02115
USA

Hall BM 1300
Department of Medicine
Division of Nephrology
Stanford University Medical Center
Stanford
California 94305
USA

Hara Y 1003
Tokyo Women's Medical College
Tokyo, Japan

Harris K 1155
Washington University School of Medicine
Department of Medicine, Renal Division
St Louis
Missouri 63110, USA

Heller J 75
Institute for Clinical and Experimental Medicine
Prague
Czechoslovakia

Heyman SN 937
Department of Medicine
Hadassah University Hospital
Mount Scopus
Jerusalem, Israel

Higashihara E 1138
Department of Urology
Faculty of Medicine
The University of Tokyo
7-3-1 Hongo, Bunkyo-ku
Tokyo 113
Japan

Hirsch F 462
Hôpital Broussais
INSERM U28
96 rue Didot
Paris, France

Hofbauer K 896
Division of Hypertension
University Hospital
CH-1011 Lausanne
Switzerland

Hoedemaeker Ph J 409
Department of Pathology
University of Leiden
PO Box 9603
2300 RC Leiden
The Netherlands

Holdsworth SR 523
Monash University
Department of Medicine
Prince Henry's Hospital
Melbourne
Australia

Holz FG 37
I Physiologisches Institut
Universität Heidelberg
Heidelberg
FGR

Horáček V 75
Institute for Clinical and Experimental Medicine
Prague
Czechoslovakia

Hors-Cayla MC 637
INSERM U12
Hôpital des Enfants Malades
Paris
France

Hostetter MK 599
Department of Pediatrics
University of Minnesota
Minneapolis
Minnesota, USA

Hostetter TH 599, 1196
Department of Medicine
University of Minnesota
Box 736 UMHC
516 Delaware Street SE
Minneapolis
Minnesota 55455, USA

Ichikawa I 57
Head, Division of Pediatric Nephrology
Vanderbilt University School of Medicine
21st and Garland Avenue
Nashville
Tennessee 38232, USA

Imai M 231
Department of Pharmacology
National Cardiovascular Center
Research Institute
5-7-1 Fujishirodai, Suita
Osaka 565, Japan

Jahn H 1026
Service de Néphrologie et d'Hémodialyse
Université Louis Pasteur
Strasbourg
France

Johnson RJ 495
University of Washington
Seattle
Washington 98195
USA

Kaplan JC 637
INSERM U129
Institut de Pathologie Moléculaire
CHU Cochin
Paris
France

Kamarádová S 75
Institute for Clinical and Experimental Medicine
Prague
Czechoslovakia

Karniski LP 190
Laboratory of Epithelial Transport
Department of Internal Medicine
University of Iowa and Veterans Administration Medical Center
Iowa City
Iowa 52242
USA

Kashgarian M 552
Yale University School of Medicine
New Haven
Connecticut, USA

Keane WF 1255
University of Minnesota Medical School
Hennepin County Medical Center
Minnesota, USA

Kelley VE 1293
Evans Department of Clinical Research and Department of Medicine
The University Hospital
Boston University Medical Center
Boston
Massachussetts 02118
USA

Kelly RA 1003
Harvard Medical School
Boston
Massachusetts 02115, USA

Klahr S 1182
Washington University School of Medicine
Department of Medicine, Renal Division
St Louis
Missouri 63110
USA

Klebanoff SJ 495
University of Washington
Seattle
Washington 98195
USA

Knepper MA 317
Laboratory of Kidney and Electrolyte Metabolism
National Heart, Lung, and Blood Institute
National Institutes of Health
Bethesda
Maryland 20892
USA

Koeppen BM 304
Division of Nephrology
University of Connecticut Health Center
Farmington
Connecticut 06032
USA

Kokko JP 24
Department of Medicine
Emory University School of Medicine
1364 Clifton Road NE
Atlanta
Georgia 30322
USA

Kon V 57
Vanderbilt University School of Medicine
Nashville
Tennessee
USA

Kondo Y 231
Department of Pharmacology
National Cardiovascular Center
Research Institute
5-7-1 Fujishirodai, Suita
Osaka 565
Japan

Koseki C 231
Department of Pharmacology
National Cardiovascular Center
Research Institute
5-7-1 Fujishirodai, Suita
Osaka 565, Japan

Krensky AM 365
Stanford University
Stanford
California 94305
USA

Kriz W 3
Anatomisches Institut I
Universität Heidelberg
Im Neuenheimer Feld 307
D-6900 Heidelberg, FRG

Kuo S-M 190
Section of Nephrology
Departments of Internal Medicine and Physiology
Yale University School of Medicine
New Haven
Connecticut 06510
USA

Kurokawa K 541
Fourth Department of Internal Medicine
The University of Tokyo School of Medicine
3-28-6 Mejirodai, Bunkyo-ku
Tokyo 112
Japan

Landers DV 365
Department of Pediatrics
Stanford University
Stanford
California 94305
USA

Lange MA 402
Metabolic Diseases Branch
National Institute of Diabetes and Digestive and Kidney Diseases
National Institutes of Health
Bethesda
Maryland 20892
USA

Leckie B 884
MRC Blood Pressure Unit
Western Infirmary
Glasgow
G11 6NT
United Kingdom

Lee HW 816
WHO Collaborating Centre for Virus Reference and Research (HFRS)
The Institute for Viral Diseases
Korea University
Seoul, Korea

Lever AF 884
MRC Blood Pressure Unit
Western Infirmary
Glasgow
G11 6NT
United Kingdom

Leviel F 275
Hôpital Louis Mourier
92701 Colombes, France

Lockwood CM 637
Department of Medicine
Royal Postgraduate Medical School
Hammersmith Hospital
Ducane Road
London
United Kingdom

Lopez-Hilker S 1067
The Renal Division
Department of Medicine
Washington University School of Medicine
St Louis
Missouri 63100, USA

Maack T 123
Department of Physiology
Cornell University Medical College
1300 York Avenue
New York
NY 10021, USA

Madsen KM 587
Laboratory of Experimental Morphology
University of Florida College of Medicine
Gainesville
Florida 32610, USA

Maher JF 1284
Nephrology Division
Department of Medicine
Uniformed Services University of the Health Sciences
4301 Jones Bridge Road
Bethesda
Maryland 20814-4799
USA

Mahony JF 1341
Department of Renal Medicine
Royal North Shore Hospital
St Leonards
NSW 2065
Australia

Malluche HH 1082
Division of Nephrology, Bone and Mineral Metabolism
University of Kentucky
Lexington
Kentucky, USA

Maroni BJ 1003
Emory University School of Medicine
Atlanta
Georgia 30322, USA

Martin K 1067
The Renal Division
Department of Medicine
Washington University School of Medicine
St Louis
Missouri 63110, USA

Mason J 955
Physiology Department
University of Munich and
Sandoz
Renal Research
CH-4002 Basel
Switzerland

Massry SG 1038
Division of Nephrology
LAC/USC Medical Center
1200 North State Street, Room 4250
Los Angeles
California 90033
USA

Mathew TH 1368
Renal Unit
The Queen Elizabeth Hospital
Woodville South, 5011
South Australia

Matsunaga H 541
Fourth Department of Internal Medicine
The University of Tokyo School of Medicine
3-28-6 Mejirodai, Bunkyo-ku
Tokyo 112, Japan

May RC 1003
Emory University School of Medicine
Atlanta
Georgia 30322, USA

Menè P 98
Department of Medicine
Case Western Reserve University
Cleveland
Ohio, USA

Mercier O 275
Hôpital Louis Mourier
92701 Colombes, France

Méry JP 802
Hôpital Bichat
Department of Nephrology
75018 Paris, France

Mickisch O 1126
University of Pathology
Im Neuenheimer Feld 220/221
D-6900 Heidelberg, FRG

Mistry C 1268
Department of Renal Medicine
Manchester Royal Infirmary
Manchester
M13 9WL
United Kingdom

Mitch WE 1003
Renal Division
Emory University School of Medicine
Atlanta
Georgia 30322
USA

Moe O 1319
Division of Nephrology
Toronto Western Hospital
ECW 7-042
399 Bathurst Street
Toronto
Ontario M5T 2S8
Canada

Mogensen CE 729
Second University Clinic of Internal Medicine
Kommune Hospitalet
DK-8000 Aarhus C
Denmark

Molony DA 268
Division of Nephrology
Department of Internal Medicine
University of Texas Medical School
PO Box 20708
Houston
Texas 77225, USA

Morris PJ 1326
Nuffield Department of Surgery
University of Oxford
John Radcliffe Hospital
Oxford
OX3 9DU
United Kingdom

Morrissey J 1067
The Renal Division
Department of Medicine
Washington University School of Medicine
St Louis
Missouri 63100, USA

Moss J 790
Charing Cross and Westminster Medical School
Fulham Palace Road
London
United Kingdom

Moullier P 509
Department of Immunology
Research Institute of Scripps Clinic
10666 North Torrey Pines Road
La Jolla
California 92037, USA

Murphy JR 1293
Department of Medicine
Brigham and Women's Hospital
Harvard Medical School
Boston
Massachusetts 02115
USA

Myers BD 977
Division of Nephrology
Stanford University School of Medicine
Stanford
California 94305
USA

Nakhoul NL 213
Department of Cellular and Molecular Physiology
Yale University School of Medicine
New Haven
Connecticut 06510
USA

Nanni Costa A 1042
Institute of Nephrology and Dialysis
St Orsola University Hospital
via Massarenti 9
40138 Bologna
Italy

Nath KA 599
Department of Internal Medicine
University of Minnesota
Minneapolis
Minnesota
USA

Navar LG 46
Department of Physiology and Biophysics
Nephrology Research and Training Center
University of Alabama at Birmingham
Birmingham
Alabama 35294
USA

Naveh-Many T 1076
Nephrology Services
Hadassah University Hospital
Ein Karem
Jerusalem
Israel

Nicod P 896
Division of Hypertension
University Hospital
CH-1011 Lausanne
Switzerland

Noël LH 637
Département de Néphrologie
Hôpital Necker
Paris
France

Nonoguchi H 317
Laboratory of Kidney and Electrolyte Metabolism
National Heart, Lung and Blood Institute
National Institutes of Health
Bethesda
Maryland 20892
USA

Nussberger J 896
Division of Hypertension
University Hospital
CH-1011 Lausanne
Switzerland

Okuda T 541
Fourth Department of Internal Medicine
The University of Tokyo School of Medicine
3-28-6 Mejirodai, Bunkyo-ku
Tokyo 112
Japan

Packer RK 304
George Washington University
Washington DC
USA

Paillard M 275
Metabolic and Renal Unit and Kidney and Electrolyte Laboratory
Université Paris VII
Hôpital Louis Mourier
92701 Colombes
France

Paoletti E 1011
Istituto Scientifico di Medicina
Interna
Section of Nephrology
Viale Benedetto XV, 6
16132 Genova
Italy

Parekh N 37
I Physiologisches Institut
Universität Heidelberg
Heidelberg
FRG

Pelletier L 462
Hôpital Broussais
INSERM U28
96 rue Didot
Paris
France

Pence T 1255
University of Minnesota Medical
School
Hennepin County Medical Center
Minnesota
USA

Pepys MB 761
MRC Acute Phase Protein Research
Group
Royal Postgraduate Medical School
Hammersmith Hospital
Ducane Road
London
W12 0HS
United Kingdom

Peterson PK 1255
University of Minnesota Medical School
Hennepin County Medical Center
Minnesota
USA

Phan S 532
Departments of Internal Medicine and
Pathology
University of Michigan
Ann Arbor
Michigan
USA

Preisig PA 202
Department of Internal Medicine
University of Texas Health Science Center
at Dallas
Southwestern Medical School
5323 Harry Hines Boulevard
Dallas
Texas 75235-9030, USA

Prevost P 1333
Unité INSERM U93
Hôpital Saint Louis
Paris, France

Prigent A 275
Hôpital Louis Mourier
92701 Colombes, France

Purkerson ML 1155
Washington University School of Medicine
Department of Medicine, Renal Division
St Louis
Missouri 63110, USA

Quigg RJ 481
Renal Section, The University Hospital
75 East Newton Street
Boston
Massachusetts 02118, USA

Ram CVS 907
Department of Internal Medicine
University of Texas Health Science Center
at Dallas
5323 Harry Hines Boulevard
Dallas
Texas 75235-9030, USA

Rasch R 744
Department of Cell Biology
Institute of Anatomy
University of Aarhus
DK-8000 Aarhus C
Denmark

Raymond KH 964
University of Texas Health Science Center,
San Antonio
Audie L Murphy Veterans Administration
Hospital
San Antonio
Texas, USA

Rector FC Jr 196
Cardiovascular Research Institute
University of California, San Francisco
San Francisco
California 94143-0532, USA

Rees L 989
Department of Paediatrics
United Medical and Dental Schools of
Guy's and St Thomas's Hospitals
Guy's Hospital
London
SE1 9RT
United Kingdom

Reeves WB 268
Division of Nephrology
Department of Internal Medicine
University of Texas Medical School
PO Box 20708
Houston
Texas 77225, USA

Reid G 860
Urology Research
Bell Wing G-631
200 Elizabeth Street
Toronto
Ontario
M5G 2C4
Canada

Reinherz EL 355
Laboratory of Immunobiology
Dana-Farber Cancer Institute
Department of Medicine
Harvard Medical School
Boston
Massachusetts, USA

Ritz E 1126
University of Heidelberg
Im Neuenheimer Feld 220/221
D-6900 Heidelberg
FRG

Robaudo C 1011
Istituto Scientifico di Medicina Interna
Section of Nephrology
Viale Benedetto XV, 6
16132 Genova, Italy

Roberts JA 844
Department of Urology
Tulane University School of Medicine
New Orleans
Louisiana 70112
and Delta Regional Primate Research Center
Covington
Lousiana 70422, USA

Rosen S 937, 945
Department of Pathology
Beth Israel Hospital
Harvard Medical School
330 Brookline Avenue
Boston
Massachusetts 02215, USA

Rosivall L 46
Department of Pathophysiology
Semmelweis University Medical School
Nagyvárad tér 4
Budapest H-1089, Hungary

Ruben de Campione MM 109
Heart Institute Research Centre
Ottawa Civic Hospital
1053 Carling Avenue
Ottawa
Ontario K1Y 4E9
Canada

Russell GI 917
Department of Medicine
Clinical Sciences Building
Leicester Royal Infirmary
PO Box 65
Leicester
LE2 7LX
United Kingdom

Saffioti S 1011
Istituto Scientifico di Medicina Interna
Section of Nephrology
Viale Benedetto XV, 6
16132 Genova, Italy

Sahai A 384
3914 Taubman Health Care Center
University of Michigan
Ann Arbor
Michigan 48109-0364, USA

Sakai T 3
Department of Anatomy
Faculty of Medicine
University of Tokyo
Tokyo 113
Japan

Salant DJ 481
Evans Memorial Department of Clinical Research and Department of Medicine
The University Hospital
Boston University Medical Center
Boston
Massachusetts, USA

Salvidio G 441
State University of New York at Buffalo
and Renal Research Laboratory of the Buffalo General Hospital
Buffalo
New York, USA

Sands JM 317
Laboratory of Kidney and Electrolyte Metabolism
National Heart, Lung, and Blood Institute
National Institutes of Health
Bethesda
Maryland 20892, USA

Sapin C 462
Hôpital Broussais
INSERM U28
96 rue Didot
Paris, France

Savage COS 637
Department of Medicine
Royal Postgraduate Medical School
Hammersmith Hospital
Ducane Road
London
United Kingdom

Schafer JA 294
Nephrology Research and Training Center
Departments of Physiology and Biophysics and Medicine
University of Alabama at Birmingham
Birmingham
Alabama 35294, USA

Schild L 179
Department of Physiology
Yale University School of Medicine
333 Cedar Street
New Haven
Connecticut 06510, USA

Schlatter E 294
Albert-Ludwigs-Universität
Physiologisches Institut, Lehrstuhl II
Herman-Herder-Strasse 7
7800 Freiburg, FRG

Schmitz A 729
Second University Clinic of Internal Medicine
Kommunehospitalet
DK-8000 Aarhus C
Denmark

Schrier RW 663
Department of Medicine
University of Colorado School of Medicine
Denver
Colorado 80262, USA

Schuster VL 283
Department of Medicine
University of Iowa
and Veterans Administration Medical Center
Iowa City
Iowa 52242, USA

Scoggins BA 869
Howard Florey Institute of Experimental Physiology and Medicine
University of Melbourne
Melbourne
Victoria
Australia

Selwood NH 1276
EDTA Registry
St Thomas' Hospital
London, SE1 7EH
United Kingdom

Semple P 884
MRC Blood Pressure Unit
Western Infirmary
Glasgow G11 6NT
United Kingdom

Sheil AGP 1341
Division of Transplant Surgery
Royal North Shore Hospital
St Leonards
NSW 2065
Australia

Silver J 1076
Hebrew University Medical School
Nephrology Services
Hadassah University Hospital
Ein Karem
Jerusalem
Israel

Sinniah R 558
Department of Pathology
National University of Singapore
Singapore

Sissons JGP 781
Department of Medicine
Royal Postgraduate Medical School
Ducane Road
London
W12 0HS
United Kingdom

Sraer J 87
INSERM 64
Hôpital Tenon
Paris
France

Star RA 304
Southwestern Medical School
Dallas
Texas
USA

Slatopolsky E 1067
The Renal Division
Department of Medicine
Washington University School of Medicine
St Louis
Missouri 63110
USA

Stefoni S 1042
Institute of Nephrology and Dialysis
St Orsolo University Hospital
via Massarenti 9
40138 Bologna, Italy

Stein JH 964
University of Texas Health Science Center, San Antonio
Audie L Murphy Veterans Administration Hospital
San Antonio
Texas, USA

Steinhausen M 37
I Physiologisches Institut
Universität Heidelberg
Heidelberg, FRG

Sterzel RB 552
Yale University School of Medicine
New Haven
Connecticut
USA

Striker GE 402
Metabolic Diseases Branch
National Institute of Diabetes and Digestive and Kidney Diseases
National Institutes of Health
Bethesda
Maryland 20892
USA

Striker LJ 402
Metabolic Diseases Branch
National Institute of Diabetes and Digestive and Kidney Diseases
National Institutes of Health
Bethesda
Maryland 20892
USA

Strom TB 613, 1293
Charles A Dana Research Institute
Harvard Thorndike Laboratory of the Beth Israel Hospital
Harvard Medical School
Boston
Massachusetts 02215
USA

Sugino N 1229
Department of Medicine
Kidney Center
Tokyo Women's College
Tokyo, Japan

Swales JD 917
Department of Medicine
Clinical Sciences Building
Leicester Royal Infirmary
PO Box 65
Leicester
LE2 7LX
United Kingdom

Szpiro-Tapia S 637
INSERM U12
Hôpital des Enfants Malades
Paris, France

Tamminen-Möbius T 854
University Children's Hospital
Essen, FRG

Tang M-J 384
Internal Medicine
3914 Taubman Health Care Center
University of Michigan
Ann Arbor
Michigan 48109-0364, USA

Taniguchi J 231
Department of Pharmacology
National Cardiovascular Center
Research Institute
5-7-1 Fujishirodai, Suita
Osaka 565, Japan

Tannen RL 384
Internal Medicine (Nephrology)
3914 Taubman Health Care Center
University of Michigan
Ann Arbor
Michigan 48109-0364
USA

Taugner R 46
Department of Physiology I
University of Heidelberg
Heidelberg D-6900
FRG

Thomson S 453
University of California
San Diego School of Medicine
and Veterans Administration Medical Center
San Diego
California
USA

Thurston H 917
Department of Medicine
Clinical Sciences Building
Leicester Royal Infirmary
PO Box 65
Leicester
LE2 7LX
United Kingdom

Tipping PG 523
Monash University
Department of Medicine
Prince Henry's Hospital
Melbourne
Victoria
Australia

Tisher CC 587
Division of Nephrology, Hypertension and Transplantation
University of Florida
Box J-224, JHMHC
Gainesville
Florida 32610
USA

Tizianello A 1011
Istituto Scientifico di Medicina Interna
Section of Nephrology
University of Genoa
Viale Benedetto XV, 6
16132 Genova
Italy

Tolins JP 599
Department of Internal Medicine
University of Minnesota
Minneapolis
Minnesota
USA

Ulich TR 618
Department of Pathology
University of California
Irvine Medical Center
101 City Drive, South
Orange
California 92668
USA

van de Vyver FL 1086
University of Utrecht
Laboratory for Bone Metabolism
Utrecht
The Netherlands

Van Doren K 402
Metabolic Diseases Branch
National Institute of Diabetes and Digestive and Kidney Diseases
National Institutes of Health
Bethesda
Maryland 20892
USA

Vangelista A 1042
Institute of Nephrology and Dialysis
St Orsola University Hospital
via Massarenti 9
40138 Bologna
Italy

van Ypersele de Strihou C 802
University of Louvain
Medical School
Cliniques Universitaires St-Luc
Department of Nephrology
1200 Brussels
Belgium

Visser WJ 1086
University of Utrecht
Laboratory for Bone Metabolism
Utrecht
The Netherlands

Waeber B 896
Division of Hypertension
University Hospital
CH-1011 Lausanne
Switzerland

Waldherr R 1126
Department of Pathology
University of Heidelberg
Im Neuenheimer Feld 220/221
D-6900 Heidelberg
FRG

Walser M 1155
Department of Pharmacology and Molecular Sciences
Johns Hopkins University School of Medicine
725 North Wolfe Street
Baltimore
Maryland
USA

Webb D 884
MRC Blood Pressure Unit
Western Infirmary
Glasgow
G11 6NT
United Kingdom

Whitworth JA 869
Department of Nephrology
The Royal Melbourne Hospital
Victoria 3050
Australia

Wiggins R 532
Departments of Internal Medicine and Pathology
University of Michigan
Ann Arbor
Michigan
USA

Wilson CB 453, 509, 618
Department of Immunology
Research Institute of Scripps Clinic
10666 North Torrey Pines Road
La Jolla
California 92037
USA

Wing AJ 1232, 1276
United Medical and Dental Schools
St Thomas' Hospital
London, SE1 7EH
United Kingdom

Woodrow DF 790
Charing Cross and Westminster Medical School
Department of Histopathology
Fulham Palace Road
London
W6 8RF
United Kingdom

Yamamoto T 509
Department of Immunology
Research Institute of Scripps Clinic
10666 North Torrey Pines Road
La Jolla
California 92037
USA

Yamashita N 541
Fourth Department of Internal Medicine
The University of Tokyo School of Medicine
3-28-6 Mejirodai, Bunkyo-ku
Tokyo 112
Japan

Yared A 57
Vanderbilt University School of Medicine
Nashville
Tennessee
USA

Yoshioka T 57
Vanderbilt University School of Medicine
Nashville
Tennessee
USA

Yoshitomi K 231
Department of Pharmacology
National Cardiovascular Center Research Institute
5-7-1 Fujishirodai, Suita
Osaka 565, Japan

Zeidel ML 145
Harvard Medical School
Boston
Massachusetts
USA

Zhou X-J 441
State University of New York at Buffalo
and Renal Research Laboratory of the Buffalo General Hospital
Buffalo
New York
USA

Zimmerhackl LB 69
Department of Pediatrics
Philipps-University
D-3550 Marburg, FRG

1993 NATIONAL ELECTRICAL CODE®

INTERPRETIVE DIAGRAMS

1993 EDITION

A Publication of

Los Angeles County, Chapter
401 Shatto Place
Los Angeles,
CA 90020
(213) 487-7313

PRINTED AND MARKETED BY

BNi Building News

3055 Overland Avenue, Los Angeles, CA 90034
(310) 202-7775

Foreword

The National Electrical Code is the recognized national standard for safe and efficient electrical installations, endorsed, adopted and enforced by the majority of building authorities in the United States.

Researched, edited and updated every three years by a broad committee representative of the most advanced technical leadership of the electrical industry, this code is published and promulgated by the National Fire Protection Association, headquartered in Quincy, Massachusetts.

This Interpretive Diagrams Manual, based upon the 1993 edition of the National Electrical Code, had its origin in triennial similar interpretive diagrams manuals, based upon earlier editions of the National Electrical Code, published by the Los Angeles County Chapter of the National Electrical Contractors Association. This book seeks to visually explain and interpret the key provisions of the National Electrical Code as seen through the eyes of an electrical inspector who might be called upon to inspect and approve such installations.

Special acknowledgements and thanks are expressed to the following electrical inspectors who contributed their time and expertise to the preparation and review of this book: [from the County of Los Angeles, Department of Public Works, Constantine S. Golovko, chief electrical inspector; from the City of Los Angeles, Tim Taylor, chief of the Mechanical Bureau; Department of Building and Safety, Gary Wilson and Mickey McQuire; from the City of San Diego, Tom Trainor, chief electrical inspector; from the City and County of San Francisco, Steve Young, chief electrical inspector].

A special thanks to Scott Cline for assuming the task of drafting the revised diagrams.

The diagrams and commentary in this book have been carefully and diligently prepared and reviewed by the foregoing inspectors and by LA/NECA's Codes and Standard Committee as well as the code committees in other NECA chapters, as well as local inspectors in their respective areas. The diagrams show not only approved electrical apparatus installations, but in some cases those not in compliance with the electrical codes noted. In some cases, where pertinent, there are specific references to the individual codes of local jurisdictions such as Los Angeles City and Los Angeles County.

The publishers wish to emphasize that this publication is unofficial. Accordingly, the final responsibility for code interpretations rests with the governmental body or authority having legal jurisdiction. Therefore, NECA and/or the publisher can assume no responsibility for anything that may happen as a result of following the diagrams and commentary herein; nor for any errors or omissions.